Fighting the COVID-19 Pandemic

Edited by Manal Mohammad Baddour

Published in London, United Kingdom

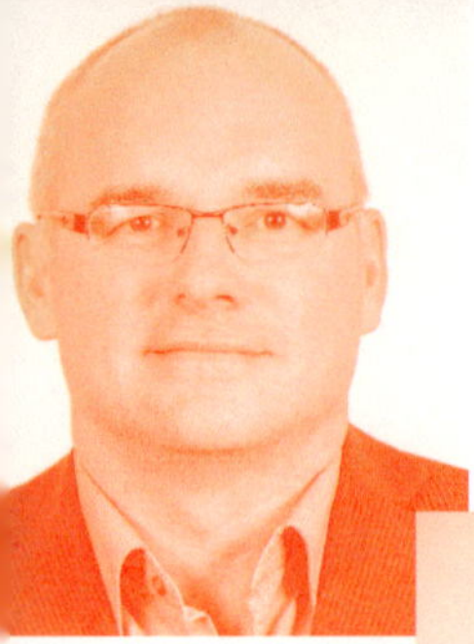
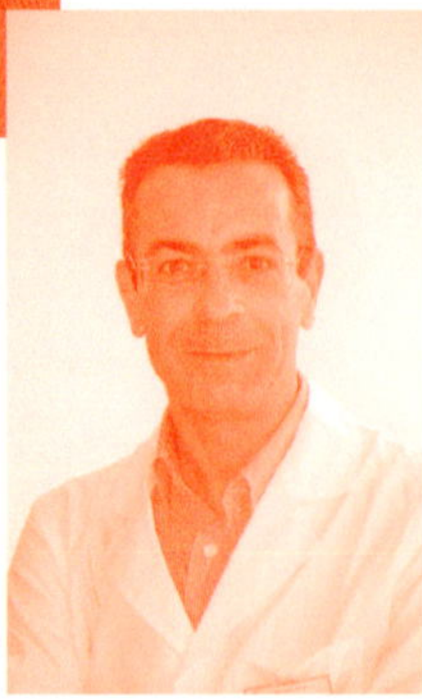
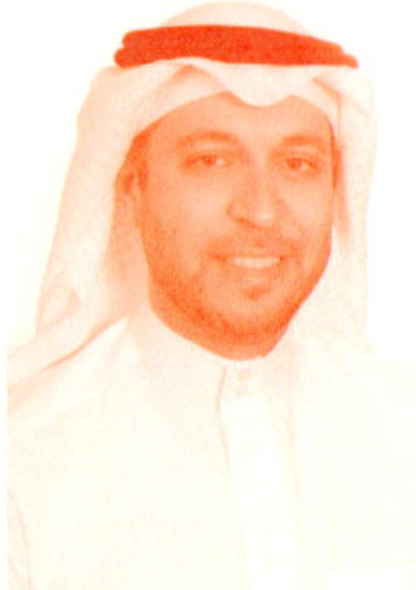
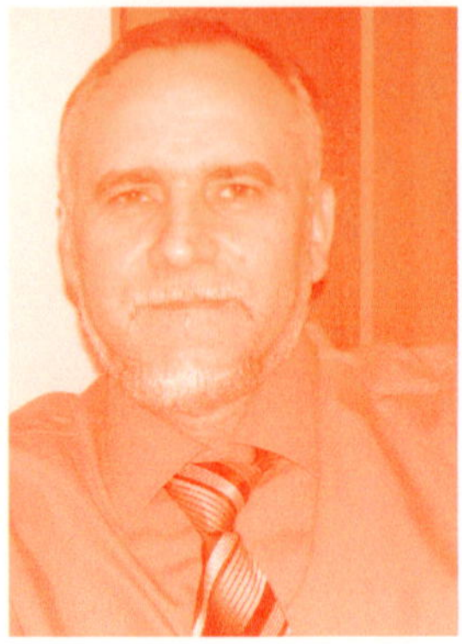
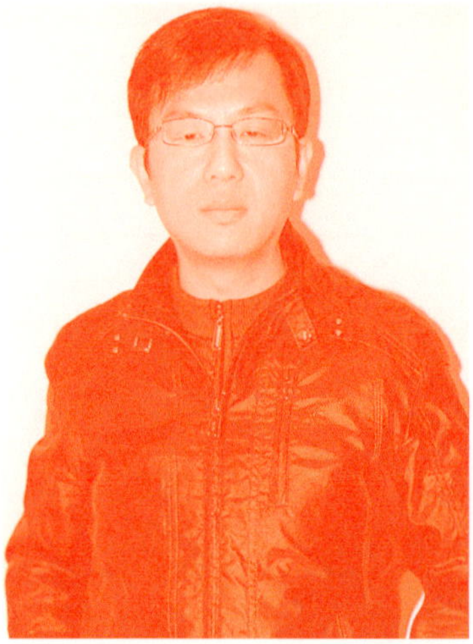
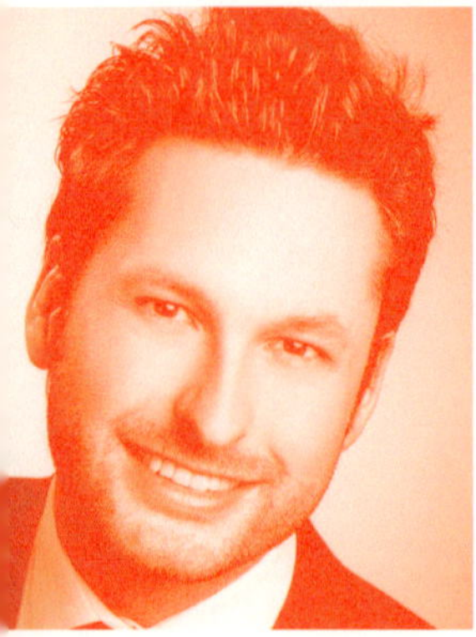
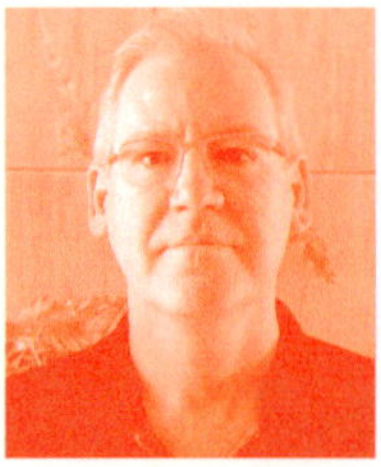

IntechOpen

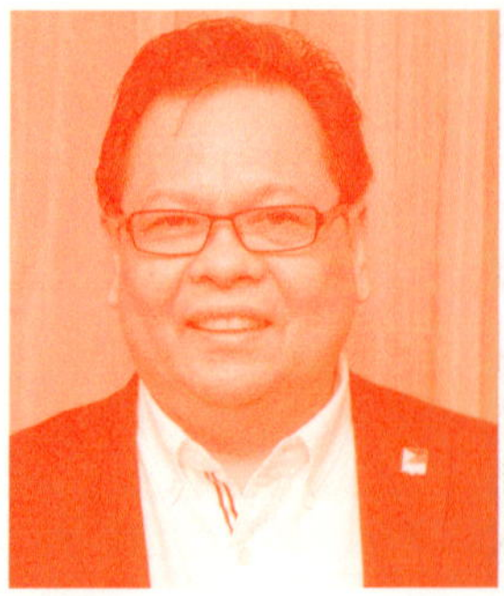
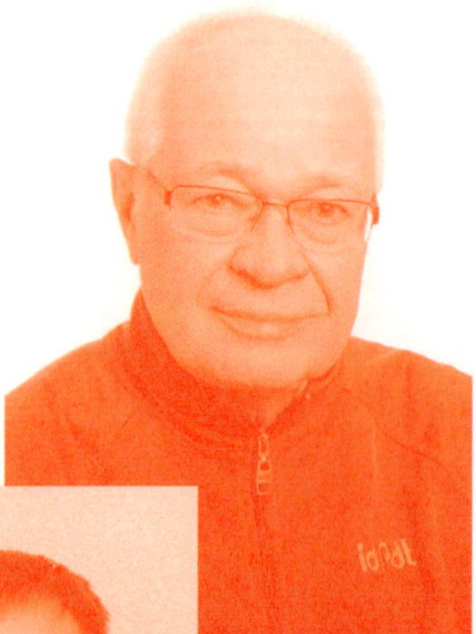
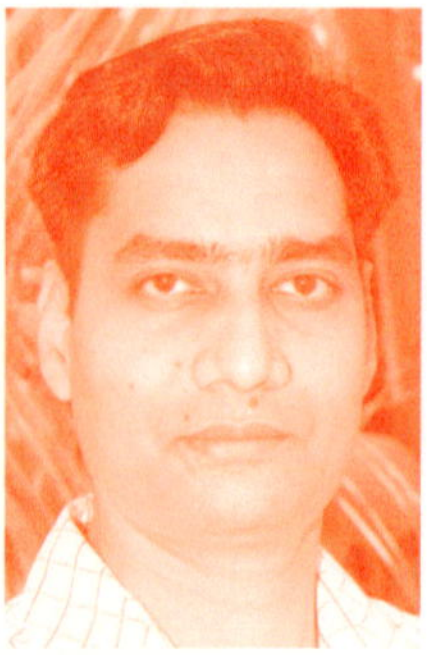
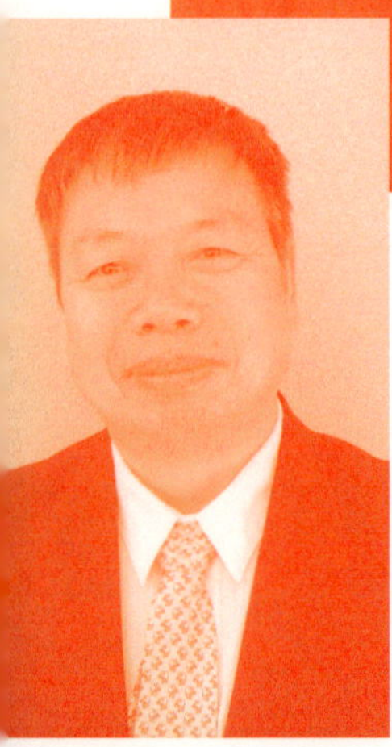
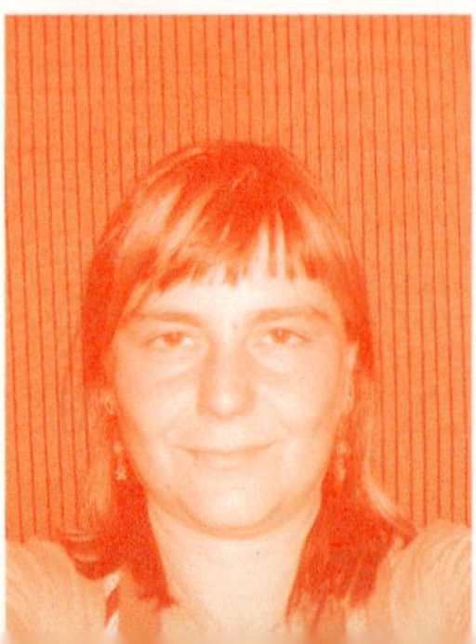
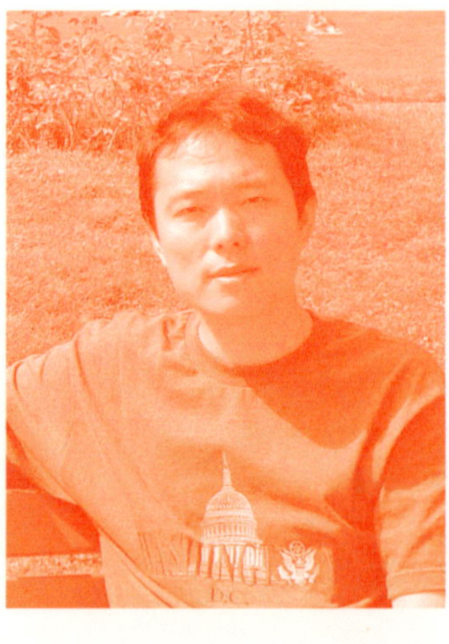

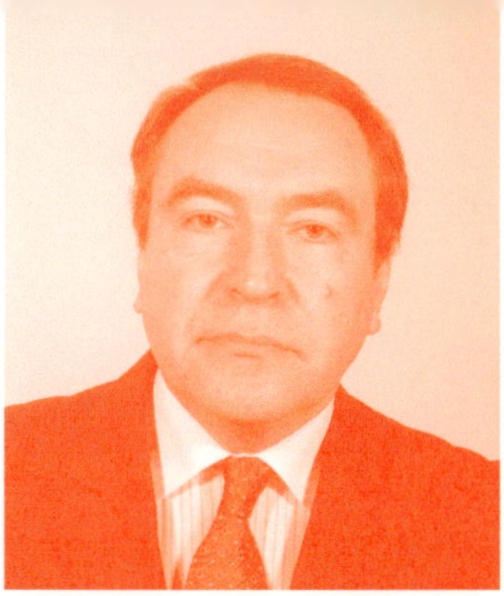
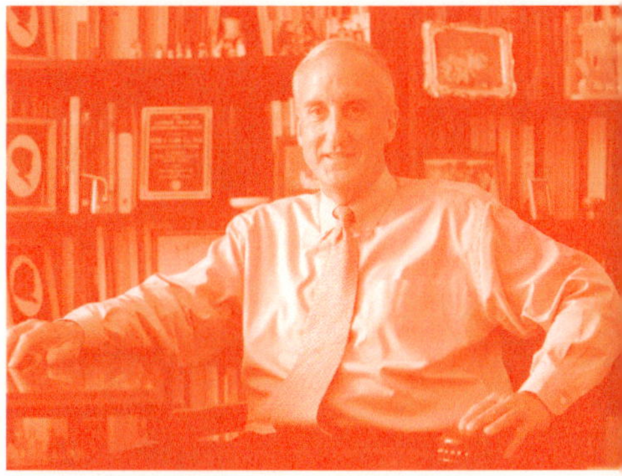
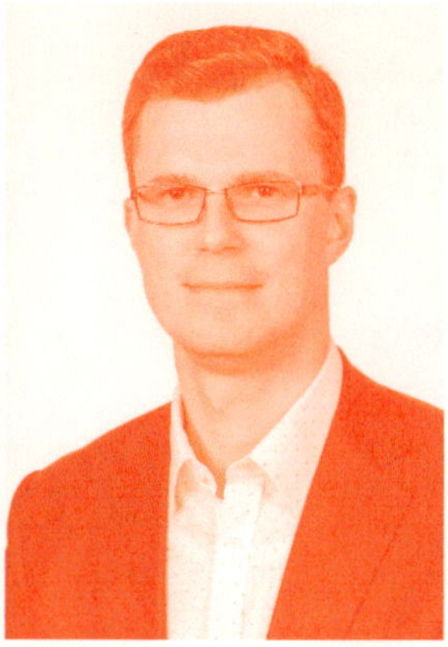
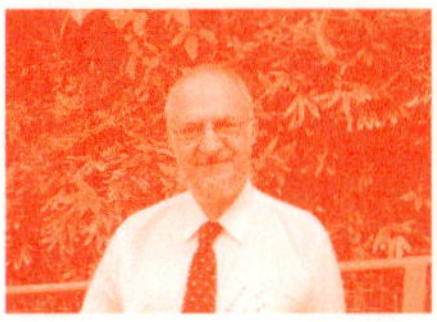
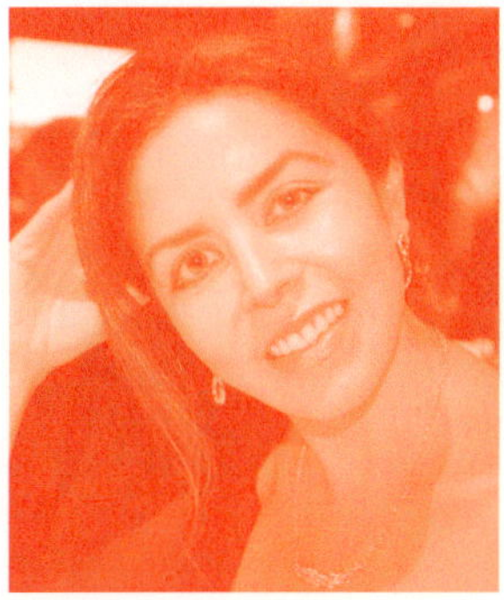

Supporting open minds since 2005

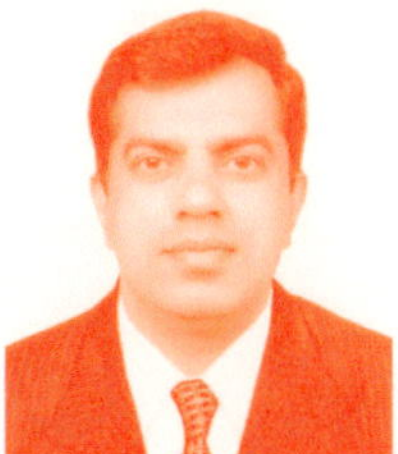
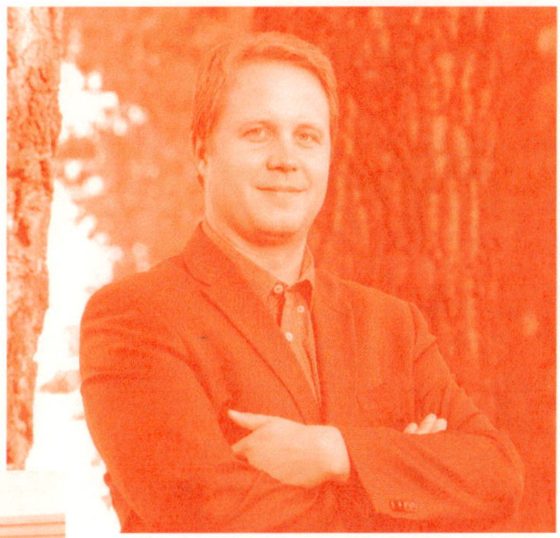
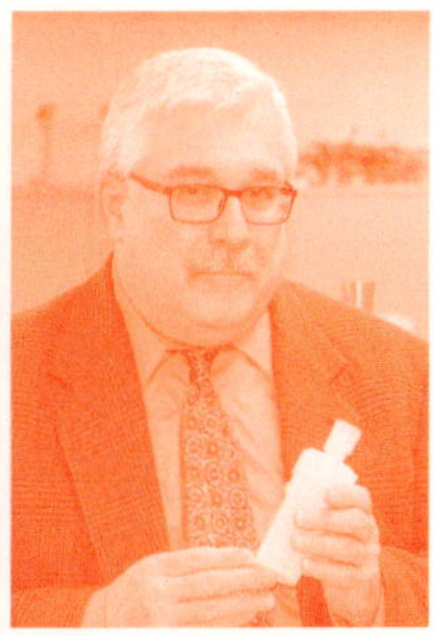
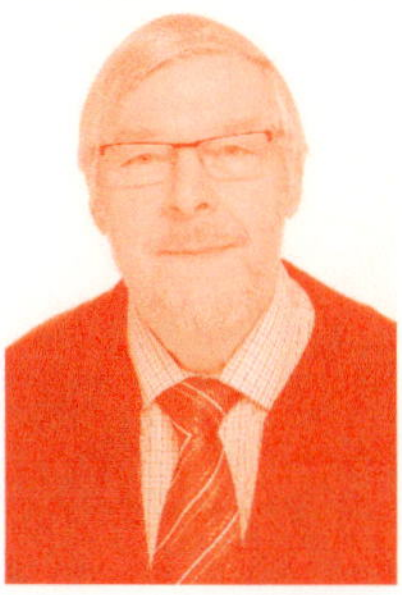
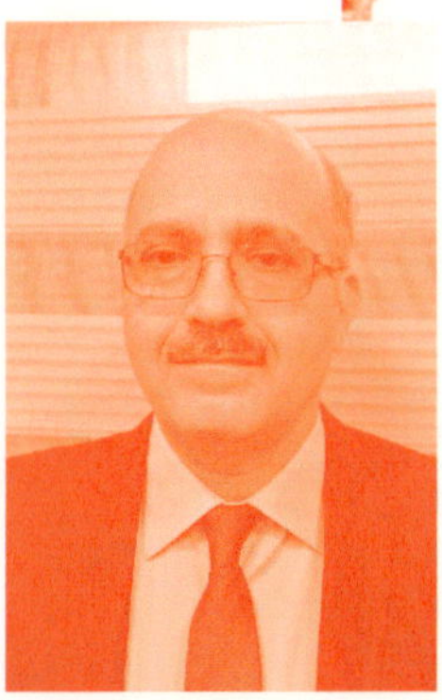
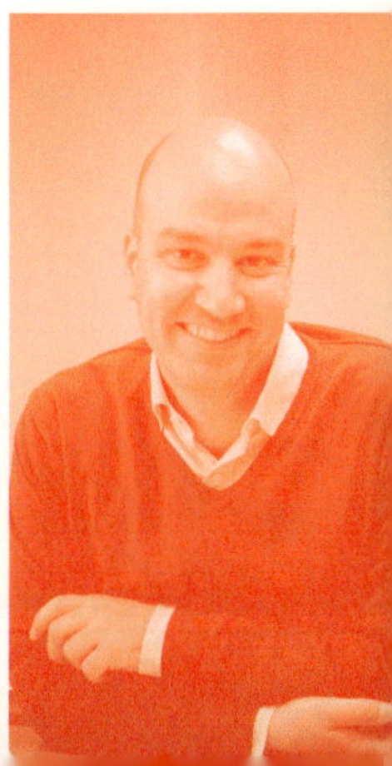
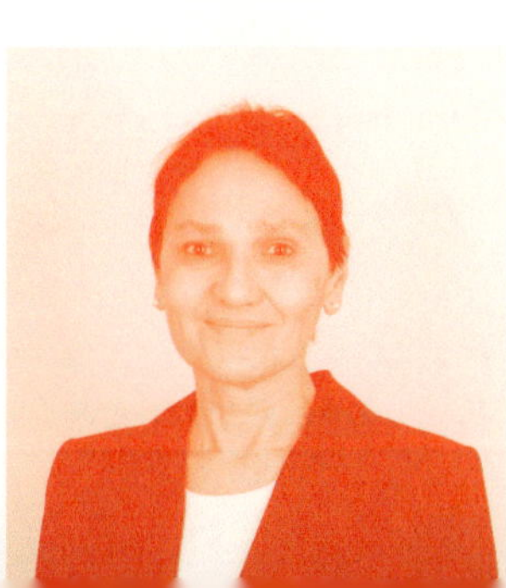

Fighting the COVID-19 Pandemic
http://dx.doi.org/10.5772/intechopen.94676
Edited by Manal Mohammad Baddour

Contributors
Valentina Opancina, Kristijan Krstic, Predrag Sazdanovic, Nebojsa Zdravkovic, Radisa Vojinovic, Ruzica Radojevic Marjanovic, Vicente Enrique Machaca Arceda, Miguel Angel Machaca Arceda, Pamela Claudia Laguna Laura, John Zizzo, Jucier Gonçalves Junior, Gislene Farias De Oliveira, Modesto Leite Rolim-Neto, Estelita Lima Cândido, Maanasa Rajagopalan, Hemant Bherwani, Prasan Kumar Panda, Mayank Kapoor, Vivek Mohanty, Harpreet Kaur, Sushruti Kaushal, Nihal Seden, Raghunath Satpathy, Prangya Ranjan Rout, Mohamed A Abdullah Jaber, Hisyovi Cardenas Suri, David Jimomila Bening, Benjamín Demah Nuertey, Obeta Mark M. Uchejeso, Jwanse I. Rinpan, Mantu E. Chongs, Maureen O. Ekpere-Ezeugwu, ayse erturk, Moez Guettari, Ahmed El Aferni, Iana Simova, Denislava Hristova, Hristina Tzanovska, Denis Nikolov, Diliana Iakova, Aniuta Ivanova, Maria-Magdalena Pintova, Ognyan Matkov, Todor Samardjiev, Vladimir Kornovski, Jordan Krasnaliev, Todor Kundurzhiev, Nikolay Dimitrov, Toni Vekov, Pavlin Pavlov, Ricardo Wesley Alberca, Heloisa Amaral Gaspar, Claudio Oliveira Flauzino, Olabode Omotoso, Gbenga Ojo, John Teibo, Jitendra D. Lakhani, Sajani Kapadia, Rohit Chordiya, Roop Gill, Som J. Lakhani, Fermín Jesús Jesus González-Melado, María Luisa Di Pietro, Sara Palermo, Alejandro López-Escobar, Sara Jimeno, Alejandro Peixoto, Sara Velázquez, Salvador I. García-Adasme, Paula Sol Ventura Wichner, sarika jain, Manish Yadav, Mohammed S.B. Huda, Ritwika Mallik, Aman Sachdeva, Arup Saha, Ayodele Oluwaseun Ajayi, Olawale Peter Odeleye, Oluwabukola Atinuke Popoola, Ugur Kostakoglu, Ilknur Esen Yildiz, Nur Hursoy, Sevda Ozdemir Al, Songul Ozyurt, Neslihan Ozcelik, Hatice Beyazal Polat, Aysegul Copur Cicek

First published in London, United Kingdom, 2021 by IntechOpen
IntechOpen is the global imprint of INTECHOPEN LIMITED, registered in England and Wales, registration number: 11086078, 5 Princes Gate Court, London, SW7 2QJ, United Kingdom
Printed in Croatia

British Library Cataloguing-in-Publication Data
A catalogue record for this book is available from the British Library

Additional hard and PDF copies can be obtained from orders@intechopen.com

Fighting the COVID-19 Pandemic
Edited by Manal Mohammad Baddour
p. cm.
Print ISBN 978-1-83968-216-2
Online ISBN 978-1-83968-217-9
eBook (PDF) ISBN 978-1-83968-246-9

For EU product safety concerns:
IN TECH d.o.o., Prolaz Marije Krucifikse Kozulić 3, 51000 Rijeka, Croatia, info@intechopen.com or visit our website at intechopen.com.

Meet the editor

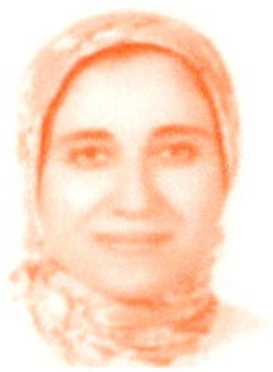

Manal Mohammad Baddour is a Professor of Medical Microbiology and Immunology in the Faculty of Medicine, Alexandria University, Egypt. She obtained a Ph.D. in Microbiology and Immunology from the same university in 1995. Dr. Baddour was ranked first among high school examinees in Saudi Arabia in 1979. She has also been listed in the Marquis Who's Who in the World 2009 and in the Academic Keys Who's Who list for Medicine Higher Education. She has held several positions including secretary general of the Permanent Scientific Committee for Promotion of Professors and Associate Professors in Medical Microbiology and Immunology, Egypt. She is also an editor and reviewer for numerous scientific journals. She has edited or authored several books and has thirty-six journal publications to her credit. She is an assessor for promotion files of faculty members from Egyptian, Jordanian, and Saudi Arabian universities. Dr. Baddour is a member of several organizations including the Gerson Lehrman Group for Healthcare & Biomedical Council; Society for General Microbiology, England; Egyptian Society for Medical Microbiology; Egyptian Association of Immunologists; Egyptian Society for Infection Control; Egyptian Medical Syndicate; Alexandria Medical Syndicate Council; African Association of Physiological Sciences, South Africa; and African Regional Training Network for Medical and Allied Health Sciences, South Africa.

Contents

Preface **XIII**

Section 1
The Virus and Epidemiology **1**

Chapter 1 **3**
Knowing Our Rival–Coronaviridae: The Virus Family
by Maanasa Rajagopalan

Chapter 2 **17**
COVID-19: An Updated Insight of the Pandemic
by Raghunath Satpathy and Prangya Ranjan Rout

Chapter 3 **35**
COVID-19 Pandemic: Analysis and Statistics of Confirmed Cases
by Vicente Enrique Machaca Arceda, Miguel Angel Machaca Arceda and Pamela Claudia Laguna Laura

Chapter 4 **51**
Demographic, Clinical and Radiological Features of Healthcare Workers and Two Index Cases That Were Infected with COVID-19 (SARS-Cov-2)
by Ayse Erturk, Ugur Kostakoglu, Ilknur Esen Yildiz, Nur Hursoy, Sevda Ozdemir Al, Songul Ozyurt, Neslihan Ozcelik, Hatice Beyazal Polat and Aysegul Copur Cicek

Chapter 5 **69**
Coronavirus Disinfection Physical Methods
by Moez Guettari and Ahmed El Aferni

Chapter 6 **89**
Immune Response to COVID-19
by Ricardo Wesley Alberca

Section 2
Manifestations of Disease **111**

Chapter 7 **113**
Clinical Characteristics of COVID-19 Infection
by Mohamed Abdullah Jaber

Chapter 8 123
Loss of Smell and Taste as Clinical Onset of COVID-19
by Nihal Seden

Chapter 9 133
Cardiovascular System and SARS-CoV-2: Etiology, Physiopathology and Clinical Presentation: A Systematic Review
by Jucier Gonçalves Júnior, Estelita Lima Cândido, Gislene Farias de Oliveira and Modesto Leite Rolim Neto

Chapter 10 149
Post COVID-19 Conditions and the Cardiovascular System
by Iana Simova, Denislava Hristova, Hristina Tzanovska, Denis Nikolov, Diliana Iakova, Anyuta Ivanova, Maria-Magdalena Pintova, Pavlin Pavlov, Ognyan Matkov, Todor Samardjiev, Vladimir Kornovski, Jordan Krasnaliev, Todor Kundurzhiev, Nikolay Dimitrov and Toni Vekov

Chapter 11 173
COVID-19 and Type 2 Diabetes Mellitus
by Ritwika Mallik and Mohammed S.B. Huda

Chapter 12 185
Pregnancy and COVID-19
by Sushruti Kaushal and Harpreet Kaur

Chapter 13 197
Neurological Involvement in COVID-19
by Valentina Opancina, Kristijan Krstic, Predrag Sazdanovic, Nebojsa Zdravkovic, Ruzica Radojevic Marjanovic and Radisa Vojinovic

Chapter 14 215
"Neurocovid": An Analysis of the Impact of Covid-19 on the Older Adults. Evolving Psychological and Neuropsychological Understanding
by Sara Palermo

Chapter 15 229
Consequences of the SARS-CoV-2 Pandemic on Mental Health: Integrative Review
by Jucier Gonçalves Júnior, Gislene Farias de Oliviera and Modesto Leite Rolim-Neto

Chapter 16 241
COVID-19 in India: Problems, Challenges and Strategies (Psychological Aspects)
by Sarika Jain and Manish Yadav

Chapter 17 263
COVID-19 and Multiorgan Dysfunction Syndrome
by Jitendra D. Lakhani, Sajni Kapadia, Rohit Choradiya, Roop Preet Gill and Som J. Lakhani

Chapter 18 289
COVID-19 and Catastrophic Antiphospholipid Syndrome
by Hisyovi Cardenas Suri, David Jimomila Bening and Benjamín Demah Nuertey

Section 3
Diagnosis and Management 299

Chapter 19 301
Fighting COVID-19: The Medical Laboratory Involvement
by Obeta M. Uchejeso, Jwanse I. Rinpan, Mantu E. Chongs and Maureen O. Ekpere-Ezeugwu

Chapter 20 317
Evolution of Diagnostic Methods and Prevalence Detection of COVID-19: A Review
by Hemant Bherwani

Chapter 21 333
Usefulness of the Hemogram in COVID-19
by Sara Jimeno, Alejandro Peixoto, Sara Velázquez, Paula Sol Ventura, Salvador I. García Adasme and Alejandro López-Escobar

Chapter 22 347
COVID-19 Vaccine: A Way Out of Crisis
by Aman Sachdeva and Arup Saha

Chapter 23 357
Myths: Barriers to Fighting the COVID-19 Pandemic
by Olabode Omotoso, Teibo John and Gbenga Ojo

Chapter 24 369
Myths Surrounding Covid-19 Vaccine Candidates: A Guide to Fight Back
by John Zizzo

Chapter 25 385
Covid-19 Vaccines and Institutional Trust
by Fermín Jesús González-Melado and María Luisa Di Pietro

Chapter 26 397
Pharmacotherapy for COVID-19: A Ray of Hope
by Mayank Kapoor, Prasan Kumar Panda and Vivek Mohanty

Chapter 27 419
Home Care as a Safe Alternative during COVID-19 Crisis
by Heloisa Amaral Gaspar and Claudio Oliveira Flauzino

Chapter 28 429
Tackling COVID-19 through the One Health Approach
by Ayodele Oluwaseun Ajayi, Olawale Peter Odeleye and Oluwabukola Atinuke Popoola

Preface

What are coronaviruses? What is SARS-CoV-2? What is its origin? Why did it suddenly appear? How does it cause disease? How do these viruses spread? How can the surrounding environment be decontaminated? How does our body respond and fight back? Who gets complications and why?

How can we diagnose these infections? What are the different diagnostic modalities?

What are the proposed treatment options? When do we treat and who do we treat?

Why are there so many vaccine candidates? Why is there reluctance and hesitancy to vaccination efforts? What are the myths and barriers to vaccines?

What is meant by a "one-health approach" and how does it affect human health?

Over three sections, this book, *Fighting the COVID-19 Pandemic*, tackles these questions and more.

The first section deals with the coronavirus, highlighting its properties and the demographic features of the pandemic. Additionally, it examines how we can target the virus through our immune systems in vivo and through methods of decontamination in vitro.

The second section talks about the different manifestations of the disease in various clinical cohorts including pregnant females, diabetics, and persons with cardiovascular morbidities. It examines the effect of the coronavirus on the nervous system, senses of taste and smell, and mental health. The chapter highlights the association of the virus with multiorgan dysfunction and catastrophic antiphospholipid antibody syndrome.

The third section discusses the role of the medical laboratory in diagnosis, and evaluates diagnostic methods such as the hemogram. Prevention relies on vaccines in addition to precautionary measures against exposure, yet many myths are barriers to vaccination efforts. A decline in institutional trust serves to perpetuate myths and vaccine hesitancy. As such, this section also outlines the role of pharmacotherapeutics and discusses options for home care, with an introduction to the possible role of the "one-health approach" in tackling such situations.

The book represents the current situation. As time goes on and the situation changes and evolves, some of the information presented herein may become obsolete.

Manal Mohammad Baddour
Faculty of Medicine,
Medical Microbiology and Immunology Department,
Alexandria University,
Alexandria, Egypt

Section 1

The Virus and Epidemiology

Chapter 1

Knowing Our Rival–Coronaviridae: The Virus Family

Maanasa Rajagopalan

Abstract

This chapter will describe the biological nature of viruses belonging to the Coronaviridae family. Coronavirus disease or COVID-19 which, with its ever-expanding attack around the globe has become the topic of discussion of the current era. The disease is caused by a SARS-CoV-2 virus which belongs to the Coronaviridae family. This family of the virus has a history of pandemic significance through its attacks of SARS and MERS since the year 2000. They are known to have affinity towards respiratory tract and any disease that erupts out of their group have caused mild and severe respiratory infections globally. Thus, understanding the virus by learning the characteristics of its familial strain will help us to combat their attack even after mutation in the future. This chapter also discusses the pathogenesis of each virus organism in this family, as well as their clinical characteristics and diagnostics, in order to understand their disease-causing pattern and the efficacy of vaccination in mitigating the worst outcomes of the disease.

Keywords: The Virus Family, Coronaviridae, SARS-CoV, Pandemics, Vaccination

1. Introduction

Coronaviruses have historically been the most common type of virus that has caused global pandemics. This virus family began its first outbreak as a mild endemic common cold in 1892 but quickly evolved into a viral pandemic that affected millions of people. The four major strains of human coronaviruses that have spread across the world, evolving from a common cold to a severe respiratory tract disease, are NL63, 229E, OC43, and HKU1 [1]. The majority of them are spread by zoonotic transmission from bats, cats, and camels through droplets or direct contact. However, SARS-CoV, MERS-CoV, and SARS-CoV-2 (a different strain of SARS-CoV) were the key causes of the three pandemics that occurred in the last two decades, and their similarities and variations in nature must be recognized in order to figure out how they attack and how to combat them effectively in the future.

2. Coronaviridae–the virus

The Family of Coronaviridae has two subfamilies named ***Coronavirinae*** and ***Torovirinae***, where the Torovirus family infects vertebrates and has been isolated with gastroenteritis while Coronavirinae affects mammals with respiratory and enteric infections. Torovirinae has unique doughnut-shaped nucleocapsids which distinguish them from Coronavirinae. The current classification of coronaviruses recognizes 39 species in 27 subgenera, five genera, and two subfamilies that belong to the family Coronaviridae, suborder Cornidovirineae, order Nidovirales, and realm Riboviria [2].

The Coronavirinae family of viruses is widespread among mammals and is known to cause respiratory or enteric infections. This subfamily has four genus-group of viruses namely –

- Genus *Alphacoronavirus*

- Genus *Betacoronavirus*

- Genus *Gammacoronavirus*

- Genus *Deltacoronavirus*

Among the four genera, various disease affections by 60 virus species were found to belong to Genus *Betacoronavirus.* They were mostly isolated from bats but were also found to be from camels and sea species.

Members of the Coronavirinae family are mostly large, enveloped, single-stranded RNA viruses with genomes ranging from 25 to 32 kb and a virion of 118–136 nm in diameter. They are roughly spherical with large spike glycoproteins that extend 16–21 nm from the virus envelope. Almost two – thirds of the genome encodes a non-structural protein (nsp) required for transcription and genome replication and among the non-structural proteins, nsp – 12 forms a multiprotein complex with other CoV nsps which are synthesized as long precursor polypeptides. Ribosomes approaching the frame-shift site slip into the minus-1 reading frame almost 20–25% of the time, and a longer polyprotein called REP1b gets synthesized [3]. The RdRP (nsp12), a protein with helicase and phosphatase activities (nsp13), a protein with exonuclease and methyltransferase activities (nsp14), an endoribonuclease (nsp15), and a second methyltransferase (nsp16) are among the five additional proteins coded for by REP1b (**Figure 1**).

There are hundreds of coronaviruses of which most of them circulate among animals like pigs, camels, cats, and bats. Some of them have transmitted to humans as a result of spillover event, causing dreadful diseases.

The positive-strand RNA genome contains 7–10 open reading frames (ORF) with additional 7–10 frames lying downstream of the replicase-associated genes. The largest of these encodes is the spike protein (S) and the order of the structural proteins of the coronavirus genome is well conserved. The additional small ORFs thus lie in between or overlap the structural protein genes and are called accessory proteins which are encoded by the shortest mRNA. Previous studies on virus mutations have stated that these accessory proteins are not essential for coronavirus replication in cell culture. However, mutating the accessory protein has had a profound effect on the ability of the virus to replicate in their hosts and influence the viral pathogenesis [4].

2.1 Structural proteins of coronavirus

Viruses belonging to the family of Coronavirinae encode four structural proteins namely –

- Three membrane-associated proteins (S, M, and E)

- A single nucleocapsid (N) protein.

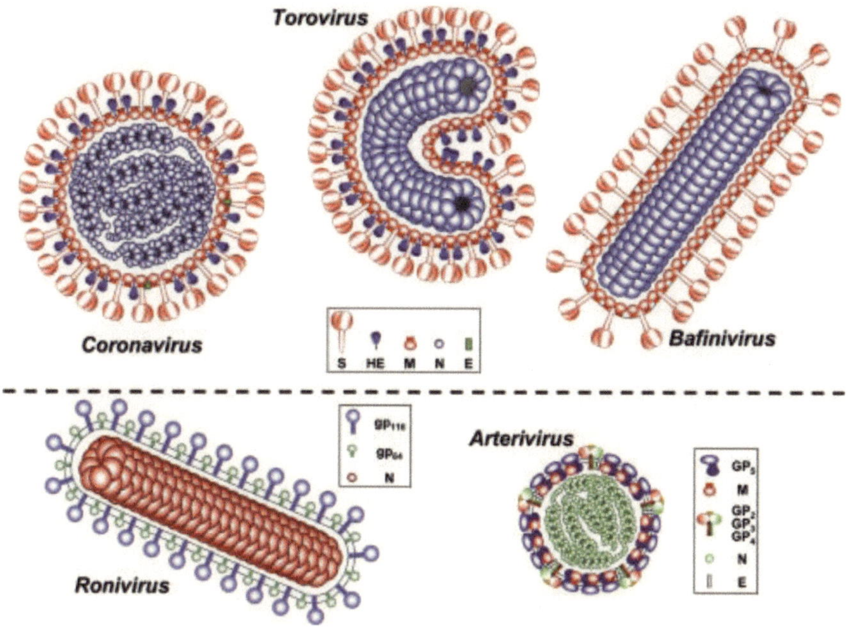

Figure 1.
Coronaviridae family. (reprinted from: Coronaviridae (Chapter-24) by MacLachlan NJ, Dubovi EJ, editors; science direct [4]).

However, some virus species belonging to the genus beta coronavirus have an additional membrane protein with Hemagglutinating and Esterase activities, called HE. Thus the order of the structural genes on the CoV genome is (HE) S, M, E, N [4].

S – CoVs have a distinctive appearance due to the **spike protein**, which forms a conspicuous projection from the virus envelope. S is glycosylated and becomes the attachment and fusion protein. Among the CoVs, there are some variations in the way S is processed (cleaved into S1 and S2 fragments) where it is often ER-associated and is altered by N-linked glycosylation.

S is partially or completely cleaved by host furin-like proteases in the ER (before an assembly of new virions) in many beta and gamma coronaviruses. The extent of proteolysis correlates with the number of highly basic residues at the S1/S2 cleavage site. The S1 (N-terminal) and S2 (C-terminal) products remain noncovalently associated.

SARS-CoV, on the other hand, does not have S cleaved during assembly or release. Instead, during entry/penetration, it is cleaved in an acidified endosome. A cleavage at the S1/S2 boundary and a second cleavage within S2 (called the S2′ cleavage site) tend to be two crucial cleavage events that function in concert to mediate fusion [5].

Also within several isolates of a single type of coronavirus, comparison of S1 sequences show that they diverge widely and are not strongly conserved, leaving us with a fair assumption that the sequence divergence is a result of host immune response. However, unlike S1, the S2 product is highly conserved across the sub-family Coronavirinae subfamily.

M – The **membrane protein** is the most abundant protein in the virion containing three hydrophobic domains and thus tightly associated with the virus envelope. It has a short ectodomain (extracellular domain) that is modified by glycosylation and plays a major role in promoting membrane curvature. Expression of M in Human Corona Virus (HCoV) – SARS (in the absence of other viral proteins) results in self-assembly and release of membrane-enveloped vesicles. M also interacts with the N and E proteins and virus-like particles are released when M is co-expressed with either N or E [6].

E – The **envelope protein** is present in the virion in very small quantities (about 20 molecules per virion), however larger amounts of E are present in infected cells. During particle formation, different CoVs have varying requirements for E, ranging from mandatory to optional. In fact, virus titres close to 1 × 106 pfu per mL have been reported for HCoV-SARS lacking the E protein. Studies show that E is a viroporin as it assembles in membranes to form ion channels and they influence the electrochemical balance in subcellular compartments [7].

N – The only protein found in the ribonucleoprotein particle is **nucleocapsid protein**. N forms homodimers and homo-oligomers and binds genomic RNA, packaging it into a long flexible nucleocapsid. In the infected cell, N localizes to the cytoplasm, and for some CoVs, N is also found in the nucleolus. N has a role in the assembly and binding as it interacts with other CoV structural proteins. It also co-localizes with replicas–transcriptase components and is required for RNA synthesis [8]. Other roles for N include modulating cell cycle (promoting cell-cycle arrest) and inhibiting host cell translation (**Figure 2**).

2.2 Viral replication

The first event in the replication cycle is the translation of the viral genome by the ribosomes in the host cell. REP1a and REP1b are translated from genomic RNA and some of the other REP1a products have transmembrane domains that serve to anchor the replication-transcription complex to cell membranes and become a pre-requisite for the synthesis of additional viral RNAs. This interaction causes the remodeling of host cell membranes to form structures for viral RNA synthesis.

The next event after translation comes the synthesis of RNA by RNA-dependent RNA polymerase (RdRP). A primer, specifically a short RNA oligonucleotide, is required by the CoV RdRP. It just so happens that the CoVs encode two separate RdRP-active proteins. The product of the nsp8 gene is thought to be a primase that can synthesize short oligonucleotides while nsp12 is the elongating polymerase. Cap synthesis is carried out by other viral nsps in the replication–transcription complex.

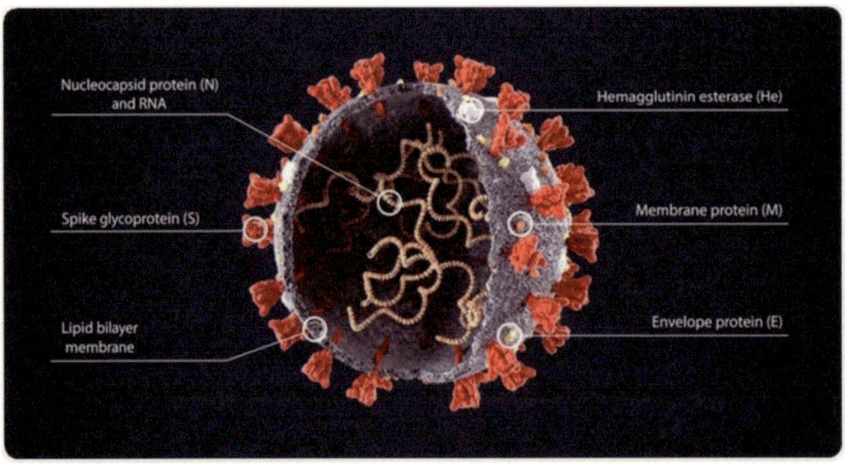

Figure 2.
Structural proteins. (reprinted from: The week: X-rays size up coronavirus protein structure at room temperature [9]).

The other two ribonucleases that are encoded are nsp14 and nsp 15, where nsp 14 is a 3′–5′ exonuclease while nsp 15 is a Nidovirales endonuclease that cleaves both single- and double-stranded RNA, cutting downstream of uridylate residues. Infected cells contain a set of subgenomic (sg) mRNAs in addition to genome-length RNA. The structural and accessory proteins are expressed using the sg mRNAs. They're all capped and polyadenylated, and all have the same 3′ end, creating a "nested set" of mRNAs. A closer examination of the sg mRNAs shows that they all have the same 70–100 nucleotides (nt) leader sequence at the 5′ end. These sequences are identical and though found on all sg mRNAs, they are found only once in the genome.

The transcription regulating sequence is formed when these leader sequences fuse with downstream sequences at short 8–9 nt motifs (TRS). A TRS is located upstream of the structural protein-coding ORFs (these are called TRS body or TRS-B). In the 5′ UTR, a TRS has been found just downstream of the leader chain. These results shed light on the unique strategy used for CoV mRNA synthesis [4].

The high degree of CoV genome recombination is most likely due to discontinuous transcription, and this form of RNA virus genome recombination is known as a copy-choice mechanism. The presence of cRNAs (negative-sense RNAs with 5′ oligo (U)) in infected cells is 0.1–0.01 times lower than that of "positive-sense" genomes and mRNAs, according to a study. This shows that the recombinants are more likely to occur during the synthesis of negative strands.

2.3 Release

Virion assembly takes place on membranes, where the N protein binds genomic RNA, which then interacts with M protein and buds into ER/Golgi membranes. M protein intends to induce the membrane curvature that drives budding by packing tightly into membranes. S and E are also Membrane proteins and are acquired during the budding phase. E protein has the ion channel activity of a viroporin, which changes cell secretory pathways to facilitate virus release. One of E's functions may be to raise the pH of the transport vesicles. The virus particles that are found in membrane-bound vesicles are released from cells by exocytosis [4].

3. Pandemics and coronaviridae

In concern to Infectious Diseases and Global Healthcare, Pandemic is a worst-case scenario spreading beyond country borders. Communicable diseases have escalated to a pandemic situation since the time of origin of the human race, where the first disease that spread across borders affecting millions of people was the Plague. Our world witnessed the spread of the Bubonic Plague, which started in Egypt and spread all over the Middle East, Roman, and Mediterranean regions.

This was then followed by other diseases like Leprosy, Small Pox, Cholera, Measles, AIDS, and Influenza draining out the health care for decades and centuries. The new addition to this series of diseases that are causing nightmare to global healthcare is SARS, MERS, and COVID-19, all caused by the family of coronavirus.

This large family of viruses is known to cause mild to moderate upper respiratory tract illnesses from the common cold to respiratory distress and failure. Among the group, three coronaviruses have emerged from animal reservoirs over the past two decades and spilled over to humans, causing three serious pandemics – SARS, MERS, and COVID-19.

Severe Acute Respiratory Syndrome (SARS) caused by SARS coronavirus emerged in 2002 and spread over all major continents affecting thousands of people which later came down and disappeared in 2004. This was followed by Middle East Respiratory Syndrome (MERS) which emerged in 2012 was caused by MERS Coronavirus, which originated from an animal reservoir in camels in Saudi Arabia. This caused severe sporadic and localized outbreaks across 27 countries, namely Algeria, Austria, Bahrain, China, Egypt, France, Greece, Germany, Islamic Republic of Iran, Italy, Jordan, Kuwait, Lebanon, Malaysia, the Netherlands, Oman, Philippines, Qatar, Republic of Korea, Kingdom of Saudi Arabia, Thailand, Tunisia, Turkey, United Arab Emirates (UAE), United Kingdom (UK), United States of America (USA), and Yemen. The disease affected millions of people across the world and continue to report its prevalence in some parts even today.

The third coronavirus that emerged out of the family is SARS-CoV-2, a novel virus that is quite similar to the SARS coronavirus. This emerged in the China Sea market in 2019 as an upper respiratory tract infection, which later spread rapidly across more than 200 countries and was soon declared as a global pandemic. The disease continues to affect millions of people, causing thousands of deaths even today.

3.1 SARS

In early 2003, a new pneumonic disease emerged as a life-threatening pandemic from the family of coronaviruses, SARS, caused by SARS – CoV virus. The disease originated in South China as an endemic upper respiratory tract infection and soon spread over various countries affecting millions of people in the United States of America, Europe, and other countries with approximately 10% mortality. The pathogenesis of the SARS CoV virus is quite complex where the genomic characterization is less similar to other known coronaviruses than the rest [10].

SARS-CoV involves a large viral RNA genome encompassing 29,727 nucleotides predicted to contain 14 ORF. The two large 5′-terminal ORF - 1a and 1b, constitute the replicase gene encoding the proteins required for viral RNA transcription and replication [9]. The remaining twelve ORFs encode the four key structural proteins, the spike (S) protein, the nucleocapsid (N) protein, the membrane (M) protein and the small envelope (E) protein, and other eight accessory proteins that are not likely to be essential in tissue culture but may provide a selective advantage in the infected host [11].

Polyprotein pp1a and pp1ab are cleaved extensively by a papain-like cysteine protease (PL2pro) and another chymotrypsin-like protease ($3CL^{pro}$) to yield a multi-subunits protein complex called “viral replicase-transcriptase”. 3CLpro functions as a pivotal protease in coronavirus polyproteins processing and controls the activities of coronavirus replication complexes [12].

Coronavirus Spike (S) protein is a type I membrane glycoprotein that has an N-terminal ectodomain, a C-terminal hydrophobic anchor and an unusual cysteine-rich domain bridging the putative junction of the anchor and the cytoplasmic tail. SARS-CoV S protein is 1255 amino acids long glycoprotein [13]. It is predicted to possess a 13 amino acid signal peptide at the N-terminus, a single ectodomain (1182 amino acids) and a transmembrane region followed by a short cytoplasmic tail (28 residues) at the C-terminus. The protein is translated as a large polypeptide, which is subsequently cleaved by virus-encoded or host-encoded proteases to produce two functional subunits, S1 and S2. S1 is known to be the peripheral fragment and S2 is the membrane-spanning fragment. Both the S1 and S2 subunits appear to cause cell fusion when expressed individually suggesting their biological activity. The N, M and E proteins also play a vital role in SARS-CoV replication and infection mechanism [14].

The virus was isolated from a variety of species, including civet cats and raccoon dogs, but none was considered to be the true source. Certain bat species were later identified as possible natural reservoirs. Direct touch, droplets, and airborne routes are all used to spread SARS to and from humans. Additional routes are suggested by viral isolation from feces and urine samples [9]. Thus, SARS began to spread through droplet transmission or contact with fomite from person to person, affecting more than 70% of patients with shortness of breath or fever and 30% of patients with severe illness that required mechanical ventilation for survival.

3.2 MERS

The first case of MERS occurred in 2012 in Jordon, UAE as a mild upper respiratory tract illness caused by MERS CoV. The virus sequence was found to be in bats and dromedary camels which soon transmitted to humans and caused one of the most dreadful pandemics of the century. Thousands of laboratory-confirmed cases and hundreds of deaths due to the disease are reported even today in the Middle East [11] and the zoonotic transmission of the virus from animals to humans was caused by a common entry receptor named dipeptidyl peptidase 4 (DPP4).

The MERS-CoV genome is 30119 nt in length and contains 10 predicted ORFs. The single-stranded, positive-sense polyadenylated RNA genome has 5′ and 3′ UTR of 278 and 300 nt in length, respectively [12]. The 5′ end of the genome is translated to yield a large polyprotein, which gets co-translationally cleaved in cis by two viral proteases into 16 functional non-structural proteins, which then work together to shape the complex machinery for viral RNA synthesis and recombination. The region downstream of ORF1b is distinguished by the presence of a diverse set of structural proteins, including the spike and envelope proteins.

The case fatality rate of MERS seemed to be higher than SARS, which is reported to be due to the high virulence of the virus and its increased attacks on the lower respiratory tract that resulted in respiratory distress and failure.

3.3 COVID-19

Severe Acute Respiratory Syndrome Coronavirus 2 (SARS-CoV-2), the virus behind the current global pandemic COVID-19 has unique variants that result in a change in transmissibility, clinical presentation, and severity causing greater impact in diagnostics, therapeutics, and vaccine measures. The disease that started as a case of flu in the city of Wuhan, China soon caught up with the global population affecting millions of people and killing thousands every day.

The first affection of COVID-19 that emerged in December 2019, was caused by a strain of beta-coronavirus. The virus showed a high nucleotide sequence homology with two bat-like - severe acute respiratory syndrome:

- bat-SL-CoVZC45
- bat-SL-CoVZXC21 (88% homology)

This strain, however, has 79.5% homology with SARS-CoV, and with MERS-CoV, it has 50% homology. SARS-CoV-2 contains a single-stranded positive RNA of 30 kilobases that encodes 10 genes. The virus enters cells by binding the angiotensin-converting enzyme 2 (ACE2), through its receptor-binding domain in the spike protein [13].

The initial strain, soon on community transmission, began to endanger the novel mutation and gave rise to a new variant, D614G substitution in the gene encoding the spike protein. This variant soon replaced the initial strain and became the dominant form of the virus circulating globally. Almost all strains of D614G mutation have a mutation in the protein responsible for replication (ORF1ab P4715L; RdRP P323L). Due to mutations in the spike protein's receptor binding domain, these variants are unlikely to reduce ACE2 binding affinity, since this would reduce the virus's fitness. V483A and G476S are mostly found in US samples, while V367F is found in samples from China, the Hong Kong Special Administrative Region, France, and the Netherlands [14].

In the evolution of SARS-CoV-2, phylogenetic research suggests population structuring. The results provide an independent test of the major clades we discovered, as well as the variants' regional expansions. Although the earliest samples from the United States seem to be from China and belong to the basal or L84S clades, clades such as D614G/Q57H, appear to be from Europe. D614G was discovered in late January in China and quickly rose to the top of the clade hierarchy. The mutation rate of $1.12*10^{-3}$ mutations per site-year is comparable to the SARS-CoV-1 mutation rate of $0.80*10^{-3}$ to $2.38*10^{-3}$ mutations per site-year [15].

From the present shreds of evidence, we can conclude that the SARS-CoV genome has evolving nature that causes serious implications to human lives. Due to this nature, the number of people with confirmed COVID-19 has been on a continuous increase for the past few months with no sign of decline and the site of affection has also been changing with every new strand. Thus, the major challenge for drug developers against COVID-19 will be to understand the biological reservoirs carrying coronaviruses and the modes of contact with the human population through trade, travel, or recreation to anticipate future risks for novel infections.

3.4 Clinical picture

Knowledge of viral dynamics and host response is essential to understand the clinical picture of any viral disease and its transition after mutations. With regard to COVID-19, this analysis holds more importance due to its serious pandemic attack in the current era.

A cohort study on 23 patients admitted to the hospital with COVID-19 reported that the viral load peaked during the first week of illness and gradually declined in the second week. This may be due to the high transmissibility of SARS-CoV-2 and the increase in IgG and IgM antibody levels [16]. The high viral load in elderly patients was also found to be associated not only with low immunity but also with high expression of the ACE2 receptor (the cell-entry receptor for SARS-CoV-2). From this study, we can conclude that the analysis of serial viral load and antibody profile is essential to understand the viral and host interactions and their transition over the virus mutations [17].

The clinical picture of the disease thus began to vary from its initial attack to the current day from simple respiratory affection to multi-system illness. However, the most common signs and symptoms even today includes –

- Fever/chills
- Cough
- Shortness of breath/breathing difficulty
- Fatigue
- Muscle/body aches

- Headache
- Loss of taste/smell
- Sore throat
- Congestion/runny nose
- Nausea
- Vomiting
- Diarrhea [18]

According to WHO, CDC, and ICMR, the signs and symptoms of COVID-19 that may appear 2–14 days after exposure to the virus are classified into different stages namely mild–moderate, severe, and critical [19].

Mild–Moderate Stage:

- Fever
- Dyspnoea
- Gastrointestinal troubles like Nausea, Vomiting
- Nasal congestion
- Sore throat
- Loss of smell
- Mild gasping for breath with Pneumonia

Severe Stage:

- High Fever
- Cough with gasping for breath
- Severe respiratory distress [$SpO_2 < 90\%$ on room air]
- Bloody expectoration
- Delirium

Children with clinical signs of Pneumonia and Central Cyanosis.

Critical Stage:

- Acute Respiratory Distress Syndrome
- Pulmonary Oedema
- Fluid overload leading to Cardiac Failure

- Sepsis with weak pulse, cold extremities.
- Reduced urinary output
- Thrombocytopenia, Hyperbilirubinemia
- Septic shock with Hypothermia and Collapse [20]

While most people with COVID-19 develop only mild (40%) or moderate (40%) disease, approximately 15% develop the severe stage that requires oxygen support, and 5% have the critical disease with complications such as respiratory failure, acute respiratory distress syndrome (ARDS), sepsis and septic shock, thromboembolism, and/or multiorgan failure including acute kidney disease and cardiac failure [21].

However, this clinical picture is found to be similar to the previous pandemic attacks of this century by the same family of viruses. SARS-CoV and MERS also started as upper respiratory tract infections and rapidly progressed towards respiratory failure, septic shock, and multi-organ failure resulting in death [22]. The incubation period for both SARS-CoV and MERS was around 2–10 days with a mean incubation period of 6.4 and 5 days respectively. Also, the meantime from the onset of illness to the hospitalization in both diseases is 4 days [23]. This shows the similarity of affection and rapidity in the progression of illness caused by any type of virus from the Coronaviridae family.

4. The future of coronaviridae

Howard Markel, a medical historian once quoted "The most predictable thing about this coronavirus is its unpredictability" when describing several pandemic outbreaks. Historically, the occurrence of a viral outbreak and its transition from a mild endemic disease to a global pandemic has been a great challenge to public health researchers and global healthcare. Apart from disease, the geography, host response, and treatment procedures have been influential in viral mutation and its pathogenicity. This is notably important to understand the future attacks of viruses from the Coronaviridae family [24].

Some infectious disease researchers, on the other hand, foresee a healthy future in which virus transmission is reduced due to increased vaccination among people. Experts are hopeful that as vaccinations reach more people, the effect of the COVID phase will lessen and help protect them from the worst possible outcomes of the disease. Current vaccination developed has proven to provide complete and effective protection against most variants of coronavirus and thus, as more people develop specific immunity on vaccination, scientists hope any attack of illness caused by this family of the virus will be of no threat more than an endemic common cold.

5. Conclusion

Since the first pandemic, which was caused by human coronavirus OC-43, one of the four coronaviruses, the existence of disease attacks by them has remained a mystery to medical professionals. The viral organism and its variants, on the other hand, have often evolved after each attack, resurfacing as a new variant of the same Coronaviridae family. To predict the emergence of any viral attack from the family Coronaviridae that has caused serious illness in the global population in the future, it is essential to understand the nature of each organism from the family Coronaviridae.

Furthermore, achieving full immunity by vaccination would aid in the fight against the disease without causing any harm to the global population.

Conflict of interest

There are no conflicts of interest.

Ethical considerations

Not Applicable.

Author details

Maanasa Rajagopalan
Independent Researcher, Chennai, Tamil Nadu, India

*Address all correspondence to: maanasarajagopal.95@gmail.com

References

[1] Raj VS, Osterhaus AD, Fouchier RA, Haagmans BL. MERS: emergence of a novel human coronavirus. Curr Opin Virol. 2014 Apr;5:58-62.

[2] Siddell SG, Walker PJ, Lefkowitz EJ, Mushegian AR, Adams MJ, Dutilh BE, et al. Additional changes to taxonomy ratified in a special vote by the International Committee on Taxonomy of Viruses (October 2018). Arch Virol. 2019 Mar 1;164(3):943-6.

[3] Astuti I, Ysrafil. Severe Acute Respiratory Syndrome Coronavirus 2 (SARS-CoV-2): An overview of viral structure and host response. Diabetes Metab Syndr. 2020;14(4):407-12.

[4] MacLachlan NJ, Dubovi EJ, editors. Chapter 24 - Coronaviridae. In: Fenner's Veterinary Virology (Fifth Edition) [Internet]. Boston: Academic Press; 2017 [cited 2021 Jun 9]. p. 435-61. Available from: https://www.sciencedirect.com/science/article/pii/B9780128009468000246

[5] Payne S. Family Coronaviridae. Viruses. 2017;149-58.

[6] Gioia M, Ciaccio C, Calligari P, De Simone G, Sbardella D, Tundo G, et al. Role of proteolytic enzymes in the COVID-19 infection and promising therapeutic approaches. Biochem Pharmacol. 2020 Dec;182:114225.

[7] J Alsaadi EA, Jones IM. Membrane binding proteins of coronaviruses. Future Virol. 2019 Apr 1;14(4):275-86.

[8] Schoeman D, Fielding BC. Coronavirus envelope protein: current knowledge. Virol J. 2019 May 27;16(1):69.

[9] The Week. X-rays size up coronavirus protein structure at room temperature [Internet]. The Week. 2020 [cited 2021 Jun 9]. Available from: https://www.theweek.in/news/health/2020/06/30/xrays-size-up-coronavirus-structure-at-room-temperature.html

[10] McBride R, van Zyl M, Fielding BC. The Coronavirus Nucleocapsid Is a Multifunctional Protein. Viruses. 2014 Aug 7;6(8):2991-3018.

[11] Gu J, Korteweg C. Pathology and Pathogenesis of Severe Acute Respiratory Syndrome. Am J Pathol. 2007 Apr;170(4):1136-47.

[12] Rota PA, Oberste MS, Monroe SS, Nix WA, Campagnoli R, Icenogle JP, et al. Characterization of a novel coronavirus associated with severe acute respiratory syndrome. Science. 2003 May 30;300(5624):1394-9.

[13] Thiel V, Ivanov KA, Putics Á, Hertzig T, Schelle B, Bayer S, et al. Mechanisms and enzymes involved in SARS coronavirus genome expression. J Gen Virol. 2003 Sep;84(Pt 9):2305-15.

[14] Anand K, Ziebuhr J, Wadhwani P, Mesters JR, Hilgenfeld R. Coronavirus main proteinase (3CLpro) structure: basis for design of anti-SARS drugs. Science. 2003 Jun 13;300(5626):1763-7.

[15] WHO. WHO | Variant analysis of SARS-CoV-2 genomes [Internet]. WHO. World Health Organization; 2020 [cited 2021 Apr 20]. Available from: http://www.who.int/bulletin/volumes/98/7/20-253591/en/

[16] Marra MA, Jones SJM, Astell CR, Holt RA, Brooks-Wilson A, Butterfield YSN, et al. The Genome sequence of the SARS-associated coronavirus. Science. 2003 May 30;300(5624):1399-404.

[17] Suresh R, Maanasa R, Karthikeyan P R, Srinivas G, Antony. Can Homoeopathy Combat COVID-19: A

Repertorial View. Glob J Res Anal. 2021 Apr;10(4):1-4.

[18] Ziebuhr J, Snijder EJ, Gorbalenya AE. Virus-encoded proteinases and proteolytic processing in the Nidovirales. J Gen Virol. 2000 Apr;81(Pt 4):853-79.

[19] CDC. Healthcare Workers [Internet]. Centers for Disease Control and Prevention. 2020 [cited 2021 Apr 21]. Available from: https://www.cdc.gov/coronavirus/2019-ncov/hcp/clinical-guidance-management-patients.html

[20] HUI DS, WONG P, WANG C. SARS: clinical features and diagnosis. Respirol Carlton Vic. 2003 Nov;8(Suppl 1):S20-4.

[21] Li W, Shi Z, Yu M, Ren W, Smith C, Epstein JH, et al. Bats are natural reservoirs of SARS-like coronaviruses. Science. 2005 Oct 28;310(5748):676-9.

[22] van den Brand JM, Smits SL, Haagmans BL. Pathogenesis of Middle East respiratory syndrome coronavirus. J Pathol. 2015 Jan;235(2):175-84.

[23] van Boheemen S, de Graaf M, Lauber C, Bestebroer TM, Raj VS, Zaki AM, et al. Genomic characterization of a newly discovered coronavirus associated with acute respiratory distress syndrome in humans. mBio. 2012 Nov 20;3(6).

[24] Chen Y, Li L. SARS-CoV-2: virus dynamics and host response. Lancet Infect Dis. 2020 May 1;20(5):515-6.

Chapter 2

COVID-19: An Updated Insight of the Pandemic

Raghunath Satpathy and Prangya Ranjan Rout

Abstract

Novel coronavirus (SARS-CoV-2) out-broke in the city of Wuhan in China and widely spread across the globe in a pandemic manner, causing societal and economic disruptions. Though the origin of the novel virus is still a debating topic, it is certain that SARS-CoV-2 acquired human to human transmission capacity. Regardless of aggressive containment and quarantine approaches, the number of confirmed cases continues to rise and being reported due to its highly infectious nature. As of the time, there is a little scope for the antiviral drugs or vaccines for the treatment of coronavirus infection; due to the vigorous mutation rate in the viral genome. However, existing anti-parasite drugs like ivermectin and chloroquine could effectively inhibit the virus has been reported. Few of the vaccines have come up with certain degree of efficacy and many are under the clinical trial phase. The research on novel coronavirus is still in the preliminary stage. In this chapter, we systematically summarize the origin, transmission route, molecular characterization, pathogenic mechanism, contagious nature, clinical symptoms, diagnosis, treatment, mutation and infection as well as prevention strategy of coronavirus disease based on the recently available literature. In addition to this, this chapter presents updated insights of the current state of knowledge pertaining to novel coronavirus and can be referred for potential future studies.

Keywords: Novel coronavirus (SARS-CoV-2), coronavirus disease, prevention strategy, transmission capacity, drug targets, treatment methods, virus structure, mutation

1. Introduction

In December 2019, Wuhan city in China became the center of origin of the novel coronavirus disease with the acronym COVID-19 outbreak that continues to spread quickly across the globe in a very short time. Due to its severe infection rate, on January 30, 2020, World Health Organization (WHO) declared COVID-19 as the public health emergency of international concern (PHEIC), followed by a worldwide pandemic declaration on March 11, 2020. As of May 5, 2020, it has spread to 220 countries with 3665403 confirmed covid-19 positive cases. The recent data (as of June 28, 2021) show that the number of countries affected by Covid-19 is 229, with a total of 181,741,361 confirmed cases of COVID-19 and 3,936,510 deaths. It is anticipated that the full extent of spreading and severity of this 2019 novel coronavirus is yet to be seen and global control of COVID-19 will be one of the toughest challenges humanity has ever faced [1, 2]. According to the international committee on taxonomy of viruses (ICTV) classifications, coronaviruses belong to the order *Nidovirales*, family *Coronaviridae*, and sub-family *Coronavirinae,* as shown in **Figure 1**. These are the largest group of viruses belonging to the *Nidovirales* order. The sub-family *Coronavirinae* is further divided into four genera, such as *Alphacoronavirus*, *Betacoronavirus*, *Gammacoronavirus*, and *Deltacoronavirus*withfour different lineages (A (*embecovirus*), B (*sarbecovirus*), C (*merbecovirus*), and D (*nobecovirus*)) of the *Betacoronavirus*genus [3, 4]. COVID-19, officially named by the WHO on February 11, 2020, is caused by the severe acute respiratory syndrome coronavirus 2 (named by ICTV), otherwise known as SARS-CoV-2. The emerging SARS-CoV-2 is a beta coronavirus of lineage B and seems to be the seventh member of the coronaviruses that infect humans, primarily targeting the respiratory system [5]. The first human coronavirus (HCoV), named B814, was isolated in 1965 from patients with common cold [6]. The other six different HCoVs include severe acute respiratory syndrome coronavirus (SARS-CoV), Middle East respiratory syndrome coronavirus (MERS-CoV), HCoV- 229E, HCoV-OC43, HCoV-NL63, and HCoV-HKU1. Among these HCoVs, HCoV-NL63 and HCoV-229E belong to *Alphacoronavirus*, HCoV-HKU1 and HCoV-OC43 belong to lineage A, SARS-CoV to lineage B, and MERS-CoV to lineage C of the *Betacoronavirus*as depicted in **Figure 1**.

HCoVs are zoonotic pathogens that originated in animals and all HCoVs are believed to have a bat origin, with the exception of *Betacoronavirus* lineage A that

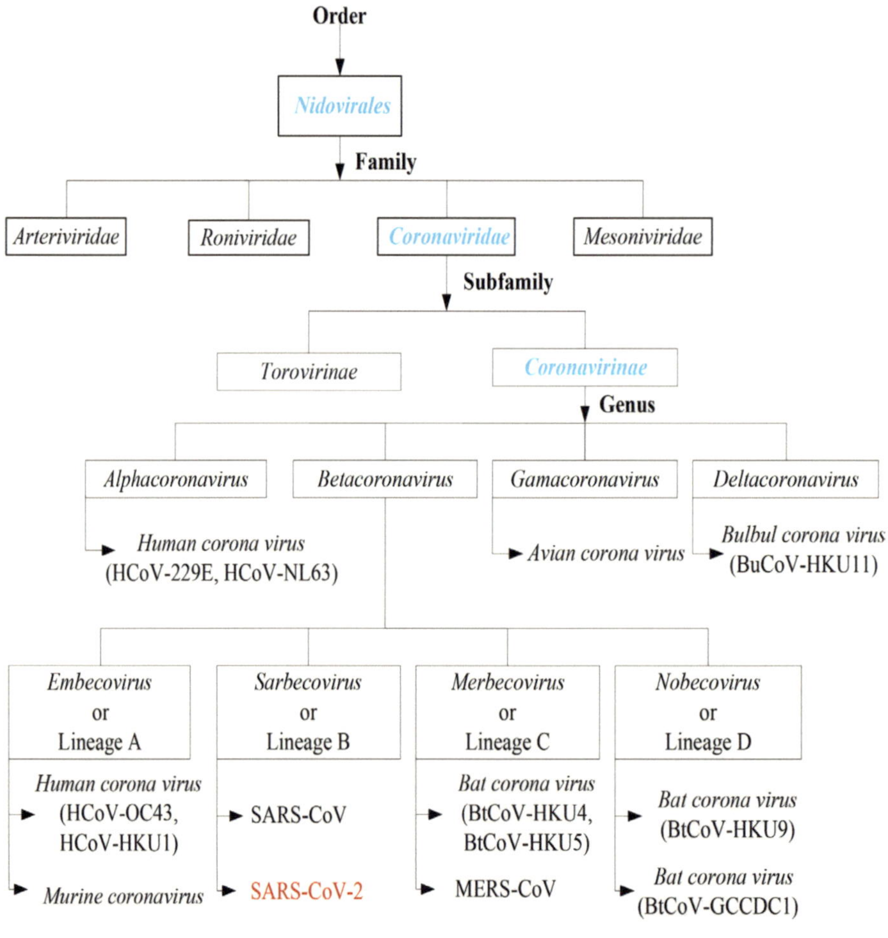

Figure 1.
Classification of novel corona virus.

may have rodent origin [7, 8]. Similar to the case of other SARS-CoVs, the bat might be the probable origin for SARS-CoV-2 as SARS-CoV-2 shares about 96% whole-genome sequence similarity with the bat coronavirus (BatCoV). The confirmed and suspected origins of HCoVs are summarized in **Figure 2**.

Zhou et al. (2020), through complete genome analysis of samples collected from COVID-19 patients, found that SARS-CoV-2 is a *Betacoronavirus* with a sequence identity of 96% with a bat coronavirus [9]. Studies of Pasteur Institute, Shanghai also highlighted that the natural hosts of SARS-CoV-2 might be the bats [10]. However, few studies also highlighted that the pangolin is expected as an intermediate host of the SARS-CoV-2 [11, 12]. Zhang et al. (2019) reported that coronavirus from the pangolin might be the origin of the SARS-CoV-2 on the basis of genome sequence identity [11]. However, the claim was rejected by Cyranoski (2020), based on the fact that the origin is not by the genomic sequence similarity but by the receptor-binding domain (RBD) of the virus that enables the virus to enter the host cell [13]. Although, the potential natural and intermediate host of the virus is not fully established, regardless of its initial transmission source, it is certain that SARS-CoV-2 acquired the capacity for human to human transmission [14]. SARS-CoV-2 is highly infectious; the entire population is generally highly susceptible to infection, and respiratory droplets through coughing and sneezing of COVID-19 patients and coming into contact with them are the primary infectious source in the population. It is even claimed by some experts that transmission during conversations through micro-droplet may possibly be the third infection route. The digestive tract can also be a potential route of infection as SARS-CoV-2 is detected in the stool and gastro-intestinal tract of COVID-19 patients, in addition to its detection in saliva, tear, urine, etc. [15, 16]. There was no evidence of transmission from mother to child during pregnancy [17]. Though based on the currently available evidence, bats are considered to be the natural hosts and pangolins are the intermediate hosts, the origin of SARS-CoV-2 necessitates further in-depth investigations.

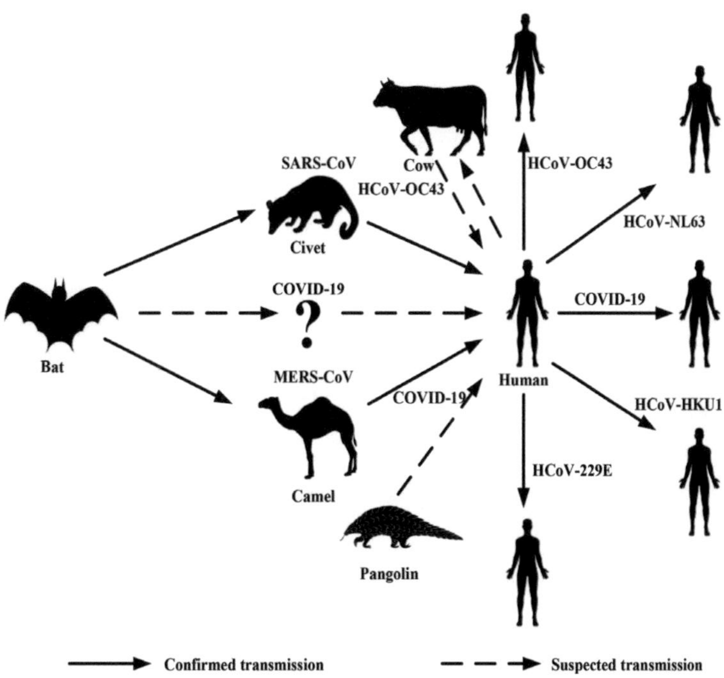

Figure 2.
Probable origin and intermediate host during interspecies transmission of the corona virus.

2. Molecular characterization and pathogenic mechanism

Coronaviruses are enveloped, spherical, or exhibit size and shape variation (pleomorphic) with a diameter in the range of 60–140 nm containing a positive sense, single-stranded RNA genome of approximately 26–32 kilobase size, the largest genome among RNA viruses [8, 18]. The genomic RNA contains multiple open reading frames (ORFs) for encoding 16 non-structural proteins (nsps) and four structural proteins like spike (S), envelope (E), membrane (M), and nucleocapsid (N). About two-thirds of genomic RNA is located in the first ORF (ORF1a/b) that helps in the translation of two polyproteins viz. pp1a and pp1ab at the 5′ end. Further, the subsequent proteolytic cleavages of polyproteins generate 16 non-structural proteins (NSP). The remaining part of the virus genome encodes the four important structural proteins, E, S, N, and M, including other accessory proteins that interfere with the host's innate immune response [19, 20]. The invariant gene order is 5'-ORF1a-ORF1b-S-E-M-N-3′, with additional small ORFs in between the structural genes for encoding accessory proteins. The term 'corona' in Latin means 'crown' under the electron microscope observation; the spike protein projections of the virus appear as a crown, hence termed as 'coronavirus' (**Figure 3a**).

3. Infection strategy

2019-nCoV is extremely contagious and with very high transmission capacity, the virus is transmitted from person to person with ease. The transmission capacity is represented based on the reproduction number symbolized as R_0 that signifies the average number of secondary cases (infectee) caused by the primary case (infector) in a population highly susceptible to infection [21]. The value $R_0 > 1$ indicates the rapid spreading of the infection whereas $R_0 < 1$ signifies the low extension capacity of the infectious disease. The R_0 value of COVID-19 is in the range of 1.4–2.5, whereas severe acute respiratory syndrome coronavirus (SARS-CoV) is 0.67–1.23 and Middle East respiratory syndrome coronavirus (MERS-CoV) is 0.29–0.8; therefore, COVID-19 could be more easily transmitted [22, 23]. However, there are cases when an infected individual will not transmit the disease to anyone or can infect far more people than the standard transmission rate and the individuals are termed as "super-spreaders" [22]. In COVID-19, for the first time in early 2020, two patients were reported to be super-spreaders. One was a British national who had infected a dozen others whereas another suspect, a South Korean woman, had infected several dozens of others. The rate of initial spread is also dependent on the serial interval, which means the time gap between the onset of illness in an infector and in an infectee. The serial interval can be estimated by linking dates of onset of illness for infector-infectee pairs. The serial interval for COVID-19 is 4.4–7.5 days, whereas the mean value for SARS-CoV was 8.4 days, indicating the rapid transmission nature of COVID-19 [24].

It is reported in the literature that SARS-CoV-2 uses angiotensin converting enzyme 2 (ACE2) as its cell surface receptor and the binding of the S protein to the ACE2 receptor is the first step of viral infection followed by fusion with the cell membrane and subsequent viral entry to the respiratory mucosa [3, 18, 25]. As demonstrated in **Figure 3b**, after entry and un-coating, the translation of ORFs from the viral genomic RNA occurs for encoding non-structural proteins. Subsequently, the nsps assemble into the replicase-transcriptase complex (RTC) to facilitate RNA replication and transcription. First of all, full-length negative-sense anti-genome is synthesized using the genomic RNA as a template, and subsequently, the negative-sense strand serves as a template for the synthesis of new genomic and sub-genomic

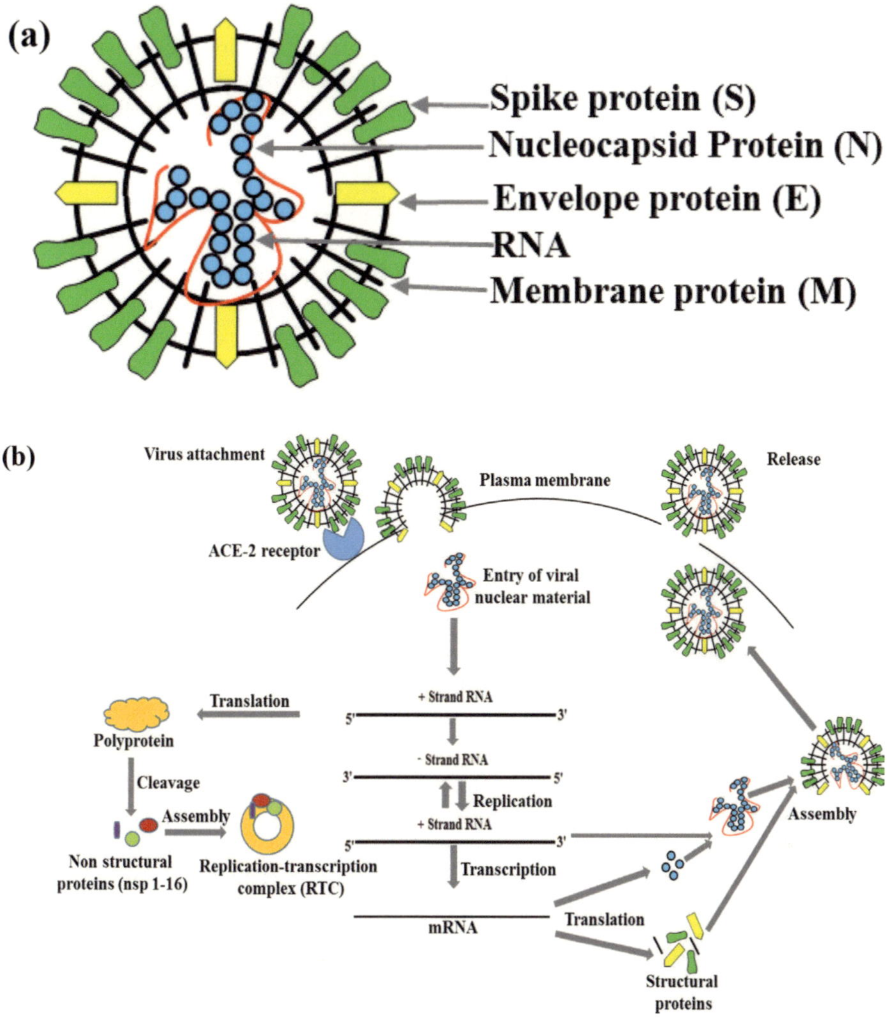

Figure 3.
(a) Basic structure of Covid-19, (b) life cycle in the host.

RNA. Sub-genomic RNAs serve as mRNAs for the translation of structural proteins. The structural proteins and viral genomic RNA assemble in the endoplasmic reticulum (ER) - Golgi intermediate compartment (ERGIC) mediated by M protein to form the mature virions. Ultimately, the virions are transported to the cell surface through smooth-wall vesicles and released by exocytosis for subsequent rounds of infection [3, 25].

4. Clinical symptoms

SARS-CoV-2 attacks the lower airway as the primary target of infection, causing a respiratory and systemic illness that subsequently progresses to a severe form of pneumonia in 10–15% of patients [26, 27]. Clinical symptoms of COVID-19 vary from asymptomatic state to critical illness, with acute respiratory distress (ARDS), acute cardiac injury, multi-organ failure (MOF) and at the end, development of small blood clots throughout the bloodstream (intravascular coagulopathy) [17, 28]. The symptoms of COVID-19 illness are cough, fever, fatigue, headache, muscle pain (myalgia), difficulty in breathing (dyspnoea), decreased lymphocytes in blood (lymphocytopenia), lower platelet count (thrombocytopenia), etc., which are indifferent from other respiratory infections [29]. However, the unique clinical symptoms of COVID-19 are runny nose (rhinorrhea), sneezing, sore throat, presence of infiltrate in the upper lobe of the lung that causes shortness of breath and subsequent decreased level of oxygen in the blood (hypoxemia), detection of viral RNA in samples of plasma, serum, whole blood, etc., (RNAemia) and sometimes gastrointestinal symptoms like diarrhea [29]. The incubation period of the virus is usually between 3 to 7 days on average, however with 1 day as the shortest and 14 days longest is observed in some circumstances. The symptoms of infection appear after the average incubation period of 5 days approximately however, the average time from onset of symptom to dyspnoea is five days, ARDS is eight days, and death is 6 to 41 days with a median of 14 days [18, 29, 30]. These periods are variable and dependent on several parameters like age and immunity of the patient, typically shorter periods are observed for patients above 70 years old [30].

5. Diagnosis and treatment

As discussed in the previous section, based on the preliminary clinical features such as fever, sore throat, and dry cough of a suspected COVID-19 infectee can be investigated to confirm the exposure history of the person. In some of the cases, this may be asymptotic, i.e., showing none of the above mentioned clinical symptoms, hence, in those cases, the detection of viral genomic material is considered as the only reliable source of COVID-19 diagnosis. The method includes taking the samples from the (suspected) infectee in the form of nasopharyngeal swab, sputum, bronchoalveolar washing, endotracheal aspirates, followed by RNA extraction and subsequent analysis by reverse transcription polymerase chain reaction (RT-PCR) for synthesis, amplification, and identification of viral nucleic acid [18, 25]. Since RT-PCR based techniques take a relatively longer time, therefore, the development of rapid diagnosis kits is on works. Clustered regularly interspaced short palindromic repeats (CRISPR) based diagnostics are such techniques believed in delivering the results within an hour without the need for sophisticated laboratory equipment. Based on this technology, SHERLOCK and DETECTR are two test methods developed by Sherlock Biosciences, and Mammoth Biosciences, respectively and waiting for clinical verifications and approvals [31]. Another sophisticated approach would be a serological assay in which the antibodies from the blood sample of the patients are analyzed to detect viral infections. Computed tomography (CT) imaging is also a highly specific and sensitive method and a chest CT scan of the patients generally shows ground-glass opacities and infiltrates [17, 18].

As of the time, there are no specific, effective and proven antiviral drugs (and/or) vaccines for the treatment of COVID-19 infection, so treatments are limited to support and palliative care only. The first-line treatment emphasizes maintaining hydration and controlling fever and cough through routine dosages of antipyretics and expectorants [32]. Patients with severe respiratory distress should be administered with supplemental oxygen. The alternative treatment is based on the use of broad-spectrum antiviral drugs like neurominidase inhibitor (oseltamivir), nucleotide analogues (remdesivir), nucleoside analogues (ganciclovir), HIV-protease inhibitors (lopinavir, ritonavir) that can reduce the virus infection [33, 34]. As per a recent report by Chen et al. (2020), the effective dosage for the treatment of COVID-19 patients includes oral administration of 75 mg oseltamivir, 500 mg lopinavir, 500 mg ritonavir twice a day and the intravenous administration of 0·25 g ganciclovir for 3–14 days [35]. Also, it is reported by many researchers that the antimalarial-drug chloroquine could effectively inhibit the virus by virtue of its immune-modulating activity [36, 37]. Deng et al. (2020) confirmed the antiviral activity of Arbidol (small indole derivative molecule) on COVID-19 patients and the antiviral activity against SARS-CoV and also it blocks the viral fusion against the influenza A and B viruses and hepatitis C viruses [10, 38]. A clinical candidate, EIDD-2801, with high therapeutic potential against the influenza virus, is in development, which can be a promising drug to be considered for the COVID-19 [39].

In addition to this, the synthetic recombinant interferons could be used for the treatment of COVID-19 based on their effectiveness against SARS-CoVs and MERS-CoVs [10]. It is also discussed that a small recommended amount of vitamin C supplementation could effectively prevent COVID-19. Convalescent plasma therapy in which plasma of patients recovered from COVID-19 enriched with virus neutralizing antibodies is administered in a prophylactic manner to prevent infection in high-risk cases could also be an effective approach to alleviate COVID-19 infection. On 31st March 2020, the first US patient received convalescent plasma therapy for the COVID-19 treatment [40]. In the latest development, Caly et al. (2020) reported that Ivermectin existing anti-parasite inhibited SARS-CoV-2 and a single treatment, reduced approximately 5000 fold viral RNA in 48 h in in-vitro [41]. However, the anti-parasitic drug is not approved by U.S Food and Drug Administration (FDA) due to lack of well-designed clinical trials. It is also recommended that the existing related vaccines for RNA virus including encephalitis B and influenza, etc., could be explored as possible alternatives until the development of an effective COVID-19 vaccine. There is an urgent need to establish a nonhuman animal model for a better understanding of the virus-host interactions and subsequent testing of potential drug/vaccines for COVID-19 infections [17].

6. Preventive measures to control the spread of the infection

Since there is limited availability of effective treatment for COVID-19, therefore, currently, *prevention* is used as a vital step in controlling the (community) spread of the infection. However, some unique features of the disease like a transmission from asymptomatic people, long incubation period, and infectivity in the incubation period even before the onset of symptoms, prolonged illness, and transmission after recovery, etc., make the preventive measures really more challenging [18]. First of all, extensive measures should be taken to limit human to human transmission with an emphasis on susceptible populations like healthcare providers and older people to prevent further transmission amplification and spread [42]. The second essential step must be the facilitation of advanced health surveillance systems along with rapid diagnostic facilities for the identification of cases. It should be followed by quarantine or isolation when necessary, with intensive care for patients and contact tracing for preventing further transmission by contacts who are infected [43]. Patients should be isolated in well ventilated room with regular decontamination, and they should follow cough and sneeze hygiene, practice hand hygiene and should be asked to wear surgical masks to prevent infection spreading. The healthcare workers attending the patients should be advised to use personal protective equipment (PPE) like gloves, N95 masks, goggles, protective suits, etc. The use of masks by healthy people though not recommended by WHO, owing to the recent finding by Japanese scientists that simple conversations in close proximity without coughs and sneeze could spread the virus through micro-droplets, it is advisable to wear masks, particularly in crowded public places [44]. Owing to the community spread nature of the virus, the government's action to ban mass gatherings is an important preventive step and locking down cities, states, provinces as part of the action plan of many governments, including India, the US, European Union, etc., will definitely be beneficial in flattening the pandemic. Physical contact with inanimate objects should be avoided since coronaviruses can remain infectious on these surfaces for up to 9 days, however, surface decontamination with ethanol (> 70%) or 0.1% sodium hypochlorite can significantly reduce the virus infectivity even within 1 min exposure time [45]. The public should avoid non-essential travel to places with ongoing transmission and the countries should strictly implement preventive measures like travel screenings and quarantining of the travelers to control further spread of the infection. In countries with resource limitations, to triage a large number of cases, the proposed simple screening algorithm by Ayebare et al. (2020), as shown in **Figure 4** can be followed for effective infection prevention and control [46].

International collaborations and co-operations are highly essential to minimize social as well as economic disruptions [43]. The government's strategy for timely education and training of hospital staff and health care providers along with awareness and counseling to the general public about the risks of COVID-19 are absolutely necessary for minimizing the spread of the infection and managing an economic downturn. However, during this crisis, personal rather than government

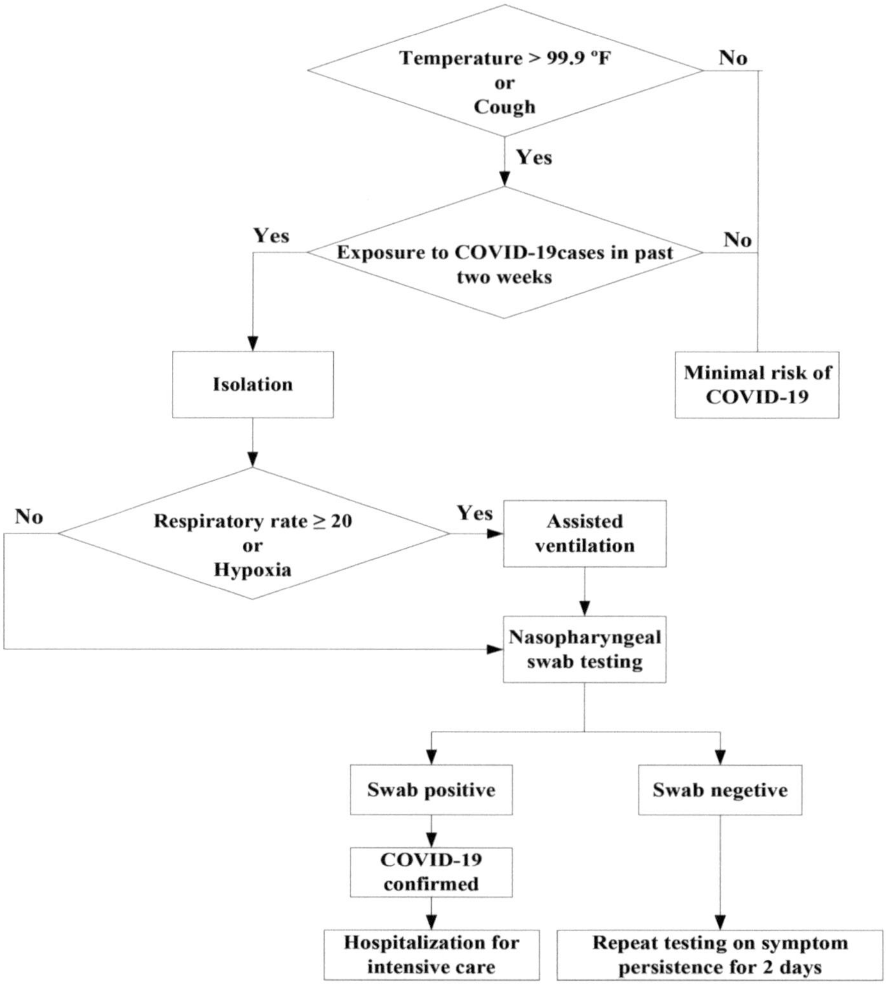

Figure 4.
Outline of infection prevention and control (IPC) strategies.

S.No	Trade name of the vaccine	Company and country	Remark
1	Comirnaty	German company BioNTech, American company Pfizer	RNA vaccine
2	Covishield	Oxford–AstraZeneca COVID-19 vaccine	viral vector vaccine
3	Sputnik V COVID-19 vaccine	Russian Gamaleya Research Institute of Epidemiology and Microbiology.	viral vector vaccine
4	BBIBP-CorV	China National Pharmaceutical Group (Sinopharm)	inactivated virus vaccine
5	Johnson & Johnson COVID-19 vaccine	Janssen Pharmaceutica and Beth Israel Deaconess Medical Center.	viral vector vaccine
6	Moderna COVID-19 vaccine	American company Moderna	RNA vaccine
7	CoronaVac	Chinese company Sinovac Biotech.	inactivated virus vaccine
8	Covaxin	Bharat Biotech, India	inactivated virus vaccine
9	Convidecia	Chinese company CanSino Biologics and the Beijing Institute of Biotechnology of the Academy of Military Medical Sciences.	viral vector vaccine
10	EpiVacCorona	Russian State Research Center of Virology and Biotechnology VECTOR	peptide vaccine
11	RBD-Dimer	Chinese company Anhui	subunit vaccine
12	WIBP-CorV	China National Pharmaceutical Group (Sinopharm)	inactivated virus vaccine
13	CoviVac	Chumakov Centre at the Russian Academy of Sciences.	inactivated virus vaccine

Table 1.
Showing developed vaccine details for Covid-19 infection.

action might be most important and individual behavior will definitely play a crucial role in infection prevention and control the spread of COVID-19. To date some of the countries have approved many anti-viral drugs as pharmacological treatment strategies for COVID-19. However, some approved COVID-19-specific vaccines are available (**Table 1**). Several companies have developed various vaccine candidates for human CoV infections which are in the clinical trial stage [47].

7. Future challenges in controlling the global pandemic

From the end of July 2020, an increase in new cases of SARS-CoV-2 infections was appeared in the different geographical territories of the European Union, confirmed about the origin of the second wave of outbreaks of these infectious diseases. On September 20, a new variant type of SARS-CoV-2, called B117, was first time identified in the United Kingdom (UK). Also, In December 2020, an unexpected rise in reported COVID-19 cases was observed due to the emergence of a new variant of SARS-CoV-2 (B.1.351) in South Africa. However, it was observed that that B117 is far more transmissible with comparatively less fatality rate [48–51]. Hence, it is important to correlate the mutation of the virus as well as the degree of pathogenicity. The existence of genetic diversity and specific mutations in the genome of SARS-CoV-2 and the virulence property has been investigated by Abdullahi, et al. In this work, they focused on the mutations of the non-structural proteins (NSPs) such as nsp 2 and nsp 3, Spike protein and RNA-dependent RNA polymerase (RdRp). The spike protein is the key determining factor for the evolution, virulence and transmission [52]. Similarly, the enhanced infection property and pathogenicity in case of SARS-CoV-2 is related to mutation at S-protein receptor-binding domain, has been studied by Padhi and Tripathi [53]. To address the significance of mutation to infection, Yao et al. conducted an experimental work by considering eleven numbers of SARS-CoV-2 viral isolates and observed that the mutations are directly related to the increase in viral load as well as a cytopathic effect [54]. Bakhshandeh et al., emphasized that the gradual accumulation of the genomic mutation in SARS-CoV-2 are having a crucial role in genetic variability of the virus. This helps the virus to escape from the host cell immunity and converts the strain in to a drug resistance virus with more deadly behavior [55]. Another recent study has uncovered that the rate of infection of novel corona virus is not only due to the mutation of the viral genome but also associated with host genetics, the genetic and epigenetic variations of the human population. For example, the ACE2 gene variation might be the key genetic factor for SARS-CoV-2 infection that facilitates the virus entry into human cells [56].

Currently, several strategies are being followed, such as contact tracing of infected people, enforcing the social distancing, maintaining the quarantine, and restricted mobility of people and use of disinfectant for self-protection purpose. However, none of these methods have proved to be effective in controlling the global pandemic caused by COVID-19. Usually, there are three basic areas that is to be emphasized more for the best control of the global pandemic [57–64].

1. Mass vaccination of the people:

2. The government of each country should take the initiative for the mass vaccination for all the people that may be the most effective way of control. However, it may be challenging as the country should cross the financial burden and human resources to develop the technology as well as the material for mass production of the vaccine. Also, international collaboration for the same may be fruitful. In addition to this, the possible long term efficacy and the side effects of the vaccine should be well-studied.Herd immunity

3. Several studies have proved that the COVID-19 infection leads to the production of antibodies in the patient against the SARS-CoV-2. So, if a large group of the population will induce resistance for the virus in their immunosystem, then it is expected that the entire population may be protected gradually, called herd immunity. However, the establishment of herd immunity in the population is determined by a large number of molecular and immunological factors. Also, frequent change in the viral genome may be another hurdle for acquiring herd immunity.Implementation of new technologies

In order to protect the human population and in the limited effective treatment strategy for COVID-19 infection, the implementation of new and effective online technologies in different sectors is desirable. These technologies will help the people in the timely response and control of epidemics in the areas of public training, education, medication, including digital surveillance systems, telemedicine, rapid identification and diagnosis devices, and prediction about the future infection.

8. Conclusion

The global impact of coronavirus disease is one of the heightening concerns of the present time. Though at this stage, it is not possible to determine the precise source of the coronavirus, however, the bats are considered as their natural hosts based on the available sequence based phylogenetic study. Genomic analysis revealed the arrangement of gene order and ORF positions. The largest genome RNA of coronavirus might be the reason behind the *intraspecies variability* and *interspecies transmission* via mutations and recombination mediated flexible genome modifications. Therefore, future outbreaks of zoonotic viruses cannot be overlooked. So, to avoid the future threat of zoonotic viral outbreaks, comprehensive measures should be planned alongside curbing this corona pandemic. In addition to this, the mutation acquired by the virus from time to time changes its pathogenicity is a concern. So a thorough study is essential to establish the relationship between the mutated forms of the virus with respect to the different geographical areas to predict the future genotypic pattern change of the virus. Further, in-depth investigations at individual protein levels of the virus are necessary to precisely predict the origin, to predict mutation mediated evolutionary selection pressure, and for a better understanding and development of the potential drug molecule binding efficacy.

Author contributions

All authors contributed equally to the conception of the study, data analysis and interpretation and drafting the article and final approval of the version to be submitted.

Conflict of interest

The authors declare that they have no known conflict of interests.

Ethical approval

Not required.

Author details

Raghunath Satpathy[1*†] and Prangya Ranjan Rout[2†]

1 School of Biotechnology, Gangadhar Meher University, Sambalpur, Odisha, India

2 Department of Biotechnology, Thapar Institute of Engineering and Technology, Patiala, Punjab, India

*Address all correspondence to: rnsatpathy@gmail.com

† Joint first authors-Contributed equally.

References

[1] Coronavirus Outbreak. [Internet].2021 Available from: https:// www.worldometers.info/coronavirus. [Accessed 2021-04-25]

[2] Lee A. Wuhan novel coronavirus (COVID-19): why global control is challenging? Public Health. 2020; 179: A1-A2. DOI: 10.1016/j.puhe.2020. 02.001, PMID 32111295.

[3] Fung TS, Liu DX. Human coronavirus: Host-Pathogen Interaction. Annu Rev Microbiol. 2019; 73:529-557. DOI: 10.1146/annurev-micro-020518-115759, PMID 31226023.

[4] Hui DS, I Azhar E, Madani TA, Ntoumi F, Kock R, Dar O, Ippolito G, Mchugh TD, Memish ZA, Drosten C, Zumla A, Petersen E. The continuing 2019-nCoV epidemic threat of novel coronaviruses to global health-The latest 2019 novel coronavirus outbreak in Wuhan, China. Int J Infect Dis. 2020; 91:264-6. DOI: 10.1016/j. ijid.2020.01.009, PMID 31953166.

[5] Zhang Y, Xu J, Li H, Cao B. A novel coronavirus (COVID-19) outbreak: a call for action. Chest. 2020; 1547; 4:99-101.DOI: 10.1016/j. chest.2020.02.014.

[6] Tyrrell DAJ, Bynoe ML. Cultivation of a novel type of common-cold virus in organ cultures. Br Med J. 1965; 1(5448):1467-70. DOI: 10.1136/ bmj.1.5448.1467, PMID 14288084.

[7] Forni D, Cagliani R, Clerici M, Sironi M. Molecular evolution of human coronavirus genomes. Trends Microbiol. 2017; 25(1):35-48. DOI: 10.1016/j. tim.2016.09.001, PMID 27743750.

[8] Su S, Wong G, Shi W, Liu J, Lai ACK, Zhou J, Liu W, Bi Y, Gao GF. Epidemiology, genetic recombination, and pathogenesis of coronaviruses. Trends Microbiol. 2016; 24(6):490-502. DOI: 10.1016/j.tim.2016.03.003, PMID 27012512.

[9] Zhou P, Yang XL, Wang XG, Hu B, Zhang L, Zhang W, Si HR, Zhu Y, Li B, Huang CL, Chen HD, Chen J, Luo Y, Guo H, Jiang RD, Liu MQ, Chen Y, Shen XR, Wang X, Zheng XS, Zhao K, Chen QJ, Deng F, Liu LL, Yan B, Zhan FX, Wang YY, Xiao GF, Shi ZL. A pneumonia outbreak associated with a new coronavirus of probable bat origin. Nature. 2020; 579(7798):270-273. DOI: 10.1038/s41586-020-2012-7, PMID 32015507.

[10] Wang LS, Wang YR, Ye DW, Liu QQ. A review of the 2019 Novel coronavirus (COVID-19) based on current evidence. Int J Antimicrob Agents. 2020; 55(6):105948. DOI: 10.1016/j.ijantimicag.2020.105948.

[11] Zhang T, Wu Q, Zhang Z. Probable pangolin origin of 2019-nCoV associated with outbreak of COVID-19. Curr Biol-*D-20-00299*. 2020.DOI: 10.2139/ssrn.3542586.

[12] Xu X, Chen P, Wang J, Feng J, Zhou H, Li X, Zhong W, Hao P. Evolution of the novel coronavirus from the ongoing Wuhan outbreak and modeling of its spike protein for risk of human transmission. Sci China (Life Sci). 2020; 63(3):457-60.DOI:10.1007/ s11427-020-1637-5, PMID 32009228.

[13] Cyranoski D. Mystery deepens over animal source of coronavirus. Nature. 2020;579(7797):18-19. DOI: 10.1038/ d41586-020-00548-w, PMID 32127703.

[14] Xu Y. Unveiling the origin and transmission of 2019-nCoV. Trends Microbiol. 2020; 28(4):239-40. DOI: 10.1016/j.tim.2020.02.001, PMID 32155431.

[15] Xiao F, Tang M, Zheng X, Li Y, He J, Hong Z, Huang S, Zhang Z, Lin X,

Fang Z, Lai R. Evidence for gastrointestinal infection of SARS-CoV-2. *medRxiv* 2020. Gastroenterology. 2020; 158(6):1831-1833.e3. DOI: 10.1053/j.gastro.2020.02.055, PMID 32142773.

[16] Xia J, Tong J, Liu M, Shen Y, Guo D. Evaluation of coronavirus in tears and conjunctival secretions of patients with SARS-CoV-2 infection. J Med Virol. 2020; 92(6):589-594. DOI: 10.1002/jmv.25725, PMID 32100876.

[17] Fenizia C, Biasin M, Cetin I, Vergani P, Mileto D, Spinillo A, Gismondo MR, Perotti F, Callegari C, Mancon A, Cammarata S, Beretta I, Nebuloni M, Trabattoni D, Clerici M, Savasi V. Analysis of SARS-CoV-2 vertical transmission during pregnancy. Nat Commun. 2020 October 12; 11(1):5128. DOI: 10.1038/s41467-020-18933-4, PMID 33046695.

[18] Singhal T. A review of coronavirus Disease-2019 (COVID-19). Indian J Pediatr. 2020; 87(4):281-6. DOI: 10.1007/s12098-020-03263-6, PMID 32166607.

[19] Sievers F, Higgins DG. Clustal Omega for making accurate alignments of many protein sequences. Protein Sci. 2018; 27(1):135-145. DOI: 10.1002/pro.3290, PMID 28884485.

[20] Kumar S, Stecher G, Li M, Knyaz C, Tamura K. MEGA X: molecular evolutionary genetics analysis across computing platforms. Mol Biol Evol. 2018; 35(6):1547-9. DOI: 10.1093/molbev/msy096, PMID 29722887.

[21] Anderson RM, Heesterbeek H, Klinkenberg D, Hollingsworth TD. How will country-based mitigation measures influence the course of the COVID-19 epidemic? Lancet. 2020; 395(10228):931-4. DOI: 10.1016/S0140-6736(20)30567-5, PMID 32164834.

[22] Trilla A. One world, one health: the novel coronavirus COVID-19 epidemic. Med Clin (Barc). 2020; 154(5):175-177. DOI: 10.1016/j.medcli.2020.02.002, PMID 32093921.

[23] Wu JT, Leung K, Leung GM. Nowcasting and forecasting the potential domestic and international spread of the 2019-nCoV outbreak originating in Wuhan, China: a modelling study. Lancet. 2020; 395(10225):689-97. DOI: 10.1016/S0140-6736(20)30260-9, PMID 32014114.

[24] Nishiura H, Linton NM, Akhmetzhanov AR. Serial interval of novel coronavirus (COVID-19) infections. Int J Infect Dis. 2020; 93:284-286. DOI: 10.1016/j.ijid.2020.02.060, PMID 32145466.

[25] Fehr AR, Perlman S. Coronaviruses: an overview of their replication and pathogenesis. Methods Mol Biol. 2015; 1282:1-23. DOI: 10.1007/978-1-4939-2438-7_1, PMID 25720466.

[26] Patel RS, Patel N, Baksh M, Zaidi A, Patel J. Clinical perspective on 2019 Novel Coronavirus Pneumonia: A Systematic Review of Published Case Reports. Cureus. 2020; 12(6):e8488. DOI: 10.7759/cureus.8488, PMID 32656006.

[27] Lai CC, Shih TP, Ko WC, Tang HJ, Hsueh PR. Severe acute respiratory syndrome coronavirus 2 (SARS-CoV-2) and coronavirus disease-2019 (COVID-19): the epidemic and the challenges. Int J Antimicrob Agents. 2020;55(3):105924. DOI: 10.1016/j.ijantimicag.2020.105924, PMID 32081636.

[28] Lippi G, Plebani M, Henry BM. Thrombocytopenia is associated with severe coronavirus disease 2019 (COVID-19) infections: A meta-analysis. Clin Chim Acta. 2020; 506:145-148. DOI: 10.1016/j.cca.2020.03.022, PMID 32178975.

[29] Rothan HA, Byrareddy SN. The epidemiology and pathogenesis of

coronavirus disease (COVID-19) outbreak. J Autoimmun. 2020; 109:102433. DOI: 10.1016/j.jaut.2020. 102433.

[30] Wang W, Tang J, Wei F. Updated understanding of the outbreak of 2019 novel coronavirus (2019-nCoV) in Wuhan, China. J Med Virol. 2020; 92(4):441-447. DOI: 10.1002/jmv.25689, PMID 31994742.

[31] Yüce M, Filiztekin E, Özkaya KG. COVID-19 diagnosis—a review of current methods. Biosens Bioelectron. 2020 Oct 24:112752. DOI: 10.7759/ cureus.8488.

[32] Wang D, Hu B, Hu C, Zhu F, Liu X, Zhang J, Wang B, Xiang H, Cheng Z, Xiong Y, Zhao Y, Li Y, Wang X, Peng Z. Clinical characteristics of 138 hospitalized patients with 2019 novel coronavirus–infected pneumonia in Wuhan, China. JAMA. 2020; 323(11):1061-9. DOI: 10.1001/ jama.2020.1585, PMID 32031570.

[33] Lu H. Drug treatment options for the 2019-new coronavirus (2019-nCoV). BioSci Trends. 2020;14(1):69-71. DOI: 10.5582/bst.2020.01020, PMID 31996494.

[34] Holshue ML, DeBolt C, Lindquist S, Lofy KH, Wiesman J, Bruce H, Spitters C, Ericson K, Wilkerson S, Tural A, Diaz G, Cohn A, Fox L, Patel A, Gerber SI, Kim L, Tong S, Lu X, Lindstrom S, Pallansch MA, Weldon WC, Biggs HM, Uyeki TM, Pillai SK, Washington State 2019-nCoV Case Investigation Team. First case of 2019 novel coronavirus in the United States. N Engl J Med. 2020; 382(10):929-936. DOI: 10.1056/NEJMoa2001191, PMID 32004427.

[35] Chen N, Zhou M, Dong X, Qu J, Gong F, Han Y, Qiu Y, Wang J, Liu Y, Wei Y, Xia J, Yu T, Zhang X, Zhang L. Epidemiological and clinical characteristics of 99 cases of 2019 novel coronavirus pneumonia in Wuhan, China: a descriptive study. Lancet. 2020; 395(10223):507-13. DOI: 10.1016/ S0140-6736(20)30211-7, PMID 32007143.

[36] Wang M, Cao R, Zhang L, Yang X, Liu J, Xu M, Shi Z, Hu Z, Zhong W, Xiao G. Remdesivir and chloroquine effectively inhibit the recently emerged novel coronavirus (2019-nCoV) in vitro. Cell Res. 2020; 30(3):269-271. DOI: 10.1038/s41422-020-0282-0, PMID 32020029.

[37] Singh AK, Singh A, Shaikh A, Singh R, Misra A. Chloroquine and hydroxychloroquine in the treatment of COVID-19 with or without diabetes: A systematic search and a narrative review with a special reference to India and other developing countries. Diabetes Metab Syndr Clin Res Rev. 2020; 14(3):241-246. DOI: 10.1016/j. dsx.2020.03.011.

[38] Deng L, Li C, Zeng Q, Liu X, Li X, Zhang H, Hong Z, Xia J. Arbidol combined with LPV/r versus LPV/r alone against Corona Virus Disease 2019: a retrospective cohort study. J Infect. 2020; 81(1):e1-e5. DOI: 10.1016/j. jinf.2020.03.002, PMID 32171872.

[39] Toots M, Yoon JJ, Cox RM, Hart M, Sticher ZM, Makhsous N, Plesker R, Barrena AH, Reddy PG, Mitchell DG, Shean RC, Bluemling GR, Kolykhalov AA, Greninger AL, Natchus MG, Painter GR, Plemper RK. Characterization of orally efficacious influenza drug with high resistance barrier in ferrets and human airway epithelia. Sci Transl Med. 2019; 11(515). DOI: 10.1126/scitranslmed.aax5866, PMID 31645453.

[40] Liu STH, Lin HM, Baine I, Wajnberg A, Gumprecht JP, Rahman F, Rodriguez D, Tandon P, Bassily-Marcus A, Bander J, Sanky C, Dupper A, Zheng A, Nguyen FT, Amanat F, Stadlbauer D, Altman DR,

Chen BK, Krammer F, Mendu DR, Firpo-Betancourt A, Levin MA, Bagiella E, Casadevall A, Cordon-Cardo C, Jhang JS, Arinsburg SA, Reich DL, Aberg JA, Bouvier NM. Convalescent plasma treatment of severe COVID-19: a propensity score–matched control study. Nat Med. 2020 Nov; 26(11):1708-13. DOI: 10.1038/s41591-020-1088-9, PMID 32934372.

[41] Caly L, Druce JD, Catton MG, Jans DA, Wagstaff KM. The FDA-approved Drug ivermectin inhibits the replication of SARS-CoV-2 in vitro. Antiviral Res. 2020; 178:104787. DOI: 10.1016/j.antiviral.2020.104787.

[42] Xiao Y, Torok ME. Taking the right measures to control COVID-19. Lancet Infect Dis. 2020; 20(5):523-524. DOI: 10.1016/S1473-3099(20)30152-3, PMID 32145766.

[43] Hellewell J, Abbott S, Gimma A, Bosse NI, Jarvis CI, Russell TW, Munday JD, Kucharski AJ, Edmunds WJ, Centre for the Mathematical Modelling of Infectious Diseases COVID-19 Working Group, Funk S, Eggo RM. Feasibility of controlling COVID-19 outbreaks by isolation of cases and contacts. Lancet Glob Health. 2020; 8(4):e488-e496. DOI: 10.1016/S2214-109X(20)30074-7, PMID 32119825.

[44] Ningthoujam R. COVID 19 can spread through breathing, talking, study estimates. Curr Med Res Pract. 2020; 10(3):132-3.DOI: 10.1016/j.cmrp.2020.05.003, PMID 32391407.

[45] Kampf G, Todt D, Pfaender S, Steinmann E. Persistence of coronaviruses on inanimate surfaces and its inactivation with biocidal agents. J Hosp Infect. 2020; 104(3):246-251. DOI: 10.1016/j.jhin.2020.01.022, PMID 32035997.

[46] Ayebare RR, Flick R, Okware S, Bodo B, Lamorde M. Adoption of COVID-19 triage strategies for low-income settings. Lancet Respir Med. 2020; 8(4):e22. DOI: 10.1016/S2213-2600(20)30114-4, PMID 32171063.

[47] Forni G, Mantovani A, COVID-19 Commission of Accademia Nazionale dei Lincei, Rome. COVID-19 vaccines: where we stand and challenges ahead. Cell Death Differ. 2021; 28(2):626-39. DOI: 10.1038/s41418-020-00720-9, PMID 33479399.

[48] Bontempi E. The Europe second wave of COVID-19 infection and the Italy "strange" situation. Environ Res. 2021;193:110476. DOI: 10.1016/j.envres.2020.110476.

[49] Duong D. What's important to know about the new COVID-19 variants? BMJ. 2021 2021; 372:n359. DOI: 10.1136/bmj.n359 (Published 05 February 2021) Cite this as: BMJ 2021; 372.

[50] Fontanet A, Autran B, Lina B, Kieny MP, Karim SSA, Sridhar D. SARS-CoV-2 variants and ending the COVID-19 pandemic. Lancet. 2021;397(10278):952-4. DOI: 10.1016/S0140-6736(21)00370-6, PMID 33581803.

[51] Volz E, Mishra S, Chand M, Barrett JC, Johnson R, Geidelberg L, Hinsley WR, Laydon DJ, Dabrera G, O'Toole Á, Amato R. Transmission of SARS-CoV-2 lineage B. 2021;1.1. 7 in England: Insights from linking epidemiological and genetic data. medRxiv:2020-12.DOI: 10.1101/2020.12.30.20249034.

[52] Abdullahi IN, Emeribe AU, Ajayi OA, Oderinde BS, Amadu DO, Osuji AI. Implications of SARS-CoV-2 genetic diversity and mutations on pathogenicity of COVID-19 and biomedical interventions. J Taibah Univ Med Sci. 2020 Jul 10; 15(4):258-264. DOI: 10.1016/j.jtumed.2020.06.005, PMID 32837505.

[53] Padhi AK, Tripathi T. Can SARS-CoV-2 accumulate mutations in the S-protein to increase pathogenicity?. ACS Pharmacol Transl Sci. 2020;3(5):1023-6. DOI: 10.1021/acsptsci.0c00113, PMID 33073197.

[54] Yao HP, Lu X, Chen Q, Xu K, Chen Y, Cheng L, Liu F, Wu Z, Wu H, Jin C, Zheng M, Wu N, Jiang C, Li L. Patient-derived mutations impact pathogenicity of SARS-CoV-2. SSRN Journal. 2020 Jan 1. DOI: 10.2139/ssrn.3578153.

[55] Bakhshandeh B, Jahanafrooz Z, Abbasi A, Goli MB, Sadeghi M, Mottaqi MS, Zamani M. Mutations in SARS-CoV-2; Consequences in structure, function, and pathogenicity of the virus. Microb Pathog. 2021; 154:104831. DOI: 10.1016/j.micpath.2021.104831.

[56] Choudhary S, Sreenivasulu K, Mitra P, Misra S, Sharma P. Role of genetic variants and gene expression in the susceptibility and severity of COVID-19. Ann Lab Med. 2021; 41(2):129-38. DOI: 10.3343/alm.2021.41.2.129, PMID 33063674.

[57] Chen WH, Strych U, Hotez PJ, Bottazzi ME. The SARS-CoV-2 vaccine pipeline: an overview. Curr Trop Med Rep. 2020; 7(2):1-4. DOI: 10.1007/s40475-020-00201-6, PMID 32219057.

[58] Forni G, Mantovani A, COVID-19 Commission of Accademia Nazionale dei Lincei, Rome. COVID-19 vaccines: where we stand and challenges ahead. Cell Death Differ. 2021; 28(2):626-39. DOI: 10.1038/s41418-020-00720-9, PMID 33479399.

[59] Azizi H, Esmaeili ED. Challenges and potential solutions in the development of COVID-19 pandemic control measures. New Microbes New Infect. 2021; 40:100852. DOI: 10.1016/j.nmni.2021.100852.

[60] Haynes BF, Corey L, Fernandes P, Gilbert PB, Hotez PJ, Rao S, Santos MR, Schuitemaker H, Watson M, Arvin A. Prospects for a safe COVID-19 vaccine. Sci Transl Med. 2020; 12(568). DOI: 10.1126/scitranslmed.abe0948, PMID 33077678.

[61] Musa TH, Ahmad T, Khan M, Haroon H, Wei P. Global outbreak of 2019-nCoV, a new challenge? J Infect Dev Ctries. 2020; 14(3):244-245. DOI: 10.3855/jidc.12530, PMID 32235083.

[62] Randolph HE, Barreiro LB. Herd immunity: understanding COVID-19. Immunity. 2020; 52(5):737-741. DOI: 10.1016/j.immuni.2020.04.012, PMID 32433946.

[63] Kang H, Wang Y, Tong Z, Liu X. Retest positive for SARS-CoV-2 RNA of ”recovered” patients with COVID-19: persistence, sampling issues, or re-infection? J Med Virol. 2020; 92(11):2263-5. DOI: 10.1002/jmv.26114, PMID 32492212.

[64] Budd J, Miller BS, Manning EM, Lampos V, Zhuang M, Edelstein M, Rees G, Emery VC, Stevens MM, Keegan N, Short MJ, Pillay D, Manley E, Cox IJ, Heymann D, Johnson AM, McKendry RA. Digital technologies in the public-health response to COVID-19. Nat Med. 2020; 26(8):1183-92. DOI: 10.1038/s41591-020-1011-4, PMID 32770165.

Chapter 3

COVID-19 Pandemic: Analysis and Statistics of Confirmed Cases

Vicente Enrique Machaca Arceda,
Miguel Angel Machaca Arceda
and Pamela Claudia Laguna Laura

Abstract

Coronavirus COVID-19 started in December 2019, and it has spread rapidly across China and the whole world. In this chapter, we analyzed the number of confirmed cases in US, India, France, Russia and Brazil. Additionally, we took into account Latin American countries like Argentina, Colombia, Peru, Chile and Mexico. We noticed, how some countries got a low death rate, despite its high number of confirmed cases (US). Additionally, it is interesting, how some countries with a high percentage of obesity got the highest death rate (Mexico). Also, we noticed a decreasing number in confirmed cases after a intensive vaccination plan (US). Finally, we evaluated Weibull Long Short-Term Memory (W-LSTM) and Multiplicative Trend Exponential Smoothing (MTES) to predict confirmed cases, in this case, W-LSTM showed a more realistic forecasting.

Keywords: Coronavirus, COVID-19, Analysis, Forecasting, LSTM, MTES

1. Introduction

Coronavirus COVID-19 pandemic started in December 2019 in Wuhan, China. This virus has high viral infectivity [1], so it has spread rapidly across China and other countries. Furthermore, 140,849,925 confirmed cases and 3,013,217 deaths were reported in the whole world until the last April 20th [2].

This new coronavirus made huge strain on the health system around the world forcing to establish decisions like quarantines and social distances in a effort to contain the spread of the virus [3]. Some countries with high incomes like United Kingdom, Italy, Spain and United States of America had to take measures such as hiring retired health personnel to assist battle infections.

Also, countries like United States agreed with car and weapon manufacturers to provide ventilators to help in the pandemic fight. The situation in countries with low and middle incomes were challenged, because they already have poor and weak health systems before COVID-19. They had limited financial resources, unavailable medications and inadequate health personnel, also in these countries exist a gap on the socio-economic. A person of higher socio-economic standing are more likely to have access to quality health services and medications [4].

Since the identification of SARS-CoV-2 virus, the scientific community was starting to develop over 300 vaccines projects, 40 of them are now on undergoing clinical evaluation, 10 of these are in Phase III and 3 of them have passed the phase

III with effective outcomes. The existing data propound that the vaccine candidates can reduce the spread of the pandemic protecting individuals. On the other hand, the fast development of vaccines candidates carries with some unresolved issues (only time could clarify). Moreover, technical and ethical problems were added with the production of billions of doses [5]. Despite, there are dozens of potential vaccine candidates [6], the herd immunity has not achieved yet.

Nowadays, the scientist communities are publishing several papers of studies about COVID-19. For instance, a research team had published an analysis of confirmed cases with Multiplicative Trend Exponential Smoothing (MTES) and Long Short-Term Memory (LSTM) [7]. Nonetheless, other researchers made a comparison with Auto-Regressive Integrated Moving Average (ARIMA), Nonlinear Autoregression Neural Network (NARNN) and LSTM to predict the confirmed cases of Denmark, Belgium, Germany, France, United Kingdom, Finland, Switzerland and Turkey, they concluded that LSTM was the most accurate model [8]. In addition, LSTM had been used to predict the trends and possible ended time of COVID-19 [9]. Also, other research used LSTM to predict the cumulative recovered, fatalities and confirmed cases [10].

In this Chapter, we analyzed the evolution of COVID-19. We took into account countries with the major number of confirmed cases like US, India, France, Russia and Brazil. Additionally, we took into account Latin American countries like Argentina, Colombia, Peru, Chile and Mexico. We analyzed the evolution of confirmed cases, deaths, the effects of vaccination and finally, we evaluated some models to forecast the number of confirmed cases.

2. Analysis of confirmed cases and deaths

In this section, we analyzed the number of confirmed cases and deaths in some countries. We focused on countries like US, India, France, Russia and Brazil, because, they got the major number of confirmed cases around the world. Additionally, we focused in the some Latin American countries like Argentina, Colombia, Peru, Chile and Mexico. They also, got the highest number of confirmed cases in Latin America.

2.1 American countries

The number of confirmed cases, varies from each country to another. For example in **Figure 1**, we showed the evolution of confirmed cases in top countries with the major impact. In this case, United States (US), shows an increasing curve

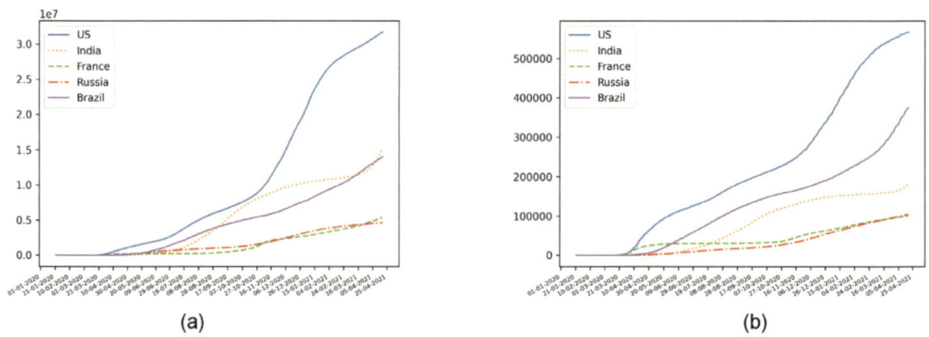

Figure 1.
Evolution of confirmed and deaths in US, India, France, Russia and Brazil. (a) Confirmed cases. (b) Deaths.

with 31,786,856 confirmed cases until April-20th. Furthermore, in **Figure 2**, we plotted the confirmed cases and deaths per million inhabitants. This shows a more realistic overview.

An interesting point is related to the differences between, confirmed cases and deaths in some countries. For instance, despite US got the major number of infected people, it has 1.77 of mortality rate (see **Table 1**), meanwhile France and Russia got 2.23 and 2.00 respectively. This difference between countries, could be related to the vaccinations, medical system, population's social behavior, etc. For example, meanwhile US has 5262 hospitals, Peru has 390, there is a huge difference. So, it is not adequate to use just one metric to measure the pandemic impact, we need to evaluate other metrics in order to understand this COVID-19 pandemic.

Brazil represents another interesting case. Brazil, has the highest public cost of health services in Latin America but it has 2.48% of death rate (the highest). The Brazil's president played a key role in the severity of the virus, at the beginning of the pandemic, he overestimated the virus.

2.2 Latin American countries

Additionally, in **Figures 3** and **4**, we shows the confirmed cases and deaths in Latin American countries. In this case, Mexico has an interesting behavior, this country got a death rate of 8.85 (see **Table 1**). According to some researches, the severity of COVID-19 is positively correlated with several factors, such as age and coexisting diseases. Moreover, obesity is considered as the main risk factor [11–13].

Obesity, is the key problem in Mexico. According to some surveys in 2000, 2006, 2012, and 2018, the adult obesity increased 42.2%. Moreover, the latest national survey (2018), concluded that 40.2% female adults and 36.1% male adults

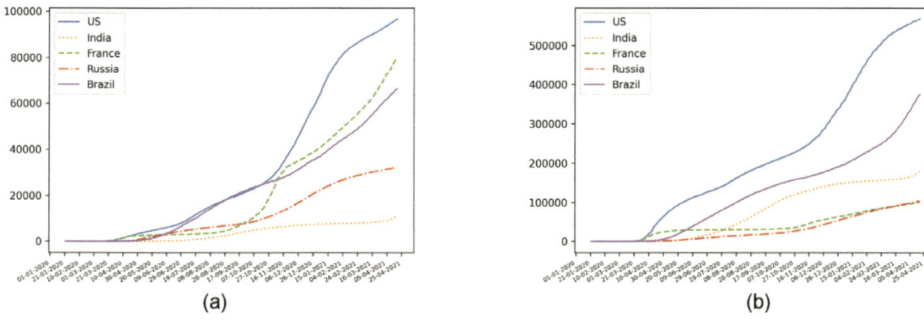

Figure 2.
Evolution of confirmed and deaths per million habitants in US, India, France, Russia and Brazil. (a) Confirmed cases. (b) Deaths.

Country	Death rate (%)[a]	Country	Death rate (%)[a]
US	1.77	Argentina	2.46
India	1.39	Colombia	2.61
France	2.23	Peru	3.52
Russia	2.00	Chile	2.47
Brazil	**2.48**	**Mexico**	**8.85**

[a]*We compute death rate as the mean of each day from 01 to 01-2021 to 20-04-2021.*

Table 1.
Death rate for US, India, France, Russia, Brazil, Argentina, Colombia, Peru, Chile and Mexico.

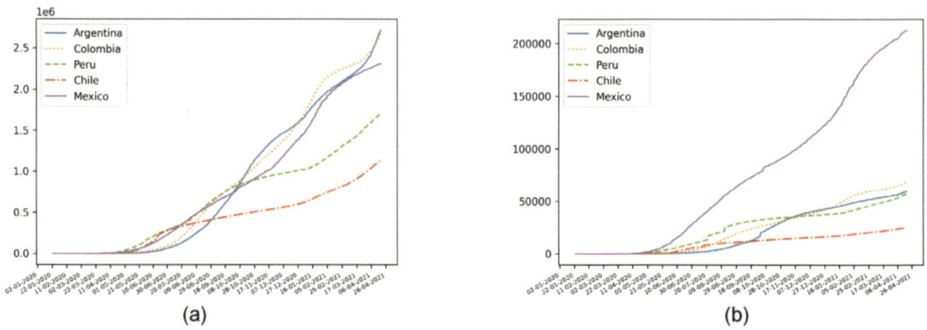

Figure 3.
Evolution of confirmed and deaths in Argentina, Colombia, Peru, Chile and Mexico. (a) Confirmed cases. (b) Deaths.

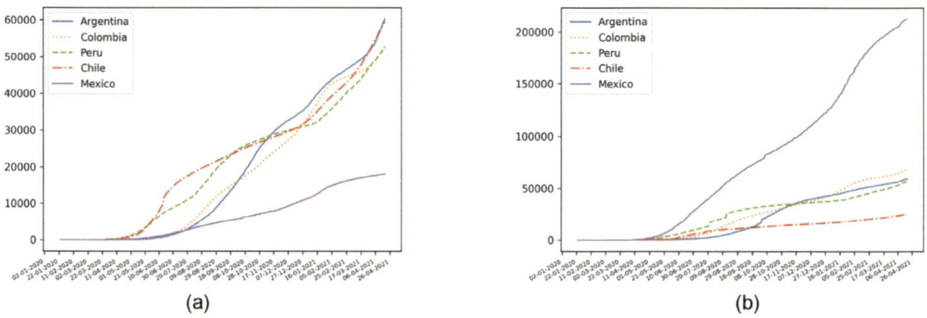

Figure 4.
Evolution of confirmed and deaths per million habitants in Argentina, Colombia, Peru, Chile and Mexico. (a) Confirmed cases. (b) Deaths.

suffer from obesity. More alarming, only 23.5% of the adult population had a healthy weight ($BMI <= 25kg/m^2$) [14].

3. Vaccination against COVID-19

In this section, we review the main COVID-19 vaccination projects. The effects of virus variants and the impact of vaccination in US, India, France, Russia, Brazil, Argentina, Colombia, Peru, Chile and Mexico.

3.1 COVID-19 variants

Unfortunately, like other viruses, COVID-19 virus evolves over time. Normally, when the virus replicates, it makes copies of itself with little changes (mutations), a virus with one or more mutations is call a"variant" of the original virus. Moreover, the US government inter agency group developed a Variant Classification scheme: Variant of Interest (VOI), Variant of Concern (VOC) and Variant of High Consequence (VOHC) [15]. In **Table 2**, we describe each variant.

In **Table 3**, we resumed the VOI variant of COVID-19, some of them present a reduced neutralization by antibody treatments and convalescent and post-vaccination sera [16–19]. In **Table 4**, VOC variant are presented, for instance B.1.1.7 and B.1.351 have approximately 50% increased transmission [20, 21].

Variant type	Description[a]
VOI	"A variant with specific genetic markers that have been associated with changes to receptor binding, reduced neutralization by antibodies generated against previous infection or vaccination, reduced efficacy of treatments, potential diagnostic impact, or predicted increase in transmissibility or disease severity"
VOC	"A variant for which there is evidence of an increase in transmissibility, more severe disease (e.g., increased hospitalizations or deaths), significant reduction in neutralization by antibodies generated during previous infection or vaccination, reduced effectiveness of treatments or vaccines, or diagnostic detection failures."
VOHC	"A variant of high consequence has clear evidence that prevention measures or medical countermeasures (MCMs) have significantly reduced effectiveness relative to previously circulating variants."

[a]*The definition of each variant was extracted from Centers for Disease Control and Prevention [15].*

Table 2.
COVID-19 variant classification proposed by US government inter agency group.

Variant name	First detected	Variant name	First detected
B.1.526	United States (New York) - November 2020	B.1.526.1	United States (New York) - October 2020
B.1.525	United Kingdom/Nigeria - December 2020	P.2	Brazil - April 2020

Table 3.
COVID-19 VOI variants detected.

Variant name	First detected	Variant name	First detected
B.1.1.7	United Kingdom	P.1	Japan/Brazil
B.1.351	South Africa	B.1.427	United States (California)
B.1.429	United States (California)		

Table 4.
COVID-19 VOC variants detected.

Variants B.1.427 and B.1.429 have 20% increased transmissibility [22]. Moreover, all of VOC variants presents a reduction in neutralization by convalescent and post-vaccination sera. In order to see a detailed description of each variant, visit: SARS-CoV-2 Variant Classifications and Definitions [15].

3.2 Vaccination projects

In order to fight this pandemic, global vaccine development efforts have been accelerated. Clinical development consist of three phases. In Phase I, a small group of people receive the vaccine. In Phase II, the vaccine is delivered for people whose characteristics such as age and physical health are similar to which ones the new vaccine is intended. Finally, in Phase III, the vaccine is given to thousands of people and tested for efficacy and safety [23].

Approximately, there are 56 verified effective vaccines candidates for COVID-19, produced in China, North America, Europe and Australia [24]. Furthermore, thanks to new technologies, it is possible to develop different types of vaccines. In

Vaccine type	Description
DNA vaccine	"DNA vaccines consist in delivering genes or fragments of it, encoding immunogenic antigens to the host's cells by using DNA plasmids as a vector" [25]. Some of these candidates focused in the development of a synthetic DNA-based SARS-CoV-2 S protein [23].
RNA vaccine	RNA vaccines contains RNA, when it is introduced into a tissue, acts as a messenger RNA (mRNA), then it cause the cells to build the foreign protein and stimulate an adaptive immune response [26].
Sub-unit vaccine	A sub-unit vaccine delivers some antigens to the immune system without introducing pathogen particles [27]
Vector-based vaccines	"Viral vectors are commonly utilized together with virus vaccines, in which the genome of one virus is applied to transmit the antigen of another virus, facilitating the advancement of platform system for the creation of viruses" [24].
Inactivated SARS-CoV-2 vaccine	It is another candidate that simulates production of antibodies in rats, mice, rabbits and primates [23].

Table 5.
COVID-19 vaccine types.

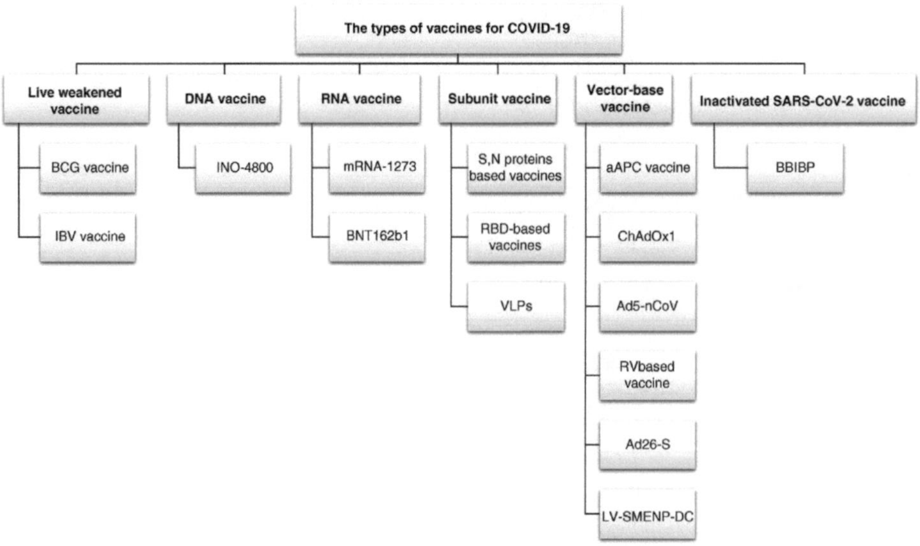

Figure 5.
Types of vaccines for COVID-19. Source: [23].

Table 5, we present the vaccine types for COVID-19. Finally, in **Figure 5**, we present the most important vaccines types against COVID.

3.3 The impact of vaccination

In order to evaluate the impact of vaccination, we analyzed, how the number of total people vaccinated affects the number of confirmed cases and deaths. We took data from a data-set that store information about vaccinations [28] and other that daily store information about the number of confirmed cases and deaths around the world [29]. For instance, in **Figure 6**, we present the relation between the total number of people vaccinated and the total number of confirmed cases and deaths. In this plot, we evaluated US, India, France, Russia and Brazil. Moreover, we

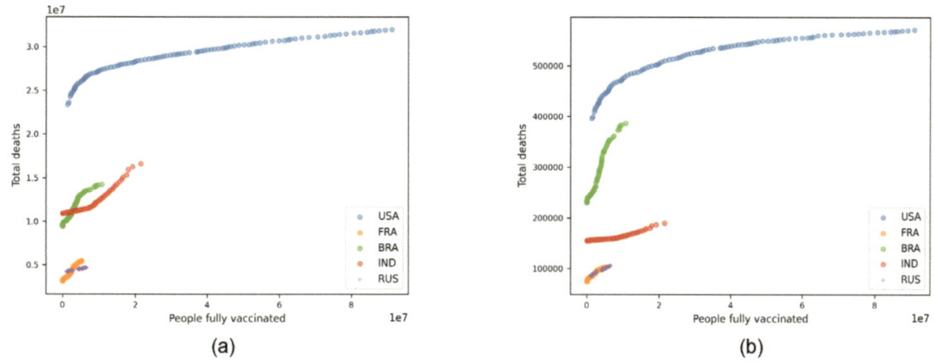

Figure 6.
The effect of vaccination in total confirmed cases and deaths in US, India, France, Russia and Brazil. (a) Confirmed cases. (b) Deaths.

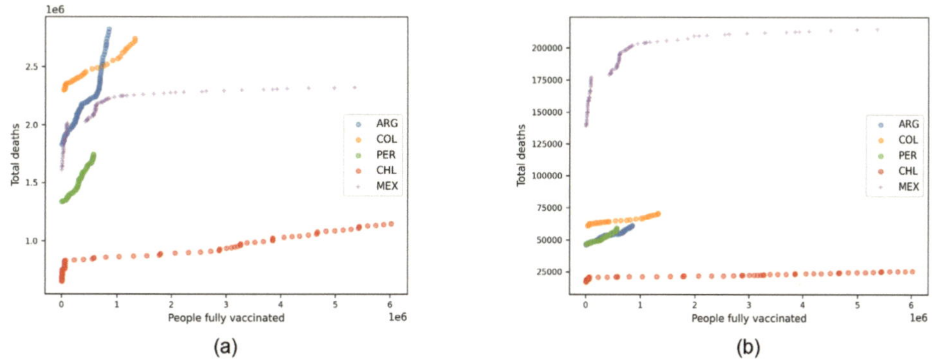

Figure 7.
The effect of vaccination in total confirmed cases and deaths in Argentina, Colombia, Peru, Chile and Mexico. (a) Confirmed cases. (b) Deaths.

noticed the differences between some countries (US is the country with the major number of people vaccinated). Furthermore, we noticed how the number of confirmed cases and deaths were reduced since the vaccination started.

Latin American countries, present a similar behavior. In **Figure 7**, we plotted, how the number of people vaccinated, affect the number of confirmed cases and deaths. In this case, Chile and Mexico are the leaders of vaccination in Latin America. Moreover, the number of confirmed cases and death seems to decrease in this countries.

4. Forecasting COVID-19 confirmed cases

In this section, we evaluated the accuracy of some methods to predict the confirmed cases of COVID-19. In this case we choose Multiplicative Trend Exponential Smoothing (MTES) and Long Short-Term Memory (LSTM), as it was proposed in a previous work [7].

4.1 Multiplicative trend exponential smoothing

The MTES method [30] is usually known to predict non-seasonality data as modeling with a trend in a multiplicative way, differing from the Hold (additive trend) method that considered the trend in a additive way [31]. It's known that on the real world the majority series have multiplicative trends. The MTES method works with two smoothing parameters designing the local growth rate by smoothing successive divisions from the local level [32].

4.2 Long short-term memory

LSTM is a recurrent neural network [33]. This network introduces the concepts of memory cells (**Figure 8**), this unit is composed of a cell, an input gate, an output gate and a forget gate. This cell remembers values over time intervals, then the other gates regulate the flow of information.

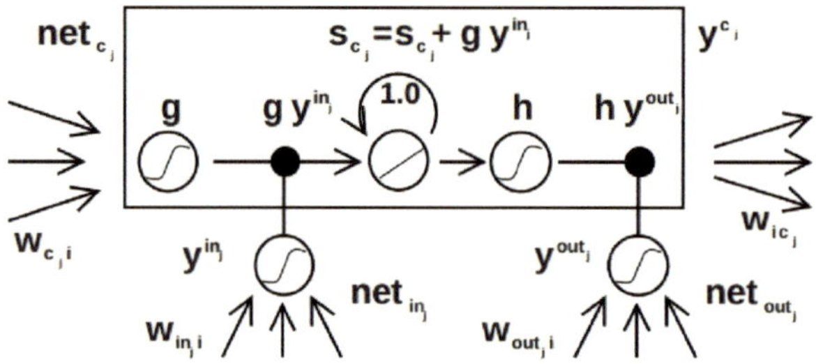

Figure 8.
Architecture of memory cell c_j and its gate units in_j, out_j. Source: [33].

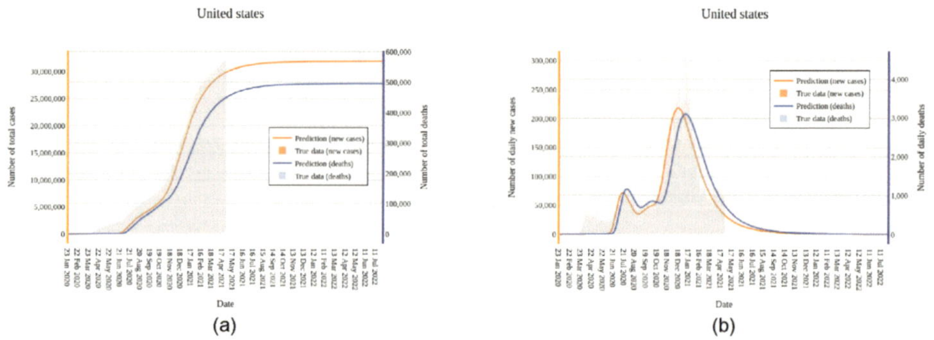

Figure 9.
Prediciton of total and daily confirmed cases in United States, using LSTM. (a) Total confirmed cases. (b) Daily confirmed cases.

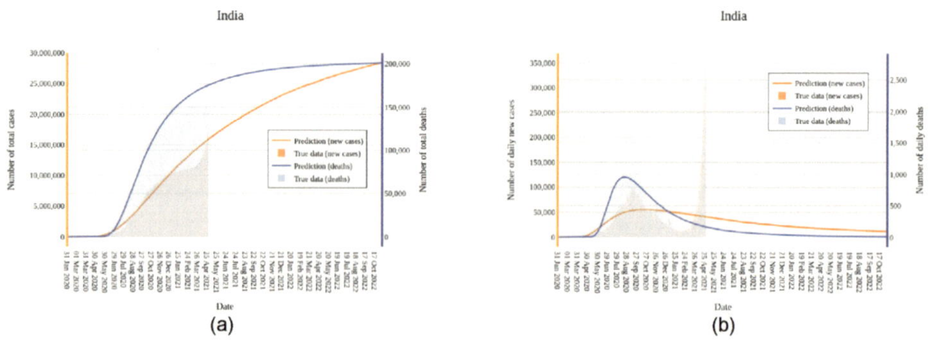

Figure 10.
Prediciton of total and daily confirmed cases in India, using LSTM. (a) Total confirmed cases. (b) Daily confirmed cases.

4.3 Forecasting results

For prediction, we used a Weibull based Long-Short-Term-Memory approach (W-LSTM) [34]. According to the author of W-LSTM, the model outperformed ARIMA and other LSTM variants. Moreover, the network got 82% of accuracy. In **Figures 9–12**, we show the predictions of total confirmed cases and daily cases for

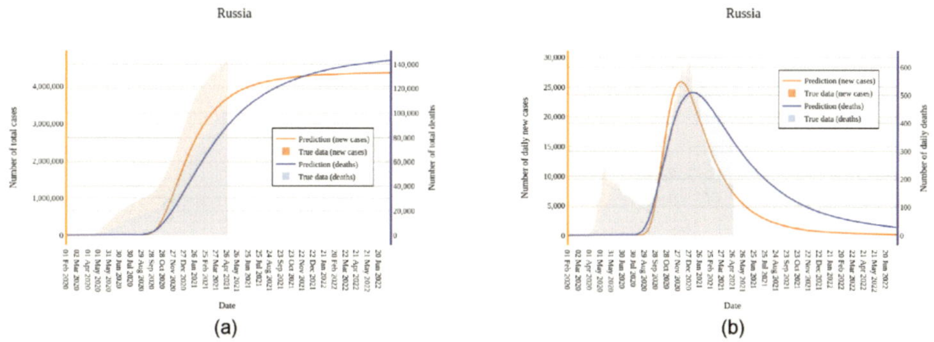

Figure 11.
Prediciton of total and daily confirmed cases in Russia, using LSTM. (a) Total confirmed cases. (b) Daily confirmed cases.

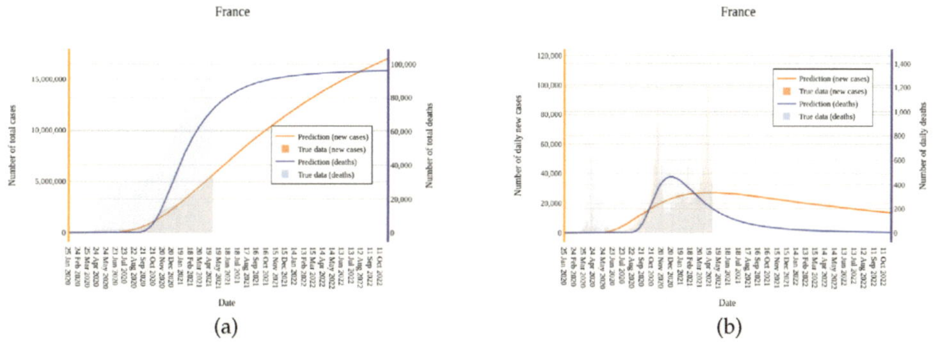

Figure 12.
Prediciton of total and daily confirmed cases in France, using LSTM. (a) Total confirmed cases. (b) Daily confirmed cases.

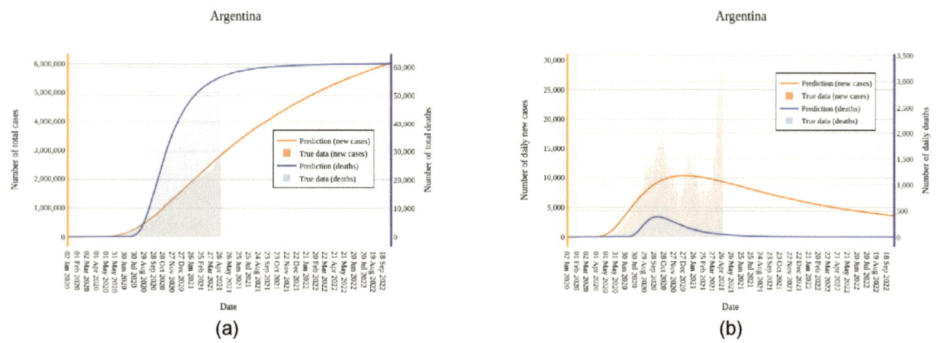

Figure 13.
Prediciton of total and daily confirmed cases in Argentina, using LSTM. (a) Total confirmed cases. (b) Daily confirmed cases.

US, India, Russia and France. Additionally, in **Figures 13–17**, we present the predictions for Latin American countries.

In **Figure 18a**, we plotted the total confirmed cases predictions for US, India, Russia, France and Brazil, using MTES algorithm. Additionally, In **Figure 18b**, we plotted the total confirmed cases predictions for Peru, Argentina, Colombia, Chile and Mexico. We know that, MTES is usually well used for short time series

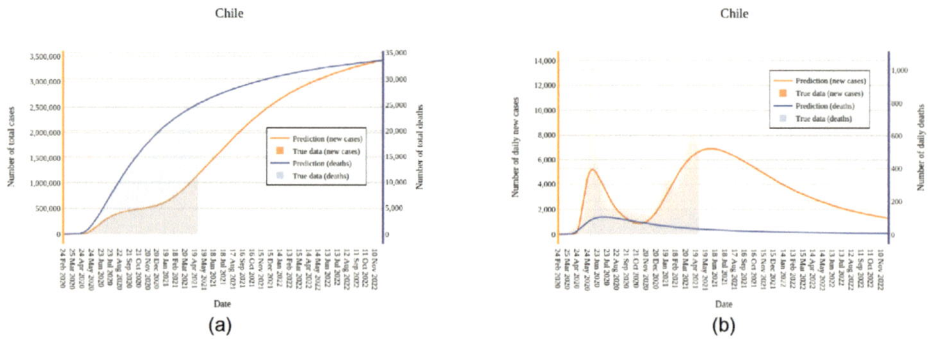

Figure 14.
Prediciton of total and daily confirmed cases in Chile, using LSTM. (a) Total confirmed cases. (b) Daily confirmed cases.

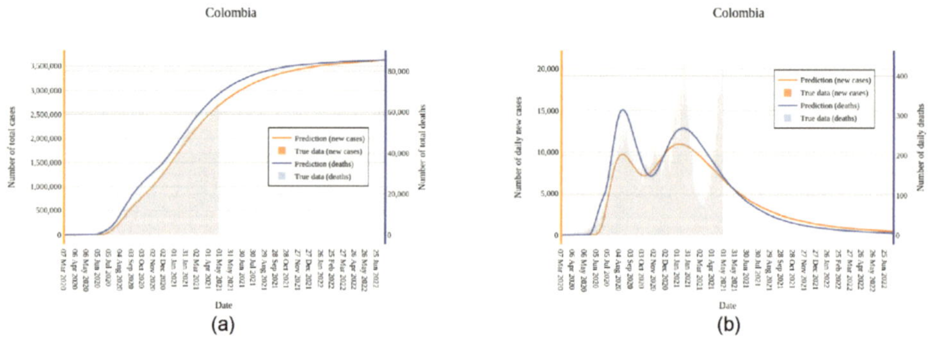

Figure 15.
Prediciton of total and daily confirmed cases in Colombia, using LSTM. (a) Total confirmed cases. (b) Daily confirmed cases.

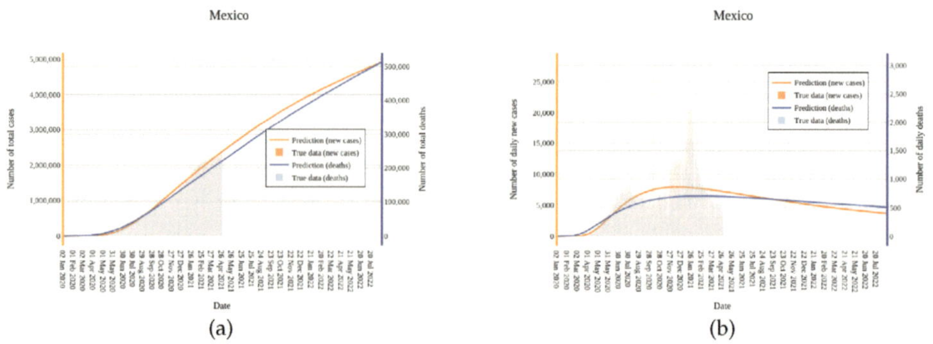

Figure 16.
Prediciton of total and daily confirmed cases in Mexico, using LSTM. (a) Total confirmed cases. (b) Daily confirmed cases.

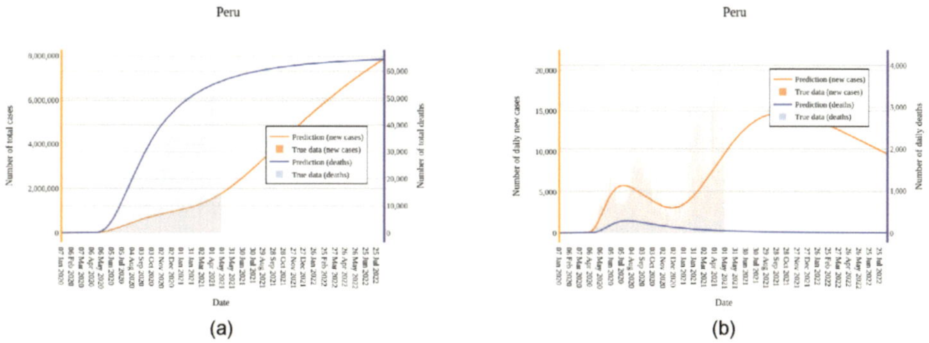

Figure 17.
Prediciton of total and daily confirmed cases in Peru, using LSTM. (a) Total confirmed cases. (b) Daily confirmed cases.

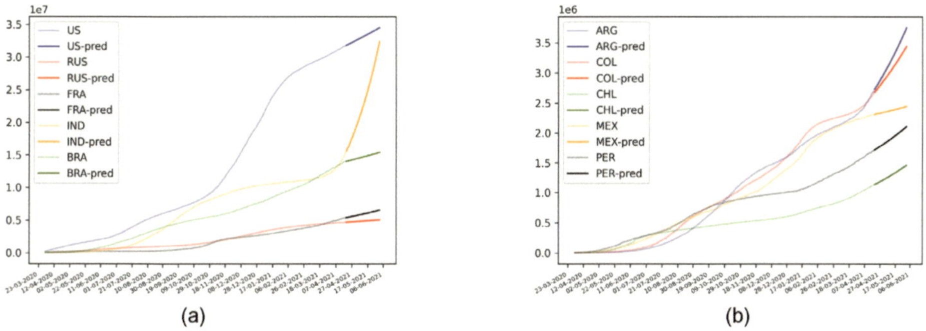

Figure 18.
Prediciton of total and daily confirmed cases in Peru, using LSTM. (a) Predicitons for US, India, Russia, France and Brazil. (b) Predictions for Peru, Argentinca, Colombia, Chile and Mexico.

prediction. For that reason, the India confirmed cases predictions shows an increased trend, due to the increasing behavior during the last weeks.

5. Conclusions

The coronavirus COVID-19 pandemic caused strain on all the world getting abundant deaths and forcing lock downs to contain the spread. However, the scientific community was not left behind because it was developed a lot of projects like vaccines candidates, analysis of the confirmed cases, and forecast of confirmed cases and deaths.

The behavior and evolution of confirmed cases is different for each country. Moreover, there are several factors that increase or mitigate the COVID-19 evolution like: population, health system, social behavior and the overestimation of some authorities. Moreover, in order to evaluate the impact of the pandemic, we need to evaluate the number of confirmed cases, population, deaths, etc. For instance, despite US has the major number of confirmed cases, it has a low death rate of 1.77%.

The death rate, is a good metric to evaluate the impact of COVID-19 over population. For example, we noticed that Mexico has the highest death rate in this study (8.85%). After review, we found out, that the reason of this high death rate, is the percentage of over weighted people in Mexico (40.2% for males and 36.1% for females). According to researches, obesity is considered the main risk factor of death by COVID-19.

Additionally, we reviewed the variants and vaccination projects for COVID-19. Thankfully, we only have VOI and VOC variants. Furthermore, there are several vaccination projects around the world. Some countries, like US has started a massive vaccination plan, as a consequence, the number of confirmed cases and deaths, show a decreasing behavior.

Finally, we made some predictions. We used W-LSTM and MTES to predict the total and daily confirmed cases in US, India, Russia, France, Argentina, Colombia, Chile, Peru and Mexico. According to the results, W-LSTM showed a more realistic prediction than MTES.

Nomenclature

ARG	Argentina
BRA	Brazil
COL	Colombia
CHL	Chile
IND	India
FRA	Francia
LSTM	Long Short-Term Memory
PER	Peru
RUS	Russia
US	United States
UK	United Kingdom
USA	United States of America
VOI	Variant of Interest
VOC	Variant of Concern
VOHC	Variant of High Consequence

Author details

Vicente Enrique Machaca Arceda[1*†], Miguel Angel Machaca Arceda[2†] and Pamela Claudia Laguna Laura[2†]

1 Universidad La Salle, Arequipa, Perú

2 Universidad Nacional de San Agust'in, Arequipa, Perú

*Address all correspondence to: vmachacaa@ulasalle.edu.pe

† These authors contributed equally.

References

[1] İsmail Kırbaş, A. Sözen, A. D. Tuncer, and F. Şinasi Kazancıoğlu, "Comparative analysis and forecasting of covid-19 cases in various european countries with arima, narnn and lstm approaches," *Chaos, Solitons and Fractals*, vol. 138, p. 110015, 2020.

[2] Google, "Google news covid-19," https://news.google.com/covid19/map?hl=en-US&gl=US&ceid=US:en, accessed: 2020-28-04.

[3] H. Legido-Quigley, N. Asgari, Y. Y. Teo, G. M. Leung, H. Oshitani, K. Fukuda, A. R. Cook, L. Y. Hsu, K. Shibuya, and D. Heymann, "Are high-performing health systems resilient against the covid-19 epidemic?" *The Lancet*, vol. 395, no. 10227, pp. 848–850, 2020.

[4] I. A. Kretchy, M. Asiedu-Danso, and J.-P. Kretchy, "Medication management and adherence during the covid-19 pandemic: perspectives and experiences from low-and middle-income countries," *Research in social and administrative pharmacy*, vol. 17, no. 1, pp. 2023–2026, 2021.

[5] G. Forni and A. Mantovani, "Covid-19 vaccines: where we stand and challenges ahead," *Cell Death & Differentiation*, vol. 28, no. 2, pp. 626–639, 2021.

[6] Covid-19 vaccine tracker. [Online]. Available: https://www.sciencedirect.com/science/article/pii/S0277953620308613

[7] M. M. Arceda, P. L. Laura, and V. M. Arceda, "Forecasting time series with multiplicative trend exponential smoothing and lstm: Covid-19 case study," in *Proceedings of the Future Technologies Conference*. Springer, 2020, pp. 568–582.

[8] İ. Kırbas¸, A. Sözen, A. D. Tuncer, and F. S¸. Kazancıoğlu, "Comparative analysis and forecasting of covid-19 cases in various european countries with arima, narnn and lstm approaches," *Chaos, Solitons & Fractals*, vol. 138, p. 110015, 2020.

[9] V. K. R. Chimmula and L. Zhang, "Time series forecasting of covid-19 transmission in canada using lstm networks," *Chaos, Solitons & Fractals*, vol. 135, p. 109864, 2020.

[10] K. ArunKumar, D. V. Kalaga, C. M. S. Kumar, M. Kawaji, and T. M. Brenza, "Forecasting of covid-19 using deep layer recurrent neural networks (rnns) with gated recurrent units (grus) and long short-term memory (lstm) cells," *Chaos, Solitons & Fractals*, vol. 146, p. 110861, 2021.

[11] W. Dietz and C. Santos-Burgoa, "Obesity and its implications for covid-19 mortality," *Obesity*, vol. 28, no. 6, pp. 1005–1005, 2020.

[12] N. Sattar, I. B. McInnes, and J. J. McMurray, "Obesity is a risk factor for severe covid-19 infection: multiple potential mechanisms," *Circulation*, vol. 142, no. 1, pp. 4–6, 2020.

[13] A. M. Rychter, A. Zawada, A. E. Ratajczak, A. Dobrowolska, and I. Krela-Kaźmierczak, "Should patients with obesity be more afraid of covid-19?" *Obesity Reviews*, vol. 21, no. 9, p. e13083, 2020.

[14] S. Barquera and J. A. Rivera, "Obesity in mexico: rapid epidemiological transition and food industry interference in health policies," *The Lancet Diabetes & Endocrinology*, vol. 8, no. 9, pp. 746–747, 2020.

[15] CDC, "Sars-cov-2 variant classifications and definitions," 2021.

[16] S. Jangra, C. Ye, R. Rathnasinghe, D. Stadlbauer, H. Alshammary, A. A.

Amoako, M. H. Awawda, K. F. Beach, M. C. Bermúdez-González, R. L. Chernet *et al.*, "Sars-cov-2 spike e484k mutation reduces antibody neutralisation," *The Lancet Microbe*, 2021.

[17] W. F. Garcia-Beltran, E. C. Lam, K. S. Denis, A. D. Nitido, Z. H. Garcia, B. M. Hauser, J. Feldman, M. N. Pavlovic, D. J. Gregory, M. C. Poznansky *et al.*, "Multiple sars-cov-2 variants escape neutralization by vaccine-induced humoral immunity," *Cell*, 2021.

[18] Regeneron, "Fact sheet for health care providers emergency use authorization (eua) of regen-cov."

[19] E. Lilly and Company, "Fact sheet for health care providers emergency use authorization (eua) of bamlanivimab and etesevimab."

[20] N. G. Davies, S. Abbott, R. C. Barnard, C. I. Jarvis, A. J. Kucharski, J. D. Munday, C. A. Pearson, T. W. Russell, D. C. Tully, A. D. Washburne *et al.*, "Estimated transmissibility and impact of sars-cov-2 lineage b. 1.1. 7 in england," *Science*, vol. 372, no. 6538, 2021.

[21] C. A. Pearson, T. W. Russell, N. Davies, A. J. Kucharski, C. C.-. working group, W. J. Edmunds, R. M. Eggo *et al.*, "Estimates of severity and transmissibility of novel south africa sars-cov-2 variant 501y. v2," *Preprint at https://cmmid. github. io/topics/covid19/sa-novel-variant. html*, 2021.

[22] X. Deng, M. A. Garcia-Knight, M. M. Khalid, V. Servellita, C. Wang, M. K. Morris, A. Sotomayor-González, D. R. Glasner, K. R. Reyes, A. S. Gliwa *et al.*, "Transmission, infectivity, and antibody neutralization of an emerging sars-cov-2 variant in california carrying a l452r spike protein mutation," *medRxiv*, 2021.

[23] CDC, "Vaccines and immunizations," 2021.

[24] S. H. Shahcheraghi, J. Ayatollahi, A. A. Aljabali, M. D. Shastri, S. D. Shukla, D. K. Chellappan, N. K. Jha, K. Anand, N. K. Katari, M. Mehta *et al.*, "An overview of vaccine development for covid-19," *Therapeutic Delivery*, vol. 12, no. 3, pp. 235–244, 2021.

[25] M. M. Silveira, G. M. S. G. Moreira, and M. Mendonc¸a, "Dna vaccines against covid-19: Perspectives and challenges," *Life sciences*, p. 118919, 2020.

[26] S. Pascolo, "Vaccination with messenger rna (mrna)," *Toll-like receptors (TLRs) and innate immunity*, pp. 221–235, 2008.

[27] M. Mort, A. Baleta, F. Destefano, J. G. Nsubuga, C. Vellozzi, U. Mehta, R. Pless, S. A. Abdoellah, P. Yosephine, S. Karolina *et al.*, "Vaccine safety basics: learning manual," World Health Organization, Tech. Rep., 2013.

[28] B. Hasell J., Mathieu E., "A cross-country database of covid-19 testing," in *Sci Data*, 2020, p. 345.

[29] G. L. Dong E, Du H, "An interactive web-based dashboard to track covid-19 in real time," in *Lancet Inf Dis*, 2020, pp. 533–534.

[30] C. C. Pegels, "Exponential forecasting: some new variations," *Management Science*, pp. 311–315, 1969.

[31] C. C. Holt, "Forecasting trends and seasonals by exponentially weighted averages. carnegie institute of technology," Pittsburgh ONR memorandum, Tech. Rep., 1957.

[32] J. W. Taylor, "Exponential smoothing with a damped multiplicative trend," *International journal of Forecasting*, vol. 19, no. 4, pp. 715–725, 2003.

[33] S. Hochreiter and J. Schmidhuber, "Long short-term memory," *Neural*

computation, vol. 9, no. 8, pp. 1735–1780, 1997.

[34] S. Tuli, S. Tuli, R. Verma, and R. Tuli, "Modelling for prediction of the spread and severity of covid-19 and its association with socioeconomic factors and virus types," *Biomedical Research and Clinical Reviews*, vol. 1, 2020.

Chapter 4

Demographic, Clinical and Radiological Features of Healthcare Workers and Two Index Cases That Were Infected with COVID-19 (SARS-Cov-2)

Ayse Erturk, Ugur Kostakoglu, Ilknur Esen Yildiz, Nur Hursoy, Sevda Ozdemir Al, Songul Ozyurt, Neslihan Ozcelik, Hatice Beyazal Polat and Aysegul Copur Cicek

Abstract

To evaluate the index cases leading to the transmission of healthcare workers (HCWs) in Rize/Turkey Recep Tayyip Erdogan University Faculty of Medicine Education and Research Hospital with COVID-19 infection and the clinical features of infected HCWs. The first two COVID-19 test positive patients treated at Rize/Turkey between 10.03.2020 and 12.04.2020 and HCWs those who examined these two patients whose COVID-19 PCR test results were positive were included in this study. In Rize/Turkey, the first and second cases of positive COVID-19 which was recorded on 13.03.2020 on 25.03.2020, 27 HCWs (female, 63%, n = 17 and male, 37%, n = 10 and the mean age was 33.2 ± 6.9 years) who contacted during the treatment of these cases and became COVID-19 positive were examined. The median of symptom duration (days) of the HCWs was 5 days (range: 0–17 days). Fever, 55.6% (n = 15); malaise, 44.4% (n = 12); cough, 40.7% (n = 11); sore throat, 33.3% (n = 9); myalgia, 33.3% (n = 9); dyspnea, 14.8% (n = 4); diarrhea, 22.2% (n = 6); vomiting, 14.8% (n = 4); anosmia, 18.5% (n = 5); ageusia, 22.2% (n = 6) and headache, 37% (n = 10) of the cases. The rates of headache in female HCWs infected with COVID-19 were found to be significantly higher compared to men (52.9%). None of them had severe clinical situation requiring intensive care follow-up or acute respiratory distress syndrome (ARDS). Laboratory measurements of HCWs were carried out at the first when they had symptoms and when they recovered, and results were compared accordingly. The thorax computerized tomography (CT) findings of HCWs were normal in 74.1% (n = 20) of total. HCWs were initially affected by the COVID-19 pandemic. Early measures provided by the Health authorities, access to diagnosis and treatment, and the young age average in HCWs prevented severe outcomes such as severe clinical course and mortality at the beginning of the outbreak.

Keywords: COVID-19, healthcare workers, transmission, pandemic

1. Introduction

COVID 19 continues to threaten health of the humankind [1, 2]. COVID-19 is transmitted by close contact and droplets among people. However, airborne contamination may be possible under certain conditions and environments in which procedures or supportive treatments that produce aerosols are performed [3]. Those who are most at risk of getting this disease are those who have contact with the patient or those who provides care for them. Therefore, the protection of HCWs is considered as one of the top priorities [4–6].

In all countries with COVID-19 pandemic, the caught unaware staff was effective in the transmission, since the transmission dynamics of the COVID-19 virus was not fully known at the onset of the outbreak [7, 8]. With the reporting of the first cases, the protective equipment has been widespread used. The initial case diagnosis in our country were made with guides in the form of a history of international contact and clinical definitions [8, 9]. Recently, as of September 2020, 601 HCWs were positive for the COVID-19 test during the onset of the outbreak, and then it was reported as 7,428 health workers had been infected, which is around 6.5 percent of the total number of cases [10].

The cases reported by our HCWs in the first week concurrently with the general course of the country, there was no history of traveling abroad and there had not been aware of suspected contacts. The fact that there were 27 HCWs in the first month and the first two index cases and 4 HCWs in the second month supported this outcome. During the epidemy, HCWs are under tremendous stress. Working with personal protective equipment (PPE) and performing specific procedures are cumbersome and were not convenient [11, 12]. Despite all these difficulties it was necessity to use highly protective respirators such as N95 or P2/FFP2/FFP3 for HCWs. Employees' occupational health and safety should be given high priority and a uniform policy should be applied to use personal protective equipment to prevent infection [7].

We aimed to identify the clinical features of 27 HCWs who were in contact with the first two index cases infected with COVID-19 and compare them with previous studies.

2. Material and methods

After the first index cases were diagnosed, filiation and evaluation of concurrent symptomatic applicants were performed at the Infectious Diseases clinic. Retrospectively, clinical findings were classified as severe (1–14 days), moderate (1–7 days), and mild (no hospitalization days), considering the duration of symptoms, length of hospital stay, and treatment practices. Patients with possible SARS-CoV-2 infection were examined via real-time RT-PCR and next-generation sequencing laboratory techniques. This study was approved by the Ministry of Health of Turkey, Scientific Research Ethics Committee No: Ayse Erturk-2020-05-11T12_27_08 and local ethics committee RTEU Faculty of Medicine Rize/Turkey – No: 2020/82.

2.1 Statistical analysis

SPSS 17.0 (Chicago Inc., 2008) program was used in the analysis. Categorical variables were expressed in terms of frequency (n) and percent (%) and in arithmetic mean, standard deviation, median, minimum and maximum values. While the Student t-test was used for comparison of continuous distributors with normal distribution, those without normal distribution were analyzed with the Mann–Whitney U test. Pearson-$\chi 2$ and Fisher's exact tests were used for categorical variables. Paired-t test and Wilcoxon signed rank tests were used to compare the first and second levels of laboratory measurement parameters. $P < 0.05$ was accepted as the level of significance.

3. Results

3.1 Features of index cases (patients)

Characteristics of a 75-year-old female patient who was reported as the first COVID-19 test positive patient in Rize on 13.03.2020, and a 69-year-old male patient who was positive on the tracheal aspirate COVID-19 test on 25.03.2020 were summarized as follows:

3.1.1 The Index patient 1

75 years-old, women. Place of birth and living: Rize province. The first-degree relative lives in Istanbul province. With the symptoms of fever, cough, shortness of breath, vomiting, chest pain, F.T was admitted to emergency service of Rize State Hospital on 10.03.2020 and she was hospitalized with diagnoses of primary hypertension (HT), congestive heart failure (CHF), acute sub-endocardial myocardial infarction (MI), non-ST elevated acute myocardial infarction (AMI), and acute renal failure (ARF). On 13.03.20, she was transferred to the RTEU Training and Research Hospital Cardiology service. On 13.03.2020, the patient's nasopharyngeal COVID-19 sampling was performed. The patient was started on hydroxychloroquine 2x400 mg loading and 2x200 mg/day maintenance doses (po), azithromycin 1x500 mg/day (po), oseltamivir 2x30 mg/day (po), and piperacillin-tazobactam 4x3.375 g (1.5 flacon) iv treatment. On the date of 22.03.2020, she was transferred 1st stage coronary intensive care unit and intubated due to the deterioration in general condition, unconsciousness, hypotension, bradycardia, cyanosis, and decreased urine output.

Radiologically, there was no apparent opacity on the The posteroanterior (PA) chest X-ray dated 16.03.2020 (**Figure 1a**). Newly developed opacities in the right lung were noticeable on the control radiography dated 23.03.2020 (**Figure 1b**). In the IV contrast-free axial CT section dated 24.03.2020, ground-glass opacities (GGOs) were observed in the upper lobes, and an endobronchial intubation tube was present in the trachea (**Figure 1c**).

On 25.03.2020 and 29.03 2020, patient's endotracheal aspirate (ETA)-COVID-19 test resulted in positive. There was no overseas contact history. However, there was, a history of contact with the positive case (daughter), who was living in Istanbul and detected her positivity in RTEU hospital. Unfortunately, patient died on 30.03.2020.

While being followed up in the cardiology service and coronary intensive care unit, the staff working in these units was thought to have been transmitted.

3.1.2 The Index patient 1 and the expanse GGOs on CT

Radiologically, there was no apparent opacity on the PA chest X-ray dated 16.03.2020 (**Figure 1a**). Newly developed opacities in the right lung were noticeable on the control radiograph dated 23.03.2020 (**Figure 1b**). In the IV contrast-free axial CT section dated 24.03.2020, GGOs were observed in the upper lobes, and an endobronchial intubation tube was present in the trachea (**Figure 1c**).

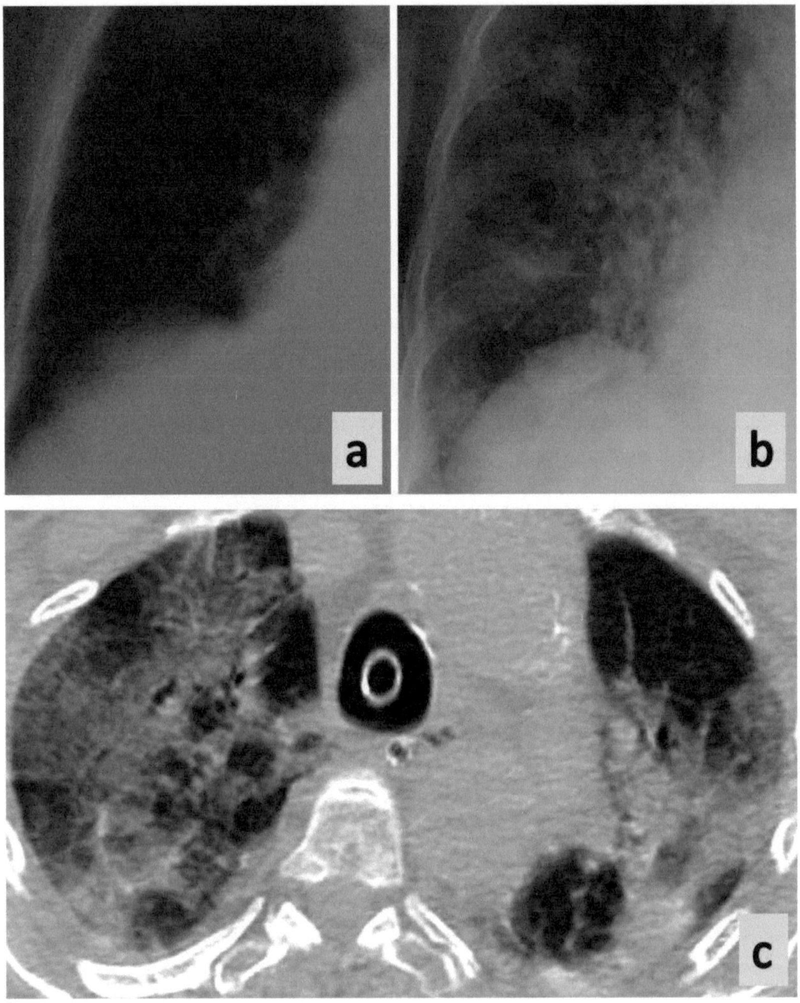

Figure 1.
(a–c) Radiologically, there was no apparent opacity on the PA chest X-ray dated 16.03.2020 (a). Newly developed opacities in the right lung were noticeable on the control radiograph dated 23.03.2020 (b). In the IV contrast-free axial CT section dated 24.03.2020, GGOs were observed in the upper lobes, and an endobronchial intubation tube was present in the trachea (c).

3.1.3 The Index patient 2

69 years-old, male. On 16.03.2020, he was hospitalized to the Pulmonology clinic with the diagnoses of hyperlipidemia, essential (primary) hypertension (HT), atherosclerotic heart disease, pacemaker use, and myalgia. There were 20 packs per month of smoking history for 25 years. The patient, whose preliminary diagnosis of viral pneumonia was interned, had a history of cough and sputum for 2 months, and had a fever since the last 3 days, lymphopenia, higher levels of CRP and D-dimer. SO_2 levels were around 80 receiving with 6 lt/min O_2 support and his tachypnea continued.

With prediagnosis of COVID-19, the nasopharyngeal (NF)-COVID-19 test performed on the same day was negative and this negativity continued the second NF-COVID-19 test carried on 20.03.2020. Patients' endotracheal aspirate (ETA)-COVID-19 test examined on 24.03.2020 was also negative.

Radiological findings of the patient were the following; Peripheral ground-glass areas were detected in the axial Pulmonary CT Angiography section dated

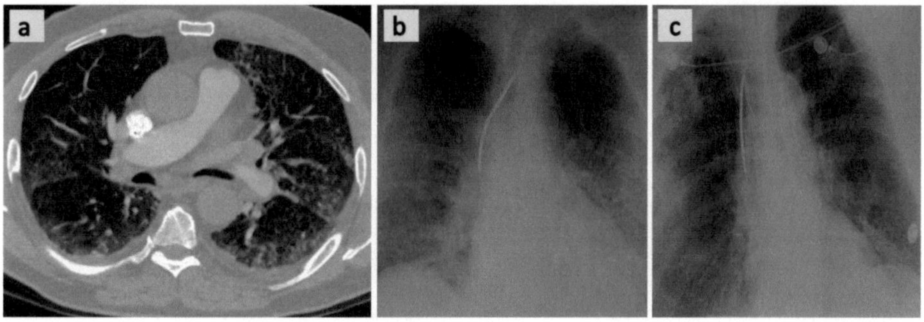

Figure 2.
(a-c) Radiological findings of the patient was the following; peripheral GGOs were detected in the axial pulmonary CT angiography section dated 19.03.2020 (a). Reticulonodular opacities were present on the PA chest x-ray of the same date (b). Newly developed opacities were detected in both lung upper lobes on the control graph taken on 4.04.2020. Electrodes and pacemaker were displayed in the left pectoral region (c).

19.03.2020 (**Figure 2a**). Reticulonodular opacities were present on the PA chest x-ray of the same date (**Figure 2b**). Newly developed opacities were detected in both lung upper lobes on the control graph taken on 4.04.2020 (**Figure 2c**).

On 25.03.2020, the patient's ETA COVID-19 test was found as positive and the case was recorded as the second COVID-19 case of Rize province. The patient diagnosed by COVID-19 via clinical and radiological imaging findings and was given hydroxychloroquine 2x400 mg loading and 2x200 mg/day maintenance doses (po), azithromycin 1x500 mg/day (po), oseltamivir 2x30 mg/day (po), piperacillin tazobactam 4x3.375 g (1.5 flacons) iv route. He, unfortunately, died on 10.04.2020.

While the patient was followed up by clinics of pulmonology and infectious diseases, it was thought that the personnel working in these units caught infection.

3.1.4 The Index patient 2 and the expanse peripheral GGOs on CT

Radiological findings of the patient was the following; Peripheral GGOs were detected in the axial Pulmonary CT Angiography section dated 19.03.2020 (**Figure 2a**). Reticulonodular opacities were present on the PA chest x-ray of the same date (**Figure 2b**). Newly developed opacities were detected in both lung upper lobes on the control graph taken on 4.04.2020. Electrodes and pacemaker were displayed in the left pectoral region (**Figure 2c**).

3.2 Demographic and clinical features of health personnel

COVID-19 positive health workers among them were 27 and 63% (n = 17) of them were women and 37% (n = 10) were men and the mean age was 33.2 ± 6.9 years. Of 55.6% (n = 15) cases were from Coronary ICU, 25.9% (n = 7) of them from Cardiology, and 18.5% (n = 5) of them from Infectious diseases clinic's personnel. Occupational distributions of cases were follows; 51.9% (n = 14) were nurses, 29.6% (n = 8) were doctors, 11.1% (n = 3) were cleaning staff and 7.4% (n = 2) were secretaries. Male doctors were found to be significantly higher than female doctors (70% vs. 5.9%, $p < .001$, Fisher's exact test, see (**Table 1**).

Clinically, patients with symptoms including at least one symptom were 74.1% (n = 20). None of the HCWs had comorbidity. While 63% of the cases (n = 17) had a mild clinical level, 29.6% (n = 8) were of moderate and 7.4% (n = 2) were severe. None of them had severe clinical outcome and acute respiratory distress syndrome

	Total	Females	Males	Statistics	
	n = 27	n = 17	n = 10	t, z, or $\chi 2$	p value
Age (years)[a]	33.2 (6.9)	32.3 (6.8)	34.7 (7.3)	−.838	.410
Occupations, n (%)				15.901*	.000
Nurse	14 (51.9)	13 (76.5)	1 (10.0)		
Doctor	8 (29.6)	1 (5.9)	7 (70.0)		
Cleaning stuff	3 (11.1)	1 (5.9)	2 (20.0)		
Sekretary	2 (7.4)	2 (11.8)	0		
Working service, n (%)				1.318*	.647
Coronary	15 (55.6)	8 (47.1)	7 (70.0)		
Cardiology	7 (25.9)	5 (29.4)	2 (20.0)		
Infectious diseases	5 (18.5)	4 (23.5)	1 (10.0)		
First PCR positivity (day)[b]	2 (0–7)	3 (0–7)	0 (0–4)	−1.594	.111
1st PCR negativity (day)[b]	7 (0–12)	8 (0–12)	6 (5–10)	−1.384	.167
2nd PCR negativity (day)[b]	10 (7–15)	10 (7–15)	10 (7–15)	−.627	.531
Symptom presence (at least one), n (%)	20 (74.1)	13 (76.5)	7 (70.0)	.137*	1.00
COVID-contact, n (%)				2.830*	.124
Knew	11 (40.7)	9 (52.9)	2 (20.0)		
Not-knew	16 (59.3)	8 (47.1)	8 (80.0)		
Hospitalization (day)[b]	0 (0–15)	0 (0–14)	0 (0–15)	−.116	.908
Clinic severity, n (%)				1.478*	.578
Good	17 (63.0)	12 (70.6)	5 (50.0)		
Moderate	8 (29.6)	4 (23.5)	4 (40.0)		
Severe	2 (7.4)	1 (5.9)	1 (10.0)		
Symptoms duration (day)[b]	5 (0–17)	4 (0–13)	7 (0–17)	−1.295	.195
Symptoms presence, n (%)					
Fever	15 (55.6)	9 (52.9)	6 (60.0)	.127*	1.00
Cough	11 (40.7)	5 (29.4)	6 (60.0)	2.440*	.224
Sore throat	9 (33.3)	5 (29.4)	4 (40.0)	.318*	.683
Shortness of breath	4 (14.8)	2 (11.8)	2 (20.0)	.338*	.613
Miyalgia	9 (33.3)	6 (35.3)	3 (30.0)	.079*	1.00
Malaise	12 (44.4)	19 (58.8)	2 (20.0)	3.844*	.107

	Total	Females	Males	Statistics	
	n = 27	n = 17	n = 10	t, z, or $\chi 2$	p value
Headache	10 (37.0)	9 (52.9)	1 (10.0)	4.979*	**.042**
Diarrhea	6 (22.2)	5 (29.4)	1 (10.0)	1.373*	.363
Vomiting	4 (14.8)	4 (23.5)	0	2.762*	.264
Loss of smell	5 (18.5)	3 (17.6)	2 (20.0)	.023*	1.00
Loss of taste	6 (22.2)	4 (23.5)	2 (20.0)	.045*	1.00
Smoking (Yes), n (%)	5 (18.5)	0	5 (50.0)	10.432*	**.003**
CT findings (Yes), n (%)	7 (25.9)	4 (23.5)	3 (30.0)	.137*	1.00
Reversed halo (Yes), n (%)	2 (7.4)	1 (5.9)	1 (10.0)	.156*	1.00
Frosted-glass opacity (Yes), n (%)	7 (25.9)	4 (23.5)	3 (30.0)	.137*	1.00
Consolidation (Yes), n (%)	1 (3.7)	0	1 (10.0)	1.765*	.370
Bilaterally involvement (Yes), n (%)	2 (7.4)	0	2 (20.0)	3.672*	.128
Peripheral and dorsal (Yes), n (%)	7 (25.9)	4 (23.5)	3 (30.0)	.137*	1.00
Middle and lower zones (Yes), n (%)	5 (18.5)	3 (17.6)	2 (20.0)	.023*	1.00

[a]*Mean (standard deviation)*
[b]*Median (minimum-maximum)*
**Fisher's exact test*
CT: computerized tomography.

Table 1.
Descriptives of health personnel infected with COVID-19 in terms of gender.

(ARDS) requiring intensive care follow-up. While 40.7% (n = 11) of the cases knew COVID-contact, 59.3% (n = 16) did not. The hospitalization value (days) of the patients was in the range 0–15.

The findings were classified as severe (1–14 days), moderate (1–7 days), and mild (no hospitalization days) considering the duration of symptoms, length of hospital stay, and treatment practices. Milddefines, very close to asymptomatic patients who received only hydroxychloroquine therapy whereas moderate defines, symptomatic findings were evident, those who received hydroxychloroquine and azithromycin therapy followed in hospital and severe means, respiratory symptoms were severe, supportive therapy- receiving oxygen, hydroxychloroquine- azithromycin and favipiravir therapy.

While the CT findings of the HCW were normal in 74.1% (n = 20), the appearance of ground glass was found in 25.9% (n = 7), reversed halo or atoll sign was found in 7.4% (n = 2), consolidation was present in 3.7% of the cases (n = 1). Bilaterally involvement was detected in 7.4% of the cases (n = 2), peripheral and dorsal involvement in 25.9% of the cases (n = 7). The involvement of the middle and sub-zones was detected in 18.5% (n = 5) of the cases. Especially in the female gender, 76.5% (n = 13) of them had normal CT findings (see **Table 1**).

3.3 Comparison of laboratory measurements

The laboratory measurements of the patients in the first week of admission were compared with the test results when the patients were discharged from the hospital or re-admitted for control (second week). Laboratory measurements of HCWs were carried out at the first when they had symptoms and the second when they healed, and results were compared. A significant reduction was found between the mean PLT (238.3 vs. 204.310^3/μL; z = −2.858, p = .004), MPV (10.0 vs. 9.5 fL; z = −2.161, p = .031), CRP (2.9 vs. 1 g/dL; z = −2.490, p = .013), Hgb (13.5 vs. 13.1 g/dL; z = −2.300, p = .021), LDH (91.1 vs. 47.2 U/L; z = −4.542, p < .001), CK (77 vs. 60 U/L; z = −3.340, p = .001), CK-MB (0.8 vs. 0.5 mg/mL; z = −2.212, p = .027), troponin (all second examinations were < 3.2, z = −2.032, p = .042), ferritin (151.7 vs. 95 ng/mL; z = −2.822, p = .005) levels whereas a significant increase was found the mean albumin (43.8 vs. 44.4 g/L; z = −2.000, p = .046), K^+ (4.1 vs. 4.3 mmol/L; t(26) = −2.213, p = .036) and Na^+ (137.5 vs. 138.2 mmol/L; t(26) = −2.174, p = .039) levels. The D-dimer had increased in 2 poor-clinical findings of HCWs, but their mean values were within normal limits (see **Table 2**).

	Laboratory measurements[a]		**Statistics**	
	First	**Second**	**paired-t or z**	**p value**
WBC (10^3/μL) (N: 4–10)	6.3 (1.3)	6.3 (1.5)	−.102	.919
NE (%) (N: 50–70)	61.5 (9.7)	58.4 (8.8)	−1.765	.078
LY (%) (N: 20–40)	31.4 (9.8)	28.9 (8.5)	−1.105	.269
N/L ratio	2.3 (1.6)	2.2 (0.8)	−.288	.773
PLT (10^3/μL) (N: 100–400)	238.3 (43.0)	204.3 (46.5)	−2.858	.004
MPV (fL) (N: 6.5–12)	10.0 (1.1)	9.5 (0.8)	−2.161	.031
PDW (fL) (N: 15–17)	16.0 (0.3)	16.1 (0.3)	−.345	.730
Hb (g/dL) (N: 10–16)	13.5 (1.1)	13.1 (1.2)	−2.300	.021
APTT (sec) (N: 26–38)	29.1 (2.4)	28.7 (1.9)	−.170	.865
PT (sec) (N: 12–16.5)	13.7 (2.5)	13.1 (0.7)	−.787	.432
CRP (mg/L)[b] (N: 0–5)	2.9 (0.4–114)	1 (0.3–16.7)	−2.490	.013
AST (U/L) (N: 0–35)	21.4 (5.7)	20.4 (6.7)	−.994	.320
ALT (U/L) (N: 0–35)	19.8 (0.9)	23.6 (11.7)	−1.828	.068
LDH (U/L) (N: 0–248)	191.1 (56.1)	47.2 (4.0)	−4.542	.000
Albumin (g/L) (N: 35–52)	43.8 (3.3)	44.4 (2.9)	−2.000	.046
K (mmol/L)[a] (N: 3.5–5.1)	4.1 (0.4)	4.3 (0.4)	−2.213	.036
Na (mmol/L)[a] (N: 136–146)	137.5 (2.4)	138.2 (1.9)	−2.174	.039
Cre (mg/dL) (N: 0.51–0.95)	0.6 (0.1)	0.6 (0.1)	−.294	.769
CK (U/L)[b] (N: 0–145)	77 (55–684)	60 (35–136)	−3.340	.001
CK-MB (mg/mL) (N: 0–3.1)	0.8 (0.6)	0.5 (0.1)	−2.212	.027
Troponin (pg/mL)[b] (N: 0–15.6)	<3.2 (<3.2–7.9)	<3.2	−2.032	.042
D-dimer (μgFEU/mL) (N: 0–0.5)	<.25 (<.25–0.3)	<.25	−1.890	.059
Sedim (mm/hour) (N: 0–20)	19.2 (17.9)	13.1 (7.7)	−1.298	.194
Ferritin (ng/mL) (N: 21.8–274.6)	151.7 (115.7)	95.0 (38.8)	−2.822	.005

[a]*Mean (standard deviation)*
[b]*Median (minimum-maksimum)*
N: normal reference range; WBC: White blood cell; NE: neutrophil; LY: lymphocyte; N/L: neutrophil/lymphocyte; PLT: platelet.

Table 2.
Comparison of the first and second values of laboratory measurements.

3.4 Imaging findings

3.4.1 The HCW with the worst clinical findings and the expanse GGOs on CT

44 year old male patient, it was noteworthy that in the first examination (**Figure 3a**), the GGOs observed in the lower lobe of the left lung expanded in the control examination on iv non-contrasted axial CT images obtained with an interval of 4 days (**Figure 3b**). In the control evaluation in the ground glass area (**Figure 3c**) located in the left lobe lower lobe posterobasal segment, fibrous bands developed (**Figure 3d**).

3.4.2 The HCW with good clinical findings and the halo sign on CT

41 year old female patient, in the CT images of 31.03.2020 (**Figure 4a**) and 5.05.2020 (**Figure 4b**), the minimum-intensity-projection coronal cross-sectional CT images show different areas of involvement. Right lung lower lobe findings (**Figure 4a**) declined in control, but consolidation developed with a reverse halo sign in posterobasal (**Figure 4b**).

3.4.3 The HCW with asymptomatic clinical findings and the minimal peripheral GGOs on CT

34-year-old female patient, peripheral small-sized GGOs are observed in the iv non-contrasted axial CT images obtained every 10 days apart (**Figure 5a**). The GGOswere diminished but new ground glass areas developed (**Figure 5b**).

4. Discussion

In many countries, especially China, which is the country where the COVID-19 epidemic was first seen, the healthcare professionals became the “frontline” occupational group struggling against COVID-19 [13–15]. According to the first date of February 11, 2020, 1716 Chinese HCWs have been reported to have COVID-19 infection when the first 15 affected cases were reported in Wuhan [13]. On February 17, 2020, the CDC weekly report reported that a total of 3,019 Chinese HCWs were infected with severe acute respiratory syndrome coronavirus 2 (SARS-CoV-2) and 1,716 of them were confirmed with COVID-19. As of February 20, ten health workers died [16]. Reasons why healthcare professionals get an increasing number of infections were the following; 1) People who are unaware of the disease and epidemic are transmitted to HCWs who do not have protective clothing when they return to their place of residence, 2) Inadequate protective equipment supply especially for primary HCWs in primary care, and 3) Computed tomography (CT) scan results before COVID-19 case definition criteria are not specified and then it was later seen as sudden changes in the criteria [13, 14].

After the first case reported in Turkey and the Ministry of Health have published the management and treatment algorithm guides. The possible case and the definite case definitions were made by them and HCWs were informed. The use of protective equipment was recommended by the Governments [17, 18]. In the Rize province, which was 1150 km away since the first cases originated from Istanbul, 16 (59.3%) of the HCWs did not have awareness about index cases. The use of surgical masks was widespread among the staff, but the mask use of the patient and accompanying people to patients weremissing, and the highly protective respiratory mask

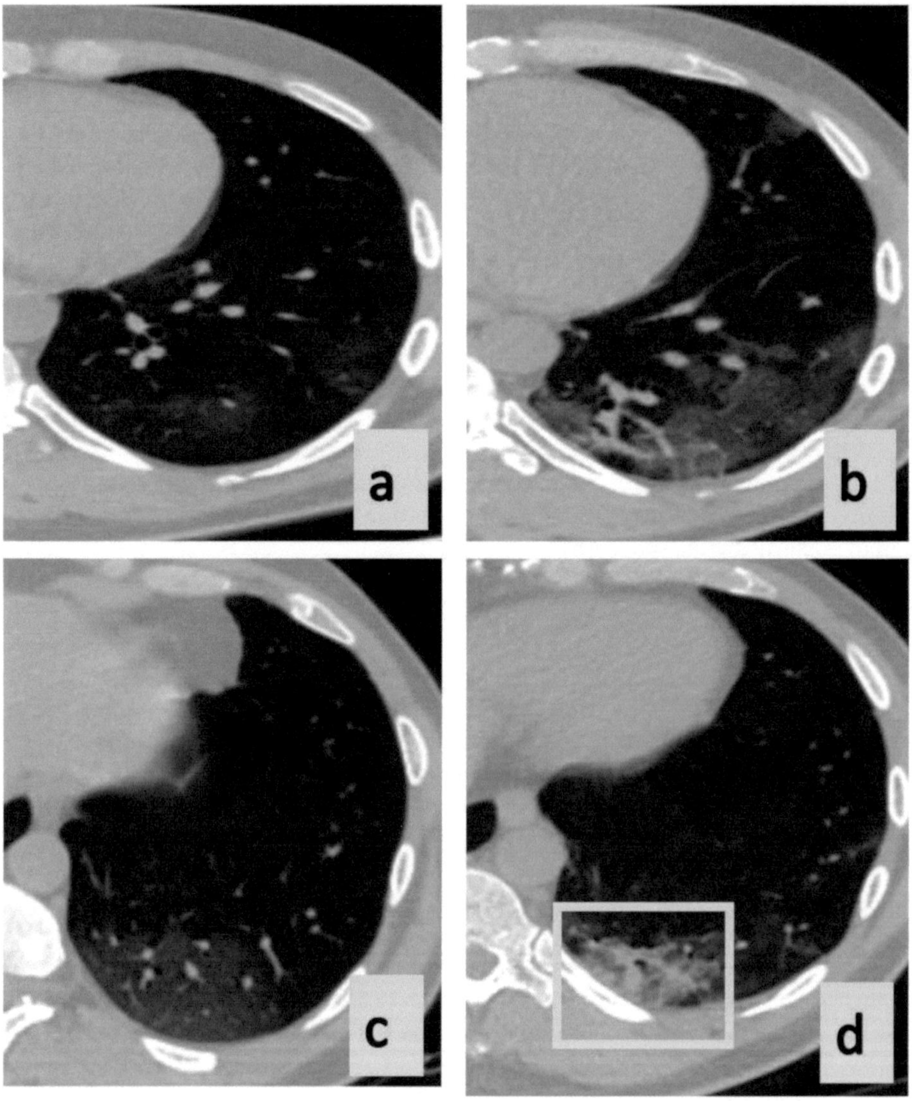

Figure 3.
(a-d) 44 year old male patient, it was noteworthy that in the first examination (a), the GGOs observed in the lower lobe of the left lung expanded in the control examination on iv non-contrasted axial CT images obtained with an interval of 4 days (b). In the control evaluation in the ground glass area (c) located in the left lobe lower lobe posterobasal segment, fibrous bands developed (d).

was used in case of intubation. While 63% of the cases (n = 17) had a mild clinical level, 29.6% (n = 8) were moderate and 7.4% (n = 2) were severe. Index 2 case had comorbidities and died but there was no severe clinical condition such as ARDS or death among the medical staff which were in contact with her.

In our study, the mean age of the total 27 HCW was 33.2 ± 6.9 years. The median age was 39 (IQR: 32–48.5 years) in studies conducted in health workers in China [19] the age ranges of 72 HCWs, 33 of whom were at high-risk Section 39 and general departments were 21–66 years [13]. It was similar to the report showing the age of 41 (IQR: 32–52 years) from Zhejiang province in the first studies [20]. The average age in the local study of Wuhan, the starting place of the outbreak, was 56 (IQR: 42–68 years) [21]. In another study conducted in Wuhan, the average age was 49.0 (IQR 41.0–58.0) [22]. In our study, 63% (n = 17) of the 27 health personnel were

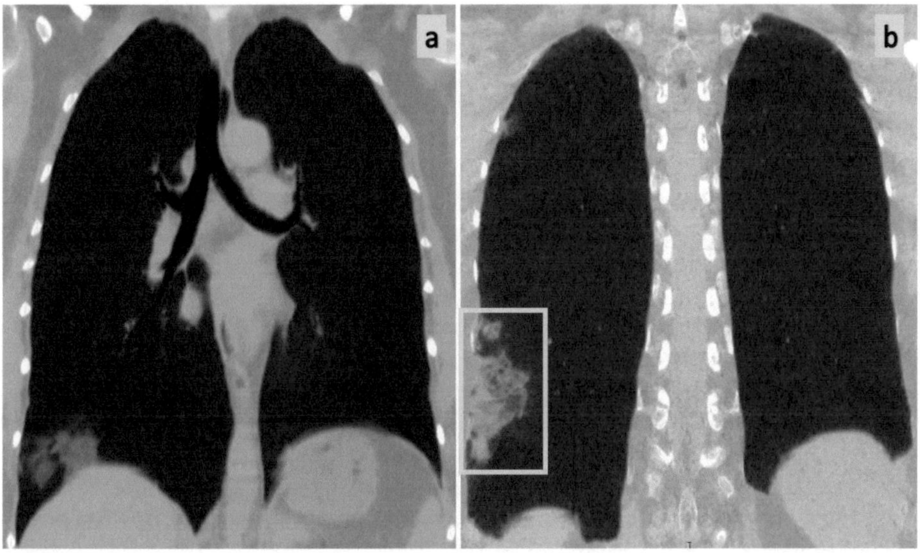

Figure 4.
(a-d) 41 year old female patient, in the CT images of 31.03.2020 (a) and 5.05.2020 (b), the minimum-intensity-projection coronal cross-sectional CT images show different areas of involvement. Right lung lower lobe findings (a) declined in control, but consolidation developed with a reverse halo sign in posterobasal (b).

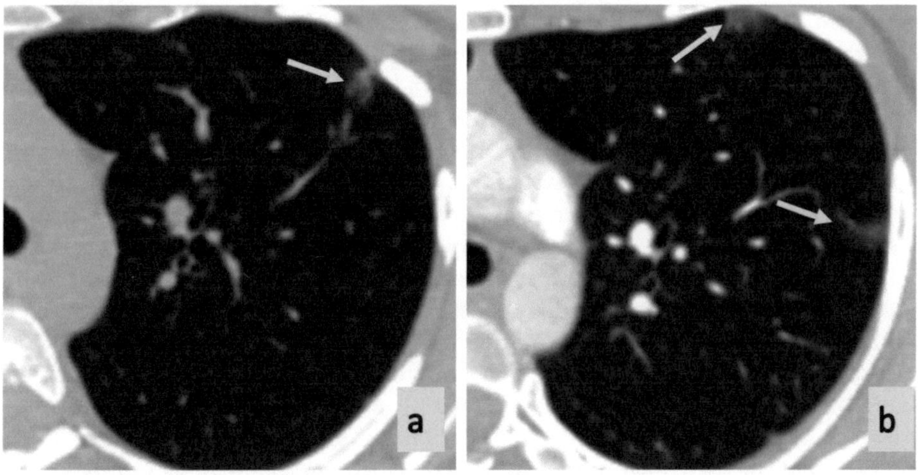

Figure 5.
(a, b) 34-year-old female patient, peripheral small-sized GGOs are observed in the iv non-contrasted axial CT images obtained every 10 days apart (a). The GGOswere diminished but new ground glass areas developed (b).

female and 37% (n = 10) were male and Wang et al. reported that female patients constituted the majority of all cases (61.25%), the male ratio was (38.75%) [19]. Ran et al. showed that the genders were similar ($\chi 2$ = 2.243, p = 0.134) [13]. In other studies conducted in Wuhan, most of the infected patients were men 30/41 (73%), and (54.3%) were male [15, 21], respectively. Most of our HCW cases were high-risk departments workers, such as coronary intensive care. It was found similar to the study conducted in Wuhan [13]. In our study, 51.9% (n = 14) of the infected profession group were female nurses and 13 (76.5%) were among the nurses. It was similar to the work of Wang et al. [19] the ratio as 41/80 (51.25%). In the comparison between doctors in our study, male doctors were found to be significantly higher than female doctors (70% vs. 5.9%, p < .001). It was observed that thorax CT findings were normal in the female gender.

In our study, none of the healthcare professionals had comorbidity. The clinic of 63% (n = 17) of the cases was followed up with outpatient home isolation. Wang D et al., also constituted a significant number of HCWs in the majority of non-intensive care patients (p < .001) [21]. However, having a non-intensive care follow-up suggested that they were clinically mild. In previous studies, it was shown that this infection may cause severe clinical picture in non-comorbid patients, however hypertension, diabetes, cardiovascular, chronic obstructive pulmonary diseases, liver, and kidney failure are risk-causing comorbidities [15, 19–21].

The most common clinical symptoms in our study were present in 55.6% (n = 15) of fever and 40.7% (n = 11) of cough, respectively, less than the signs of fever and cough in previous studies [15, 19–21]. Chinese cases showed more severe clinical. Fever was seen at a relatively low rate in the European studies which were more extensive studies and they included mild to moderate COVID-19 (45.7% and 48%) [23, 24]. The cough was reported at high rates in European studies (63.2 and 80%) [22, 23]. Shortness of breath was present in 14.8% of the cases (n = 4), which was less than the previous study results [15, 21–23]. In our study, the complaint of malaise was present in 44.4% of the cases (n = 12) and myalgia in 33.3% (n = 9), this rate was higher than that of the health workers in Wuhan-China [19] compared to other studies [15, 20–23] was less. The low levels of these findings may be since most of the clinical conditions are good-moderate or the number of cases was limited. According to clinical studies in Asia [15, 19–21], the most common symptoms were fever, cough, shortness of breath, muscle pain, arthralgia, headache, diarrhea. With the spread of COVID-19 in Europe, he emphasized a new atypical presentation of the disease: smell and taste dysfunction [22–27].

In our study, anosmia was detected in 18.5% of the cases (n = 5) and complaints about the sense of taste in 22.2% of the cases (n = 6). Taste and smell tests were not performed, only the presence of symptoms was said by the staff themselves, similar to the previous studies [24]. The rate of anosmia in Europe was shown to be in 201 patients (14.2%) [22]. Even in a more comprehensive study of 2428 patient series, 74% of the 80 subjects tested were positive despite limited access. Cases; only 51% reported their symptoms as cough or fever, while 16% reported it as isolated anosmia as an isolated symptom [25]. Another recent study reported that anosmia was recorded in 73% of patients and the first symptom in 26.6% before the diagnosis of COVID-19 [26]. In the European study (54.2%) there was a taste impairment [22]. In a study of 417 mild to moderate COVID-19 patients in European hospitals, 85.6% and 88.0% of the patients reported smell and taste impairment and a significant relationship between both disorders (p < 0.001) [23]. It has been argued that the reason for sensory loss may be due to neurotropic and neuroinvasive coronaviruses [27]. In our study, headache complaints were found in 37% of the cases (n = 10), and headache rates in female HCWs infected with COVID-19 were found to be significantly higher than men (52.9% vs. 10%, p = .042, Fisher's exact test). All other complaints except for headaches were found in male and female workers at similar rates (p > .05 for all).

While it was 21/62 (34%) (2021) close to our study in Zhejiang provincial, it was lower in studies from Wuhan; The most comprehensive study on 138 patients Wang D et all. Headache was 6.5% in 9 people in total (15, 19–21). But in the more extensive European mild to moderate Coronavirus Disease 2019 study, this rate was much higher. The most common symptom was reported asheadache (70.3%) [22]. Diarrhea, another symptom in our study, was in 22.2% (n = 6) of the cases. In two studies [19, 21] involving health workers in China (80 and 138 cases), it was 18.75% and 10.1%, respectively, in other studies, the rate was reported to be much (3–8%)

less [15, 20]. In European studies, it was 473/1420 (38.1%) [22] and 50% [23]. In our study, vomiting was reported in 14.8% of the cases (n = 4), less in Chinese studies [21, 22], and in European studies at a similar rate [22, 23].

As laboratory parameters; WBC, neutrophil, and lymphocyte levels were normal. However, the decrease in PLT, MPV, hemoglobin levels in the first and last measurements in hospital admission was found significant.

From the place where the outbreak and clinical findings were severe, for instance, Huang C. et al. reported 25% leukopenia and 63% lymphopenia [15]. In the Chinese HCWs study, 19 of 80 patients (23.75%) had leukopenia and 38 (47.5%) had lymphopenia [19]. In the Zhejiang province study, there was leukopenia and 42% lymphopenia at 31% at the time of admission [20]. Wang et al. showed that although the total of 138 patients was within normal limits, white blood cell and neutrophil counts were significantly higher in intensive care patients [21]. In our study, neutrophil/lymphocyte rate (NLR) was normal, as the clinical well-being ratio of HCWs was high. In the study in which they compared mild type and severe-critical patient groups in China, NLR was the most useful prognostic factor affecting prognosis in patients with a severe disease with COVID-19 pneumonia. In the severe group, the blood neutrophil count was higher than in the mild group, the blood lymphocyte count was significantly lower, and the bacterial infection rate increased significantly [28]. When the results of many studies in China were evaluated, high NLR was argued to be an independent prognostic biomarker for COVID-19 patients [29, 30]. Studies were reporting that MPV was elevated during the active period of some viral infection [31, 32]. In our study, it was noteworthy that the HCW was higher than the values of the first measurement MPV levels were higher than that of recovery period measurement (10.0 vs. 9.5; $z = -2.161$, $p = .031$).

In our study, mild elevation was found in two patients with moderate to severe pneumonia signs, and total D-dimer measurements were in the normal range and were similar to some Chinese studies [19, 20], but were high in intensive care patients in China [15, 21, 33]. Tang N et al. [34] showed that abnormal coagulation results, especially markedly elevated D-dimer and fibrin degradation product FDP, are common in deaths with new coronavirus pneumonia NCP (34).PLT levels were within normal limits in all studies, including intensive care patients [15, 19–21, 33]. Lippi G and Plebani M [33], reported that the country where the epidemic spread, increased C-reactive protein (CRP) and lactate dehydrogenase (LDH) in their letters, which summarize abnormal laboratory parameters, which are prognostic biomarkers in studies in most Wuhan studies in China, were shown as negative prognoses. In our study, a significant difference was found between the median value of the first and second CRP (g/dL) levels (2.9 vs. 1). Another significant difference was found between the mean first and second LDH (U/L) levels (91.1 vs. 47.2). A significant difference was found between the mean values of first and second albumin (g/L) levels in our cases (43.8 vs. 44.4). The value of troponin levels in the second measurement was found to be <3.2 in all cases. Although our cases showed clinically good to moderate clinics [34], they were consistent with the study. We found a significant difference between the first and second median CK (U/L) levels (77 vs. 60). A significant difference was found between the first CK-MB (mg/mL) of the cases and the second CK-MB (0.8 vs. 0.5). There was a significant difference between the mean values of the first ferritin (ng/mL) and the second ferritin (151.7 vs. 95).

Computed Tomography (CT) can help in diagnosis and differential diagnosis in patients with COVID-19 [35] and is particularly high when evaluated with serial CT images. RT-PCR provides a chance to catch 93% of negative patients earlier [36] history of contact, clinical findings, and imaging findings were considered more sensitive in the diagnosis of COVID-19 [36]. Typical radiological findings of COVID-19 pneumonia have been reported as interstitial inflammation, ground-glass opacities, crazy paving appearance, and bilateral or multiple lobular or subsegmental widespread consolidation [19–21, 35–37]. In our study, pneumonia findings and CT findings were seen in 7 persons (25.9%) and in 20 subjects (74.1%), there was no CT involvement. The clinical progresses was good in HCWs at the beginning of the outbreak.

While not being aware of the cases initially caused contamination by contact, it may be related to the aerosol contact formed later by intubation. Nevertheless, the timely implementation of protective measures prevented negative consequences. The clinical reflection severity of the contamination was low, the radiological reflection was moderate, and the laboratory reflections were partly significant in HCWs. Acute respiratory distress syndrome (ARDS) was not seen in any healthcare worker.

In conclusion, HCWs are a respected professional group that must be at the forefront of the epidemic and the center of the risk. The risk decreases when the virus load is reduced using PPE. It would be also crucial to ensure that complete PPE, including the electrical air purification device, is fitted, providing a negative pressure isolation ward environment that prevents patients from spreading to the rest of the infectious pathogen.

Declaration of conflict of interest

All authors declare that there is no any type of conflict of interest regarding this study.

Author details

Ayse Erturk[1*], Ugur Kostakoglu[1], Ilknur Esen Yildiz[1], Nur Hursoy[2], Sevda Ozdemir Al[1], Songul Ozyurt[3], Neslihan Ozcelik[3], Hatice Beyazal Polat[4] and Aysegul Copur Cicek[5]

1 Department of Infectious Diseases and Clinical Microbiology, Faculty of Medicine, Recep Tayyip Erdogan University, Rize, Turkey

2 Department of Radiology, Faculty of Medicine, Recep Tayyip Erdogan University, Rize, Turkey

3 Department of Chest Diseases, Faculty of Medicine, Recep Tayyip Erdogan University, Rize, Turkey

4 Department of Internal Medicine, Faculty of Medicine, Recep Tayyip Erdogan University, Rize, Turkey

5 Department of Medical Microbiology, Faculty of Medicine, Recep Tayyip Erdogan University, Rize, Turkey

*Address all correspondence to: ayseace25@gmail.com

References

[1] World Health Organization. Statement on these secondmeeting of the International Health Regulations (2005) Emergency Committee regarding the outbreak of novel coronavirus (SARS-CoV-2), Available from: https://www.who.int/news-room/detail/30-05-2021-

[2] World Health Organization. WHO Director-General's opening remarks at the media briefing on COVID-19 – 11 March 2020. Available from: https://www.who.int/newsroom/commentaries/detail/modes-of-transmission-of-virus-causing-COVID-19-implications-for-ipc-precaution-recommendations

[3] Ferioli M, Cisternino C, Leo V, Pisani L, Palange P, Nava S. Protecting healthcare workers from SARS-CoV-2 infection: practical indications. Eur Respir Rev. 2020 Apr 3;29(155). pii: 200068. doi: 10.1183/16000617.0068-2020.

[4] Information for Healthcare Professionals about Coronavirus (COVID-19) Available from: https://www.cdc.gov/coronavirus/2019-ncov/hcp/infection-control.html

[5] Wang J, Zhou M, Liu F. Reasons for healthcare workers becoming infected with novel coronavirus disease 2019 (COVID-19) in China. J Hosp Infect. 2020 Mar 6. pii: S0195-6701(20)30101-8. doi: 10.1016/j.jhin.2020.03.002.

[6] Chang, Xu H, Rebaza A, Sharma L, Dela Cruz CS. Protecting health-care workers from subclinical coronavirus infection. Lancet Respir Med. 2020 Mar;8(3):e13. doi: 10.1016/S2213-2600(20)30066-7.

[7] Chughtai AA, Seale H, Islam MS, et al. Policies on the use of respiratory protection for hospital health workers to protect from coronavirus disease (COVID-19). Int J Nurs Stud. 2020 Mar 13; 105:103567.

[8] World Health Organization. Available from: https://www.who.int/docs/default-source/coronaviruse/situation-reports/20200312-sitrep-52-COVID-19.pdf?sfvrsn=e2bfc9c0_4

[9] Patel A, Jernigan DB; 2019-nCoV CDC Response Team. Initial Public Health Response and Interim Clinical Guidance for the 2019 Novel Coronavirus Outbreak-United States, December 31, 2019-February 4, 2020. MMWR Morb Mortal Wkly Rep. 2020 Feb 7;69(5):140-146. doi: 10.15585/mmwr.mm6905e1. Available from: https://www.trtworld.com/turkey/turkey-has-lowest-COVID-19-death-rate-in-europe-health-minister-says-35877

[10] Turkey has lowest COVID-19 death rate in Europe, health minister says Available from: https://www.trtworld.com/turkey/turkey-has-lowest-COVID-19-death-rate-in-europe

[11] Infection Control Guidance for Healthcare Professionals about Coronavirus (COVID-19) Available from: https://www.cdc.gov/coronavirus/2019-ncov/hcp/infection-control.html

[12] Wong JEL, Leo YS, Tan CC. COVID-19 in Singapore-Current Experience: Critical Global IssuesThat Require Attention and Action. JAMA. 2020 Feb 20. doi: 10.1001/jama.2020.2467.

[13] Ran L,ChenX,Wang Y, et al. Risk Factors of Healthcare Workers with Corona Virus Disease 2019: A Retrospective Cohort Study in a Designated Hospital of Wuhan in China. Clin Infect Dis. 2020 Mar 17. pii: ciaa287. doi: 10.1093/cid/ciaa287.

[14] Xiang YT, Jin Y, Wang Y, Zhang Q, Zhang L, Cheung T. Tribute to health

workers in China: A group of respectable population during the outbreak of the COVID-19. Int J BiolSci. 2020 Mar 15;16(10):1739-1740. doi: 10.7150/ijbs.45135.eCollection 2020.

[15] Huang C, Wang Y, Li X, Ren L, Zhao J, Hu Y, Zhang L, Fan G, Xu J, Gu X, Cheng Z, Yu T, Xia J, Wei Y, Wu W, Xie X, Yin W, Li H, Liu M, Xiao Y, Gao H, Guo L, Xie J, Wang G, Jiang R, Gao Z, Jin Q, Wang J, Cao B. Clinical features of patients infected with 2019 novel coronavirus in Wuhan, China. Lancet. 2020 Feb 15;395(10223):497-506. doi: 10.1016/S0140-6736(20)30183-5.

[16] The Novel Coronavirus Pneumonia Emergency Response Epidemiology Team. Vital surveillances: the epidemiological characteristics of an outbreak of 2019 novel coronavirus diseases (COVID-19)- China, 2020. 2020: Available from: http://weekly.chinacdc.cn/en/article/id/e53946e2-c6c4-41e9-9a9b-fea8db1a8f51

[17] T.C SağlıkBakanlığıCOVID-19 (SARS-CoV2 enfeksiyonu) rehberiAvailable from: https://www.sanko.edu.tr/wp-content/uploads/2020/03/COVID-19_RehberiV5-25Subat2020-1.pdf

[18] COVID-19 SağlıkPersonelineYönelik SıkçaSorulanSorularAvailable from: https://COVID19bilgi.saglik.gov.tr/tr/sss/saglik-personeli.html

[19] Wang X, Liu W, Zhao J, Lu Y, Wang X, Yu C, Hu S, Shen N, Liu W, Sun Z, Li W. Clinical characteristics of 80 hospitalized frontline medical workers infected with COVID-19 in Wuhan, China. J Hosp Infect. 2020;S0195-6701(20)30194-8. doi:10.1016/j.jhin.2020.04.019

[20] Xu, X. W. et al. Clinical findings in a group of patients infected with the 2019 novel coronavirus (SARS-Cov-2) outside of Wuhan, China: retrospective case series. Bmj 368368, m606, doi:10.1136/bmj.m606 (2020).

[21] Wang D, Hu B, Hu C, Zhu F, Liu X, Zhang J, Wang B, Xiang H, Cheng Z, Xiong Y, Zhao Y, Li Y, Wang X, Peng Z. Clinical Characteristics of 138 Hospitalized Patients With 2019 Novel Coronavirus-Infected Pneumonia in Wuhan, China. JAMA. 2020 Feb 7. doi: 10.1001/jama.2020.1585.

[22] Lechien JR, Chiesa-Estomba CM, Place S, Van Laethem Y, Cabaraux P, Mat Q, Huet K, Plzak J, Horoi M, Hans S, Barillari MR, Cammaroto G, Fakhry N, Martiny D, Ayad T, Jouffe L, Hopkins C, Saussez S; COVID-19 Task Force of YO-IFOS. Clinical and Epidemiological Characteristics of 1,420 European Patients with mild-to-moderate Coronavirus Disease 2019. J Intern Med. 2020 Apr 30. doi: 10.1111/joim.13089.

[23] Lechien JR, Chiesa-Estomba CM, De Siati DR, Horoi M, Le Bon SD, Rodriguez A, Dequanter D, Blecic S, El Afia F, Distinguin L, Chekkoury-Idrissi Y, Hans S, Delgado IL, Calvo-Henriquez C, Lavigne P, Falanga C, Barillari MR, Cammaroto G, Khalife M, Leich P, Souchay C, Rossi C, Journe F, Hsieh J, Edjlali M, Carlier R, Ris L, Lovato A, De Filippis C, Coppee F, Fakhry N, Ayad T, Saussez S. Olfactory and gustatory dysfunctions as a clinical presentation of mild-to-moderate forms of the coronavirus disease (COVID-19): a multicenter European study. Eur Arch Otorhinolaryngol. 2020 Apr 6. doi: 10.1007/s00405-020-05965-1.

[24] Giacomelli A, Pezzati L, Conti F, Bernacchia D, Siano M, Oreni L, Rusconi S, Gervasoni C, Ridolfo AL, Rizzardini G, Antinori S, Galli M. Self-reported olfactory and taste disorders in SARS-CoV-2 patients: a cross-sectional study. Clin Infect Dis. 2020 Mar 26. pii: ciaa330. doi: 10.1093/cid/ciaa330.

[25] Hopkins C, Surda P, Kumar N. Presentation of newonset anosmia during the COVID-19 pandemic. Rhinology. 2020 Apr 11. doi: 10.4193/Rhin20.116.

[26] Kaye R, Chang CWD, Kazahaya K, Brereton J, Denneny JC 3rd. COVID-19 Anosmia Reporting Tool: Initial Findings. Otolaryngol Head Neck Surg. 2020 Apr 28:194599820922992. doi: 10.1177/0194599820922992.

[27] Xydakis MS, Dehgani-Mobaraki P, Holbrook EH, Geisthoff UW, Bauer C, Hautefort C, Herman P, Manley GT, Lyon DM, Hopkins C. Smell and taste dysfunction in patients with COVID-19. Lancet Infect Dis. 2020 Apr 15. pii: S1473-3099(20)30293-0. doi: 10.1016/S1473-3099(20)30293-0.

[28] Liu J, Liu Y, Xiang P, et al. Neutrophil-to-Lymphocyte Ratio Predicts Severe Illness Patients with 2019 Novel Coronavirus in the Early Stage. medRxiv; 2020. DOI: 10.1101/2020.02.10.20021584.

[29] Henry BM, Lippi G, Plebani M. Laboratory abnormalities in children with novel coronavirus disease 2019. Clin Chem Lab Med. 2020 Mar 16. pii:/j/cclm.ahead-of-print/cclm-2020-0272/cclm-2020-0272.xml. doi: 10.1515/cclm-2020-0272.

[30] Ai-Ping Yang, Jianping Liu, Wenqiang Tao, Hui-ming Li The diagnostic and predictive role of NLR, d-NLR and PLR in COVID-19 patients Int Immunopharmacol. 2020 Apr 13: 106504. doi: 10.1016/j.intimp.2020.106504

[31] Akın F, Sert A, Arslan Ş. Mean platelet volume in children with hepatitis A. J Health PopulNutr. 2016;35(1):32

[32] Han X, Xu P, Duan X, Liu Y, Zhang J, Xu H. High mean platelet volume-to-platelet count ratio as a diagnostic maker for increased risk of liver function damage in pediatric patients with infectious mononucleosis in China. Exp Ther Med. 2019 Dec;18(6):4523-4527. doi: 10.3892/etm.2019.8104.

[33] Lippi G, Plebani M. Laboratory abnormalities in patients with COVID-2019 infection. Clin Chem Lab Med. 2020 Mar 3. pii: /j/cclm.ahead-of-print/cclm-2020-0198/cclm-2020-0198.xml. doi: 10.1515/cclm-2020-0198.

[34] Tang N, Li D, Wang X, Sun Z. Abnormal coagulation parameters are associated with poor prognosis in patients with novel coronavirus pneumonia. J ThrombHaemost. 2020 Apr;18(4):844-847. doi: 10.1111/jth.14768.

[35] Pan F, Ye T, Sun P, et al. Time Course of Lung Changes On Chest CT During Recovery From 2019 Novel Coronavirus (COVID-19) Pneumonia. Radiology, 200370, 2020.

[36] Ai T, Yang Z, Hou H, et al. Correlation of Chest CT and RT-PCR Testing in Coronavirus Disease 2019 (COVID-19) in China: A Report of 1014 Cases. Radiology, In Press (2020;xx:xx). https://pubs.rsna.org/doi/full/10.1148/radiol.2020200642

[37] Bernheim A, Mei X, Huang M, Yang Y, Fayad ZA, Zhang N, Diao K, Lin B, Zhu X, Li K, Li S, Shan H, Jacobi A, Chung M. Chest CT Findings in Coronavirus Disease-19 (COVID-19): Relationship to Duration of Infection. Radiology. 2020 Feb 20:200463. doi: 10.1148/radiol.2020200463.

Chapter 5

Coronavirus Disinfection Physical Methods

Moez Guettari and Ahmed El Aferni

Abstract

Since 2019, the spread of the Coronavirus pandemic becomes the global health crisis. To fight the pandemic, several measures were adopted such as: Hygiene measure, massive test, social distancing, quarantine and distancing. Disinfection is an important operation in the fight against the spread of Corona virus pandemic. The disinfection methods are of chemical and physical type. In this work, we focused our interest to the physical methods. These methods are classified in three principal categories: irradiation techniques, heat treatment and mechanical techniques. All the different aspect of techniques are exposed in this chapter. The efficiency of the used techniques is also discussed.

Keywords: Covid-19, disinfection, irradiation, heat treatment, mechanical treatment

1. Introduction

The COVID-19 pandemic is the global health crisis, with 133 991 203 infected persons and 2 903 728 deaths in the world until 09/04/2021 [1]. The virus responsible for the disease is mostly transmitted through aerosols. To fight the pandemic spread, several measures have been adopted such as the disinfection. This operation consists in reducing the number of microorganisms: viruses, bacteria, fungi… Eliminating all microorganisms is called sterilization [2]. Disinfection techniques are classified in two categories: Chemicals and physical types [3–6]. Applying a chemical agents such as acids, Alcohols, Aldehydes,Alkalis, Biguanides, Halogens, Oxidizing agents and Quaternary ammonium compounds, permits to disinfect surfaces and medical devices [4, 6]. Al-Sayah [6] has shown that the used chemical agents have excellent biocidal activity within a short time, easy to use and low toxicity. However, if chemical agents' concentration is high, the medical devices can be damaged and risk toxic effects on the technician [7]. Since 1908, Chick-and Watson have proposed a model to study the kinetics disinfection of water chlorination [8]. This model was refined by taking into account the disinfection process such as dissipating/volatile disinfectant [9–13]. The physical disinfection methods are classified in three categories: **(1)** Mechanical, **(2)** thermal treatment and **(3)** radiation effect [14]. The mechanical treatments include disinfection of surfaces by ultra-sound, plasma treatment and detergent action. Using ionizing or non-ionizing radiation (UV light, X rays, gamma rays, electron beam and heavy metals) is an important technique to disinfect surface. The efficiency of treatment depends on the penetration depth of the radiation; this is due to the wave length [15, 16]. The

IntechOpen

thermal treatment consists of heating or cooling medical devices. In this context, cold plasma was considered as an emergent disinfection technology [16]. Heating infected medical devices by using steam under pressure or autoclave is a routine procedure in health care. In this chapter, we focus our interest on the disinfection physical methods used to fight Coronavirus spread. As we have mentioned previously, in a first step the different disinfection categories are discussed and so their efficiency and limitations are reported.

2. Irradiation techniques

The radiation includes non-ionizing radiation, such as UV rays, infrared rays,... etc. and ionizing radiation, such as α-β particles, neutrino, X-rays, −rays, the two last radiation are considered as indirectly ionizing radiations. The most common irradiation techniques used for killing Corona virus are UVC and -X rays.

2.1 UVC irradiation

2.1.1 The germicide lamps

UV light spectrum is ranged between 400 and 100 nanometers. It can be divided in three categories: UVA (400–315 nm), UVB (315–280 nm) and UVC (280–100 nm). The UV radiations are emitted by the sun, but UVC does not reach the earth's surface due to the ozone layer in the atmosphere. The UVC is known as a powerful radiation to inactivate microbes and virus especially for the wavelength 254 nm. This type of radiation is produced artificially by the so called Germicidal lamps and microbes as it reported by several authors [3, 16–18]. The disinfection efficiency depends on lamp placement, mixing degree of room air, room configuration, lamp age air movement patterns and relative humidity, RH. Considering respectively, N_0 and N, the number of initial micro-organisms at t = 0 s, and at a given time t. According to Kaniho and Ohgaki [17], N and N_0 can be connected by the following Equation [17]:

$$N(t) = N_0 e^{-ZI.t} \tag{1}$$

Where, Z($cm^2/\mu Ws$) and I($\mu W/cm^2$) are respectively the microorganism susceptibility factor and the UVC lamp intensity. Several authors [18, 19], have shown that the susceptibility parameters depends RH, where UVC effectiveness decreases with increasing relative humidity [19]. In practice, the dose received by microorganisms by surface unity is considered to estimate the efficiency of a lamp. In fact the dose, *D*, is calculated according Eq. **(2)**:

$$D = It \tag{2}$$

Where, I ($\mu W/cm^2$) and t(s), are respectively the UVC lamp intensity and the irradiation time. The required dose to inactivate 90% of microorganisms is denoted D90. We report in **Table 1**, required dose, D90, to inactivate bacteria in different conditions and medium (water, surface, air-low RH and air-high RH).

The SARS-CoV-2 inactivation dose corresponds to D90 = 7 J/m^2 [21, 22], its susceptibility is 3 times greater than common cold virus (Influenza). Recently, Heilingloh et al. [23] have shown that the UVC required dose for complete inactivation of a high infected sample after 9 min of irradiation corresponds to 10,48 J/m^2. The sample was at a distance 3 cm of the UVC source.

D90(J/m²)				
Bacteria	**Water**	**Surface**	**Air-Low RH**	**Air-High RH**
Bacillus subtilis spores	131	88	95	89
Eschenchia coli	26	22	5	11
Mecobacterium bovis BCG	—	22	13	33

Table 1.
The required D90 values of some bacteria in different conditions and medium [20].

2.1.2 The Corona-virus inactivation process

UV-C (254 nm) is the most effective germicidal region of the UV spectrum. In fact, the UVC light is absorbed by DNA and RNA, causing photochemical damage and fusion of pyrimidines. The pyrimidine dimmers interrupt transcription and replication of RNA and DNA and so inactivate the virus [24]. The different devices using UVC technique revolve around the disinfection unit type, where complementary devices are used to ensure maximum efficiency. Certain devices can be mobile or ordered. The device types are discussed in the next sections.

2.1.3 UVC devices

2.1.3.1 Conventional lamps and UVC-LEDs

The UVC radiation is generated by artificial sources, which we called disinfection unity. It includes lamps and UVC-Lamps. The lamps contain a gas, mercury or xenon, or a mixture of gases such as xenon-mercury (in small quantity), however UVC-LEDs are manufactured from semiconductors [25, 26]. The UVC-LEDs are an alternative to conventional lamps due to their compact size and energy saving. However, their cost is relatively high, light emitting (UVC-LEDs can be continuous or pulsed.Several authors have reported that pulsed UVC-LEDs are more effective then continuous and conventional lamps [27–29].

2.1.3.2 Reflective wall and humidifiers

To enhance the inactivation virus effectiveness, reflective wall and humidifiers are used as complementary devices. In fact, several authors [27–32], have shown that using reflective walls reduce the inactivation microorganism's time. On the other hand, Woo et al. [33], have shown that using deionized water as humidifier enhance the disinfection effectiveness.

2.1.3.3 Chemical disinfectant

Usually, disinfectant devices are combined with chemical disinfectants and were used to inactivate microorganisms in hospitals. Usual lamps and/or UVC-LEDs were used with gaseous ozone and hydrogen peroxide vapor. Several authors [34, 35], have shown that using chemical agents, such as hydrogen peroxide vapor, in addition to conventional UVC treatment permit more effective disinfection.

2.1.3.4 Mobile and automated UVC devices

Disinfecting robot is an emerging technology used to fight against the spread of Covid-19 in public transport, hospitals and any closed areas. However, it requires a mastery of mechanics, electronics and programming. In fact, the mobile UVC device, Tru-D, has been shown to be more efficient than the static device and inactivate microorganisms within a period between three and four hours [36]. It was also shown that the used robot is quicker than chemical agents such as hydrogen peroxide. In this context, Bentancor and Vidal [37], have used a programmed device to communicate with the robot using Bluetooth devices and can be operated thanks to a mobile application. Recently, Guettari et al. [38] have shown that mobile robots are the most efficient device to inactivate microorganisms and developed an i-Robot UVC, this robot is essentially composed with two lamps on the top. Several sensors are integrated to measure physical parameters such as temperature and humidity to control the mobility of the robot to detect motion and to avoid obstacles. The disinfection time is monitored by Wi-Fi.

2.1.3.5 Advantages and limitations

Using UVC (200-280 nm) radiation has been successful in inactivating various viruses. This physical technique is non-toxic, non-corrosive to medical devices and environmentally friendly, it does not have to be portable. The disinfection time is reduced when complementary devices are used. However, this type of radiation is not highly penetrating and it may be ineffective of masks. Handling this type of radiation presents a significant danger for the human health. Primary skin cancers can manifested after a long period. So, the ICNIRP have reported the limit values for exposure to this kind of radiation [39].

2.2 Gamma rays irradiation

2.2.1 Virus inactivation

When Cobalt 59, the natural state of Cobalt, is bombarded with neutrons, it produces a synthetic radioactive isotope of Cobalt-60, which decays by beta disintegration to the stable Nickel-60. The gamma emission obeys the following Equation [40]:

$$^{59}_{27}Co + n \rightarrow {}^{60}_{27}Co \rightarrow {}^{60}_{28}Ni + e^{-} + gamma.irradiation \qquad (3)$$

The Gamma irradiation emitted by Cobalt 60 was performed sterilization in food science and to develop vaccine [41]. In fact, the treatment consists to irradiate products until 50 kGy and it known as bio-security of food. The required doses depend on the nature of microorganisms (bacteria, virus, pathogens and parasites).

Family virus	Virus structure	Presence of envelop	Diameter (nm)	D90	
				Minimum	Maximum
Adenoviridae	Double stranded-DNA	No	70-90	3.5	5.61
Birnaviridae	Double stranded-RNA	No	60	6.2	10
Coronovirdae	Single stranded-RNA	Yes	120-160	<2	3.6
Flaviviriadae	Single stranded-RNA	Yes	40-60	1.8	8.6

Table 2.
The required D90 (maximum and minimum) values of some virus and their properties [42].

The required dose to inactivate 90% of microorganisms depends on environmental factors such as water content, media and temperature. The process of inactivation consists to induce damage in intercellular acids as a physicochemical damage in a single-strand break or double-strand break. Two processes can damage the DNA: **(1)** direct energy deposition;**(2)** secondary interactions with surrounding water molecules which permitting the formation of OH^- free radicals. The irradiation susceptibility of virus is lower than other microorganisms; this is due to their low dimension. The estimated dose D90 (minimum and maximum) to inactivate various virus was reported in **Table 2**. The structure, size and the presence of envelop was also indicated.

2.2.1.1 The target theory

The inactivation of viruses by irradiation is perfectly described by the target theory. In fact, the hit probability P for N targets to be hit n times by radiation is described according the following equation:

$$P = \left[1 - e^{-\nu D}\sum_{k=0}^{n-1}\frac{(\nu D)^k}{k!}\right]^N \tag{4}$$

Where D and, ν are respectively, the radiation dose and the target volume. The single-hit-single-target model corresponds to one targets, n = 1, and to be high one time by radiation, n = 1. So, the hit probability is reduced to Eq. **(5)**.

$$P = 1 - e^{-\nu D} \tag{5}$$

The quantity, νD is connected to the fluence, F(particles/cm^2), and the inactivation cross section, $\sigma(cm^2)$, according the following Equation [41]:

$$\nu D = FD \tag{6}$$

2.2.1.2 Corona virus inactivation by gamma irradiation

In a recent work, Feldmann et al. [43], have studied the effect of gamma irradiation on infected tissues with Coronavirus. They have used doses ranged between 10 kGy and 40 kGy and found that the virus was completely inactivated at 10 kGy and recommend a 20 kGy dose. Several authors [44–46], have studied the disinfection of N-95 masks. These masks are designed to filter 95% of particles of size 0.3 μm. However, in this doses range (10 kGy-20 kGy), radiation can damage the masks tissues because of the cross linking and/or scissioning polymer [47]. It was shown also that the inactivation of Coronavirus depends on the infected medium, which can reduce the required D90 doses to 0.5 kGy [48].

2.2.1.3 Advantages and limitations

Gamma ray irradiation produce uniform dose and can travel through the surface due to their highly penetration depth. The technique does not induce an increasing of temperature; the disinfection time is about few minutes in maximum. However, gamma radiation requires an adequate and expansive device. This method can damage medical devices.

3. Heat treatment

3.1 Heat treatment as major method for SARS-CoV-2inactivation

Since the onset of the Covid-19 pandemic, the influence of temperature has been the subject of intensive discussion among epidemiologists about its influence on the dynamics of the spread of the virus on the one hand and its inactivation on the other hand. Such a debate seemed obvious given that heating has long been considered as the acquired effects of this thermodynamic parameter as well as on the physico-chemical properties of biological macromolecules (proteins, enzymes, etc.) and microorganisms (viruses, parasites). From this point of view, the change in temperature could induce changes of conformational nature, the destruction (and formation) of chemical bonds, changes in physical phases which result in variations of a functional nature. Moreover, virologists have raised questions about the ability of high temperatures to destroy chemical bonds within the SARS-CoV-2 virus and to cause morphological variations in order to be able to inactivate its functions or reduce its virulence. Several works has been conducted in this regard to highlight how heating can help combat the Covid-19 pandemic. In this section we present the most uplifting among them [49–53].

3.2 Heating to inactivate the virus

From the first months of the pandemic, typical studies were carried out to observe the direct impact of an increase in temperature on the stability of SARS-CoV-2. They revealed that SARS-CoV-2 keeps its stability for 24 hours at a temperature of 37° C, On the other hand, heating up to 56° C for 30 minutes succeeded in inactivating the virus. However, such process preserved the stability of viral RNA in both human sera and sputum samples.

Te Faye and his collaborators [54] published a work in which they introduced a predictive thermodynamic model, based on the rate of a first order reaction and Arrhenius law. This model makes it possible to correlate data related to contamination and disinfection using heating. Their results provided very relevant information to help on the disinfection of protective equipment such as masks. For example, they have shown that exposing N95-type masks for 3 minutes can reduce the viral load of SARS-CoV-2 by almost 99%.

Batejat et al. [49] subjected cells infected with SARS-CoV-2 to 3 different temperatures and varying the heating time from 30 seconds to 60 minutes. They observed that SARS-CoV-2 could be inactivated in less than 30 minutes, 15 minutes and 3 minutes at 56° C, 65° C and 95° C respectively.

3.3 Thermal inactivation improves RNA quality

Based on what we quoted in the previous section on the heating power to inactivate the SARS-CoV-2, it seems evident that several laboratories would uses heating to reduce the risk of catching up with the virus.

Since virologists analyze the existence of viruses by conventional PCR and RT-PCR tests, a polymerase technique based on the extraction of virus RNA. So, to get the best results from PCR test, it is essential to have the virus RNA of better quality. In this context, questions were raised about the effect of heating on the quality of results obtained. Hemati et al. [50] exposed 36 samples from COVID - 19 patients to thermal inactivation (60° C for 30 min). The results were surprising and very satisfactory. In fact, heating increased significantly the concentration of the extracted RNAs.

3.4 The use of microwave for hospital disinfection

Another problem that raises concern in relation to combating the harmful effects of Covid 19 lies in the level of waste treatment, especially hospital waste of all kinds (medicine excretion, active component of drugs and metabolite, chemicals, residues of pharmaceuticals,,). It is also known that an important part of this waste is discharged into hospital wastewater, so the problem of disinfecting this water is an important challenge. For this, Wang et al. [51] have suggested several physical disinfection technologies of hospital wastes and wastewater to mitigate the virus spread in China. Among them, they used microwaves of frequencies between (2,450 $\pm$ 50) MHz and (915 $\pm$ 25) MHz in order to reach temperature of disinfection. Indeed, the heat of disinfection is generated by molecular vibrations in the medium traversed by the microwaves.

According to Ohtsu et al. [52], Microwave disinfection technology is an energy efficient technique, in which heat loss is relatively slow, fast acting. It is also characterized by its low environmental pollution since there will be no residues and toxic products left after disinfection.

3.5 Solar heating to inactivate the SARS-CoV-2

Wang et al. [53] have proposed a simple, economic and ecological technique, which makes it possible to disinfect places with very high population density in which social distance is practically inapplicable, namely, cars, busses and other means of public transport (**Figure 1**).

The technique called "Solar heating for the deactivation of heat-sensitive pathogens", it is based on a simple direct exposure of cars to the sun heat for a few minutes during which the air temperature rises from 30°C to temperatures ranged between 50°C and 60°C. Wang and his coworkers [53] have assumed that this simple technique has already proven its effectiveness in in agronomy to kill weeds and soil pathogens. So, therefore it can be applied in the fight against covid-19 as a method of surfaces decontamination. The reported results of Wang et al. confirmed that hot air passively generated by Solar heating in enclosed spaces is an effective disinfection method with benefits without additional costs and chemicals. However, the disadvantage of this method is its dependence to hot climates. For this

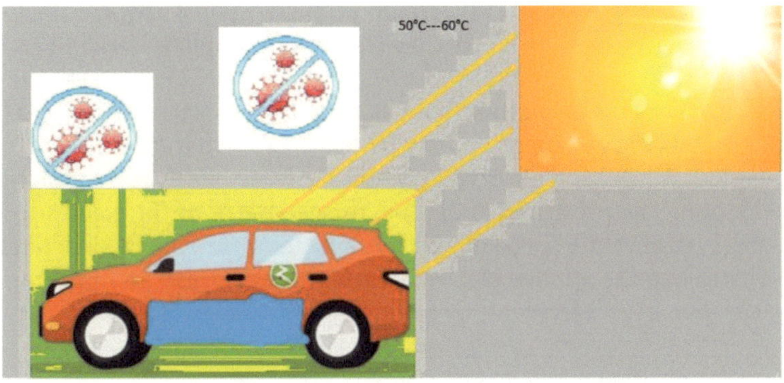

Figure 1.
Schematic representation of car exposed to solar heat.

reason, they assumed that the use of heaters in parking places could be a solution to overcome this handicap.

3.6 Dry heat for masks disinfection

Faced with the shortage of means of protection against covid-19 namely protective masks, Rubio-Romero published a paper review [55] in which he discussed the characteristics of the different types of disposable masks, considered as an alternative. To do this, he detailed the various methods of disinfection, in particular the physical methods of disinfection of deposited masks. Among these methods, he focused on dry heat disinfection. From this perspective, the main challenge was to guarantee total disinfection of the masks at temperatures over 56°C without affecting their filtering capacity. Based on this, both the Spanish Ministry of Labor and Social Economy and the International Medical Center of Beijing indicate that FFP respirators maintain their filtration efficiency after being disinfected at 70° C for 30 min.

3.7 Use of cold plasma for SARS-CoV-2 inactivation

Plasma is formed when a gas is subjected to a potential difference high enough to ionize molecules. As a result, the main properties of a plasma (electrical conductivity, etc.) depend essentially on the density of electrons but also on their volume fraction. The latter is directly influenced by temperature. Typically, the best known of plasmas is that of nuclear reactions, which is subjected to high temperatures of up to K. For this reason, plasma at ambient temperatures is called cold plasma or non-thermal plasma. At this temperature scale, cold plasma does find several industrial applications.

Cold plasma can be generated by applications of voltages ranging from 100 V up to a few kilovolts in direct current, and for radio frequencies in alternating current. In addition, this can only occur under very specific pressure conditions (a pressure between 1 Pa and 10^5 Pa).

3.7.1 Cold plasma as a disinfection technology

For years, cold plasma has been used to decontaminate and disinfect surfaces of steel, plastics, textiles ... It is also used to decontaminate some liquids and also air.

The disinfection technique is often known as «One Atmosphere Uniform Glow Discharge Plasma (OAUGDP)". The advantage of this technique is that it provides both uniform and low power density, which protects against any kind of damage to contaminated surfaces. This property gives it a strong implication in the medical field [56].

Several factors are involved in influencing the effectiveness of cold plasma disinfection. In this regard, mention may be made of the nature of the reactive species provided; it has been observed [57] that the use of oxygen species can support oxidation. The pressure conditions, the geometry of the electrodes ... It has also been observed that the speed of reactive species improves the inactivation of microbes. Increasing the applied electrical difference can play an important role in increasing the density of electrons, or even reactive species (**Figure 2**).

3.7.2 Mode of inactivation of microorganisms by OAUGDP

The mechanism of action of plasma on microorganisms is based on two simultaneous effects. The first effect is a thermal effect, which causes volatilization of cell

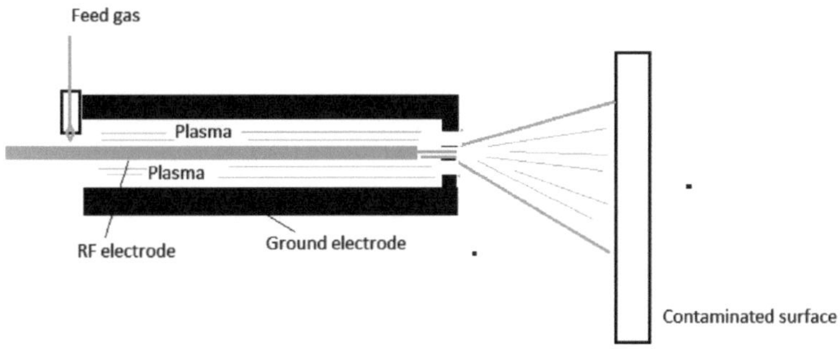

Figure 2.
The atmospheric pressure plasma jet (APPJ) as designed by Hermann et al. [57].

membranes due to its exposure to plasma gas. This facilitates the exchange of proteins between the intracellular and extracellular media. The second effect is the result of the decomposition of organic and inorganic compounds by reactive species from plasma such as ozone, hydroxyl groups, nitric oxides ... [56].

3.7.3 Application of cold plasma in the fight against Covid-19 pandemic

First, many researchers have considered using cold plasma to enhance surface decontamination procedures. All of them have been based on their power of microbial decontamination of materials, surfaces proven for a very long time. As example,Bekeschus et al. published a paper [58] recommending the use of cold plasma in the disinfection of contaminated surfaces, liquids... They do, however, advise caution when using it on human tissues in order to minimize its negative effects on the body. Indeed, it is known that the viral load of SARS-CoV-2 is channeled initially from the mouth then the throat before reaching the lungs. Given that the plasma generates the formation of ozone (O3) and nitrogen oxide (NOx). These two gases are essential for the inactivation of pathogens, but they are toxic to the lungs if they accumulate in high quantities. Therefore, it was necessary to be careful about the triggering of toxicological reactions produced by the gas in the plasma.

Otherwise, since SARS-CoV-2 has shown its ability to stabilize for hours on different types of surfaces such as metals, plastics and cardboard. This paralyzes the efforts to destroy transmission chains. For this purpose, Chen and his coworkers [59] at the University of California have reported excellent results on their work conducted on the inactivation of coronavirus Sars-Cov-2 using cold atmospheric plasma by targeting surfaces of leather, plastics and some metals.. They used an atmospheric plasma gas fed with argon. The characteristics of the atmospheric pressure plasma Jet (APPJ) (**Figure 2**) device used are as follows:

- An input power of approximately 12 W.
- The flow rates for the argon (Ar) and helium (He) plasmas were 6.4 l / min and 16.5 l / min, respectively.
- The discharge voltages for (Ar) and (He) feed gases were 16.8 kV and 16.6 kV.

Thus, they exposed surfaces contaminated by SARS-CoV-2 to cold argon and helium gases. Then compared to surfaces not exposed to gases [59]. The findings were so promising: they observed that the treatment with argon gas inactivated all the viruses for the different surfaces within a period of less than 180 seconds.

4. Ultrasound technology: a promising alternative for decontamination

Since its appearance, SARS-CoV-2 has gained a consensus among virologists on its very specific properties in relation to its high capacity for mutation and its speed of propagation. As a result, scientists have always sought to improve the efficiency of methods of disinfecting surfaces in order to decontaminate them from suspensions carrying the virus. From this perspective, ultrasound can represent an effective physical method. Indeed, the mechanical action of ultrasound on the suspensions of contaminated surfaces will be able to clean them while avoiding the side effects and dangers associated with the use of disinfection chemicals.

4.1 Principle of ultrasonic disinfection

Widely used in the medical field, Ultrasounds are mechanical sound waves, which translate the propagation of acoustic energy in the form of pressure waves. Their frequency range exceeds that of the frequencies of audible sound waves (above 16 kHz). The acoustic intensity I represents the flow of the acoustic power Ps through a surface A. Considering that the pressure amplitude is denoted by "*p*", the different parameters characterizing the propagation of an ultrasonic one are linked by the equation:

$$I = \frac{P_s}{A} = \frac{p^2}{\rho c} = \frac{p^2}{Z} \tag{7}$$

Where ρ is the density of the medium, ε is the amplitude of the ultrasound, ω is the angular speed (ω = 2πf where f is the frequency), is the speed of sound. The equation can be reduced to the following form:

$$I = \varepsilon^2 \omega^2 Z \tag{8}$$

With Z is the acoustic impedance defined by the product ρ × c. During their propagation through different interfaces (air / water for example), ultrasound can undergo either reflections, attenuations or even diffusions. An attenuation coefficient is thus introduced to describe the effect of this passage on the characteristics of the wave transmitted by an interface. For example, for ultrasounds of frequency 20 kHz, the coefficient of their attenuation through a distance of 24 cm is equal to 2. 10^7 cm^{-1}. since the difference in impedance is very slight between water and biological cells (approximately 5%), the transmission of ultrasound through biological cells is fluid. This perfectly explains their great use in diagnostic and therapeutic ultrasound [60].

4.2 Uses of ultrasound in wastewater disinfection

First, ultrasound was used to disinfect wastewater. The process of ultrasonic disinfection mainly relies on cavitation. Indeed, cavitation is a kind of concentration of energy in well-localized areas in a fluid. This cavitation leads to the creation of very extreme physical conditions (temperatures between 1726.85°C and 4726.85°C, pressures between 1800 atm and 3000 atm) [60]. These conditions cause the appearance of effects directly related to disinfection.

The first is a sonochemical effect which results in the destruction of chemical bonds in water. Thus, several types of free radicals are formed. The second effect is the sonoluminescence effect, which characterizes the emission of photons by excitation of gases.

When the collapse of the water bubbles is produced in the vicinity of a solid surface, a jet of particles will be emitted with a high velocity (up to 300 m / S), thus causing very strong mechanical effects such as the wave acoustic shock, sound emission... damage to this surface by these different physical effects contributes to disinfection [61]. According to Gibson et al. [60], the contribution of sonoluminescence and sonochemical effects to disinfection is very negligible in comparison with the mechanical and thermal effects.

4.3 Factors influencing droplet cavitation

Knowing that wastewater contains many types of particles, their interactions with ultrasound do not occur in the same way. Which can alter the cavitation process. For this, several factors must be taken into consideration. The most important of these is the nucleation of the droplets. This nucleation can be affected by the surface tension of liquid S. In fact, in a vapor pressure liquid, the critical pressure necessary to increase the bubble radius of radius R is expressed by the following equation:

$$P_{cr} = P_v - 2\frac{S}{R} \tag{9}$$

Moreover, for a droplet deposited on a liquid surface, the surface tension also depends on the contact angle of this droplet with the surface, which generally varies between 0 (hydrophobic substances) and 180° (hydrophilic substances):

$$P_{cr} = P_v - 2\frac{S\sin\theta}{R} \tag{10}$$

From an energetic point of view, the cavitation process can be altered by failure in one of the energy conversion steps. According to Löning et al. [62], the energy conversion process follows the following Scheme:

$$E_{EL} \rightarrow E_{HF} \rightarrow E_{TH} \rightarrow E_{CAV} \rightarrow E_{DOS} \rightarrow E_{EFF}$$

Where E_{EL} is the input of electrical energy, E_{HF} is the energy of ultrasound, E_{TH} is the power of input into the fluid, E_{CAV} is the energy of droplet cavitation, E_{DOS} is the energy determined by dosimetry, and E_{EFF} is the energy expended on a specific effect.

4.4 Mechanical effects of ultrasound

Gibson et al. [60] have summarized the main conclusions in relation to the mechanical effects of ultrasound in the form of a few points:

- Droplet disturbance is more noticeable at low ultrasound frequencies.
- Ultrasound has the ability to degrade polymer chains (lipids, proteins, etc.), especially for high molecular masses.
- The mechanical action of ultrasound can lead to cell lysis.

4.5 Surfactants (detergents) as main actors for disinfection

From a structural standpoint, the SARS-CoV-2 virus is made up of a viral wall layer that is composed of a lipoprotein envelope that wraps RNA in its interior (**Figure 3**).

To kill the virus, material is required to damage the inside of the envelope. It cannot be destroyed only by water, and therefore needs another ingredient: alcohol or surfactant as proposed by WHO [63].

Surfactants are amphiphilic molecules, composed of a polar part (hydrophilic) and another non polar part (hydrophobic) (**Figure 4**).

The hydrophilic–lipophilic balance (HLB) was introduced to measure the predominance of each of these two characters. According to Davies et al. [65, 66], its value can be determined from the following relation:

$$HLB = \sum \text{hydrophilic groups} - \sum \text{hydrophobic groups} + 7 \tag{11}$$

This chemical structure gives surfactants a double affinity, sometimes to polar compounds and sometimes to nonpolar compounds (**Figure 5**). From a physical point of view, surfactants act as agents to attenuate the surface tension between two immiscible phases, promoting the dispersion of one into the other.

Generally, surfactant molecules are classified according to the properties of their polar part, two main families are distinguished:

- Ionic surfactants: anionic and cationic.
- Nonionic surfactants: amphoteric and dipolar.

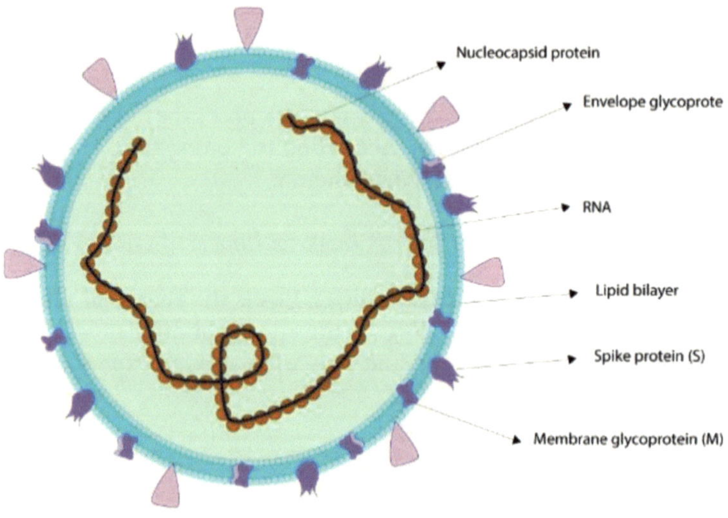

Figure 3.
Structure of the coronavirus (Sars-CoV2) [63].

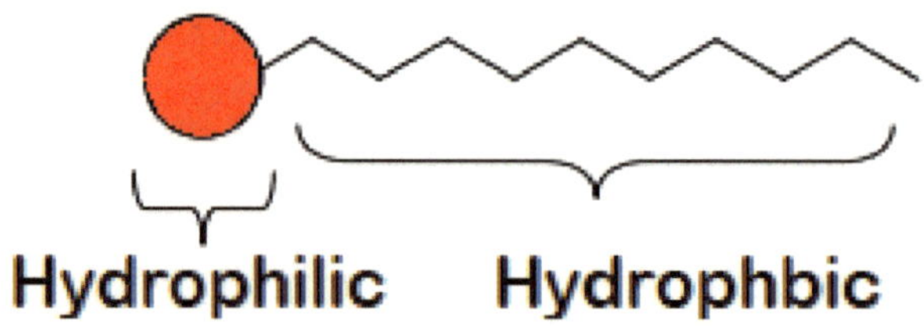

Figure 4.
Chemical structure of surfactant molecules.

A surfactant's detergency strength measures its ability to work on the soil to remove it. Every type of soil, whether fatty, solid, etc., can actually build physical connections with surfactant molecules. These interactions can be either hydrophilic (or else hydrophobic) interactions, or attractive electrostatic interactions. As a result, the detergency mechanism operates according to the different types of loads of dirt on one side and surfactant on the other side. Positive surfactants attract negatively charged soils, which they will partially neutralize. The positive part of the surfactant therefore binds to the negative part of the soil. A positively charged surfactant is interested in negatively charged soils. However, an agent (+) will not have any influence on a soiling (+) since both repel each other [67].

For long time, the soap is known for its very powerful detergent power. For this, since the Covid-19 emergence, the world health organization (WHO) recommended firstly to use it as first weapon against the virus by washing hands several times along the day. Other detergents, such as laundry detergents, are made in synthetics but they are all molecular in the same kind.

Soap is composed of fats, oils, and fatty acids. A hydrophilic polar head and a hydrophobic carbon chain, which have an affinity to organic compounds and consequently to fatty substances, constitute the molecular structure of soap.

When the soap molecules are added to the water, the hydrophobic tails orient towards the air to avoid contact with the water molecules. To bring them into

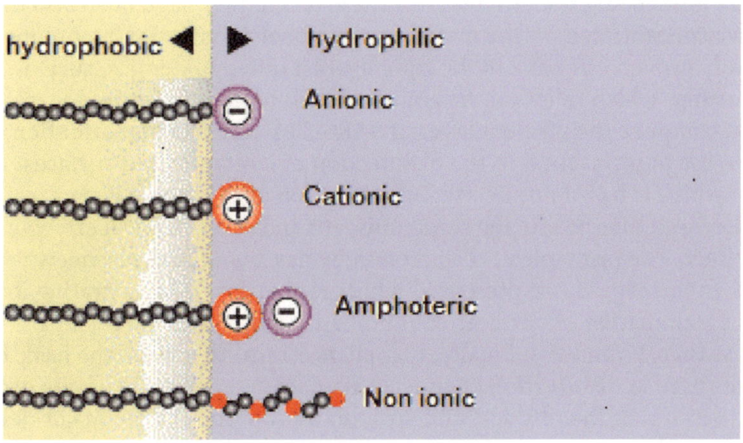

Figure 5.
Classes of surfactant molecules.

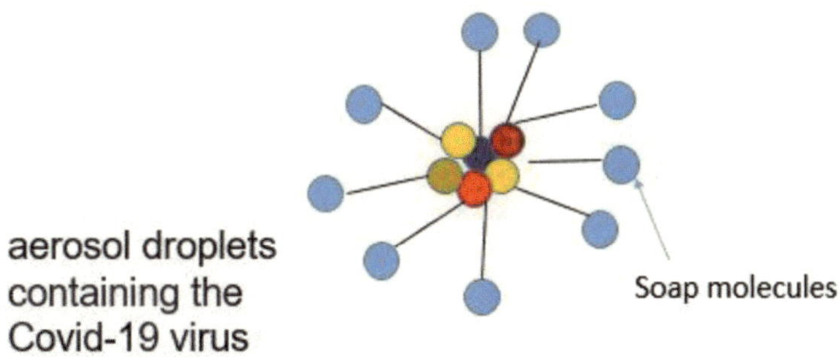

Figure 6.
Soap action on aerosol droplets containing SARS-CoV-2.

contact with the fatty compounds, mechanical action is necessary, in particular rubbing. Once in contact with the fats, the soap molecules surround it on all sides, thus forming spherical micelles (**Figure 6**). In order to decontaminate surfaces containing aerosols carrying SARS-CoV-2. A large concentration of soap molecules must be spread by rubbing the entire surface.

5. Conclusion

In the fight against a new virological epidemic, the most traditional approach is immune system development, which gives the immune system the ability to identify and attack the virus once it has entered the body. This can only be accomplished by manufacturing vaccines. However, waiting for the vaccine to be produced may cost us the lives of millions of people in a pandemic characterized by a very large spread rate such as covid-19. The use of disinfection methods (along with barrier precautions) remains the most promising way to combat this pandemic.

In this context, we have presented in this chapter the main physical methods used to disinfect contaminated surfaces. Initially, special emphasis was placed on methods based on electromagnetic irradiations, specifically ultraviolet UV radiation and gamma radiation. The required doses, capable of inactivating the virus and used in the production of disinfection devices such as UVC lamps, were presented. The parameters influencing the efficiency of these techniques have been also discussed. Second, we concentrated on the use of conventional disinfection techniques that have already proven effective in the fight against other epidemics, such as disinfection by heating, which relies on the ability of high temperatures to destroy the lipid bonds that comprise the virulent layer of SARS-CoV-2. Particular attention has been paid to the use of ultrasound in the disinfection of contaminated surfaces, this technique which is based on the mechanical action of ultrasonic waves manifested by cavitation and thus producing sonolumiscent and sonochemical effects and also a thermal effect. The principle of disinfection by gas jets of cold plasma was then described. In this regard, we presented bibliographic data demonstrating its efficacy in the decontamination of surfaces contaminated with SARS-CoV-2 in a short period (less than 2 minutes). Finally, it appears critical to discuss the basic chemical compounds used in disinfection chemicals, namely detergents. We have dedicated a section to describing the physical and structural properties of the major detergents.

We believe that, in the absence of an effective medical treatment, the bibliographical review study on various disinfection procedures represents, at this time, the best kits for both medical personnel and policymakers in the fight against this new pandemic.

Acknowledgements

The authors gratefully acknowledge financial support from the Tunisian Ministry of Education, Research, and Technology.

Conflict of interest

The authors declare that they have no known competing financial interests or personal relationships that could have appeared to influence the work reported in this paper.

Author details

Moez Guettari* and Ahmed El Aferni
Materials and Fluids Laboratory, Preparatory Institute for Engineering studies of Tunis, University of Tunis, Tunisia

*Address all correspondence to: gtarimoez@yahoo.fr

References

[1] COVID-19 Dashboard by the Center for Systems Science and Engineering (CSSE) at Johns Hopkins University (JHU) (2020). https://coronavirus.jhu.edu/map.html.

[2] Developments in Aquaculture and Fisheries Science Volume. 2002. 33, Pages 183-192 https://doi.org/10.1016/S0167-9309(02)80013-8

[3] Otto C, Zahn S, Rost F, Zahn P, Jaros D, Rohm H. Physical Methods for Cleaning and Disinfection of Surfaces. Food Eng Rev, 2011; 3:171-188. DOI: 10.1007/s12393-011-9038-4

[4] Darnella M E R, Subbaraob K, Feinstonea S M, Taylora D R. Inactivation of the coronavirus that induces severe acute respiratory syndrome, SARS-CoV. J Virol Methods, 2004; 121:85–91. doi:10.1016/j.jviromet.2004.06.006

[5] Mojarad N, Khalili Z, Aalaei S (2017) A Comparison of the efficacy of mechanical, chemical, and microwave radiation methods in disinfecting complete dentures. Dent Res J (Isfahan); 2017; 14: 131–136

[6] Al-Sayah MH. Chemical disinfectants of COVID-19: An overview. J Water Health. (2020) 18:843–848. https://doi.org/10.2166/wh.2020.108

[7] https://www.gov.nu.ca/sites/default/files/files/15_%20Reprocessing%20of%20Medical%20Equipment%20-%20March%205%20-%20low%20res(1).pdf

[8] Chick H. An investigation of the laws of disinfection. J Hyg. 1908; 8: 092-158.

[9] Hom LW. Kinetics of Chlorine Disinfection in an Ecosystem. J SanitEngDivAsce, 1970;98:183-194

[10] HomLWKinetics of chlorine disinfection in an ecosystem.J SanitEngDivAsce. 1972. 98: 183-194

[11] Lambert RJW and Johnston MD. Disinfection kinetics: a new hypothesis and model for the tailing of log-survivor/time curves, J ApplMicrobiol. 2000; 88: 907-913.

[12] Prokop A, and Humphrey AE. Kinetics of Disinfection. Disinfection ed. New York. (1970)

[13] MichaPeleg. Applied Microbiology and Biotechnology. 2021; 105:539–549. https://doi.org/10.1007/s00253-020-11042-8

[14] Otto C, Zahn S, Rost F, et al. Physical Methods for Cleaning and Disinfection of Surfaces. Food Eng Rev. 2011. 3:171–188. https://doi.org/10.1007/s12393-011-9038-4

[15] Akikazu Sakudo, Yoshihito Yagyu, and Takashi Onodera· Disinfection and Sterilization Using Plasma Technology: Fundamentals and Future Perspectives for Biological Applications. Int J Mol Sci. 2019 ; 20(20): 5216. doi: 10.3390/ijms20205216

[16] Filipić A, Gutierrez-Aguirre I, Primc G, et al. Cold Plasma, a New Hope in the Field of Virus Inactivation. Trends Biotechnol. 2020. 38:1278–1291. https://doi.org/10.1016/j.tibtech.2020.04.003

[17] Kamiko N and Ohgaki S. RnaColiphage Ob As ABioindicator of the ultraviolet disinfection efficiency. WafSci Tech. 1989. 21: 227-231

[18] Ko G, First MW, Burge HA. Influence of relative humidity on particle size and UV sensitivity of Serratiamarcescens and Mycobacterium bovis BCG aerosols. Tuber Lung Dis. 2000. 80: 217-228. https://doi.org/10.1054/tuld.2000.0249

[19] Mcdevitt JJ, Rudnick SN and Radonovich L. Aerosol Susceptibility of

Influenza Virus to UV-C Light.Appl Environ Microbiol. 2012. 78: 1666 –1669. DOI: 10.1128/AEM.06960-11

[20] https://books.google.tn/books?id=ReqUM_XNGjoC&printsec=frontcover&hl=fr#v=onepage&q&f=false

[21] Jingwen C, Li L, Hao W. Review of UVC-LED Deep Ultraviolet Killing New NCP Coronavirus Dose In Technology Sharing. (Hubei Shenzi Technology Co., Ltd). 2020.

[22] Walker CM, Ko G. Effect of ultraviolet germicidal irradiation on viral aerosols. Environ SciTechnol. 2007. 41,5460-5465.

[23] Heilingloh CS, Aufderhorst UW, Schipper L, et al. Susceptibility of SARS-CoV-2 to UV irradiation. Am J Infect Control. 2020. 48:1273–1275. https://doi.org/10.1016/j.ajic.2020.07.031

[24] Storm N, McKay LGA, Downs SN, et al. Rapid and complete inactivation of SARS-CoV-2 by ultraviolet-C irradiation. Sci Rep. 2020. 10:1–5. https://doi.org/10.1038/s41598-020-79600-8

[25] Harris TR, Pagan JG andBatoni P. Optical and Fluidic Co-Design of a UV-LED Water Disinfection Chamber. ECS Transactions. 2012. 45, 221st ECS Meeting, May 6 – May 10, Seattle, WA, 17

[26] Nyangaresi PO, Qin Y, Chen G, Zhang B, Lu Y, Shen L. Effects of single and combined UV-LEDs on inactivation and subsequent reactivation of *E. coli* in water disinfection.Water Rese. 2018. 147: 331-341. https://doi.org/10.1016/j.watres.2018.10.014

[27] McDonald KF, Curry RD, Clevenger TE, Unklesbay K, Eisenstark A, Golden J, and R. D. Morgan .A Comparison of Pulsed and Continuous Ultraviolet Light Sources for the Decontamination of Surfaces. Ieee T Plasma Sci. 2000. 28: 1581-1587

[28] Stibich M, Stachowiak J, Tanner B, Berkheiser M, Moore L, Raad I, Chemaly R. F (2011) Evaluation of a Pulsed-Xenon Ultraviolet Room Disinfection Device for Impact on Hospital Operations and Microbial Reduction. Infect Control HospEpidemiol. 32: 286–288. DOI: 10.1086/658329.

[29] Song L, Li W, Li JHL, Li T, Gu D, and Tang H. Development of a Pulsed Xenon Ultraviolet Disinfection Device for Real-Time Air Disinfection in Ambulances. HindJ Healthc Eng. 2020. 1-5. DOI: 10.1155/2020/6053065

[30] Rutala WA, Gergen MF, Tande BM, Weber DJ. Rapid Hospital Room Decontamination Using Ultraviolet (UV) Light with a Nanostructured UV-Reflective Wall Coating. Infect Control HospEpidemiol. 2013. 34: 527-529. DOI: 10.1086/670211

[31] Krishnamoorthy G and Tande BM. Improving the effectiveness of ultraviolet germicidal irradiation through reflective wall coatings: Experimental and modeling based assessments. Indoor Built Environ.2014. 1-15. https://doi.org/10.1177/1420326X14547785

[32] Sung M, Kato S, Kim YM and M. Harada. Disinfection performance of ultraviolet germicidal irradiation systems for the microbial contamination on an evaporative humidifier Hvac&R Res.2011. 17: 22-30. DOI: 10.1080/10789669.2010.541540

[33] Woo MH, Grippin A, Anwar D, Smith T, Wu CY, Wander JD. Effects of Relative Humidity and Spraying Medium on UV Decontamination of Filters Loaded with Viral Aerosols. Appl Environ Microbiol. 2012. 78: 5781–5787. doi: 10.1128/AEM.00465-12

[34] Anderson DJ, Chen LF, Weber DJ, Moehring RW, Lewis SS, Triplett PF, Blocker M, Becherer P, Schwab JC,

Knelson LP, et al. The benefits of enhanced terminal room (BETR) disinfection study: A prospective, cluster randomized, multicenter, crossover study to evaluate the impact of enhanced terminal room disinfection on acquisition and infection caused by multidrug-resistant organisms. Lancet Infect Dis. 2017. 389:805–814. https://doi.10.1016/S0140-6736(16) 31588-4

[35] Haddad LE, Ghantoji SS, Stibich M, Fleming JB, Segal C, Ware KM, Chemaly RF. Evaluation of a pulsed xenon ultraviolet disinfection system to decrease bacterial contamination in operating rooms. BMC Infect Dis. 2017. 17: 672-677. doi: 10.1186/s12879-017-2792-z

[36] Mahida N, Vaughan N, Boswell T. First UK evaluation of an automated ultraviolet-C room decontamination device (Tru-DTM) J Hosp Infect. 84: 332-335. DOI: 10.1016/j.jhin.2013.05.005

[37] Bentancor M and Vidal S (2018) Programmable and low-cost ultraviolet room disinfection device. HardwareX. 2013. 4: 1-13.https://doi.org/10.1016/j.ohx.2018.e00046

[38] Guettari M, Gharbi I and Hamza S. UVC disinfection robot. *Environ SciPollut Res* 2020. https://doi.org/10.1007/s11356-020-11184-2

[39] Gharbi I, Guettari M, Chroudi A, Touati H, Hamza S. Disinfection Technology in Hospitals: Harmful effects of UVC. LA TUNISIE MEDICALE - 2020 ;Vol 98 (06): 434-441

[40] Sanglier Contreras G, Robas Mora M, Jimenez Gomez P. Gamma radiation in aid of the population in Covid-19 type pandemics. Contemporary Engineering Sciences, Vol. 13, 2020, no. 1, 113-129. doi: 10.12988/ces.2020.91456

[41] Durante M, Schulze K, Incerti S, et al. Virus Irradiation and COVID-19 Disease. Front Phys (2020) 8:1–7. https://doi.org/10.3389/fphy.2020.565861.

[42] Gamma irradiation as a treatment to address pathogens of animal biosecurity concern available at agriculture.gov.au/ba.

[43] Lea DE. Action of Radiations on Living Cells. New York, NY: Cambridge University Press (1947).

[44] Hartzell JD, Aronson NE, Weina PJ, et al. Positive rK39 serologic assay results in US servicemen with cutaneous leishmaniasis. Am J Trop Med HyG. 2008; 79:843–846. https://doi.org/10.4269/ajtmh.2008.79.843

[45] Jinia AJ, Sunbul NB, Meert CA, et al. Review of Sterilization Techniques for Medical and Personal Protective Equipment Contaminated with SARS-CoV-2. IEEE Access. 2020. 8:111347–111354. https://doi.org/10.1109/ACCESS.2020.3002886

[46] Cramer A, Tian E, Yu SH, et al. Disposable n95 masks pass qualitative fit-test but have decreased filtration efficiency after cobalt-60 gamma irradiation. medRxiv. 2020; 10–14. https://doi.org/10.1101/2020.03.28.20043471

[47] Man D et al., "Sterilization of disposable face masks by means of dry and steam sterilization processes ; an alternative in case of acute mask shortages due to COVID-19," J. Hosp. Infect., 2020, doi: https://doi.org/10.1016/j.jhin.2020.04.001

[48] IAEA, "Trends in Radiation Sterilization of Health Care Products," 2008. [Online]. Available: https://www.iaea.org/publications/7691/trends-in-radiationsterilization-of-health-care-products

[49] Yap TF, Liu Z, Shveda RA, Preston DJ. A predictive model of the temperature-dependent inactivation of coronaviruses. ApplPhysLett. 2020;117:. https://doi.org/10.1063/5.0020782

[50] Batéjat C, Grassin Q, Manuguerra JC, Leclercq I. Heat inactivation of the severe acute respiratory syndrome coronavirus 2. bioRxiv. 2020: 6–10. https://doi.org/10.1101/2020.05.01.067769

[51] Hemati M, Soosanabadi M, Ghorashi T, et al. Thermal inactivation of COVID-19 specimens improves RNA quality and quantity. J Cell Physiol. 2020. https://doi.org/10.1002/jcp.30206

[52] Wang J, Shen J, Ye D, et al. Disinfection technology of hospital wastes and wastewater: Suggestions for disinfection strategy during coronavirus Disease 2019 (COVID-19) pandemic in China. Environ Pollut. 2020: 262:114665. https://doi.org/10.1016/j.envpol.2020.114665

[53] Ohtsu Y, Onoda K, Kawashita H, Urasaki H. A comparison of microwave irradiation, electric, and hybrid heating for medical plastic-waste treatment. J Renew Sustain Energy. 2011. 3:1–8. https://doi.org/10.1063/1.3600706

[54] Jebri S et al., “Effect of gamma irradiation on bacteriophages used as viral indicators,” Water Res., vol. 47, no. 11, pp. 3673– 3678, 2013, doi: 10.1016/j.watres.2013.04.036.

[55] Wang X, Sun S, Zhang B, Han J. Solar heating to inactivate thermal-sensitive pathogenic microorganisms in vehicles: application to COVID-19. Environ ChemLett. 2020. 19: https://doi.org/10.1007/s10311-020-01132-4

[56] Rubio-Romero JC, Pardo-Ferreira M del C, Torrecilla-García JA, Calero-Castro S. Disposable masks: Disinfection and sterilization for reuse, and non-certified manufacturing, in the face of shortages during the COVID-19 pandemic. SafSci. 2020. 129:104830. https://doi.org/10.1016/j.ssci.2020.104830

[57] Otto C, Zahn S, Rost F, et al. Physical Methods for Cleaning and Disinfection of Surfaces. Food Eng Rev. 2011. 3:171–188. https://doi.org/10.1007/s12393-011-9038-4

[58] Herrmann HW, Henins I, Park J, Selwyn GS. Decontamination of chemical and biological warfare (CBW) agents using an atmospheric pressure plasma jet (APPJ). Phys Plasmas. 1999. 6:2284–2289. https://doi.org/10.1063/1.873480

[59] Bekeschus S, Kramer A, Suffredini E, et al. Gas Plasma Technology—An Asset to Healthcare During Viral Pandemics Such as the COVID-19 Crisis? IEEE Trans Radiat Plasma Med Sci. 2020. 4:391–399. https://doi.org/10.1109/trpms.2020.3002658

[60] Chen Z, Garcia G, Arumugaswami V, Wirz RE. Cold atmospheric plasma for SARS-CoV-2 inactivation. Phys Fluids. 2020: 32: https://doi.org/10.1063/5.0031332

[61] Gibson JH, Yong DHN, Farnood RR, Seto P. A literature review of ultrasound technology and its application in wastewater disinfection. Water Qual Res J Canada. 2008. 43:23–35. https://doi.org/10.2166/wqrj.2008.004

[62] Brennen CH. Phase Change, Nucleation and Cavitation. 1995. p. 15–47. In Cavitation and Bubble Dynamics. Oxford University Press, Oxford.

[63] Löning JM, Horst C, Hoffmann U. Investigations on the energy conversion in sonochemical processes. UltrasonSonochem. 2002. 9:169–179. https://doi.org/10.1016/S1350-4177(01)00113-4

[64] Fitria H, Mutaqin I. Role of disinfectant in reducing Covid-19 outbreak. International Journal of Applied Science and Research review. 2019. 1:1–5.

[65] Shereen MA, Khan S, Kazmi A, et al. COVID-19 infection: Origin, transmission, and characteristics of human coronaviruses. J AdvRes. 2020. 24:91–98. https://doi.org/10.1016/j.jare.2020.03.005

[66] Davies J.T., Emulsion Type. I. Physical Chemistry of, Gas/Liquid Liq. Interfaces. 1957. 426–438:

[67] Massicotte et al., Disinfectants and disinfection in hygiene and sanitation: Fundamental principles. 2009. https://publications.msss.gouv.qc.ca/msss/document-000859/

Chapter 6

Immune Response to COVID-19

Ricardo Wesley Alberca

Abstract

The severe acute respiratory syndrome coronavirus-2 (SARS-CoV-2) invades the host's cells via the angiotensin-converting enzyme 2 (ACE2) and transmembrane protease serine 2 (TMPRSS2). ACE2 and TMPRSS2 molecules are highly expressed on the respiratory tract but are also expressed in other organs such as kidneys, heart, and intestine, which could partially explain the multiple organ infection, damage, and failure. During the COVID-19 disease course, patients may develop a dysregulation in the immune response, with an exacerbated production of pro-inflammatory molecules and hypercoagulation, which can collaborate to the increase in tissue damage and death. This chapter will cover general aspects of the innate and adaptive immune response during COVID-19, the impact of comorbidities on the immune response to SARS-CoV-2, and the immune response generated by COVID-19 vaccines.

Keywords: SARS-CoV-2, COVID-19, immunology, immune response, inflammation

1. Introduction

SARS-CoV-2 has four main structural proteins: the spike protein (S protein), the nucleocapsid protein (N protein), the matrix protein (M Protein), and envelope protein (E protein) [1, 2]. The SARS-CoV-2 infection starts when the virion enters the host's cell, through the connection between the viral S protein and the ACE2 receptor and TMPRSS2 on the host's cells, similarly to severe acute respiratory syndrome coronavirus-1 (SARS-CoV-1) [3].

ACE2 and TMPRSS2 are highly expressed in the lungs, partially explaining the high incidence of respiratory disorders. Nevertheless, ACE2 and TMPRSS2 are expressed in many other different organs in the human body, such as the brain, heart, liver, kidney, colonic epithelial cells, intestine luminal cells, and small intestinal enterocytes [4], with reports of SARS-CoV-2 infection on multiple organs [5]. In addition, SARS-CoV-2 may generate a systemic and exacerbated inflammatory response named "cytokine storm", which can lead to viral sepsis [6].

Several systemic biomarkers have been associated with the progression of the disease, such as creatinine, urea, C-reactive protein, ferritin, lactate dehydrogenase, and D-dimers in the blood, increase in the neutrophil-to-lymphocyte ratio, and reduction in platelet count in the blood [7–15]. During COVID-19 the increase in blood levels of chemokines and cytokines increases the pro-inflammatory stimulus and recruitment of immune cells to the infection site. Several risk factors contribute to the disease's severity, such as comorbidities and co-infections [16–18] In this chapter, the current knowledge about the innate and adaptative immune response during COVID-19 and the influence of comorbidities will the reviewed.

2. Innate immune response to SARS-CoV-2

Upon infection by SARS-CoV-2 several chemokines (CCL2, CCL3, CCL4, CCL5, CXCL8, CXCL9, and CXL10) and pro-inflammatory cytokines (IFN-γ, TNF, IL-1, IL-6, IL-12) are released, these molecules will induce cell activation, migration, and infiltration of the infected tissue by innate immune cells like monocytes and neutrophils and further activate local cells such as resident macrophages [19]. These cells will further increase the local production of pro-inflammatory mediators, which could result in tissue damage, such as alveolar damage, formation of edema, and reduced lung capacity. In addition, cytokines can generate a systemic effect, resulting in damage to other organs (kidney, liver, spleen, among others) [20]. An increase in circulating pro-inflammatory monocytes and nonclassical monocytes are commonly observed in COVID-19 patients [21, 22].

Concomitantly, the number of neutrophils in the blood increases, and the infiltration of neutrophils to the infected tissue. Upon infiltration, neutrophils release inflammatory mediators, cytokines, and neutrophil extracellular traps (NETs) which can further increase tissue injury and cellular death [23, 24]. The local production of pro-inflammatory factors, viral particles, and cellular death induces the activation of macrophage and dendritic cells (DCs), which will further increase the production of cytokines and chemokines and antigen presentation [20, 25] DCSs are commonly referred to as professional antigen-presenting cells (APCs) and integrate innate and adaptive immune response. In COVID-19 they can uptake SARS-CoV-2 viral particles, be activated, migrate to lymphatic tissue, initiate antigen presentation, and trigger adaptive immune response. Nevertheless, DCs can also be infected by SARS-CoV-2 [26], reducing quantitatively, generating functional impairment, and lower lymphocyte immune response [27].

The complement system has also been implicated in the pathogenesis of COVID-19. The activation of C3 and C5 complement components are correlated with disease severity and lung biopsy from severe COVID-19 patients presented high C3-fragment content [28]. C3-deficient mice are partially protected from respiratory dysfunction after SARS-CoV-1 infection, exhibiting less inflammatory infiltrate in the lungs, reduced production of cytokines and chemokines, but similar viral load in the lung tissue as Wild Type mice [29]. Importantly, treatment with anti-C5a antibodies resulted in clinical improvement in COVID-19 patients [28]. Indicating a possible use of complement-inhibitor to ameliorate lung injury in COVID-19 patients.

The role of eosinophils and basophils in COVID-19 is yet to be fully comprehended. To the moment, a negative correlation is established between circulating eosinophil and basophil count and COVID-19 severity, with patients exhibiting an increase in those cells upon SARS-CoV-2 clearance [30, 31]. Mast cells (MCs) may also play a role in COVID-19, since they can be activated by viral products and release chemokines, cytokines, and inflammatory mediators, increasing vascular permeability and cellular infiltrate [32]. A few reports have indicated that COVID-19 inflammatory syndrome is in many aspects similar to Mast cell activation disease [32, 33].

The frequency of mononuclear and polymorphonuclear myeloid-derived suppressor cells also increases in the blood, but not in the lungs, of COVID-19 patients according to the severity [15, 34]. Importantly, these cells do maintain their immunosuppressive functions in COVID-19 patients [35].

The hyperinflammatory state is also accompanied by a dysregulated anti-inflammatory state, with an increased early IL-10 production, which could curb the anti-viral immune response [36], and impaired T cells (CD4+ and CD8+) and T regulatory cells function [37].

3. Adaptive immunity in COVID-19

Patients with moderate and severe COVID-19 commonly present a reduction in circulating lymphocytes (T cells, B cells, natural killer cells). T CD4+ and T CD8+ cells are reduced in moderate COVID-19 patients and further reduced in more severe patients, with or without a significant change in CD4+/CD8+ ratio [38, 39]. A few reports have identified patients with a specific reduction in CD8+ cells, which is associated with poor prognosis [38]. The reduction of B cells and innate lymphocytes, like NK cells, has also been reported, but to the moment are not currently associated with severity or prognosis [40].

The mechanism for the reduction in lymphocytes is still under investigation, several reports indicate that exhaustion and apoptosis may be the primary causes of lymphopenia [41], and one report indicating direct lymphocyte infections by SARS-CoV-2 [42]. Due to the central role of lymphocytes on anti-SARS-CoV-2 immune response, several interventions to modulate the T cell proliferation or apoptosis are also being investigated [43].

Although the reduced T cell count in the blood of COVID-19 patients may reflect the recruitment to infected tissue or be influenced by the use of steroid treatment to curb the inflammation, some studies have also reported significant T cell reduction in secondary lymphoid organs of patients infected with SARS-CoV-2 [44].

Even with the reduction in lymphocytes, T cell receptor analysis indicated that COVID-19 patients do present an increase in SARS-CoV-2-specific T-cells [45]. Proliferation markers, such as Ki67, and activation markers, such as CD28 and HLA-DR, are increased in both CD4+ and CD8+ cells, including activated, effector, and memory T-cells, in COVID-19 patients in comparison to recovered patients and non-COVID-19 patients [46]. Several reports identified an increased expression of exhaustion and inhibition-associated markers in circulating T cells such as CD39, CTLA4, LAG3, NKG2A, PD-1, and TIM3 [47].

In summary, these results indicate an expansion and overactivation of CD4+ and CD8+ T-cells that could lead to unresponsiveness or cell death. This appears to be true since even with a highly activated profile, CD8+ T cells from COVID-19 patients have a reduced cytokine production after in vivo stimulation [41].

CD4+ T cells may have a dual role in COVID-19, reports have identified that patients with higher activation markers on CD4+ cells have a poor prognosis, and others have identified that patients with higher T helper 1 profile (Th1) present a less severe disease [46, 48]. SARS-CoV-2-specific Th1 cells have been identified, but patients with profiles associated with SARS-CoV-2-specific Th2 and Th17 response have also been identified [49]. Another investigation has also identified an increase in transforming growth factor-β (TGFβ)-producing T cells in COVID-19 patients [50]. CD4+ FOXP3+ T regulatory cells increase during the disease but suffer a reduction in critically ill patients, which could corroborate the hyperactivation of the immune system [47, 50].

3.1 Antibodies and B CELLS

The Production of Antibodies, especially SARS-CoV-2-specific IgM and IgG, have been used as a diagnostic tool for COVID-19, although the presence of virus-specific IgG antibodies does indicate viral clearance [51]. Anti-SARS-CoV-2 antibodies may block and neutralize SARS-CoV-2 and prevent COVID-19 development.

Importantly, reports have identified that asymptomatic, moderate, and severe COVID-19 present different IgM and IgG production courses and may vary in quantity. Severe COVID-19 patients produce anti-SARS-CoV-2 IgG earlier in comparison to moderate patients, and asymptomatic and mild patients produce less neutralizing antibodies in comparison to moderate and severe COVID-19 patients [52].

More importantly, serum antibody titers rapidly decay after COVID-19, with conflicting reports with antibody titers decaying after a few months post-diagnosis [53, 54]. Nevertheless, antigen-specific memory B cells [55], T cells, and other components of the immunological memory remain effective and can be detected in convalescent patients [52, 56]. As memory cells can rapidly respond upon subsequent antigen encounter (infection), some degree of long-term immunity is expected [57].

Since SARS-CoV-2 S protein is necessary for the infection, neutralizing antibodies against this protein could in theory prevent the infection [2]. Both S-protein and N-protein specific IgM and IgG increase after the infection by SARS-CoV-2 [58], with S-protein IgG having a negative correlation with inflammatory markers in COVID-19 patients [58].

COVID-19 patients present a rapid increase in SARS-CoV-2-specific IgM, IgA, and IgG, commonly observed around a week after the infection [51, 59], however, comorbidities may impact not only on the inflammatory response during COVID-19 but also antibody production, reports identified patients with human immunodeficiency virus (HIV) presenting a delayed SARS-CoV-specific IgM and IgG production [60, 61].

4. Comorbidities and severe COVID-19

Several comorbidities have been described as risk factors for the progression of COVID-19 into a severe, critical, and lethal stage. The first reports have identified advanced age, systemic arterial hypertension, and Diabetes Mellitus with a higher hospitalization and severity for COVID-19 patients [62–64]. Comorbidities may influence COVID-19 severity via an increase in pro-inflammatory response, coagulatory disorders, or different ACE2 expression [65–67]. Investigations confirmed that old age, systemic arterial hypertension, Diabetes Mellitus [68], obesity [16], alcohol consumption [69], smokers and chronic obstructive pulmonary disease (COPD) [70], heart disease, liver disease and kidney disease [71], cancer [72, 73], immunodeficiencies, transplanted patients [74], and co-infections [17, 74] are in fact risk factor for severe COVID-19 and increase death risk and the presence of two or more comorbidities further increase the death risk [75]. We will review the impact of the most common comorbidities associated with poor COVID-19 prognosis and their influence on the anti-SARS-CoV-2 immune response.

4.1 Old age

The majority of the fatal cases of COVID-19 occurred in elderly individuals [76, 77]. Several facts may explain this phenomenon, such as the accumulations of other comorbidities, immunosenescence, and inflammaging.

Immunosenescence is defined as a decline in the immune system function, characterized by the reduction in qualitative and quantitative responses to infections, neoplasia, and vaccination [78]. With age, the production of naïve lymphocytes (T and B cells) is reduced, and the function of innate immune cells is weakened, therefore negatively impacting the immune response during infections [78]. Concomitantly, the elderly develop a chronic low-grade systemic inflammation, named inflammaging.

The low-grade pro-inflammatory state is characterized by the increase in serum inflammatory mediators, such as C-reactive protein, IL-1, IL-6, and TNF [79, 80], which is associated with an impaired and dysregulated immune response.

In summary, accumulations of other comorbidities such as systemic arterial hypertension and Diabetes Mellitus, immunosenescence, and inflammaging present in elderly patients are likely to contribute to the poorer outcome in COVID-19 [81].

4.2 Systemic arterial hypertension

Systemic Arterial Hypertension is common among hospitalized COVID-19 patients and is associated with higher severity of the disease and mortality [15, 82, 83]. The initial hypothesis for this was that Systemic Arterial Hypertension and the drugs commonly used for its control, like renin–angiotensin–aldosterone system (RAAS) inhibitors that increase expression of ACE2, increasing the susceptibility to SARS-CoV-2 [68]. However, a recent report has not identified an association between the use of RAAS inhibitors and increased severity or death in COVID-19 patients [84].

Other explanations are related to the modulations of ICAM and E-selectin, which are increased in systemic arterial hypertension and can be downregulated by dexamethasone [85, 86]. Dexamethasone treatment during COVID-19 can reduce the death rate in patients receiving both invasive and non-invasive mechanical ventilation [87]. Although no investigation on the modulation of ICAM and E-selecin has been performed, these results further support that the reduction of inflammation during COVID-19 can improve the patients' outcome [87].

4.3 Metabolic diseases (type 1 and 2 diabetes mellitus and obesity)

Diabetes Mellitus (DM), obesity, and metabolic syndrome increase the levels of circulating pro-inflammatory cytokines in comparison to lean people. This low-grade inflammation is lower than individuals with infections but can influence cellular metabolism and immune response [88, 89]. Obesity affected the frequency and ratio of CD8+ and CD4+ T cells, inducing an increase in inflammatory macrophages [90] and reduces the frequency of T regulatory cells, therefore favoring a more pro-inflammatory profile [91]. In obesity, there is a great increase in memory T cell in the adipose tissue, that upon infection can generate pancreatitis, and increase mortality [92]. Similar to inflammaging, obesity is also characterized by low-grade inflammation, with an increase in the production of chemokines and cytokines by the adipose tissue [92]. Obesity is also associated with several risk factors for COVID-19 such as respiratory dysfunctions, type 2 Diabetes Mellitus (DM2), and hypertension [16].

The type of Diabetes Mellitus is rarely described in COVID-19 investigations [93]. A recent investigation compared the mortality rate among type 1 Diabetes Mellitus (DM1) and DM2 patients during SARS-Co-V-2 infection. The unadjusted mortality rate per 100 000 was 27 for non-DM, 138 in DM type 1 (DM1) and 260 in DM2, the adjusted data verified that the odds ratios of COVID-19-related deaths were 3.51 in DM1 and 2.03 in DM2 [94]. Concluding that both DM types present a greater risk of death by COVID-19 [94].

An important factor is that poor glycemic control can influence the disease course [95], this is supported by several manuscripts that described the deleterious effect of elevated blood glucose levels on the immune response to COVID-19 and DM2 patients with better glycemic control presented a lower death rate in comparison with COVID-19 DM2 patients with hyperglycemia [96–98]. Diabetic patients also present a low-grade inflammation with an increase in pro-inflammatory cytokines and reactive oxygen species, but an impaired inflammatory response to microbial products [99, 100].

Non-diabetic patients with COVID-19 can also present hyperglycemia [15], and is associated with an increased incidence of severe illness and death risk [101]. Several drugs used for the control of inflammation can modify or induce hyperglycemia during COVID-19 hospitalization [102], which could affect the anti-SARS-CoV-2 immune response. A few manuscripts have hypothesized COVID-19 causes alterations of glucose metabolism, via direct SARS-CoV-2 infection of the pancreatic beta cells [103, 104]. Importantly, metabolic alterations have been described in COVID-19 patients, with and without DM, developing ketosis and ketoacidosis [105]. In a case report, a 29 years old patient, non-DM with a normal glucose level was diagnosed with COVID-19. Two weeks after recovered from COVID-19 was diagnosed with DM1 [106].

Therefore, COVID-19 may also represent a risk factor for the development of DM. A related point to consider is that DM patients may have long-term consequences from COVID19, with an increase in the need for daily insulin [107]. Currently, there is no explanation for this phenomenon, but COVID-19-mediated gastrointestinal dysbiosis could be a factor since the microbiota can influence the development or aggravate metabolic disorders [108]. Also, metformin, a drug commonly used by DM2 patients, may cause alteration on the gut microbiota and impact their anti-SARS-CoV-2 immune response [109, 110].

4.4 Chronic obstructive pulmonary disease (COPD), smoking, and other respiratory disorders

Chronic obstructive pulmonary disease (COPD) affects millions of people worldwide. COPD is characterized by progressive and irreversible airflow limitation due to structural alterations on the small airways. Smoking is the leading cause of COPD, due to the increase in inflammation and pulmonary remodeling [111]. Smoking and COPD are known to increase the risk for respiratory infections [112, 113]. Smokers and COPD patients have been identified among hospitalized COVID-19 patients since early reports [83]. COPD and smoking have been associated with an increased incidence, severity, and poor prognosis in COVID-19 [70, 114–116].

A common component in tobacco cigarettes and electronic smoking devices is nicotine, which can downregulate Interferon regulatory factor 7 and curb antiviral immune response [117]. COPD patients have a reduction in the expression of type I and type II interferons, and interferon-stimulated genes, therefore having a reduced antiviral response resulting in frequent respiratory exacerbations [118].

Other mechanisms postulated for the increase in susceptibility among those patients are the increase in lung inflammation and oxidative stress [119] and increase in the expression of the ACE2 receptor, SARS-CoV-2 entry receptor, in COPD and Smokers [120].

Interestingly, allergic asthma characterized by a Th2 immune response, with increased production of IL-4, IL-5 and IL-13, is associated with a reduction of the expression of ACE2 receptor [65]. And asthma is associated with a reduction in the severity of COVID-19 [121, 122]. It is important to highlight that non-allergic asthma or neutrophilic asthma increases the production of IL-17 in the lungs, which increases ACE2 expression, therefore possibly increasing the risk for severe COVID-19 [123].

Other respiratory diseases such as bronchiectasis, sarcoidosis, idiopathic pulmonary fibrosis, and lung cancer are also associated with an increase in COVID-19 severity, but further investigations are needed to understand the immune mechanism [124].

Since asthma, smoking and COPD are also commonly associated with other comorbidities, this could further increase the COVID-19 severity and death risk in these populations [125, 126].

4.5 Neoplasia (cancer)

Cancer patients are regarded as more vulnerable to severe COVID-19, due to the direct immunosuppression caused by the tumor or indirectly by the antitumor treatment [127, 128]. Patients with hematological malignancies, such as leukemia and lymphoma, have an exacerbated cellular proliferation with a reduction in the immune response, increasing the susceptibility to infections [129].

Location and cancer stage can also impact COVID-19 development. A recent report among patients with cancer identified that lung cancer, gastrointestinal cancer, and breast cancer are the most common [130]. Patients with stage IV cancer also account for a high number of COVID-19-infected patients [130, 131]. Cancer patients with COVID-19 also have an increase in hospitalization duration and severity [130, 131].

In addition to immune suppression, hospitalized cancer patients or patients undergoing frequent hospital visits may be at great risk for SARS-CoV-2 infection, increasing the necessity for precautionary measures [132, 133].

4.6 Immunodeficiencies

Immunodeficiencies are uncommon and chronic disorders of the immune system, that hinders the ability to develop an appropriate immune response, leading to deficient, exacerbated, or absent response to an infection or disease [134]. The immunodeficiency can be localized in any cell or structure of the immune system, compromising barrier immunity, innate immunity, or adaptive immune.

Immunodeficiency disorders can be divided into primary and secondary immunodeficiencies. Primary immunodeficiencies are a consequence of genetic defects, and secondary immunodeficiencies are caused by external or environmental factors, such as nutritional disorders or HIV [135].

The most common primary immunodeficiency is the common variable immunodeficiency that affects the patients' ability to mount an appropriate humoral response during infection [136]. These patients are commonly treated with immunoglobulin replacement [137]. A recent case report identified a patient with common variable immunodeficiency and severe COVID-19, that was successfully treated with COVID-19 convalescent plasma [138]. Although it is important to highlight that convalescent plasma treatment has controversial results, even when applied at the beginning of the infection and with high titers of neutralizing antibodies [139–141].

Reports of patients with primary and secondary immunodeficiencies identified an increase in severity and mortality due to COVID-19 in these patients in comparison with available data on COVID-19 [142, 143]. Also, patients with immunodeficiencies can present other comorbidities, further increasing the death risk by COVID-19 and increased risk for the development of secondary infections during hospitalization [142, 143]. Certain immunodeficiencies compromise specific anti-viral immune responses, for example, TLR7 gene defect, with compromised type I and II interferon production, are linked to severe COVID-19 in young individuals [144].

A common secondary immunodeficiency AIDS, the one caused by HIV, can compromise the anti-viral immune response during COVID-19. Patients with low CD4+ count have a higher severity and mortality risk compared with patients with normal CD4+ count [145]. In patients with HIV viral suppression, other comorbidities may increase patients' death risk during COVID-19 [30, 145].

4.7 Co-infections

Bacteria and viral co-infections and secondary infection in COVID-19 patients are important factors in the patients' treatment and outcome [146]. Co-pathogens included bacteria, fungi, parasites and viruses can modulate patients' immunity and also curb the anti-SARS-CoV-2 immune response [146]. Patients with invasive mechanical ventilation are at greater risk for bacterial co-infections [17, 147], also several patients report diarrhea without gastrointestinal SARS-CoV-2 infection, which could be a secondary gastrointestinal infection or microbiota dysbiosis [108].

Co-infections can increase the susceptibility to severe COVID-19, by an increase in the hyper inflammation or hypercoagulation status [74, 148]. Few reports have investigated the impact of parasites on COVID-19, such as leishmaniasis, toxoplasmosis, malaria, and Chagas disease [148–151]. Clinical manifestations of those diseases are usually associated with an increased and unregulated type 1 pro-inflammatory response, similar to COVID-19 [151]. In fact, a few case reports identified that chagasic patients with COVID-19 present an exacerbated inflammatory response, with a high lethality [74, 148]. This represents a further difficulty in the treatment of COVID-19, since the combination of drugs for the treatment of COVID-19 and the co-infections, the immune response to the co-infections and possible comorbidities need to be equated.

5. COVID-19 vaccines

COVID-19 vaccines are currently the only prophylactic/curative treatment for COVID-19, since drug repurposing and monoclonal antibodies trials had limited success, and investigations with convalescent plasma have conflicting results [87, 139–141, 152, 153]. Several vaccines are currently developed and in developing. Due to the high demand for a COVID-19 vaccine, significant advances in vaccine technologies have been made in the last year. Currently, 3 types of vaccines are being administered worldwide: inactivated virus vaccines (IVV) [154], vaccines that use mRNA with lipid nanoparticle (LNP) delivery systems [155], and vaccines containing DNA delivered within non-replicating recombinant adenovirus (AdV) vector systems [156]. AdV and mRNA vaccines aim to induce the production of SARS-CoV-2 S protein and induces the production of neutralizing antibodies [139, 141, 153].

All vaccines can induce the recognition of the viral antigen (immunogen) and also serve as an adjuvant to boost the immune response, the immunogen is recognized by innate immunity receptors such as toll-like receptors 3 and 7, RIG-I, and NOD2 inducing cellular activation and the production of interferons. This process will also induce the migration of DCs to secondary lymphoid organs and prime SARS-CoV-2-specific T cells [139, 141, 153]. Further questions regarding the effectiveness of vaccines are still going to be investigated, especially the long-term immunity and efficacy against new variants.

6. Conclusions

COVID-19 is a hyperinflammatory and hypercoagulation syndrome, with a hallmark increase in inflammatory mediators such as C-reactive protein, creatinine, urea, cytokines, and chemokines in the blood, with an increase in the neutrophil count and reduction in lymphocyte and platelet count. These processes lead to a dysregulated immune response that can be lethal. The overall mortality ratio is still unknown but is higher in patients with comorbidities. Patients with common and rare comorbidities may present differences in the immune response in comparison to healthy individuals.

The COVID-19 pandemic is a hallmark of world history, this systemic disease killed millions, raised ethical dilemmas, and put science and immunology on the daily lives of millions worldwide. Immunological investigations have helped the development of treatments and vaccines for this disease, but many questions are still left to be answered. The current knowledge is limited, but never in the previous history so many researchers around the world were focused on investigations on one disease. Several technologies developed and tested during this pandemic may bring light to other diseases, such as the new technologies in vaccine development and treatments.

Acknowledgements

Ricardo Wesley Alberca has a fellowship from Fundação de Amparo à Pesquisa do Estado de São Paulo (FAPESP), Grant Number: 19/02679-7.

Author details

Ricardo Wesley Alberca
University of São Paulo, São Paulo, Brazil

*Address all correspondence to: ricardowesley@usp.br

References

[1] Hu B, Guo H, Zhou P, Shi ZL. Characteristics of SARS-CoV-2 and COVID-19 [Internet]. Vol. 19, Nature Reviews Microbiology. Nature Research; 2021 [cited 2021 Apr 26]. p. 141-54. Available from: www.nature.com/nrmicro

[2] Batra M, Tian R, Zhang C, Clarence E, Sacher CS, Miranda JN, et al. Role of IgG against N-protein of SARS-CoV2 in COVID19 clinical outcomes. Sci Rep [Internet]. 2021 Dec 1 [cited 2021 Apr 24];11(1):3455. Available from: https://doi.org/10.1038/s41598-021-83108-0

[3] Astuti I, Ysrafil. Severe Acute Respiratory Syndrome Coronavirus 2 (SARS-CoV-2): An overview of viral structure and host response. Diabetes Metab Syndr Clin Res Rev [Internet]. 2020 Jul 1 [cited 2021 Apr 19];14(4):407-12. Available from: /pmc/articles/PMC7165108/

[4] Dong M, Zhang J, Ma X, Tan J, Chen L, Liu S, et al. ACE2, TMPRSS2 distribution and extrapulmonary organ injury in patients with COVID-19. Biomedicine and Pharmacotherapy. 2020.

[5] Puelles VG, Lütgehetmann M, Lindenmeyer MT, Sperhake JP, Wong MN, Allweiss L, et al. Multiorgan and Renal Tropism of SARS-CoV-2. The New England journal of medicine. 2020.

[6] Liu D, Wang Q, Zhang H, Cui L, Shen F, Chen Y, et al. Viral sepsis is a complication in patients with Novel Corona Virus Disease (COVID-19). Med Drug Discov. 2020 Dec 1;8:100057.

[7] Xie G, Ding F, Han L, Yin D, Lu H, Zhang M. The role of peripheral blood eosinophil counts in COVID-19 patients. Allergy [Internet]. 2020 Jul 13 [cited 2020 Jul 30]; all. 14465. Available from: https://onlinelibrary.wiley.com/doi/abs/10.1111/all.14465

[8] Tan L, Wang Q, Zhang D, Ding J, Huang Q, Tang YQ, et al. Lymphopenia predicts disease severity of COVID-19: a descriptive and predictive study. Vol. 5, Signal Transduction and Targeted Therapy. 2020.

[9] Huang C, Wang Y, Li X, Ren L, Zhao J, Hu Y, et al. Clinical features of patients infected with 2019 novel coronavirus in Wuhan, China. Lancet. 2020;395(10223):497-506.

[10] Qin C, Zhou L, Hu Z, Zhang S, Yang S, Tao Y, et al. Dysregulation of immune response in patients with COVID-19 in Wuhan, China. Clin Infect Dis. 2020;

[11] Jamal MH, Doi SA, AlYouha S, Almazeedi S, Al-Haddad M, Al-Muhaini A, et al. A biomarker based severity progression indicator for COVID-19: the Kuwait prognosis indicator score. Biomarkers [Internet]. 2020 Nov 16 [cited 2021 Mar 20];25(8):641-8. Available from: https://www.tandfonline.com/doi/full/10.1080/1354750X.2020.1841296

[12] Singh N, Anchan RK, Besser SA, Belkin MN, Cruz MD, Lee L, et al. High sensitivity Troponin-T for prediction of adverse events in patients with COVID-19. Biomarkers [Internet]. 2020 Nov 16 [cited 2021 Mar 20];25(8):626-33. Available from: https://www.tandfonline.com/doi/full/10.1080/1354750X.2020.1829056

[13] Salvatici M, Barbieri B, Cioffi SMG, Morenghi E, Leone FP, Maura F, et al. Association between cardiac troponin I and mortality in patients with COVID-19. Biomarkers [Internet]. 2020 Nov 16 [cited 2021 Mar 20];25(8):634-40. Available from: https://www.

tandfonline.com/doi/full/10.1080/1354750X.2020.1831609

[14] Peiró ÓM, Carrasquer A, Sánchez-Gimenez R, Lal-Trehan N, del-Moral-Ronda V, Bonet G, et al. Biomarkers and short-term prognosis in COVID-19. Biomarkers [Internet]. 2021 Feb 17 [cited 2021 Mar 20];26(2):119-26. Available from: https://www.tandfonline.com/doi/full/10.1080/1354750X.2021.1874052

[15] Alberca RW, Andrade MM de S, Castelo Branco ACC, Pietrobon AJ, Pereira NZ, Fernandes IG, et al. Frequencies of CD33+ CD11b+ HLA-DR− CD14− CD66b+ and CD33+ CD11b+ HLA-DR− CD14+ CD66b− cells in peripheral blood as severity immune biomarkers in COVID-19. Front Med. 2020;7:654.

[16] Alberca RW, Oliveira L de M, Branco ACCC, Pereira NZ, Sato MN. Obesity as a risk factor for COVID-19: an overview. Crit Rev Food Sci Nutr [Internet]. 2020 [cited 2020 Jul 30]; Available from: https://www.tandfonline.com/doi/abs/10.1080/10408398.2020.1775546

[17] Lansbury L, Lim B, Baskaran V, Lim WS. Co-infections in people with COVID-19: a systematic review and meta-analysis. J Infect. 2020;

[18] Alberca GGF, Solis-Castro RL, Solis-Castro ME, Alberca RW. Coronavirus disease–2019 and the intestinal tract: An overview. World J Gastroenterol [Internet]. 2021 Apr 7 [cited 2021 Mar 31];27(13):1255-66. Available from: https://www.wjgnet.com/1007-9327/full/v27/i13/1255.htm

[19] Khalil BA, Elemam NM, Maghazachi AA. Chemokines and chemokine receptors during COVID-19 infection [Internet]. Vol. 19, Computational and Structural Biotechnology Journal. Elsevier B.V.; 2021 [cited 2021 Apr 22]. p. 976-88. Available from: /pmc/articles/PMC7859556/

[20] Temgoua MN, Endomba FT, Nkeck JR, Kenfack GU, Tochie JN, Essouma M. Coronavirus Disease 2019 (COVID-19) as a Multi-Systemic Disease and its Impact in Low- and Middle-Income Countries (LMICs). SN Compr Clin Med [Internet]. 2020 Sep [cited 2021 Apr 22];2(9):1377-87. Available from: /pmc/articles/PMC7371790/

[21] Ekşioğlu-Demiralp E, Alan S, Sili U, Bakan D, Ocak İ, Yürekli R, et al. Peripheral innate and adaptive immune cells during COVID-19: Functional neutrophils, pro-inflammatory monocytes and half-dead lymphocytes [Internet]. medRxiv. medRxiv; 2020 [cited 2021 Apr 13]. p. 2020.08.01.20166587. Available from: https://doi.org/10.1101/2020.08.01.20166587

[22] Stephenson E, Reynolds G, Botting RA, Calero-Nieto FJ, Morgan MD, Tuong ZK, et al. Single-cell multi-omics analysis of the immune response in COVID-19. Nat Med [Internet]. 2021 Apr 20 [cited 2021 Apr 22];1-13. Available from: http://www.nature.com/articles/s41591-021-01329-2

[23] Radermecker C, Detrembleur N, Guiot J, Cavalier E, Henket M, d'Emal C, et al. Neutrophil extracellular traps infiltrate the lung airway, interstitial, and vascular compartments in severe COVID-19. J Exp Med [Internet]. 2020 Dec 7 [cited 2021 Apr 13];217(12). Available from: https://doi.org/10.1084/jem.20201012

[24] Veras FP, Pontelli MC, Silva CM, Toller-Kawahisa JE, de Lima M, Nascimento DC, et al. SARS-CoV-2-triggered neutrophil extracellular traps mediate COVID-19 pathology. J Exp Med [Internet]. 2020 Dec 7 [cited 2021 Apr 13];217(12). Available from: /pmc/articles/PMC7488868/

[25] Meidaninikjeh S, Sabouni N, Marzouni HZ, Bengar S, Khalili A, Jafari R. Monocytes and macrophages in COVID-19: Friends and foes [Internet]. Vol. 269, Life Sciences. Elsevier Inc.; 2021 [cited 2021 Apr 22]. p. 119010. Available from: /pmc/articles/PMC7834345/

[26] Borges RC, Hohmann MS, Borghi SM. Dendritic cells in COVID-19 immunopathogenesis: insights for a possible role in determining disease outcome [Internet]. Vol. 40, International Reviews of Immunology. Taylor and Francis Ltd.; 2021 [cited 2021 Apr 22]. p. 108-25. Available from: https://www.tandfonline.com/action/journalInformation?journalCode=iiri20

[27] Zhou R, To KKW, Wong YC, Liu L, Zhou B, Li X, et al. Acute SARS-CoV-2 Infection Impairs Dendritic Cell and T Cell Responses. Immunity. 2020 Oct 13;53(4):864-877.e5.

[28] Gao T, Hu M, Zhang X, Li H, Zhu L, Liu H, et al. Highly pathogenic coronavirus N protein aggravates lung injury by MASP-2-mediated complement over-activation [Internet]. medRxiv. medRxiv; 2020 [cited 2021 Apr 23]. p. 2020.03.29.20041962. Available from: https://doi.org/10.1101/2020.03.29.20041962

[29] Gralinski LE, Sheahan TP, Morrison TE, Menachery VD, Jensen K, Leist SR, et al. Complement activation contributes to severe acute respiratory syndrome coronavirus pathogenesis. MBio [Internet]. 2018 Sep 1 [cited 2021 Apr 23];9(5):1753-71. Available from: http://mbio.asm.org/

[30] Alberca R, Aoki V, Sato M. COVID-19 and HIV: Case reports of 2 co-infected patients with different disease courses. World Acad Sci J [Internet]. 2020 Nov 26 [cited 2020 Dec 3];3(1):4. Available from: http://www.spandidos-publications.com/10.3892/wasj.2020.75

[31] Xie G, Ding F, Han L, Yin D, Lu H, Zhang M. The role of peripheral blood eosinophil counts in COVID-19 patients. Allergy [Internet]. 2020 Jul 13 [cited 2020 Aug 2];all.14465. Available from: https://onlinelibrary.wiley.com/doi/abs/10.1111/all.14465

[32] Afrin LB, Weinstock LB, Molderings GJ. Covid-19 hyperinflammation and post-Covid-19 illness may be rooted in mast cell activation syndrome. Vol. 100, International Journal of Infectious Diseases. Elsevier B.V.; 2020. p. 327-32.

[33] Brock I, Maitland A. Mast Cells and COVID-19: a case report implicating a role of mast cell activation in the prevention and treatment of Covid-19. 2021 Mar 16 [cited 2021 Apr 23]; Available from: https://doi.org/10.21203/rs.3.rs-330667/v2

[34] Falck-Jones S, Vangeti S, Yu M, Falck-Jones R, Cagigi A, Badolati I, et al. Functional monocytic myeloid-derived suppressor cells increase in blood but not airways and predict COVID-19 severity. J Clin Invest [Internet]. 2021 Mar 15 [cited 2021 Apr 26];131(6). Available from: https://doi.org/10.1172/JCI144734DS1

[35] Agrati C, Sacchi A, Bordoni V, Cimini E, Notari S, Grassi G, et al. Expansion of myeloid-derived suppressor cells in patients with severe coronavirus disease (COVID-19). Cell Death Differ. 2020;

[36] Lu L, Zhang H, Dauphars DJ, He YW. A Potential Role of Interleukin 10 in COVID-19 Pathogenesis [Internet]. Vol. 42, Trends in Immunology. Elsevier Ltd; 2021 [cited 2021 Apr 22]. p. 3-5. Available from: https://doi.org/10.1016/j.it.2020.10.012

[37] Qin C, Zhou L, Hu Z, Zhang S, Yang S, Tao Y, et al. Dysregulation of Immune Response in Patients With

Coronavirus 2019 (COVID-19) in Wuhan, China. Clin Infect Dis. 2020;71(15):762-8.

[38] Urra JM, Cabrera CM, Porras L, Ródenas I. Selective CD8 cell reduction by SARS-CoV-2 is associated with a worse prognosis and systemic inflammation in COVID-19 patients. Clin Immunol [Internet]. 2020 Aug 1 [cited 2021 Apr 22];217:108486. Available from: /pmc/articles/PMC7256549/

[39] Zhang H, Wu T. CD4+T, CD8+T counts and severe COVID-19: A meta-analysis [Internet]. Vol. 81, Journal of Infection. W.B. Saunders Ltd; 2020 [cited 2021 Apr 22]. p. e82-4. Available from: /pmc/articles/PMC7305716/

[40] Tavakolpour S, Rakhshandehroo T, Wei EX, Rashidian M. Lymphopenia during the COVID-19 infection: What it shows and what can be learned [Internet]. Vol. 225, Immunology Letters. Elsevier B.V.; 2020 [cited 2021 Apr 22]. p. 31-2. Available from: /pmc/articles/PMC7305732/

[41] Zheng M, Gao Y, Wang G, Song G, Liu S, Sun D, et al. Functional exhaustion of antiviral lymphocytes in COVID-19 patients [Internet]. Vol. 17, Cellular and Molecular Immunology. Springer Nature; 2020 [cited 2021 Apr 22]. p. 533-5. Available from: https://doi.org/10.1038/s41423-020-0402-2

[42] Pontelli MC, Castro IA, Martins RB, Veras FP, Serra L La, Nascimento DC, et al. Infection of human lymphomononuclear cells by SARS-CoV-2 [Internet]. Vol. 7, bioRxiv. bioRxiv; 2020 [cited 2021 Apr 22]. p. 2020.07.28.225912. Available from: https://doi.org/10.1101/2020.07.28.225912

[43] Lee J, Park SS, Kim TY, Lee DG, Kim DW. Lymphopenia as a biological predictor of outcomes in COVID-19 patients: A nationwide cohort study. Cancers (Basel) [Internet]. 2021 [cited 2021 Apr 22];13(3):1-15. Available from: https://pubmed.ncbi.nlm.nih.gov/33530509/

[44] Kaneko N, Kuo HH, Boucau J, Farmer JR, Allard-Chamard H, Mahajan VS, et al. Loss of Bcl-6-Expressing T Follicular Helper Cells and Germinal Centers in COVID-19. Cell. 2020 Oct 1;183(1):143-157.e13.

[45] Gutierrez L, Beckford J, Alachkar H. Deciphering the TCR Repertoire to Solve the COVID-19 Mystery [Internet]. Vol. 41, Trends in Pharmacological Sciences. Elsevier Ltd; 2020 [cited 2021 Apr 26]. p. 518-30. Available from: https://doi.org/10.1016/j.tips.2020.06.001

[46] Mathew D, Giles JR, Baxter AE, Oldridge DA, Greenplate AR, Wu JE, et al. Deep immune profiling of COVID-19 patients reveals distinct immunotypes with therapeutic implications. Science (80-) [Internet]. 2020 Sep 4 [cited 2021 Apr 26];369(6508). Available from: /pmc/articles/PMC7402624/

[47] Chen Z, John Wherry E. T cell responses in patients with COVID-19. Nat Rev Immunol [Internet]. 2020 Sep 1 [cited 2021 Apr 6];20(9):529-36. Available from: www.nature.com/nri

[48] Chen G, Wu D, Guo W, Cao Y, Huang D, Wang H, et al. Clinical and immunologic features in severe and moderate forms of Coronavirus Disease 2019. medRxiv. 2020;

[49] Weiskopf D, Schmitz KS, Raadsen MP, Grifoni A, Okba NMA, Endeman H, et al. Phenotype and kinetics of SARS-CoV-2-specific T cells in COVID-19 patients with acute respiratory distress syndrome. Sci Immunol [Internet]. 2020 Jun 26 [cited 2021 Apr 26];5(48). Available from: https://immunology.sciencemag.org/content/5/48/eabd2071

[50] Wang W, Su B, Pang L, Qiao L, Feng Y, Ouyang Y, et al.

High-dimensional immune profiling by mass cytometry revealed immunosuppression and dysfunction of immunity in COVID-19 patients. Cell Mol Immunol [Internet]. 2020 Jun 1 [cited 2021 Apr 26];17(6):650-2. Available from: https://doi.org/10.1038/s41423-020-0447-2

[51] Chong Y, Ikematsu H, Tani N, Arimizu Y, Watanabe H, Fukamachi Y, et al. Clinical significance of SARS-CoV-2-specific IgG detection with a rapid antibody kit for COVID-19 patients. Influenza Other Respi Viruses. 2020;

[52] Alberca GGF, Alberca RW. What is the long-term clinical significance of anti-SARS-CoV-2-specific IgG? Influenza and other Respiratory Viruses. Blackwell Publishing Ltd; 2020.

[53] Ibarrondo FJ, Fulcher JA, Goodman-Meza D, Elliott J, Hofmann C, Hausner MA, et al. Rapid Decay of Anti-SARS-CoV-2 Antibodies in Persons with Mild Covid-19. The New England journal of medicine. 2020.

[54] Self WH, Tenforde MW, Stubblefield WB, Feldstein LR, Steingrub JS, Shapiro NI, et al. Decline in SARS-CoV-2 Antibodies After Mild Infection Among Frontline Health Care Personnel in a Multistate Hospital Network—12 States, April–August 2020. MMWR Morb Mortal Wkly Rep [Internet]. 2020 Nov 27 [cited 2021 Apr 24];69(47):1762-6. Available from: http://www.cdc.gov/mmwr/volumes/69/wr/mm6947a2.htm?s_cid=mm6947a2_w

[55] Hartley GE, Edwards ESJ, Aui PM, Varese N, Stojanovic S, McMahon J, et al. Rapid generation of durable B cell memory to SARS-CoV-2 spike and nucleocapsid proteins in COVID-19 and convalescence. Sci Immunol [Internet]. 2020 Dec 22 [cited 2021 Apr 6];5(54). Available from: http://immunology.sciencemag.org/

[56] Dan JM, Mateus J, Kato Y, Hastie KM, Yu ED, Faliti CE, et al. Immunological memory to SARS-CoV-2 assessed for up to 8 months after infection. Science (80-) [Internet]. 2021 Feb 5 [cited 2021 Apr 6];371(6529). Available from: https://doi.org/10.1126/science.abf4063

[57] Alberca GGF, Alberca RW. What is the long-term clinical significance of anti-SARS-CoV-2-specific IgG? Influenza and other Respiratory Viruses. 2020.

[58] Sun B, Feng Y, Mo X, Zheng P, Wang Q, Li P, et al. Kinetics of SARS-CoV-2 specific IgM and IgG responses in COVID-19 patients. Emerg Microbes Infect [Internet]. 2020 Jan 1 [cited 2021 Apr 24];9(1):940-8. Available from: /pmc/articles/PMC7273175/

[59] Yu HQ, Sun BQ, Fang ZF, Zhao JC, Liu XY, Li YM, et al. Distinct features of SARS-CoV-2-specific IgA response in COVID-19 patients. European Respiratory Journal. 2020.

[60] Vizcarra P, Pérez-Elías MJ, Quereda C, Moreno A, Vivancos MJ, Dronda F, et al. Description of COVID-19 in HIV-infected individuals: a single-centre, prospective cohort. Lancet HIV. 2020;7(8):e554-64.

[61] Wang M, Luo L, Bu H, Xia H. One case of coronavirus disease 2019 (COVID-19) in a patient co-infected by HIV with a low CD4+ T-cell count. Int J Infect Dis. 2020;96:148-50.

[62] Zhang J jin, Dong X, Cao Y yuan, Yuan Y dong, Yang Y bin, Yan Y qin, et al. Clinical characteristics of 140 patients infected with SARS-CoV-2 in Wuhan, China. Allergy Eur J Allergy Clin Immunol. 2020;75(7):1730-41.

[63] Li X, Xu S, Yu M, Wang K, Tao Y, Zhou Y, et al. Risk factors for severity and mortality in adult COVID-19

inpatients in Wuhan. J Allergy Clin Immunol. 2020;

[64] Zhou F, Yu T, Du R, Fan G, Liu Y, Liu Z, et al. Clinical course and risk factors for mortality of adult inpatients with COVID-19 in Wuhan, China: a retrospective cohort study. Lancet. 2020;395(10229):1054-62.

[65] Castelo Branco ACC, Sato MN, Alberca RW. The possible dual role of the ACE2 receptor in asthma and SARS-COV2 infection. Front Cell Infect Microbiol. 2020;10:537.

[66] Merad M, Martin JC. Pathological inflammation in patients with COVID-19: a key role for monocytes and macrophages [Internet]. Vol. 20, Nature Reviews Immunology. Nature Research; 2020 [cited 2021 Apr 8]. p. 355-62. Available from: www.nature.com/nri

[67] Wolff D, Nee S, Hickey NS, Marschollek M. Risk factors for Covid-19 severity and fatality: a structured literature review. Infection. 2020.

[68] Fang L, Karakiulakis G, Roth M. Are patients with hypertension and diabetes mellitus at increased risk for COVID-19 infection? [Internet]. Vol. 8, The Lancet Respiratory Medicine. Lancet Publishing Group; 2020 [cited 2021 Apr 6]. p. e21. Available from: /pmc/articles/PMC7118626/

[69] Alberca RW, Rigato PO, Ramos YÁL, Teixeira FME, Castelo Branco ACC, Fernandes IG, et al. Clinical characteristics and survival analysis in frequent alcohol consumers with COVID-19. Front Nutr. 2021;8:260.

[70] Alberca RW, Lima JC, Oliveira EA de, Gozzi-Silva SC, Ramos YÁL, Andrade MM de S, et al. COVID-19 Disease Course in Former Smokers, Smokers and COPD Patients. Front Physiol. 2021;

[71] Cheng Y, Luo R, Wang K, Zhang M, Wang Z, Dong L, et al. Kidney disease is associated with in-hospital death of patients with COVID-19. Vol. 97, Kidney International. 2020. p. 829-38.

[72] Lee LYW, Cazier JB, Starkey T, Briggs SEW, Arnold R, Bisht V, et al. COVID-19 prevalence and mortality in patients with cancer and the effect of primary tumour subtype and patient demographics: a prospective cohort study. Lancet Oncol [Internet]. 2020 Oct 1 [cited 2021 Apr 6];21(10):1309-16. Available from: www.thelancet.com/oncology

[73] Derosa L, Melenotte C, Griscelli F, Gachot B, Marabelle A, Kroemer G, et al. The immuno-oncological challenge of COVID-19. Nat Cancer [Internet]. 2020 Oct 2 [cited 2021 Apr 6];1(10):946-64. Available from: https://doi.org/10.1038/s43018-020-00122-3

[74] Gozzi-Silva SC, Benard G, Alberca RW, Yendo TM, Teixeira FME, Oliveira L de M, et al. SARS-CoV-2 Infection and CMV Dissemination in Transplant Recipients as a Treatment for Chagas Cardiomyopathy: A Case Report. Trop Med Infect Dis [Internet]. 2021 Feb 10 [cited 2021 Feb 19];6(1):22. Available from: https://www.mdpi.com/2414-6366/6/1/22

[75] Sousa BLA, Sampaio-Carneiro M, de Carvalho WB, Silva CA, Ferraro AA. Differences among Severe Cases of Sars-CoV-2, Influenza, and Other Respiratory Viral Infections in Pediatric Patients: Symptoms, Outcomes and Preexisting Comorbidities. Clinics (Sao Paulo) [Internet]. 2020 [cited 2021 Apr 6];75:e2273. Available from: http://www.scielo.br/scielo.php?script=sci_arttext&pid=S1807-59322020000100315&lng=en&nrm=iso&tlng=en

[76] Hoffmann C, Wolf E. Older age groups and country-specific case fatality rates of COVID-19 in Europe, USA and Canada. Infection [Internet]. 2021 Feb 1 [cited 2021 Apr 24];49(1):111-6.

Available from: https://doi.org/10.1007/s15010-020-01538-w

[77] Kang SJ, Jung SI. Age-Related Morbidity and Mortality among Patients with COVID-19. Infect Chemother [Internet]. 2020 Jun 1 [cited 2021 Apr 24];52(2):154-64. Available from: /pmc/articles/PMC7335648/

[78] Fulop T, Larbi A, Dupuis G, Page A Le, Frost EH, Cohen AA, et al. Immunosenescence and inflamm-aging as two sides of the same coin: Friends or Foes? [Internet]. Vol. 8, Frontiers in Immunology. Frontiers Media S.A.; 2018 [cited 2021 Apr 24]. p. 1. Available from: /pmc/articles/PMC5767595/

[79] Franceschi C, Campisi J. Chronic inflammation (Inflammaging) and its potential contribution to age-associated diseases. Journals of Gerontology–Series A Biological Sciences and Medical Sciences. 2014.

[80] Franceschi C, Bonafè M, Valensin S, Olivieri F, De Luca M, Ottaviani E, et al. Inflamm-aging. An evolutionary perspective on immunosenescence. In: Annals of the New York Academy of Sciences [Internet]. New York Academy of Sciences; 2000 [cited 2021 Apr 24]. p. 244-54. Available from: https://pubmed.ncbi.nlm.nih.gov/10911963/

[81] Pietrobon AJ, Teixeira FME, Sato MN. I mmunosenescence and Inflammaging: Risk Factors of Severe COVID-19 in Older People [Internet]. Vol. 11, Frontiers in Immunology. Frontiers Media S.A.; 2020 [cited 2021 Apr 24]. p. 2728. Available from: www.frontiersin.org

[82] Wu C, Chen X, Cai Y, Xia J, Zhou X, Xu S, et al. Risk Factors Associated with Acute Respiratory Distress Syndrome and Death in Patients with Coronavirus Disease 2019 Pneumonia in Wuhan, China. JAMA Intern Med. 2020;

[83] Guan W, Ni Z, Hu Y, Liang W, Ou C, He J, et al. Clinical characteristics of coronavirus disease 2019 in China. N Engl J Med. 2020;382(18):1708-20.

[84] de Abajo FJ, Rodríguez-Martín S, Lerma V, Mejía-Abril G, Aguilar M, García-Luque A, et al. Use of renin–angiotensin–aldosterone system inhibitors and risk of COVID-19 requiring admission to hospital: a case-population study. Lancet [Internet]. 2020 May 30 [cited 2021 Apr 24];395(10238):1705-14. Available from: www.bifap.org

[85] De Caterina R, Ghiadoni L, Taddei S, Virdis A, Almerigogna F, Basta G, et al. Soluble E-selectin in essential hypertension: A correlate of vascular structural changes. Am J Hypertens [Internet]. 2001 Mar 1 [cited 2021 Apr 24];14(3):259-66. Available from: https://academic.oup.com/ajh/article-lookup/doi/10.1016/S0895-7061(00)01276-0

[86] Jilma B, Blann AD, Stohlawetz P, Eichler HG, Kautzky-Willer A, Wagner OF. Dexamethasone lowers circulating E-selectin and ICAM-1 in healthy men. J Lab Clin Med [Internet]. 2000 [cited 2021 Apr 24];135(3):270-4. Available from: https://pubmed.ncbi.nlm.nih.gov/10711866/

[87] Dexamethasone in Hospitalized Patients with Covid-19—Preliminary Report. N Engl J Med. 2020;

[88] Moutschen MP, Scheen AJ, Lefebvre PJ. Impaired immune responses in diabetes mellitus: Analysis of the factors and mechanisms involved. Relevance to the increased susceptibility of diabetic patients to specific infections [Internet]. Vol. 18, Diabete et Metabolisme. 1992 [cited 2021 Apr 25]. p. 187-201. Available from: https://europepmc.org/article/med/1397473

[89] Daryabor G, Atashzar MR, Kabelitz D, Meri S, Kalantar K. The

Effects of Type 2 Diabetes Mellitus on Organ Metabolism and the Immune System [Internet]. Vol. 11, Frontiers in Immunology. Frontiers Media S.A.; 2020 [cited 2021 Apr 25]. p. 1582. Available from: www.frontiersin.org

[90] Nishimura S, Manabe I, Nagasaki M, Eto K, Yamashita H, Ohsugi M, et al. CD8+ effector T cells contribute to macrophage recruitment and adipose tissue inflammation in obesity. Nat Med [Internet]. 2009 Aug [cited 2021 Apr 25];15(8):914-20. Available from: https://pubmed.ncbi.nlm.nih.gov/19633658/

[91] Wagner NM, Brandhorst G, Czepluch F, Lankeit M, Eberle C, Herzberg S, et al. Circulating regulatory T cells are reduced in obesity and may identify subjects at increased metabolic and cardiovascular risk. Obesity [Internet]. 2013 Mar [cited 2021 Apr 25];21(3):461-8. Available from: https://pubmed.ncbi.nlm.nih.gov/23592653/

[92] Misumi I, Starmer J, Uchimura T, Beck MA, Magnuson T, Whitmire Correspondence JK. Obesity Expands a Distinct Population of T Cells in Adipose Tissue and Increases Vulnerability to Infection. CellReports [Internet]. 2019 [cited 2021 Apr 25];27:514-524.e5. Available from: https://doi.org/10.1016/j.celrep.2019.03.030

[93] Liang X, Xu J, Xiao W, Shi L, Yang H. The association of diabetes with COVID-19 disease severity: evidence from adjusted effect estimates. Hormones. 2020.

[94] Barron E, Bakhai C, Kar P, Weaver A, Bradley D, Ismail H, et al. Associations of type 1 and type 2 diabetes with COVID-19-related mortality in England: a whole-population study. Lancet Diabetes Endocrinol. 2020;

[95] Lei M, Lin K, Pi Y, Huang X, Fan L, Huang J, et al. Clinical Features and Risk Factors of ICU Admission for COVID-19 Patients with Diabetes. J Diabetes Res. 2020;2020.

[96] Palaiodimos L, Chamorro-Pareja N, Karamanis D, Li W, Zavras PD, Chang KM, et al. Diabetes is associated with increased risk for in-hospital mortality in patients with COVID-19: a systematic review and meta-analysis comprising 18,506 patients. Hormones. 2020;

[97] Ceriello A. Hyperglycemia and COVID-19: What was known and what is really new? [Internet]. Vol. 167, Diabetes Research and Clinical Practice. Elsevier Ireland Ltd; 2020 [cited 2021 Apr 24]. p. 108383. Available from: /pmc/articles/PMC7445137/

[98] Zhu L, She ZG, Cheng X, Qin JJ, Zhang XJ, Cai J, et al. Association of Blood Glucose Control and Outcomes in Patients with COVID-19 and Pre-existing Type 2 Diabetes. Cell Metab. 2020;

[99] Berbudi A, Rahmadika N, Tjahjadi AI, Ruslami R. Type 2 Diabetes and its Impact on the Immune System. Curr Diabetes Rev [Internet]. 2019 Oct 28 [cited 2021 Apr 24];16(5):442-9. Available from: /pmc/articles/PMC7475801/

[100] Mooradian AD, Reed RL, Meredith KE, Scuderi P. Serum levels of tumor necrosis factor and IL-1α and IL-1β in diabetic patients. Diabetes Care [Internet]. 1991 [cited 2021 Apr 24];14(1):63-5. Available from: https://pubmed.ncbi.nlm.nih.gov/1991438/

[101] Sachdeva S, Desai R, Gupta U, Prakash A, Jain A, Aggarwal A. Admission Hyperglycemia in Non-diabetics Predicts Mortality and Disease Severity in COVID-19: a Pooled Analysis and Meta-summary of Literature. SN Compr Clin Med. 2020;

[102] Wang A, Zhao W, Xu Z, Gu J. Timely blood glucose management for

the outbreak of 2019 novel coronavirus disease (COVID-19) is urgently needed. Diabetes Res Clin Pract. 2020;

[103] Hamming I, Timens W, Bulthuis MLC, Lely AT, Navis GJ, van Goor H. Tissue distribution of ACE2 protein, the functional receptor for SARS coronavirus. A first step in understanding SARS pathogenesis. J Pathol. 2004;

[104] Pinto BG, Oliveira AE, Singh Y, Jimenez L, Goncalves AN, Ogava RL, et al. ACE2 Expression is Increased in the Lungs of Patients with Comorbidities Associated with Severe COVID-19. medRxiv. 2020;

[105] Li J, Wang X, Chen J, Zuo X, Zhang H, Deng A. COVID-19 infection may cause ketosis and ketoacidosis. Diabetes, Obes Metab. 2020;

[106] Marchand L, Pecquet M, Luyton C. Type 1 diabetes onset triggered by COVID-19. Acta Diabetol. 2020;

[107] Akter F, Mannan A, Mehedi HMH, Rob MA, Ahmed S, Salauddin A, et al. Clinical characteristics and short term outcomes after recovery from COVID-19 in patients with and without diabetes in Bangladesh. Diabetes Metab Syndr Clin Res Rev. 2020;

[108] Alberca GGF, Solis-Castro RL, Solis-Castro ME, Alberca RW. Coronavirus disease–2019 and the intestinal tract: An overview. World J Gastroenterol [Internet]. 2021 Apr 7 [cited 2021 Apr 24];27(13):1255-66. Available from: https://www.wjgnet.com/1007-9327/full/v27/i13/1255.htm

[109] Vallianou NG, Stratigou T, Tsagarakis S. Metformin and gut microbiota: their interactions and their impact on diabetes. Hormones. 2019.

[110] Zuo T, Zhang F, Lui GCY, Yeoh YK, Li AYL, Zhan H, et al. Alterations in Gut Microbiota of Patients With COVID-19 During Time of Hospitalization. Gastroenterology. 2020;

[111] Marsh S, Aldington S, Shirtchiffe P, Weatherall M, Beasley R. Smoking and COPD: What really are the risks? [1] [Internet]. Vol. 28, European Respiratory Journal. European Respiratory Society; 2006 [cited 2020 Sep 21]. p. 883-4. Available from: www.goldcopd.com.

[112] Gilca R, de Serres G, Boulianne N, Ouhoummane N, Papenburg J, Douville-Fradet M, et al. Risk factors for hospitalization and severe outcomes of 2009 pandemic H1N1 influenza in Quebec, Canada. Influenza Other Respi Viruses. 2011;

[113] Aikphaibul P, Theerawit T, Sophonphan J, Wacharachaisurapol N, Jitrungruengnij N, Puthanakit T. Risk factors of severe hospitalized respiratory syncytial virus infection in tertiary care center in Thailand. Influenza Other Respi Viruses. 2020;

[114] Dai M, Tao L, Chen Z, Tian Z, Guo X, Allen-Gipson DS, et al. Influence of Cigarettes and Alcohol on the Severity and Death of COVID-19: A Multicenter Retrospective Study in Wuhan, China. Front Physiol [Internet]. 2020 Dec 9 [cited 2020 Dec 26];11:588553. Available from: https://www.frontiersin.org/articles/10.3389/fphys.2020.588553/full

[115] Lian J, Jin X, Hao S, Jia H, Cai H, Zhang X, et al. Epidemiological, clinical, and virological characteristics of 465 hospitalized cases of coronavirus disease 2019 (COVID-19) from Zhejiang province in China. Influenza Other Respi Viruses. 2020;

[116] Zhao Q, Meng M, Kumar R, Wu Y, Huang J, Lian N, et al. The impact of COPD and smoking history on the severity of Covid-19: A systemic review and meta-analysis. J Med Virol. 2020;

[117] Han H, Huang W, Du W, Shen Q, Yang Z, Li MD, et al. Involvement of Interferon Regulatory Factor 7 in Nicotine's Suppression of Antiviral Immune Responses. J Neuroimmune Pharmacol. 2019;

[118] Singanayagam A, Loo SL, Calderazzo M, Finney LJ, Torralbo MBT, Bakhsoliani E, et al. Antiviral immunity is impaired in COPD patients with frequent exacerbations. Am J Physiol – Lung Cell Mol Physiol. 2019;

[119] Tian Z, Zhang H, DIxon J, Traphagen N, Wyatt TA, Kharbanda K, et al. Cigarette Smoke Impairs A 2A Adenosine Receptor Mediated Wound Repair through Up-regulation of Duox-1 Expression. Sci Rep. 2017;

[120] Leung JM, Yang CX, Tam A, Shaipanich T, Hackett TL, Singhera GK, et al. ACE-2 expression in the small airway epithelia of smokers and COPD patients: implications for COVID-19. The European respiratory journal. 2020.

[121] Alberca RW, Yendo T, Aoki V, Sato MN. Asthmatic patients and COVID-19: Different disease course? Allergy. 2020;1-2.

[122] Caminati M, Lombardi C, Micheletto C, Roca E, Bigni B, Furci F, et al. Asthmatic patients in COVID-19 outbreak: Few cases despite many cases. J Allergy Clin Immunol. 2020 Jun;0(0).

[123] Alberca RW. Asthma endotypes and COVID-19. Journal of Asthma. 2020.

[124] Aveyard P, Gao M, Lindson N, Hartmann-Boyce J, Watkinson P, Young D, et al. Association between pre-existing respiratory disease and its treatment, and severe COVID-19: a population cohort study. Lancet Respir Med [Internet]. 2021 Apr [cited 2021 Apr 26];0(0). Available from: www.thelancet.com/respiratoryPublished online

[125] Cavaillè A, Brinchault-Rabin G, Dixmier A, Goupil F, Gut-Gobert C, Marchand-Adam S, et al. Comorbidities of COPD [cited 2021 Apr 25]. Available from: http://ow.ly/o5Uqu

[126] Boulet LP. Influence of comorbid conditions on asthma [Internet]. Vol. 33, European Respiratory Journal. European Respiratory Society; 2009 [cited 2021 Apr 26]. p. 897-906. Available from: www.erj.ersjournals.com/misc/

[127] Mehta V, Goel S, Kabarriti R, Cole D, Goldfi nger M, Acuna-Villaorduna A, et al. Case Fatality Rate of Cancer Patients with COVID-19 in a New York Hospital System. CANCER Discov | 935 Cancer Discov [Internet]. 2020 [cited 2021 Apr 25];10:935-76. Available from: http://cancerdiscovery.aacrjournals.org/

[128] Liu C, Zhao Y, Okwan-Duodu D, Basho R, Cui X. COVID-19 in cancer patients: risk, clinical features, and management [Internet]. Vol. 17, Cancer Biology and Medicine. Cancer Biology and Medicine; 2020 [cited 2021 Apr 12]. p. 519-27. Available from: /pmc/articles/PMC7476081/

[129] Curran EK, Godfrey J, Kline J. Mechanisms of Immune Tolerance in Leukemia and Lymphoma [Internet]. Vol. 38, Trends in Immunology. Elsevier Ltd; 2017 [cited 2021 Apr 25]. p. 513-25. Available from: /pmc/articles/PMC6049081/

[130] Dai M, Liu D, Liu M, Zhou F, Li G, Chen Z, et al. Patients with cancer appear more vulnerable to SARS-CoV-2: A multicenter study during the COVID-19 outbreak. Cancer Discov [Internet]. 2020 Jun 1 [cited 2021 Apr 25];10(6):783. Available from: https://pubmed.ncbi.nlm.nih.gov/32345594/

[131] Zhang L, Zhu F, Xie L, Wang C, Wang J, Chen R, et al. Clinical characteristics of COVID-19-infected cancer patients: a retrospective case

study in three hospitals within Wuhan, China. Ann Oncol [Internet]. 2020 Jul 1 [cited 2021 Apr 25];31(7):894-901. Available from: https://pubmed.ncbi.nlm.nih.gov/32224151/

[132] Pestana RC, Filho DC, Centrone AF, Waisbeck TMB, Rodrigues HV, Araujo SEA, et al. COVID-19 incidence and outcomes among patients with respiratory symptoms in a cancer center emergency department. Brazilian J Oncol [Internet]. 2020 [cited 2021 Apr 25];16(0):1-5. Available from: http://www.brazilianjournalofoncology.com.br/details/131/en-US/covid-19-incidence-and-outcomes-among-patients-with-respiratory-symptoms-in-a-cancer-center-emergency-department

[133] Burki TK. Cancer care in the time of COVID-19. Lancet Oncol [Internet]. 2020 May 1 [cited 2021 Apr 25];21(5):628. Available from: https://pubmed.ncbi.nlm.nih.gov/32213339/

[134] Ballow M, Notarangelo L, Grimbacher B, Cunningham-Rundles C, Stein M, Helbert M, et al. Immunodeficiencies [Internet]. Vol. 158, Clinical and Experimental Immunology. Blackwell Publishing Ltd; 2009 [cited 2021 Apr 25]. p. 14-22. Available from: /pmc/articles/PMC2801032/

[135] Sánchez-Ramón S, Bermúdez A, González-Granado LI, Rodríguez-Gallego C, Sastre A, Soler-Palacín P. Primary and Secondary Immunodeficiency Diseases in Oncohaematology: Warning Signs, Diagnosis, and Management. Front Immunol [Internet]. 2019 Mar 26 [cited 2021 Apr 25];10(MAR):586. Available from: https://www.frontiersin.org/article/10.3389/fimmu.2019.00586/full

[136] Gereige JD, Maglione PJ. Current Understanding and Recent Developments in Common Variable Immunodeficiency Associated Autoimmunity [Internet]. Vol. 10, Frontiers in Immunology. Frontiers Media S.A.; 2019 [cited 2021 Apr 25]. Available from: https://pubmed.ncbi.nlm.nih.gov/31921101/

[137] Abolhassani H, Sagvand BT, Shokuhfar T, Mirminachi B, Rezaei N, Aghamohammadi A. A review on guidelines for management and treatment of common variable immunodeficiency. Vol. 9, Expert Review of Clinical Immunology. 2013. p. 561-75.

[138] Ribeiro LC, Benites BD, Ulaf RG, Nunes TA, Costa-Lima C, Addas-Carvalho M, et al. Rapid clinical recovery of a SARS-CoV-2 infected common variable immunodeficiency patient following the infusion of COVID-19 convalescent plasma. Allergy, Asthma Clin Immunol [Internet]. 2021 Dec 1 [cited 2021 Apr 25];17(1):14. Available from: https://aacijournal.biomedcentral.com/articles/10.1186/s13223-021-00518-5

[139] Libster R, Pérez Marc G, Wappner D, Coviello S, Bianchi A, Braem V, et al. Early High-Titer Plasma Therapy to Prevent Severe Covid-19 in Older Adults. N Engl J Med. 2021;

[140] Simonovich VA, Burgos Pratx LD, Scibona P, Beruto M V., Vallone MG, Vázquez C, et al. A Randomized Trial of Convalescent Plasma in Covid-19 Severe Pneumonia. N Engl J Med. 2020;

[141] Joyner MJ, Carter RE, Senefeld JW, Klassen SA, Mills JR, Johnson PW, et al. Convalescent Plasma Antibody Levels and the Risk of Death from Covid-19. N Engl J Med. 2021;

[142] Shields AM, Burns SO, Savic S, Richter AG, Anantharachagan A, Arumugakani G, et al. COVID-19 in patients with primary and secondary immunodeficiency: The United Kingdom experience. J Allergy Clin Immunol. 2021 Mar 1;147(3):870-875.e1.

[143] Meyts I, Bucciol G, Quinti I, Neven B, Fischer A, Seoane E, et al. Coronavirus disease 2019 in patients with inborn errors of immunity: An international study. J Allergy Clin Immunol [Internet]. 2021 Feb 1 [cited 2021 Apr 25];147(2):520-31. Available from: https://pubmed.ncbi.nlm.nih.gov/32980424/

[144] Van Der Made CI, Simons A, Schuurs-Hoeijmakers J, Van Den Heuvel G, Mantere T, Kersten S, et al. Presence of Genetic Variants among Young Men with Severe COVID-19. JAMA – J Am Med Assoc [Internet]. 2020 Aug 18 [cited 2021 Apr 25];324(7):663-73. Available from: https://jamanetwork.com/

[145] Dandachi D, Geiger G, Montgomery MW, Karmen-Tuohy S, Golzy M, Antar AAR, et al. Characteristics, Comorbidities, and Outcomes in a Multicenter Registry of Patients With Human Immunodeficiency Virus and Coronavirus Disease 2019. Clin Infect Dis [Internet]. 2020 Sep 9 [cited 2021 Apr 25]; Available from: https://academic.oup.com/cid/advance-article/doi/10.1093/cid/ciaa1339/5903368

[146] Lai CC, Wang CY, Hsueh PR. Co-infections among patients with COVID-19: The need for combination therapy with non-anti-SARS-CoV-2 agents? Vol. 53, Journal of Microbiology, Immunology and Infection. Elsevier Ltd; 2020. p. 505-12.

[147] Richardson S, Hirsch JS, Narasimhan M, Crawford JM, McGinn T, Davidson KW, et al. Presenting Characteristics, Comorbidities, and Outcomes among 5700 Patients Hospitalized with COVID-19 in the New York City Area. JAMA – J Am Med Assoc. 2020;

[148] Alberca RW et al. Case Report: COVID-19 and Chagas Disease in Two Coinfected Patients. Am J Trop Med Hyg. 2020;

[149] Jankowiak Ł, Rozsa L, Tryjanowski P, Møller AP. A negative covariation between toxoplasmosis and CoVID-19 with alternative interpretations. Sci Rep [Internet]. 2020 Dec 1 [cited 2021 Apr 25];10(1):12512. Available from: https://doi.org/10.1038/s41598-020-69351-x

[150] Carvalho SFG, Vieira TM, Moura APV, Andrade MC. Should an intersection between visceral leishmaniasis endemicity and the COVID-19 pandemic be considered? [Internet]. Vol. 144, Medical Hypotheses. Churchill Livingstone; 2020 [cited 2021 Apr 25]. p. 110289. Available from: /pmc/articles/PMC7501079/

[151] Hussein MIH, Albashir AAD, Elawad OAMA, Homeida A. Malaria and COVID-19: unmasking their ties [Internet]. Vol. 19, Malaria Journal. BioMed Central Ltd; 2020 [cited 2021 Apr 25]. p. 457. Available from: https://malariajournal.biomedcentral.com/articles/10.1186/s12936-020-03541-w

[152] Ju B, Zhang Q, Ge J, Wang R, Sun J, Ge X, et al. Human neutralizing antibodies elicited by SARS-CoV-2 infection. Nature. 2020;

[153] Garibaldi BT, Wang K, Robinson ML, Zeger SL, Bandeen-Roche K, Wang MC, et al. Comparison of Time to Clinical Improvement with vs without Remdesivir Treatment in Hospitalized Patients with COVID-19. JAMA Netw Open [Internet]. 2021 Mar 24 [cited 2021 Apr 26];4(3):e213071–e213071. Available from: https://jamanetwork.com/

[154] Zhang Y, Zeng G, Pan H, Li C, Hu Y, Chu K, et al. Safety, tolerability, and immunogenicity of an inactivated SARS-CoV-2 vaccine in healthy adults

aged 18-59 years: a randomised, double-blind, placebo-controlled, phase 1/2 clinical trial. Lancet Infect Dis. 2020;

[155] Sahin U, Muik A, Derhovanessian E, Vogler I, Kranz LM, Vormehr M, et al. COVID-19 vaccine BNT162b1 elicits human antibody and TH1 T cell responses. Nature. 2020;

[156] Sadoff J, Gray G, Vandebosch A, Cárdenas V, Shukarev G, Grinsztejn B, et al. Safety and Efficacy of Single-Dose Ad26.COV2.S Vaccine against Covid-19. N Engl J Med [Internet]. 2021 Apr 21 [cited 2021 Apr 26]; NEJMoa2101544. Available from: http://www.nejm.org/doi/10.1056/NEJMoa2101544

Section 2

Manifestations of Disease

Chapter 7

Clinical Characteristics of COVID-19 Infection

Mohamed Abdullah Jaber

Abstract

The typical clinical symptoms of the patients who suffered from the novel viral pneumonia were fever, cough, and myalgia or fatigue with abnormal chest CT, and the less common symptoms were sputum production, headache, hemoptysis, and diarrhea. This new infectious agent is more likely to affect older males to cause severe respiratory diseases. Major risk factors for severe illness and mortality from COVID-19 are age, comorbidities such as: heart disease, hypertension, prior stroke, diabetes, chronic lung disease, and chronic kidney disease and associated with adverse outcomes. Loss of taste and smell preceding the onset of respiratory symptoms has been reported.

Keywords: COVID-19, Clinical, Coronavirus, SARS-CoV

1. Introduction

This chapter will discuss the clinical features of COVID-19. The epidemiology, virology, prevention, and diagnosis of COVID-19 are discussed elsewhere.

1.1 Asymptomatic infections

Asymptomatic infections have been well documented. One review estimated that 33 percent of people with SARS-CoV-2 infection never develop symptoms [1]. This estimate was based on four large population-based, cross-sectional surveys, among which the median proportion of individuals who had no symptoms at the time of a positive test was 46 percent (range 43 to 77 percent), and on 14 longitudinal studies, among which a median of 73 percent of initially asymptomatic individuals remained so on follow-up. However, there is still uncertainty around the proportion of asymptomatic infections, with a wide range reported across studies. Additionally, the definition of "asymptomatic" may vary across studies, depending on which specific symptoms were assessed.

Patients with asymptomatic infection may have objective clinical abnormalities. As an example, in a study of 24 patients with asymptomatic infection who all underwent chest computed tomography (CT), 50 percent had typical ground-glass opacities or patchy shadowing, and another 20 percent had atypical imaging abnormalities [2]. Five patients developed low-grade fever, with or without other typical symptoms, a few days after diagnosis. In another study of 55 patients with asymptomatic infection identified through contact tracing, 67 percent had CT evidence of pneumonia on admission; only two patients developed hypoxia, and all recovered [3].

As above, some individuals who are asymptomatic at the time of diagnosis go on to develop symptoms (ie, they were actually presymptomatic). In one study, symptom onset occurred a median of four days (range of three to seven) after the initial positive RT-PCR test [4].

1.2 Severity of symptomatic infection

1.2.1 Spectrum of severity and case fatality rates

The spectrum of symptomatic infection ranges from mild to critical; most infections are not severe. Specifically, disease severity may be classified as:

- Mild disease (no or mild pneumonia) was reported in 81 percent of cases.
- Severe disease (eg, with dyspnea, hypoxia, or > 50 percent lung involvement on imaging within 24 to 48 hours) was reported in 14 percent.
- Critical disease (eg, with respiratory failure, shock, or multiorgan dysfunction) was reported in 5 percent.
- The overall case fatality rate was 2.3 percent; no deaths were reported among noncritical cases.

Since many severe acute respiratory syndrome coronavirus 2 (SARS-CoV-2) infections are asymptomatic, the infection fatality rate (ie, the estimated mortality rate among all individuals with infection) is considerably lower and has been estimated by some analyses to be between 0.5 and 1 percent. Conversely, the reported case fatality rates are likely underestimates of the true case fatality rates, as many fatal infections are undiagnosed. Neither the case fatality rate nor the infection fatality rate account for the full burden of the pandemic, which includes excess mortality from other conditions because of delayed care, overburdened health care systems, and social determinants of health.

1.2.2 Risk factors for severe illness

Severe illness can occur in otherwise healthy individuals of any age, but it predominantly occurs in adults with advanced age or certain underlying medical comorbidities. Specific demographic features and laboratory abnormalities have also been associated with severe disease.

1.2.3 Increasing age

Individuals of any age can acquire SARS-CoV-2 infection, although adults of middle age and older are most commonly affected, and older adults are more likely to have severe disease.

In several cohorts of hospitalized patients with confirmed COVID-19, the median age ranged from 49 to 56 years.

Older age is also associated with increased mortality. In contrast, individuals aged 18 to 34 years accounted for only 5 percent of adults hospitalized for COVID-19 in a large health care database study and had a mortality rate of 2.7 percent; morbid obesity, hypertension, and male sex were associated with mortality in that age group.

Symptomatic infection in children and adolescents appears to be relatively uncommon; when it occurs, it is usually mild, although a small proportion experience severe and even fatal disease.

1.2.4 Comorbidities

Comorbidities and other conditions that have been associated with severe illness and mortality include Cardiovascular disease, Diabetes mellitus, Chronic obstructive pulmonary disease and other lung diseases, Cancer (in particular hematologic malignancies, lung cancer, and metastatic disease), Chronic kidney disease, Solid organ or hematopoietic stem cell transplantation, Obesity and Smoking.

1.2.5 Socioeconomic background and sex

Certain demographic features have also been associated with more severe illness. Males have comprised a disproportionately high number of critical cases and deaths in multiple cohorts worldwide. Black, Hispanic, and South Asian individuals comprise a disproportionately high number of infections and deaths due to COVID-19, likely related to underlying disparities in the social determinants of health.

1.2.6 Laboratory abnormalities

Particular laboratory features have also been associated with worse outcomes. These include, Lymphopenia, Thrombocytopenia, Elevated liver enzymes, Elevated lactate dehydrogenase (LDH), Elevated inflammatory markers (eg, C-reactive protein [CRP], ferritin) and inflammatory cytokines (ie, interleukin 6 [IL-6] and tumor necrosis factor [TNF]-alpha), Elevated D-dimer (>1 mcg/mL), Elevated prothrombin time (PT), Elevated troponin, Elevated creatine phosphokinase (CPK), Acute kidney injury. Deficiencies in certain micronutrients, in particular vitamin D, have been associated with more severe disease in observational studies.

1.2.7 Viral factors

Patients with severe disease have also been reported to have higher viral RNA levels in respiratory specimens than those with milder disease, although some studies have found no association between respiratory viral RNA levels and disease severity. Detection of viral RNA in the blood has been associated with severe disease, including organ damage (eg, lung, heart, and kidney), coagulopathy, and mortality.

1.2.8 Genetic factors

Host genetic factors are also being evaluated for associations with severe disease. One genome-wide association study identified a relationship between polymorphisms in the genes encoding the ABO blood group and respiratory failure from COVID-19 (type A associated with a higher risk) [5]. Type O has been associated with a lower risk of both infection and severe disease [6].

1.3 Incubation period

The incubation period for COVID-19 is generally within 14 days following exposure, with most cases occurring approximately four to five days after exposure. However, determinations of the incubation period can be imprecise and may differ by the method of assessing exposure and the specific calculations used for the estimate.

1.4 Initial presentation

Among patients with symptomatic COVID-19, cough, myalgias, and headache are the most commonly reported symptoms. Other features, including diarrhea, sore throat, and smell or taste abnormalities. Pneumonia is the most frequent serious manifestation of infection, characterized primarily by fever, cough, dyspnea, and bilateral infiltrates on chest imaging. Although some clinical features (in particular smell or taste disorders) are more common with COVID-19 than with other viral respiratory infections, there are no specific symptoms or signs that can reliably distinguish COVID-19. However, development of dyspnea approximately one week after the onset of initial symptoms may be suggestive of COVID-19.

The range of associated symptoms includes; Cough in 50 percent, Fever in 43 percent, Myalgia in 36 percent, Headache in 34 percent, Dyspnea in 29 percent, Sore throat in 20 percent, Diarrhea in 19 percent, Nausea/vomiting in 12 percent, Loss of smell or taste, abdominal pain, and rhinorrhea in fewer than 10 percent each.

In a meta-analysis of observational studies, the pooled prevalence estimates for smell or taste abnormalities were 52 and 44 percent, respectively (although rates ranged from 5 to 98 percent across studies) [7]. However, the rate of objective smell or taste anomalies may be lower than the self-reported rates.

Most subjective smell and taste disorders associated with COVID-19 do not appear to be permanent; in a follow-up survey of the 202 patients with COVID-19, 89 percent of those who noted smell or taste alterations reported resolution or improvement by four weeks [8].

Although not noted in the majority of patients, gastrointestinal symptoms (eg, nausea and diarrhea) may be the presenting complaint in some patients. In a systematic review of studies reporting on gastrointestinal symptoms in patients with confirmed COVID-19, the pooled prevalence was 18 percent overall, with diarrhea, nausea/vomiting, or abdominal pain reported in 13, 10, and 9 percent, respectively [9].

Nonspecific signs and symptoms, such as falls, general health decline, and delirium, have been described in older adults, particularly those over 80 years old and those with underlying neurocognitive impairments.

Dermatologic findings in patients with COVID-19 are not well characterized. There have been reports of maculopapular, urticarial, and vesicular eruptions and transient livedo reticularis. Reddish-purple nodules on the distal digits similar in appearance to pernio have also been described, mainly in children and young adults with documented or suspected COVID-19.

1.5 Acute course and complications

Symptomatic infection can range from mild to critical. Some patients with initially non-severe symptoms may progress over the course of a week. In one study of 138 patients hospitalized in Wuhan for pneumonia due to severe acute respiratory syndrome coronavirus 2 (SARS-CoV-2), dyspnea developed after a median of five days since the onset of symptoms, and hospital admission occurred after a median of seven days of symptoms [10].

1.5.1 Recovery and long-term sequelae

The time to recovery from COVID-19 is highly variable and depends on age and pre-existing comorbidities in addition to illness severity. Individuals with mild infection are expected to recover relatively quickly (eg, within two weeks) whereas many individuals with severe disease have a longer time to recovery (eg, two to three months). The most common persistent symptoms include fatigue, dyspnea, chest pain, cough, and cognitive deficits. Data also suggest the potential for ongoing respiratory impairment and cardiac sequelae. Some patients who have recovered from COVID-19 have persistently or recurrently positive nucleic acid amplification tests (NAATs) for SARS-CoV-2. Although recurrent infection or reinfection cannot be definitively ruled out in these settings, evidence suggests that these are unlikely.

2. Special populations

2.1 Pregnant and breastfeeding women

The general approach to prevention, evaluation, diagnosis, and treatment of pregnant women with suspected COVID-19 is largely similar to that in nonpregnant individuals.

2.2 Children

Symptomatic infection in children appears to be relatively uncommon; when it occurs, it is usually mild, although severe cases have been reported.

2.3 People with HIV

The impact of HIV infection on the natural history of COVID-19 is uncertain. The clinical features appear the same as in the general population. However, many of the comorbid conditions associated with severe COVID-19 (eg, cardiovascular disease) occur frequently among persons with HIV, and it is unclear whether these or other potential confounding features, rather than HIV infection itself, contribute to the risk. Low CD4 cell count may be associated with critical illness and death in patients with HIV and COVID-19.

3. Oral manifestations associated with COVID-19

Although many physicians continue to question the direct link between SARS-CoV-2 and oral disease, studies suggest that the mouth might be the most vulnerable area to this virus due to the abundance of the ACE2 (angiotensin converting enzyme) receptor in oral tissue.

The ACE2 receptor has been well-documented to be the target receptor of the SARS-CoV-2 virus and the portal of entry into the human cell. Compared with other oral tissues, cells of the salivary glands, tongue, and tonsils carry the most RNA linked to proteins that the SARS-CoV-2 virus needs to infect cells [11].

Oral manifestations associated with COVID-19 infection includes:

3.1 Gingival inflammation

Bleeding and inflammation in oral tissue have been suggested to be a result of a generalized increase in inflammation due to elevated levels of cytokines and interleukins initiated by the SARS CoV-2 virus. COVID-19 disease severity has been linked to an immune dysregulation, leading to a cytokine storm. Periodontal disease can increase levels of circulating cytokines, particularly interleukin-6 (IL-6), which has been implicated as one of the major interleukins leading to the cytokine storm [12] and periodontal disease is currently being examined as a possible contributing disease toward COVID-19 severity.

3.2 Xerostomia (dry mouth)

COVID-19 has been suggested to cause dry mouth for a variety of reasons. The most common is mouth breathing by an individual due to mask use. Mouth breathing can desiccate oral tissue especially without frequent hydration. Studies suggest that another biologic mechanism involves viral entry into the salivary glands, which are known to be abundant in the ACE2 receptor [13].

3.3 Oral ulcerations and gingival tissue breakdown

COVID-19 has been associated with vascular anomalies due to viral damage of blood vessels a process whereby the virus gains entry into the endothelial cells that line blood vessels via the ACE2 receptor and damages them. Tissue necrosis, including oral ulcerations, can be the result of vessel damage. Ulceration and tissue damage can be further exacerbated by increased inflammation and upregulation in inflammatory markers due to the SARS-CoV-2 virus [14].

3.4 Loss of taste and smell

A sudden onset in loss of taste (ageusia) and smell (anosmia) are two symptoms that can be the earliest indicators of COVID-19. An average of 47% (up to 80%) of individuals who test positive for COVID-19 can have subjective complaints of taste and smell loss, particularly in cases of asymptomatic or mild disease [15]. The mechanism behind this loss is suspected to be viral disruption of cranial nerves 1, 7, 9, and 10, as well as the supporting cells of neural transmission [16]. In addition, because the tongue has an abundance of ACE2 receptors, direct viral entry into tongue cells is possible.

4. Laboratory findings

Common laboratory findings among hospitalized patients with COVID-19 include lymphopenia, elevated aminotransaminase levels, elevated lactate dehydrogenase levels, elevated inflammatory markers (eg, ferritin, C-reactive protein, and erythrocyte sedimentation rate), and abnormalities in coagulation tests. Lymphopenia is especially common, even though the total white blood cell count can vary. On admission, many patients with pneumonia have normal serum procalcitonin levels; however, in those requiring ICU care, they are more likely to be elevated. Several laboratory features, including high D-dimer levels and more severe lymphopenia, have been associated with critical illness or mortality.

5. Imaging findings

5.1 Chest radiographs

Chest radiographs may be normal in early or mild disease. Common abnormal radiograph findings were consolidation and ground-glass opacities, with bilateral, peripheral, and lower lung zone distributions; lung involvement increased over the course of illness, with a peak in severity at 10 to 12 days after symptom onset.

Spontaneous pneumothorax has also been described, although it is relatively uncommon.

5.2 Chest CT

Although chest computed tomography (CT) may be more sensitive than chest radiograph and some chest CT findings may be characteristic of COVID-19, no finding can completely rule in or rule out the possibility of COVID-19. Chest CT in patients with COVID-19 most commonly demonstrates ground-glass opacification with or without consolidative abnormalities, consistent with viral pneumonia. In a systematic review of studies evaluating the chest CT findings in over 2700 patients with COVID-19, the following abnormalities were noted: Ground-glass opacifications, Ground-glass opacifications with mixed consolidation, adjacent pleural thickening, Interlobular septal thickening, Air bronchograms. Other less common findings were a crazy paving pattern (ground-glass opacifications with superimposed septal thickening), bronchiectasis, pleural effusion, pericardial effusion, and lymphadenopathy. Chest CT abnormalities in COVID-19 are often bilateral, have a peripheral distribution, and involve the lower lobes.

Although these findings are common in COVID-19, they are not unique to it and are frequently seen with other viral pneumonias.

As with chest radiographs, chest CT may be normal soon after the onset of symptoms, with abnormalities more likely to develop over the course of illness. However, chest CT abnormalities have also been identified in patients prior to the development of symptoms and even prior to the detection of viral RNA from upper respiratory specimens. Among patients who clinically improve, resolution of radiographic abnormalities may lag behind improvements in fever and hypoxia.

5.3 Lung ultrasound

Findings on lung ultrasound in patients with documented COVID-19 have included thickening, discontinuation, and interruption of the pleural line; B lines visible under the pleura that appear discrete, multifocal, or confluent; patchy, strip, and nodular consolidations; and air bronchogram signs in the consolidations.

6. Complications of COVID-19

Several complications of COVID-19 have been described:

6.1 Respiratory failure

Acute respiratory distress syndrome (ARDS) is the major complication in patients with severe disease and can manifest shortly after the onset of dyspnea.

6.2 Cardiac and cardiovascular complications

Other complications have included arrhythmias, myocardial injury, heart failure, and shock.

6.3 Thromboembolic complications

Venous thromboembolism (VTE), including extensive deep vein thrombosis (DVT) and pulmonary embolism (PE), is common in severely ill patients with COVID-19, particularly among patients in the intensive care unit (ICU), among whom reported rates have ranged from 10 to 40 percent. Arterial thrombotic events, including acute stroke (even in patients younger than 50 years of age without risk factors) and limb ischemia, have also been reported.

6.4 Neurologic complications

Encephalopathy is a common complication of COVID-19, particularly among critically ill patients; Stroke, movement disorders, motor and sensory deficits, ataxia, and seizures occur less frequently.

6.5 Inflammatory complications

Some patients with severe COVID-19 have laboratory evidence of an exuberant inflammatory response, with persistent fevers, elevated inflammatory markers (eg, D-dimer, ferritin), and elevated proinflammatory cytokines; these laboratory abnormalities have been associated with critical and fatal illnesses. Although these features had been likened to cytokine release syndrome (eg, in response to T cell immunotherapy), the levels of proinflammatory cytokines in COVID-19 are substantially lower than those seen with cytokine release syndrome as well as with sepsis. Other inflammatory complications and auto-antibody-mediated manifestations have been described.

Guillain-Barré syndrome may occur, with onset 5 to 10 days after initial symptoms. A multisystem inflammatory syndrome with clinical features similar to those of Kawasaki disease and toxic shock syndrome has also been described in children with COVID-19. In the rare adults in whom it has been reported, this syndrome has been characterized by markedly elevated inflammatory markers and multiorgan dysfunction (in particular cardiac dysfunction), but minimal pulmonary involvement.

6.6 Secondary infections

Secondary infections do not appear to be common complications of COVID-19 overall, the reported rate of bacterial or fungal coinfections was 8 percent; these included mainly respiratory infections and bacteremia. Several reports have described presumptive invasive aspergillosis among immunocompetent patients with ARDS from COVID-19, although the frequency of this complication is uncertain.

Autopsy studies have noted detectable SARS-CoV-2 RNA (and, in some cases, antigen) in the kidneys, liver, heart, brain, and blood in addition to respiratory tract specimens, suggesting that the virus disseminates systemically in some cases; whether direct viral cytopathic effects at these sites contribute to the complications observed is uncertain.

7. Summary

The clinical spectrum of severe acute respiratory syndrome coronavirus 2 (SARS-COV-2) infection ranges from asymptomatic infection to critical and fatal illness. The proportion of infections that are asymptomatic is uncertain, as the definition of "asymptomatic" varies across studies and longitudinal follow-up to identify those who ultimately develop symptoms is often not performed. Nevertheless, some estimates suggest that up to 40 percent of infections are asymptomatic.

Most symptomatic infections are mild. Severe disease (eg, with hypoxia and pneumonia) has been reported in 15 to 20 percent of symptomatic infections; it can occur in otherwise healthy individuals of any age, but predominantly occurs in adults with advanced age or certain underlying medical comorbidities.

Cough, myalgias, and headache are the most commonly reported symptoms. Other features, including diarrhea, sore throat, and smell or taste abnormalities, are also well described. Pneumonia, with fever, cough, dyspnea, and infiltrates on chest imaging, is the most frequent serious manifestation of infection. There are no specific clinical features that can yet reliably distinguish COVID-19 from other viral respiratory infections.

Certain laboratory features, such as lymphopenia, elevated D-dimer, and elevated inflammatory markers have been associated with severe COVID-19.

Acute respiratory distress syndrome (ARDS) is the major complication in patients with severe disease and can manifest shortly after the onset of dyspnea. Other complications of severe illness include thromboembolic events, acute cardiac injury, kidney injury, and inflammatory complications.

The possibility of COVID-19 should be considered primarily in patients with compatible symptoms, in particular fever and/or respiratory tract symptoms, who reside in or have traveled to areas with community transmission or who have had recent close contact with a confirmed or suspected individual with COVID-19. All symptomatic patients with suspected SARS-CoV-2 infection should undergo testing.

Author details

Mohamed Abdullah Jaber
College of Dentistry, Ajman University, Ajman, United Arab Emirates

*Address all correspondence to: mjaber4@hotmail.com

References

[1] Oran DP, Topol EJ. The Proportion of SARS-CoV-2 Infections That Are Asymptomatic: A Systematic Review. Ann Intern Med 2021.

[2] Hu Z, Song C, Xu C, et al. Clinical characteristics of 24 asymptomatic infections with COVID-19 screened among close contacts in Nanjing, China. Sci China Life Sci 2020; 63:706.

[3] Wang Y, Liu Y, Liu L, et al. Clinical Outcomes in 55 Patients With Severe Acute Respiratory Syndrome Coronavirus 2 Who Were Asymptomatic at Hospital Admission in Shenzhen, China. J Infect Dis 2020; 221:1770.

[4] Sakurai A, Sasaki T, Kato S, et al. Natural History of Asymptomatic SARS-CoV-2 Infection. N Engl J Med 2020; 383:885.

[5] Severe Covid-19 GWAS Group, Ellinghaus D, Degenhardt F, et al. Genomewide Association Study of Severe Covid-19 with Respiratory Failure. N Engl J Med 2020; 383:1522.

[6] Ray JG, Schull MJ, Vermeulen MJ, Park AL. Association Between ABO and Rh Blood Groups and SARS-CoV-2 Infection or Severe COVID-19 Illness: A Population-Based Cohort Study. Ann Intern Med 2021; 174:308.

[7] Tong JY, Wong A, Zhu D, et al. The Prevalence of Olfactory and Gustatory Dysfunction in COVID-19 Patients: A Systematic Review and Meta-analysis. Otolaryngol Head Neck Surg 2020; 163:3.

[8] Boscolo-Rizzo P, Borsetto D, Fabbris C, et al. Evolution of Altered Sense of Smell or Taste in Patients With Mildly Symptomatic COVID-19. JAMA Otolaryngol Head Neck Surg 2020.

[9] Cheung KS, Hung IFN, Chan PPY, et al. Gastrointestinal Manifestations of SARS-CoV-2 Infection and Virus Load in Fecal Samples From a Hong Kong Cohort: Systematic Review and Meta-analysis. Gastroenterology 2020; 159:81.

[10] Wang D, Hu B, Hu C, et al. Clinical Characteristics of 138 Hospitalized Patients With 2019 Novel Coronavirus-Infected Pneumonia in Wuhan, China. JAMA 2020; 323:1061.

[11] Huang N, Perez P, Kato T, et al. Integrated single-cell atlases reveal an oral SARS-CoV-2 infection and transmission axis. *medRxiv*. 2020;2020.10.26.20219089. doi:10.1101/2020.10.26.20219089

[12] Tanaka T, Narazaki M, Kishimoto T. Immunotherapeutic implications of IL-6 blockade for cytokine storm. Immunotherapy. 2016;8(8):959-970. doi:10.2217/imt-2016-0020

[13] Xu J, Li Y, Gan F, Du Y, Yao Y. Salivary glands: potential reservoirs for COVID-19 asymptomatic infection. J Dent Res. 2020;99(8):989.

[14] Sampson V, Kamona N, Sampson A. Could there be a link between oral hygiene and the severity of SARS-CoV-2 infections? Br Dent J. 2020;228(12): 971-975.

[15] Agyeman AA, Chin KL, Landersdorfer CB, Liew D, Ofori-Asenso R. Smell and taste dysfunction in patients with COVID-19: a systematic review and meta-analysis. Mayo Clin Proc. 2020;95(8):1621-1631.

[16] Brann DH, Tsukahara T, Weinreb C, et al. Non-neuronal expression of SARS-CoV-2 entry genes in the olfactory system suggests mechanisms underlying COVID-19–associated anosmia. *Sci Adv*. 2020;6(31):eabc5801.

Chapter 8

Loss of Smell and Taste as Clinical Onset of COVID-19

Nihal Seden

Abstract

Initially, symptoms of COVID-19 associated with Ear-Nose-Throat were thought to be flulike symptoms in the foreground. Such as fever, chills, cough, dyspnoea, myalgia, headache, sore throat. Olfactory and gustatory dysfunction was not a noticeable symptom at first. As the number of cases has risen worldwide, sudden onset hyposmia/anosmia has received increasing attention as a symptom of COVID-19. The reported incidence of anosmia varies internationally: as low as 30% in South Korea, and as high as 88% in Europe. The loss of smell that occurs in COVID-19 infection its general character is sudden onset anosmia. There is currently no specific treatment for COVID-19 related anosmia. Olfactory dysfunction can heal spontaneously. However, not a small number of patients may have permanent impairment.

Keywords: olfactory dysfunction, postviral anosmia, COVID-19 related anosmia, ENT

1. Introduction

Like all healthcare workers, Ear-Nose-Throat (ENT) specialists did not hesitate to take part in the forefront of the epidemic, and investigated the issues where they could benefit both in terms of their expertise and as primary physicians in combating the pandemic.

Initially, symptoms of COVID-19 associated with ENT were thought to be flulike symptoms in the foreground. Such as fever, chills, cough, dyspnoea, myalgia, headache, sore throat, etc. [1]. Olfactory and gustatory dysfunction was not a noticeable symptom at first. In the first studies reported from China, there were no evidence of patients with symptoms of changes and/or loss of smell and taste [2–4]. As the number of cases has risen worldwide, sudden onset hyposmia/anosmia was received increasing attention as a symptom of COVID-19. Due to the efforts of the American Academy of Otolaryngology-Head and Neck Surgery and the British Association of Otorhinolaryngology-Head and Neck Surgery, sudden onset hyposmia and anosmia were accepted as symptoms of COVID-19 by the Centers for Disease Control and Prevention (CDC) and the World Health Organization on 17 April 2020 and 4 May 2020, respectively [5–7]. The reported incidence of anosmia varies internationally: as low as 30% in South Korea, and as high as 88% in Europe [8]. Various hypotheses are on the agenda as to what might cause this difference. One hypothesis is focused on the ethnicity-host factor. A meta-analysis, reported on nearly 40,000 patients across 104 studies found that anosmia (and ageusia) is more prevalent in Caucasians than Asians (54.8 vs. 17.7%, respectively) [9]. In another hypothesis, spike protein mutations - pathogenic factor - are questioned as the cause of the difference in smell loss [10].

In a multicenter European study, a total of 357 patients (85.6%) had olfactory dysfunction related to COVID-19 infection. Among them, 284 (79.6%) patients were anosmic, and 73 (20.4%) were hyposmic. Phantosmia and parosmia were noted in 12.6% and 32.4% of the patients during the disease course, respectively [11]. As we leave behind a year of the pandemic today, the sudden onset of odor loss and taste disturbance are now among the most important ENT-related symptoms, and olfactory disorder is the best predictor of COVID-19 status of all the associated symptoms [12].

2. Pathophysiolgy

Coronaviruses are known to cause odor loss from previous studies [13]. However, the pathophysiological mechanism of COVID-19 that causes odor and taste disorders has not been fully clarified yet.

2.1 Pathophysiolgy of gustatory dysfunction

In humans, the sense of taste is carried by three cranial nerves. Facial nerve (7th cranial nerve), glossopharyngeal nerve (9th cranial nerve) and vagus (10th cranial nerve). When the terminal branches are stimulated, the sense of taste reaches to the nucleus solitarius in the brainstem and then it is carried to the thalamus. Hypogeusia can develop through the involvement of one of these three nerves, the nucleus solitarius or tract, or any of the thalamus nuclei. Angiotensin-Converting Enzyme 2 (ACE2) receptors, which allow SARS-CoV-2 to attach to the tissue, are widely expressed in the mucous membrane of the entire oral cavity, especially in the tongue [14–16]. The role of ACE2 in modulating taste perception has been emphasized in many studies analyzing the chemosensitive side effects of ACE2 inhibitors and angiotensin II blockers [16, 17]. Taste disturbance usually regresses after cessation of treatment. Also, a condition recently identified for SARS-CoV-2 is that it can bind to sialic acid receptors [18]. Sialic acid is an essential component of saliva mucin and protects glycoproteins that transport taste molecules into taste pores from early enzymatic degradation [16]. A decrease in sialic acid in saliva is associated with an increase in the threshold of taste [19]. Although it has been suggested that the deterioration in the perception of smell may also cause the loss of taste function due to the close functional link between these two chemosensory systems, the sense of taste seems to be more affected in recent publications.

2.2 Pathophysiolgy of olfactory dysfunction

Chen et al. reported that ACE2 immunohistochemical expression was 200 to 700 times greater in the sustentacular cells of the olfactory neuroepithelium than nasal or tracheal epithelia [20]. An animal study, showed increase in macrophages in the olfactory ephitelium and lamina propria after SARS-CoV-2 infection [21]. Generally, most data indicate that the main targets of SARS-CoV-2 are sustentacular cells in the olfactory epithelium [20–24].

These results show that hyposmia or anosmia is mainly caused by nasal epithelial infection and not a result of general malaise.

3. Diagnosis of olfactory and taste disorders in COVID-19

In many studies on the transmission method of the SARS-CoV-2 virus, it has been shown that this virus is transmitted by droplets. Objective olfactory tests may pose a risk of contamination and therefore require extra precaution.

Commonly used objective olfactory tests are the Connecticut Chemosensory Clinical Research Center (CCCRC) test, University of Pennsylvania Smell Identification test (UPSIT), the Sniffin' Sticks method and the Odor Stick Identification test (OSIT). The UPSIT has four "scratch and sniff" booklets that each contain 10 microcapsule fragrances. After people open the capsule, they smell the page in the booklet [25, 26]. In the CCCRC test, fragrances are offered in bottles that are not transparent [27]. Sniffin' Sticks are felt tip pens impregnated with scents that are handed to the patient to smell [28]. In the OSIT test, the researcher folds a piece of fragrant paraffin paper in half to crush the microcapsule and then offers it to the participant. The participant then opens and smells the paper [29]. For the Sniffin' Sticks and CCCRC tests, the odor threshold is considered along with the ability for odor discrimination, while discrimination alone is assessed in the UPSIT and OSIT.

As for the taste, since taste tests can be performed with disposable strips, they can be used safely in patients with taste disorders.

Many studies have been published on COVID-19 and odor disorders since the beginning of the pandemic, and because of the contamination risk, the vast majority were subjective reports based on questionnaires or self-reports [30–32]. However, in studies that will be done by performing objective odor tests on patients, reports about the importance of obtaining data started to increase; for example Leichen et al. examined 86 patients for anosmia and hyposmia rates by testing with Sniffin' Sticks test, which is a psychophysical odor test. A total of 33 (38%) patients who reported that they had a loss of smell were normosmic according to the Sniffin' Sticks test. In the anosmic group, 78.8% of the patients stated that they had a loss of smell [33]. We had managed to evaluate olfactory objectively, without any risk of contamination, by a method that we described at our study [34].

4. Clinical features

The general feature of loss of smell in COVID-19 infection is sudden onset anosmia. Gane et al., stated in their case series, the isolated sudden onset anosmia syndrome (ISOA), could be the only finding of COVID-19 without any other symptoms [35]. Usually, olfactory disorder is not accompanied by nasal congestion or rhinorrhea.

Olfactory dysfunction due to COVID-19 infection seems to effect females and young individuals more commonly.

Is this odor dysfunction completely reversible, or how long should a patient wait for full recovery of olfactory function? There have been many studies on the alleviation of the loss of smell in COVID-19 [36–45].

Complete recovery of olfactory dysfunction varies between 11-49% and up to 25% of the patients seems to show no improvement at all.

5. Treatment

There is currently no specific treatment for COVID-19 related anosmia. Olfactory dysfunction can heal spontaneously. However, not a small number of patients may have permanent impairment. Efficacy of the treatments are unknown due to lack of data; treatments targeting post-infectious olfactory dysfunction could potentially be beneficial for COVID-19. While the use of systemic steroids is not recommended in patients with odor loss, the use of spray form and long applicators has been found appropriate for nasal steroids [46]. Fragrance therapy gives successful results in postviral odor loss, especially when it is started early and used for at least three months. Therefore, in the loss of smell associated with COVID-19, fragrance therapy, including rose, lemon, clove and eucalyptus fragrances, each scent is sniffed for twenty seconds twice a day [47].

6. Other ENT related symptoms of COVID-19

In patients without pneumonia, the COVID-19 clinic is similar to some diseases frequently encountered by ENT physicians in the outpatient clinic. COVID-19 can be confused with the flu or common cold in terms of initial symptoms, causing patients to apply to the ENT clinic in the foreground. There may be serous nasal discharge, hyperemic oropharynx, watery eyes and tearing. Since hoarseness is not among the symptoms mentioned, it may be thought that there is no cause of laryngitis or findings similar to laryngitis are not found on examination. Sore throat is a common symptom of COVID-19. Most of pharyngitis or sore throat is of viral origin and these pathogens are predominantly rhinovirus, influenza, adenovirus, coronavirus (previously isolated types) and parainfluenza virus [48].

Other human corona viruses are common cause of viral pharyngitis. Considering that, Sars-CoV-2 is likely to cause pharyngitis and/or similar clinical features.

Both possibilities should be kept in mind in a patient presenting with hyperemia in the oropharynx and difficulty swallowing. Unfortunately, in the current situation, definitive diagnosis distinction can only be made by laboratory testing. The rapid progression and sudden onset of the disease should be thought-provoking for COVID-19.

It should be kept in mind that COVID-19 can also cause rhinitis. It may have similar symptoms with allergic rhinitis. Although fatigue and weakness due to sleep disturbance in allergic rhinitis are reported; muscle pain, malaise and sore throat are not expected. Watery and red eyes may occur in both diseases, but itching in the eyes, palate and nose can be a guide for allergic diseases. Likewise, flu and cold are other common diseases that can be confused with COVID-19. While runny nose is more common in colds than other diseases, in influenza and Sars-CoV-2 infection dry cough is in the foreground.

7. Conclusions

In the fight against COVID-19, it would not be wrong to say that the most important and alarming symptoms specifically to ENT are odor and taste disorders. It should be kept in mind that these deficits do not heal completely in all patients.

Conflict of interest

None.

Thanks

I dedicate this book chapter to all healthcare professionals who work devotedly in combating the epidemic, and especially to colleagues who have lost their lives.

With respect and mercy.

Author details

Nihal Seden
Ear Nose Throat Clinic, Istanbul Training and Research Hospital, University of Health Sciences, Istanbul, Turkey

*Address all correspondence to: nihalseden@hotmail.com

References

[1] Symptoms of Coronavirus. https://www.cdc.gov/coronavirus/2019-ncov/symptoms-testing/symptoms.html [Accessed: 2020-03-08]

[2] Chen N, Zhou M, Dong X, et al. Epidemiological and clinical characteristics of 99 cases of 2019 novel coronavirus pneumonia in Wuhan, China: a descriptive study. Lancet. 2020;395(10223):507-513. doi:10.1016/S0140-6736(20)30211-7

[3] Chen T, Dai Z, Mo P, et al. Clinical Characteristics and Outcomes of Older Patients with Coronavirus Disease 2019 (COVID-19) in Wuhan, China: A Single-Centered, Retrospective Study. J Gerontol A Biol Sci Med Sci. 2020;75(9):1788-1795. doi:10.1093/gerona/glaa089

[4] Guan WJ, Ni ZY, Hu Y, et al. Clinical Characteristics of Coronavirus Disease 2019 in China. N Engl J Med. 2020;382(18):1708-1720. doi:10.1056/NEJMoa2002032

[5] AAO-HNS. Anosmia, hyposmia, and dysgeusia symptoms of coronavirus disease. https://www.entnet.org/content/aao-hns-anosmia-hyposmia-and-dysgeusia-symptoms-coronavirus-disease; [Accessed: 2020-03-22]

[6] Q&A on coronaviruses (COVID-19)17 April 2020 Q&A. https://www.who.int/emergencies/diseases/novel-coronavirus-2019/question-and-answers-hub/q-a-detail/q-a-coronaviruses [Accessed: 2020-04-17]

[7] Hopkins, C., and Kumar, N. Loss of sense of smell as marker of COVID-19 infection, ENT UK. https://www.entuk.org/sites/default/files/files/Loss%20of%20sense%20of%20smell%20as%20marker%20of%20COVID.pdf (accessed 2020-3-20).

[8] Strauss SB, Lantos JE, Heier LA, Shatzkes DR, Phillips CD. Olfactory Bulb Signal Abnormality in Patients with COVID-19 Who Present with Neurologic Symptoms. AJNR Am J Neuroradiol. 2020;41(10):1882-1887. doi:10.3174/ajnr.A6751

[9] von Bartheld, C. S., Hagen, M. M., and Butowt, R. (2020). Prevalence of chemosensory dysfunction in COVID-19 patients: a systematic review and meta-analysis reveals significant ethnic differences. ACS Chem. Neurosci. 11, 2944-2961. doi:10.1021/acschemneuro.0c00460

[10] Butowt R, Bilinska K, Von Bartheld CS. Chemosensory Dysfunction in COVID-19: Integration of Genetic and Epidemiological Data Points to D614G Spike Protein Variant as a Contributing Factor. ACS Chem Neurosci. 2020;11(20):3180-3184. doi:10.1021/acschemneuro.0c00596

[11] Lechien JR, Chiesa-Estomba CM, De Siati DR, et al. Olfactory and gustatory dysfunctions as a clinical presentation of mild-to-moderate forms of the coronavirus disease (COVID-19): a multicenter European study. Eur Arch Otorhinolaryngol 2020;277(8):2251-61. https://doi.org/10.1007/s00405-020-05965-1.

[12] Menni C, Valdes AM, Freidin MB, et al. Real-time tracking of self-reported symptoms to predict potential COVID-19. Nat Med. 2020;26(7):1037-1040. doi:10.1038/s41591-020-0916-2

[13] Suzuki M, Saito K, Min Wp, et al. Identification of viruses in patients with postviral olfactory dysfunction. Laryngoscope. 2007. doi:10.1097/01.mlg.0000249922.37381.1e.

[14] Xu H, Zhong L, Deng J, et al. High expression of ACE2 receptor of 2019-nCoV on the epithelial cells of oral mucosa. Int J Oral Sci. 2020;12(1):8. Published 2020 Feb 24. doi:10.1038/s41368-020-0074-x

[15] Vaira LA, Salzano G, Fois AG, Piombino P, De Riu G. Potential pathogenesis of ageusia and anosmia in COVID-19 patients. Int Forum Allergy Rhinol. 2020;10(9):1103-1104. doi:10.1002/alr.22593

[16] Tsuruoka S, Wakaumi M, Araki N, Ioka T, Sugimoto K, Fujimura A. Comparative study of taste disturbance by losartan and perindopril in healthy volunteers. J Clin Pharmacol. 2005; 45(11):1319-1323. doi:10.1177/0091 270005280445

[17] Suliburska J, Duda G, Pupek-Musialik D. The influence of hypotensive drugs on the taste sensitivity in patients with primary hypertension. Acta Pol Pharm. 2012;69(1):121-127.

[18] Milanetti M, Miotto M, Di Rienzo L, Monti M, Gosti G, Ruocco G. In-Silico evidence for two receptors based strategy of SARS-CoV-2. ArXiv: 2003.11107.

[19] Pushpass RG, Pellicciotta N, Kelly C, Proctor G, Carpenter GH. Reduced Salivary Mucin Binding and Glycosylation in Older Adults Influences Taste in an In Vitro Cell Model. Nutrients. 2019;11(10):2280. Published 2019 Sep 24. doi:10.3390/nu11102280

[20] Chen M, Shen W, Rowan NR, Kulaga H, Hillel A, Ramanathan M Jr, Lane AP. Elevated ACE2 expression in the olfactory neuroepithelium: implications for anosmia and upper respiratory SARS-CoV-2 entry and replication. bioRxiv [Preprint]. 2020 May 9:2020.05.08.084996. doi: 10.1101/2020.05.08.084996.

[21] Bryche B, St Albin A, Murri S, et al. Massive transient damage of the olfactory epithelium associated with infection of sustentacular cells by SARS-CoV-2 in golden Syrian hamsters. Brain Behav Immun. 2020;89:579-586. doi:10.1016/j.bbi.2020.06.032

[22] Piques A, Brondel L and Pénicaud L (2021) COVID 19-Induced Smell and Taste Impairments: Putative Impact on Physiology. Front. Physiol. 11:625110. doi: 10.3389/fphys.2020.625110

[23] Kirschenbaum D, Imbach LL, Ulrich S, et al. Inflammatory olfactory neuropathy in two patients with COVID-19. Lancet. 2020;396(10245):166. doi:10.1016/S0140-6736(20)31525-7

[24] Brann DH, Tsukahara T, Weinreb C, et al. Non-neuronal expression of SARS-CoV-2 entry genes in the olfactory system suggests mechanisms underlying COVID-19-associated anosmia. Sci Adv. 2020;6(31):eabc5801. doi:10.1126/sciadv.abc5801

[25] Doty RL. Olfactory dysfunction and its measurement in the clinic and workplace. Int Arch Occup Environ Health 2006;79(4):268-82. https://doi.org/10.1007/s00420-005-0055-6.

[26] Doty RL, Shaman P, Kimmelman CP, Dann MS. University of Pennsylvania Smell Identification Test: a rapid quantitative olfactory function test for the clinic. Laryngoscope 1984; 94(2 Pt 1):176-8. https://doi.org/10.1288/00005537-198402000-00004.

[27] Cain WS, Gent JF, Goodspeed RB, Leonard G. Evaluation of olfactory dysfunction in the Connecticut Chemosensory Clinical Research Center. Laryngoscope 1988;98 (1):83-8. https://doi.org/10.1288/00005537-19880 1000-00017.

[28] Hummel T, Sekinger B, Wolf SR, Pauli E, Kobal G. 'Sniffin' sticks': olfactory performance assessed by the combined testing of odor identification, odor discrimination and olfactory threshold. Chem Senses 1997;22(1):39-52. https://doi.org/10.1093/chemse/22.1.39

[29] Kobayashi M, Reiter ER, DiNardo LJ, Costanzo RM. A new clinical olfactory function test: cross-cultural influence. Arch Otolaryngol Head Neck Surg 2007;133 (4):331-6. https://doi.org/10.1001/archotol.133.4.331.

[30] Speth MM, Singer-Cornelius T, Oberle M, Gengler I, Brockmeier SJ, Sedaghat AR. Olfactory dysfunction and Sinonasal symptomatology in COVID-19: prevalence, severity, timing, and associated characteristics. Otolaryngol Head Neck Surg 2020; 163(1):114-20. https://doi.org/10.1177/0194599820929185.

[31] Baig AM, Khaleeq A, Ali U, Syeda H. Evidence of the COVID-19 virus targeting the CNS: tissue distribution, host-virus interaction, and proposed neurotropic mechanisms. ACS Chem Nerosci 2020;11(7):995-8. https://doi.org/10.1021/acschemneuro.0c00122.

[32] Yan CH, Faraji F, Prajapati DP, Boone CE, DeConde AS. Association of chemosensory dysfunction and COVID-19 in patients presenting with influenza-like symptoms. Int Forum Allergy Rhinol 2020;10(7):806-13. https://doi.org/10.1002/alr.22579.

[33] Lechien JR, Cabaraux P, Chiesa-Estomba CM, et al. Objective olfactory evaluation of self-reported loss of smell in a case series of 86 COVID-19 patients. Head Neck 2020;42(7):1583-90. https://doi.org/10.1002/hed.26279.

[34] Seden N, Yiğit E, Yiğit Ö, Kaygısız İ. Objective evaluation of odor loss in COVID-19 and other suspected cases. Am J Otolaryngol. 2021;42(1):102761. doi:10.1016/j.amjoto.2020.102761

[35] Gane SB, Kelly C, Hopkins C. Isolated sudden onset anosmia in COVID-19 infection. A novel syndrome? Rhinology. 2020. doi: 10.4193/Rhin20.114.

[36] Amer MA, Elsherif HS, Abdel-Hamid AS, Elzayat S. Early recovery patterns of olfactory disorders in COVID-19 patients; a clinical cohort study. Am J Otolaryngol. 2020 Nov-Dec;41(6):102725. doi: 10.1016/j.amjoto.2020.102725.

[37] Hopkins C, Surda P, Whitehead E, Kumar BN. Early recovery following new onset anosmia during the COVID-19 pandemic - an observational cohort study. J Otolaryngol Head Neck Surg. 2020 May 4;49(1):26. doi: 10.1186/s40463-020-00423-8.

[38] Kosugi EM, Lavinsky J, Romano FR, et al. Incomplete and late recovery of sudden olfactory dysfunction in COVID-19. Braz J Otorhinolaryngol. 2020 July-Aug;86(4):490-496. doi: 10.1016/j.bjorl.2020.05.001.

[39] Panda S, Mohamed A, Sikka K, et al. Otolaryngologic manifestation and long-term outcome in mild COVID-19: experience from a tertiary care centre in India. Indian J Otolaryngol Head Neck Surg. 2020;1-6. doi:10.1007/s12070-020-02217-w

[40] Chiesa-Estomba CM, Lechien JR, Radulesco T, et al. Patterns of smell recovery in 751 patients affected by the COVID-19 outbreak. Eur J Neurol. 2020;27(11):2318-2321. doi:10.1111/ene.14440

[41] Le Bon SD, Pisarski N, Verbeke J, et al. Psychophysical evaluation of chemosensory functions 5 weeks after olfactory loss due to COVID-19: a prospective cohort study on 72 patients. Eur Arch Otorhinolaryngol. 2020;1-8. doi:10.1007/s00405-020-06267-2

[42] Iannuzzi L, Salzo AE, Angarano G, et al. Gaining back what is lost: recovering the sense of smell in mild to moderate patients after COVID-19. Chem Senses 2020 Dec 5;45(9):875-881. doi: 10.1093/chemse/bjaa066. PMID: 33033827; PMCID: PMC7665358.

[43] Vaira LA, Hopkins C, Petrocelli M, et al. Smell and taste recovery in coronavirus disease 2019 patients: a 60-day objective and prospective study. J Laryngol Otol. 2020;134(8):703-709. doi:10.1017/S0022215120001826

[44] Otte MS, Eckel HNC, Poluschkin L, Klussmann JP, Luers JC. Olfactory

dysfunction in patients after recovering from COVID-19. Acta Otolaryngol. 2020 Dec;140(12):1032-1035. doi: 10.1080/00016489.2020.1811999. Epub 2020 Aug 27. PMID: 32852240.

[45] Boscolo-Rizzo P, Menegaldo A, Fabbris C, Spinato G, Borsetto D, Vaira LA, Calvanese L, Pettorelli A, Sonego M, Frezza D, Bertolin A, Cestaro W, Rigoli R, D'Alessandro A, Tirelli G, Da Mosto MC, Menini A, Polesel J, Hopkins C. Six-Month Psychophysical Evaluation of Olfactory Dysfunction in Patients with COVID-19. Chem Senses. 2021 Jan 1;46:bjab006. doi: 10.1093/chemse/bjab006.

[46] Vroegop AV, Eeckels AS, Rompaey V Van, et al. COVID-19 and olfactory dysfunction – an ENT perspective to the current COVID-19 pandemic. B-ENT. 2020. doi:10.5152/b-ent.2020.20127.

[47] Whitcroft KL, Hummel T. Olfactory Dysfunction in COVID-19: Diagnosis and Management. JAMA. 2020. doi:10.1001/jama.2020.8391.

[48] Wolford RW, goyal A, Belgam Syed SY, Schaefer TJ. pharyngitis. [Updated 2020 Mar 30]. In:Statpearls [Internet]. Treasure Island (Fl): Statpearls publishing; 2020. Available from: https://www.ncbi.nlm.nih.gov/books/NBK519550/

Chapter 9

Cardiovascular System and SARS-CoV-2: Etiology, Physiopathology and Clinical Presentation: A Systematic Review

Jucier Gonçalves Júnior, Estelita Lima Cândido, Gislene Farias de Oliveira and Modesto Leite Rolim Neto

Abstract

During SARS-CoV-1 and Middle East Respiratory Distress Syndrome (MERS) outbreaks it was observed a particularly elevated incidence of cardiovascular disease among patients. With COVID-19, this correlation becomes evident again. However, the cardiovascular impacts by COVID-19 pandemic are not yet well established although publications about its potential deleterious effects are constant. Thus, aimed to carry a systematic review of the literature with meta-analysis, the following question was used as a guide: what practical contributions does the scientific literature produced in the period of 2019-2020 has to offer about the impact of the COVID-19 on cardiovascular system? A systematic review of the literature using the Virtual Health Library (VHL) and PubMed with the following descriptors: #1 "*cardiovascular disease*" [MeSH] AND #2 "*COVID-19*" [keyword], as well as their equivalents in the Portuguese and Spanish language, during the period from December 2019 to March 2020 was performed. One hundred articles were found in Pubmed and twenty-seven were selected. In VHL there are 59 articles and four were selected totaling thirty-one papers. The findings were then divided into three subcategories: Etiology, Physiopathology and Risk factors of SARS-CoV-2 in Cardiovascular System; Clinical presentation, laboratory markers and imagenological aspects of SARS-CoV-2 in cardiovascular system; and Anti-Hypertensive Drugs, Cardiovascular System and SARS-CoV-2. When it comes to the cardiovascular system, these issues are aggravated and urge as a joint commitment from researchers, medical and governmental organizations to carry out more robust studies with bold methodologies aimed at mapping prognostic factors and assertive therapeutic approaches in the management of cardiovascular complications of COVID- 19.

Keywords: cardiovascular disease, coronavirus infections, clinical medicine, systematic review

1. Introduction

According to the WHO, there has been a recent increase in the burden of cardiovascular disease (CVD), especially in low and middle-income countries [1].

It is estimated that 17.7 million people died from CVD in 2015, representing 31% of all deaths globally [2]. In 2020, CVDs are the number 1 cause of death globally, taking an estimated of 17.9 million lives each year [3, 4].

COVID-19 again brought the need to discussion an extremely relevant topic that was of concern during the SARS-CoV-1 (SARS - 2002) and Middle East Respiratory Distress Syndrome (MERS - 2013) epidemics, the increase incidence of cardiovascular disease among patients [5]. Studies show that patients with comorbidities, such as hypertension, heart failure, diabetes [6] and elderly people [7] are, among other factors, risk factor for severe illness by SARS-CoV-2. Also, COVID-19 is caused by the binding of the viral surface spike protein to the human angiotensin-converting enzyme 2 (ACE2) receptor following activation of the spike protein by transmembrane protease serine 2 (TMPRSS2) [8]. Thus, the cardiovascular impacts by COVID-19 pandemic are not yet well established although publications about its potential deleterious effects are constant.

Aimed to carry a systematic review of the literature with meta-analysis, the following question was used as a guide: what practical contributions does the scientific literature produced in the period of 2019-2020 has to offer about the impact of the COVID-19 on cardiovascular system? This review highlights that in a pandemic period, cardiovascular pathologies are risk factors from a worsening result. The pandemic prevention and control measures can also be used as a way to prevent cardiovascular diseases on the population, since fewer people exposed to the virus means less cardiovascular risk.

2. Methods

2.1 Literature review

A qualitative systematic review with meta-analysis of the literature using the Virtual Health Library (VHL), which hosts recognized databases – LILACS (Literatura Latino-americana e do Caribe em Ciências da Saúde), MEDLINE, SciELO (Scientific Electronic Library Online), and PubMed was performed. Initially, the following descriptors were used: #1 "cardiovascular disease" [MeSH] AND #2 "COVID-19" [keyword], as well as their equivalents in the Portuguese and Spanish language.

2.2 Eligibility criteria

The period reported in the literature ranged from December 2019 to March 2020 since the pandemic started in this period. Compilation of the data was performed in April 2020. Manuscript selection occurred primarily through the analysis of titles and abstracts. Article analysis followed the eligibility criteria: (1) At least a combination of the terms described in the search strategy were present in the title or words that refer to the theme; (2) Articles written in English, Portuguese or Spanish; (3) Articles addressing cardiovascular impact of COVID-19 pandemic; (4) Papers repeated in more than one database were computed only once; (5) Original papers with the full text available through in a virtual library created by the Brazilian Ministry of Health where content is restricted to authorized users - the CAPES (Coordination of Personal Improvement of Higher Level) Periodicals Portal. Thesis, dissertations, and monographs were excluded. Some articles were excluded because they generally approached other viruses/pandemics or the sample was children.

Author (Year)	Journal	Sample (Study type)	Main Findings
Guo et al. [9]	JAMA Cardiol	187 patients with confirmed COVID-19 at the Seventh Hospital of Wuhan City, China (cross sectional retrospective observational study).	During hospitalization, 66 (35.3%) patients had underlying CVD including hypertension, coronary heart disease, and cardiomyopathy, and 52 (27.8%) exhibited myocardial injury as indicated by elevated TnT levels. Patients with elevated TnT levels had more frequent malignant arrhythmias, and the use of glucocorticoid therapy (37 [71.2%] vs. 69 [51.1%]) and mechanical ventilation (41 [59.6%] vs. 14 [10.4%]) were higher compared with patients with normal TnT levels.
Clerkin et al. [8]	Circulation	(Integrative Review)	COVID-19 is caused by the Severe Acute Respiratory Syndrome Coronavirus-2 (SARS-CoV-2), which invades cells through the angiotensin converting enzyme 2 (ACE2) receptor. Among those with COVID-19, there is a higher prevalence of cardiovascular disease and more than 7% of patients suffer myocardial injury from the infection (22% of the critically ill).
Bansal [10]	Diabetes Metab Syndr	(Narrative Review)	Acute cardiac injury, defined as significant elevation of cardiac troponins, is the most commonly reported cardiac abnormality in COVID-19.
Cheng et al. [11]	Curr Cardiol Rep	(Integrative Review)	Emerging epidemiological evidence suggest cardiovascular risk factors are associated with increased disease severity and mortality in COVID-19 patients. Patients with a more severe form of COVID-19 are also more likely to develop cardiac complications such as myocardial injury and arrhythmia.
Li et al. [12]	Infection Dis Poverty	31 normal human tissues (Experimental study)	ACE2 expression levels were the highest in the small intestine, testis, kidneys, heart, thyroid, and adipose tissue, and were the lowest in the blood, spleen, bone marrow, brain, blood vessels, and muscle. ACE2 showed medium expression levels in the lungs, colon, liver, bladder, and adrenal gland
Han et al. [13]	J Cardiovasc Magn Reson	(Integrative Review)	First, continued urgent and semi-urgent care for the patients who have no known active COVID-19 should be provided in a safe manner for both patients and staff. Second, when necessary, CMR on patients with confirmed or suspected active COVID-19 should focus on the specific clinical question with an emphasis on myocardial function and tissue characterization while optimizing patient and staff safety.
Slawiński and Lewicka [14]	Kardiol Pol	(Integrative Review)	Among comorbidities in patients with COVID-19, cardiovascular disease is most commonly found. And in the most common symptoms of COVID-19 dyspnea is responsible by18.6%-59%.
Berre et al. [15]	Diagn Interv Imaging.	71-year-old man with COVID-19 pneumonia (Case Report)	A case report about concomitant acute aortic thrombosis and pulmonary embolism complicating COVID-19 pneumonia
Vignera et al. [16]	Int J Mol Sci.	(Short Communication)	Data on the experimental animal have shown that 17B-estradiol increases the expression and activity of ACE2 in both adipose tissue and kidney. Spontaneously hypertensive male mice have a higher myocardial ACE2 expression than females and its levels decrease after orchiectomy
Zhu et al. [17]	Curr Cardiol Rep	(Integrative Review)	The literature reports association between history of cardiac disease and worsened outcome during COVID infection. Development of new onset myocardial injury during COVID-19 also increases mortality.

Author (Year)	Journal	Sample (Study type)	Main Findings
Celina and Oliva [18]	Diagn Interv Imaging.	60-year-old man with COVID-19 pneumonia (Case Report)	A case report about acute pulmonary embolism complicating COVID-19 pneumonia
Gonzallez-Jamarillo, Low and Franco [19]	Eur J Epidemiol.	(Short Communication)	SARS-CoV-2 infection produces enzymatic shedding that inactivates ACE2 and prevents conversion of Ang-II. This effect could in part explain the cardiovascular and respiratory manifestations of COVID-19.
Gao et al. [20]	Respir Res	102 patients with severe COVID-19 (cross sectional observational study)	N terminal pro B type natriuretic peptide (NT-proBNP) might be an independent risk factor for in-hospital death in patients with severe COVID-19.
Rico-Mesa, White and Anderson [21]	Curr Cardiol Rep	(Integrative Review)	Worse outcomes appear to be more prevalent in patients with hypertension and diabetes mellitus (DM), possibly due to overexpression of angiotensin-converting enzyme 2 (ACE2) receptor in airway alveolar epithelial cells.
Wang and Xu [22]	Cells	17,520 testicular cells (Experimental Study)	ACE2 is predominantly enriched in spermatogonia and Leydig and Sertoli cells. Gene Set Enrichment Analysis (GSEA) indicates that Gene Ontology (GO) categories associated with viral reproduction and transmission are highly enriched in ACE2-positive spermatogonia, while male gamete generation related terms are downregulated.
Rizzo et al. [23]	Basic Res Cardiol	(Short Communication)	We might be able to target Notch also to fight heart and lung disease caused directly by SARS-CoV-2 infection and by the cytokine storm in response to the virus.
Laccarino et al. [5]	High Blood Press Cardiovasc Prev	(Short Communication)	In vitro studies are available to support the eventual role of ACE inhibitors and ARBs in both the promotion and antagonism of the disease. The available literature, indeed, presents contrasting results.
Schiffrin et al. [24]	Am J Hypertens	(Short Communication)	There is as yet no evidence that hypertension is related to outcomes of COVID-19, or that ACE inhibitor or ARB use is harmful, or for that matter beneficial, during the COVID-19 pandemic.
Tan and Aboulhousn [25]	Int J Cardiol	(Integrative Review)	COVID-19 results in mild symptoms in the majority of infected patients, but can cause severe lung injury, cardiac injury, and death.
Gupta and Misra [26]	Diabetes Metab Syndr	(Integrative Review)	Patients with COVID-19 infection have elevated natriuretic peptides, significance of which is uncertain and Cardiac troponin I levels are significantly increased in patients with severe SARS- CoV-2 infection.
Gackowski et al. [27]	Kardiol Pol	(Integrative Review)	Transesophageal echocardiography is considered an aerosol-generating procedure and should be performed only as a lifesaving procedure. Personnel should use appropriate personal protection equipment in the immediate vicinity of the patients in accordance with the relevant guidelines.
Guo et al. [28]	J Am Heart Associat	(Integrative Review)	ACE2 plays a protective role in both cardiovascular diseases and acute lung injury. For uninfected patients, we tend to believe it is unnecessary to discontinue ACEIs/ARBs given the lack of evidence to support the hypothesis that ACEIs/ARBs might lead to an increased risk of SARS-CoV-2 infection. For infected patients, although higher ACE2 expression might be associated with higher viral loads, ACEIs/ARBs should not be discontinued assertively because they can block the RAS and protect patients from the potential heart injuries in COVID-19 and might also reduce the severity of lung damage caused by the infection.

Author (Year)	Journal	Sample (Study type)	Main Findings
Sommerstein et al. [29]	J Am Heart Associât	(Integrative Review)	Cardiovascular diseases and/or their therapy, by affecting ACE2 levels, may play a pivotal role with regard to infectivity and outcome of COVID-19. Whether treatment or disease induced upregulation of ACE2 influences the course of COVID-19 urgently needs to be determined.
Meng et al. [7]	Emerg Microbes Infect.	51 patients with hypertension and COVID-19 (cross sectional retrospective study)	Patients receiving ACEI or ARB therapy had a lower rate of severe diseases and a trend toward a lower level of IL-6 in peripheral blood. In addition, ACEI or ARB therapy increased CD3 and CD8 T cell counts in peripheral blood and decreased the peak viral load compared to other antihypertensive drugs.
Vanduganathan et al. [30]	N Engl J Med	(Integrative Review)	Insufficient data are available to determine whether these observations readily translate to humans, and no studies have evaluated the effects of RAAS inhibitors in Covid-19
Chen et al. [31]	Cardiovasc Res	Human heart tissues were obtained from abandon donors in Center of Cardiovascular Treatment in China (Experimental Study)	The pericytes injury due to virus infection may result in capillary endothelial cells dysfunction, inducing microvascular dysfunction. And patients with basic heart failure disease showed increased ACE2 expression at both mRNA and protein levels, meaning that if infected by the virus these patients may have higher risk of heart attack and critically ill condition.
Fang et al. [6]	Lancet Respir Med	(Short Communication)	patients with cardiac diseases, hypertension, or diabetes, who are treated with ACE2-increasing drugs, are at higher risk for severe COVID-19 infection
Chen et al. [32]	Herz	(Short Communication)	The condition of some patients with severe SARS-CoV-2 infection patients might deteriorate rapidly with acute respiratory distress syndrome and septic shock, which is eventually followed by multiple organ failure and fulminant myocarditis
Hulot et al. [33]	Arch Cardiovasc Dis	(Short Communication)	COVID-19 can be caused palpitations and chest tightness, myocardial damage with an increase in high-sensitivity cardiac troponin I.
South et al. [34]	Am J Physiol Heart Circ Physiol	(Short Communication)	In lieu of the fact that many older patients with hypertension or other CVDs are routinely treated with RAAS blockers and statins, new clinical concerns have developed regarding whether these patients are at greater risk for SARS-CoV-2 infection, whether RAAS and statin therapy should be discontinued, and the potential consequences of RAAS blockade to COVID-19-related pathologies such as acute and chronic respiratory disease.
Abassi et al. [35]	Am J Physiol Heart Circ Physiol	(Short Communication)	In patients infected with SARS-CoV-2, ACE2 may transform to a Trojan horse. Its binding with ACE2 neutralizes the advantageous cardiac effects of this enzyme, especially in patients with heart failure.

CVD – Cardiovascular Disease; TnT – Troponin T; ACE2 - angiotensin converting enzyme 2; CMR – Magnetic Ressonance; NT-proBNP - N terminal pro B type natriuretic peptide; Ang-II- Angiotensin II; ARB - angiotensin-receptor blockers; RAAS - renin-angiotensin-aldosterone system; CD – Cluster of Differentiation.

Table 1.
Main Findings.

To ensure trustworthiness of the findings, data collection was performed, individually, by two researchers with divergences being solved by a third senior researcher.

Each sample article was thoroughly read and the information was inserted in a spreadsheet (**Table 1**), including the author, publishing year and main study findings. According to the PRISMA protocol (http://www.prisma- statement.org/).

2.3 Ethical issues

Since this is a systematic review, Resolution 510/16 of the Brazilian National Health Council (CNS) ensures the dispensation of submission to a Human Beings Research Ethics Committee.

3. Result

According to the research strategy, 101 articles were found in Pubmed and 27 were selected. In VHL, 59 articles were found and four were selected. After the eligibility criteria was applied (**Figure 1**), the results were input in **Table 1**.

The findings were then divided into three subcategories: Etiology, Physiopathology and Risk factors of SARS-CoV-2 in Cardiovascular System;

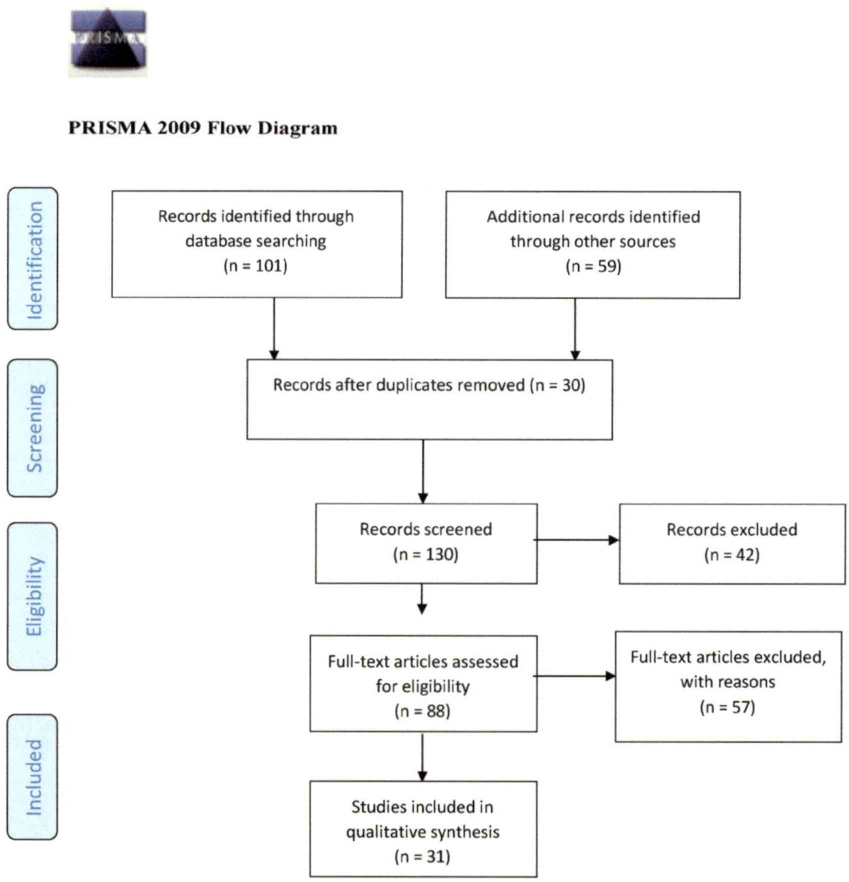

Figure 1.
PRISMA flow diagram.

Clinical presentation, laboratory markers and imagenological aspects of SARS-CoV-2 in cardiovascular system; and Anti-Hypertensive Drugs, Cardiovascular System and SARS-CoV-2.

4. Discussion

4.1 Etiology, physiopathology and risk factors of SARS-CoV-2 in cardiovascular system

SARS-CoV-2 is caused by a novel enveloped beta coronavirus that belongs to the Coronaviridae family, a group of positive strand RNA viruses causing human respiratory infections. Named after the crown shaped outer coat seen on the electron-microscopy, it was first discovered in the 1960s, receiving great attention during the 2003 SARS coronavirus (SARS-CoV) outbreak [11]. Seven species of these beta-coronaviruses are known to cause human infections, with four mainly causing mild flulike symptoms and the remaining three resulting in potentially fatal illnesses (SARS, MERS and the ongoing COVID-19) [10].

The transmission of COVID-19 occurs mainly through droplets route. However, there are theories that this can occur by fecal-oral route or/and by airborne. The average incubation time is less than six days (5.1 days), less than three percent of patients (2,5%) develop disease before the third day (2.2 days) after acquiring the virus while the rest (97,5%) develop symptoms 11.5 days after the onset of infection [27].

Although respiratory tract is the primary target for SARS-CoV-2, cardiovascular system (CVS) may get involved in several different ways [10] as destabilized coronary plaque [9], hypoxemia, systemic inflammation and enhanced myocardial oxygen demand, a direct cardiovascular injury, likely develops, initiated by binding of SARS-CoV-2 to angiotensin-converting enzyme 2 (ACE2) (**Figures 2** and **3**). This receptor is widely expressed in lungs, kidney [5] - renal tubules [26], brain, gut [34], gastrointestinal epithelium, Leydig cells in testis [22, 26], but also in the heart, where it is localized to macrophages, vascular endothelium, smooth muscle and myocytes [33].

Experimental study shows that the immune activity levels (innate immune response - NK cells and acquired immune response - B cells, CD8+ T cells and interferon response) in countless human tissues with large number of ACE2 receptors are statistical significant ($P < 0.05$, $0.27 \leq r \leq 0.78$). In the research, the following tissues obtained higher levels of CD8+ T cell - brain, blood vessels, skin and digestive system (pancreas, colon, stomach and esophagus) [3]. On the other hand, high levels of beta 17ß-estradiol have been shown to be important for increasing the number of ACE2 receptors in kidney and adipose tissues in laboratory studies. Interestingly, spontaneously hypertensive male mice, after orchiectomy, have higher levels of ACE2 than females [16].

In fact, the virus shares the ACE2 as the host cellular receptor for virus spike (S) protein according to structural analysis [31, 35] following activation by transmembrane protease serine 2 (TMPRSS2) [34]. The virus produces enzymatic shedding that inactivates ACE2 and prevents conversion of Ang-II [19]. Besides that, virus infection causes damage to pericytes and endothelial dysfunction, especially due to damage to capillary endothelial cells. The increased expression of ACE2 proteins and mRNAs in patients infected by the virus and with basic heart failure disease may have higher risk of critically ill condition and/or heart attack [31] (**Figure 2**).

Laboratory studies have suggested that other intracellular signaling pathways such as Notch could also explain the cytokine storm that ultimately induces heart

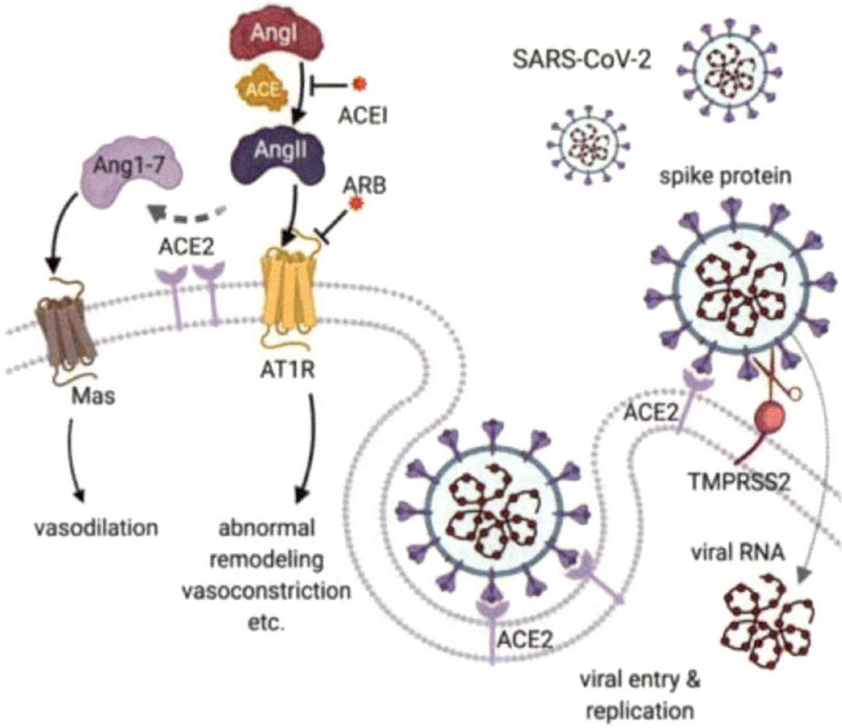

Figure 2.
The role of ACE2 in COVID-19. The spike protein of SARS-CoV-2 binds ACE2 on a cellular membrane, which triggers 1) endocytosis of the virus and subsequent sequestration of ACE2 or 2) cleavage of the viral spike protein via an enzyme TMPRSS2 leading to the entry of viral contents into the cytoplasm [adapted]. Source: Cheng et al. [11].

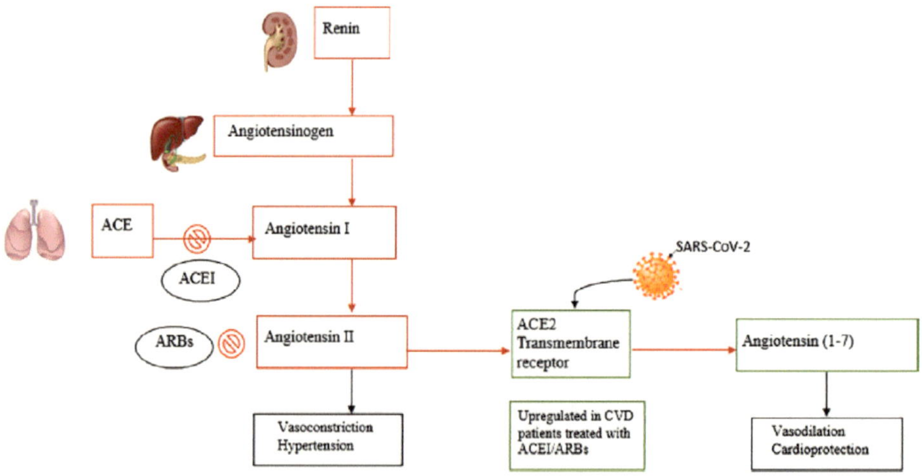

Figure 3.
Renin–angiotensin system inhibition (RAS) by Angiotensin converting enzyme/Ang-II receptor blockers (ACEI/ARBs) and SARS-CoV-2 binding to ACE2 receptors [adapted]. Source: Gonzallez-Jamarilo et al. [19].

and lung disease caused by SARS-CoV-2 direct damage to tissues [23]. Besides that, other theory is that the "cytokine storm" - term for increasing various interleukins and chemokines as TNF-α, IFN-γ, GCSF, MCP-1, MIP-1-α, IL-10, IL-6 and IL-2 contributes to cardiac injury. These situations are analogous to cardiotoxicity in the setting of CAR- T cell (chimeric antigen receptor - T cell) therapy. In this paper, left ventricular systolic dysfunction, cardiac injury and cardiovascular events (troponin elevation) post-CAR-T have been demonstrated [17].

Therefore, the exact mechanism of cardiac involvement in COVID-19 remains under investigation but it seems the SARS-CoV-2 can (a) cause cardiac injury indirectly due to a probable overwhelming immune inflammatory response and cytokine storm; (b) cause invasion of cardiomyocytes and direct damage via this process; (c) cause Severe hypoxia from acute respiratory damage caused by the virus may result in oxidative stress and myocardial injury from increased myocardial oxygen demand in the presence of severe hypoxia due to acute lung injury (ARDS) [25].

Cardiovascular disease patients are at particularly high risk for mortality from SARS-CoV-2 due to their frailty and susceptibility for a myocardial involvement [36], perhaps due to the virus's affinity for ACE2 (**Figure 3**) mainly due to the interaction with the renin-angiotensin-aldosterone system (RAAS).

RAAS has an important role in regulating blood pressure and electrolyte balance. This system compromises two pathways: ACE2/Ang (1–7)/Mas receptor and ACE/Ang II/AT1R. In physiological situations, these two metabolic pathways function harmoniously, maintaining the normal function [7] (**Figure 3**). Hence, RAAS is widely implicated in Diabetes mellitus (DM), hypertension, heart failure [21] and Coronary heart disease [29].

Patients with COVID-19 are often diagnosed with coronary artery disease (2.5–8%), diabetes (7.3%–18.8%), hypertension (15%–30.4%) and other cardiovascular disease (4%–14.6%). In addition, of the patients who had been admitted to the intensive care unit (ICU), those with cardiovascular diseases compared to those who had not had a worse prognosis [9, 14, 24].

Another fact to be considered is that COVID-19 is more aggressive in elderly patients. The literature tells us that the elderly and male have more ACE2 receptors than the general population [29]. About that, Li et al. [3] refer that, when studying the expression of ACE2 receptors in various tissues of the body and its correlation with immunogenicity, in the thyroid, lungs, adrenal gland, liver, and kidneys, ACE2 expression levels showed significant positive correlations with CD8+ T cell enrichment levels solely in males.

Finally, patients with chronic kidney and those who have received renal transplant - and have a higher cardiovascular risk - are at increased risk of COVID-19 infection and severity. Moreover, there are frequent renal function abnormalities and increased incidence of acute kidney injury in patients with COVID- 19 [26].

4.2 Clinical presentation, laboratory markers and imagenological aspects of SARS-CoV-2 in cardiovascular system

There appears to be two clinical stages to the disease. The first stage is the replicative stage, when SARS-CoV-2 is replicating over the course of several days and the patient presents with relatively mild symptoms [25] such as fever, cough, and myalgia or fatigue; less common symptoms were sputum production, headache, hemoptysis, and diarrhea [32]. The adaptive immunity stage is the second stage. The body produces antibodies against the virus and, as there is viral clearance, the antibody titers will return to baseline values and an infection solves. This creates an "Immune memory". However, a minority of patients becomes critically ill and have high mortality rates [25]. It is important to remember that some symptoms in patients with COVID-19 pneumonia suggest cardiovascular diseases. Fatigue, dyspnea, cough is typical in COVID-19, but these symptoms may also result from exacerbation of chronic heart failure [14].

Chinese study shows large number of patients (81%) with mild symptoms of COVID-19 between (no pneumonia and mild pneumonia). These patients with more aggressive symptoms, 14% has more severe clinical conditions (lung infiltrates >50% within 24 to 48 hours, partial pressure of arterial oxygen to fraction of inspired oxygen ratio < 300, blood oxygen saturation ≤ 93%, respiratory rate ≥ 30/min and dyspnea) and 5% critical medical conditions (septic shock, respiratory failure and/or multiple organ dysfunction or failure) [37]. Others publishing and anecdotal reports indicate manifestations of arrhythmia [28], cardiac arrest, acute heart failure [23] and theoretically fulminant myocarditis [17, 32].

COVID-19 virus enters cells through the angiotensin converting enzyme II (ACE2) receptor, resulting in down-regulation of ACE2 receptor function. This leads to an increase of angiotensin II activity, activation of the renin-angiotensin-aldosterone system (RAAS) following a decrease in ACE2, an increase in vasoactive, proliferative, and profibrotic Ang-II leads to cardiopulmonary damage through hemodynamic changes such as pulmonary hypertension and interstitial edema followed by respiratory failure in the most severe cases (**Figure 3**) [19].

In laboratory markers, definitive diagnosis of SARS-CoV-2 Infection is based primarily on nucleic acid amplification tests, such as real-time reverse transcriptase–polymerase chain reaction (rRT-PCR) [27].

The laboratory alterations found in COVID-19 include in descending level elevated concentrations of serum creatine kinase (7%–13.7%), total bilirubin (10.5–18%), transaminases (21–28%), D-dimer concentration (36%–46.4%), lactate dehydrogenase (41–76%), C-reactive protein (60.7–93%), thrombocytopenia (17%–36.2%) and lymphopenia (35%–82.1%). It is important to note that the first three have been rarely reported [14].

Interesting to note that elevated D-dimer values are common in COVID-19 patients, even in the absence of thrombophlebitis and acute pulmonary embolism and it seems to correlate with acute pulmonary embolism [18], arterial thrombosis, acute respiratory distress syndrome and death [15]; elevated cardiac troponin I (cTnI) levels [32] and N terminal pro B type natriuretic peptide (NT-proBNP), with the cut-off value of 88.64 pg./mL [20] are correlate with cardiovascular injury, hospitalization and death. Including, plasma TnT levels in patients with COVID-19 correlated significantly with both plasma high-sensitivity C-reactive protein levels, NT-proBNP elevation and malignant arrhythmias [20].

According to Clerkin et al. [9] the rise in elevated high sensitivity cTnI tracks with other inflammatory biomarkers (D-dimer, ferritin, interleukin-6 (IL-6), lactate dehydrogenase and elevated creatinine kinase, raising the possibility that it may reflect on cytokine storm or secondary hemophagocytic lymphohistiocytosis more than isolated myocardial injury.

Transthoracic echocardiography is routinely recommended in patients with complicated COVID-19 due to the high prevalence of heart failure or/and myocarditis. This measure is useful to differentiate dyspnea of pulmonary origin from dyspnea of cardiac origin and monitor the sequelae of ARDS. Another useful use of echocardiography in the medical practice of ICU is monitoring treatments such as extracorporeal membrane oxygenation and fluid management in shock. Ultrasound evaluation of the lung may be a sensitive marker of fluid accumulation in the interstitial space and it useful for show the most common changes present in lungs how consolidation, B-line artifacts (the earliest signs in the disease course) and pleural line abnormalities like >1 mm, loss of continuity and irregularity [27].

Cardiovascular Magnetic Resonance (CMR) is useful in mapping of the extent of myocardial injuries, impact on ventricular function and differentiating a etiologies (ischemic from non-ischemic). It stills helps in differentiating the between myocarditis and other acute myocardial injury that can elevate myocardial enzymes (eg. Troponin) and alter electrocardiographic (ECG) patterns [13].

4.3 Anti-hypertensive drugs, cardiovascular system and SARS-CoV-2

Even at the beginning of the pandemic, a publication suggested that due to hyper expression of ACE2 receptors in DM and hypertension, patients with said condition would be more likely to develop severe manifestations of COVID-19 [6] which was not confirmed with subsequent studies [21, 24, 30, 34]. At the same time, there was a theory that anti-hypertensive drugs could cause more severe cases of COVID-19, however it has been refuted. Meng et al. [27] showed that ACE inhibitors (ACEi) or angiotensin receptor-1 blockers (ARB) therapy increased CD3 and CD8 T cell counts in peripheral blood and decreased the peak viral load compared to other antihypertensive drugs and Rico-Mesa et al. [24] suggest that the effects of these drugs were positive, including ACE2 receptor blockade, disabling viral entry into the heart and lungs, and an overall decrease in inflammation secondary to ACEI/ARB.

Moreover, Societies of Hypertension affirms that in hypertensive patients with COVID-19 or at risk of COVID-19 infection, ACEi and ARBs treatment should be maintained according to the recommendations contained in the 2018 ESC/ESH guidelines [5], because blood pressure control remains an important consideration in order to reduce disease burden, even if it has no effect on susceptibility to the SARS-CoV-2 viral infection [24].

5. Final considerations

Cardiovascular diseases (CVD) are one of the most important causes of morbidity and mortality in the world being a great challenge for clinicians and researchers in the context of COVID-19. The pathophysiological explanation suggests an intimate correlation between SARS-CoV-2 protein S and ACE2 receptors, which the virus takes advantage of to increase its ability to penetrate host cells. The aggression of the cardiovascular system can be divided into three hypotheses - direct damage of the cardiomyocyte by the virus; hypoxemia due to lung injury or coronary events; or exacerbated immune response. When it comes to patients with COVID-19, the coexistence of previous cardiovascular diseases or risk factors such as hypertension, diabetes, coronary heart disease and heart failure, in addition to biochemical markers such as high troponin and pro-BNP seem to increase mortality.

Thus, when it comes to the cardiovascular system, these issues are aggravated and urge as a joint commitment from researchers, medical and governmental organizations to carry out more robust studies with bold methodologies aimed at mapping prognostic factors and assertive therapeutic approaches in the management of cardiovascular complications of COVID- 19.

Acknowledgements

The authors would like to thank Scientific Writing Lab, Medicine School – Universidade Federal of Cariri (UFCA) and the Brazilian National Council for Scientific and Technological Development (CNPq) – institution linked to the Brazilian Department of Science, Technology.

Funding

The authors declare that they have no funding.

Conflict of interests

The authors declare that they have no competing interests.

Author details

Jucier Gonçalves Júnior[1*], Estelita Lima Cândido[2], Gislene Farias de Oliveira[2] and Modesto Leite Rolim Neto[2]

1 School of Medicine, São Paulo University (USP), São Paulo, SP, Brazil

2 School of Medicine, Federal University of Cariri (UFCA), Barbalha, CE, Brazil

*Address all correspondence to: juciergjunior@hotmail.com

References

[1] Massa KHC, Duarte YAO, Chiavegatto Filho, AGV. Analysis of the prevalence of cardiovascular diseases and associated factors among the elderly, 2000-2010. Cienc Saude Colet. 2020; 24(1):105-114.

[2] WHO. Doenças Cardiovasculares. 2017. Geneva: WHO. Access in May 09, 2020. Available in: https://www.paho.org/bra/index.php?option=com_content&view=article&id=5253:doencas-cardiovasculares&Itemid=1096

[3] Li Q, et al. (2020) Early transmission dynamics in Wuhan, China, of novel coronavirus-infected pneumonia. N Engl J Med 382, 1199-1207.

[4] WHOa. Cardiovascular Disease. 2020. Geneva: WHO. Access in May 09, 2020. Available in: https://www.who.int/health-topics/cardiovascular-diseases/#tab=tab_1

[5] Laccarino et al. Renin-Angiotensin System Inhibition in Cardiovascular Patients at the Time of COVID19: Much Ado for Nothing? A Statement of Activity from the Directors of the Board and the Scientific Directors of the Italian Society of Hypertension. High Blood Press Cardiovasc Prev. 2020; 27:105-108

[6] Fang L, Karakiulakis G, Roth M. Are patients with hypertension and diabetes mellitus at increased risk for COVID-19 infection? Lancet, 2020; S2213-2600(20)30116-30118

[7] Meng et al. Renin-angiotensin system inhibitors improve the clinical outcomes of COVID-19 patients with hypertension. Emerg. Microbes Infect. 2020; 9: 760.

[8] Clerkin et al. Coronavirus Disease 2019 (COVID-19) and Cardiovascular Disease. Circulation, 2020; 6-23.

[9] Guo et al. Cardiovascular Implications of Fatal Outcomes of Patients with Coronavirus Disease 2019 (COVID-19) JAMA Cardiol. 2020a: e201017.

[10] Bansal M. Cardiovascular disease and COVID-19. Diabetes Metab Syndr.2020;14: 247e250.

[11] Cheng et al. Cardiovascular Risks in Patients with COVID-19: Potential Mechanisms and Areas of Uncertainty. Current Cardiology Reports, 2020; 22:34.

[12] Li et al. Expression of the SARS-CoV-2 cell receptor gene *ACE2* in a wide variety of human tissues. Infect Dis Poverty. 2020; 9: 45.

[13] Han et al. Society for Cardiovascular Magnetic Resonance (SCMR) guidance for the practice of cardiovascular magnetic resonance during the COVID-19 pandemic. J Cardiovasc Magn R.2020; 22:26.

[14] Sławiński G, Lewicka E.What should a cardiologist know about coronavirus disease 2019?KARDIOLOGIA POLSKA 2020; 78 (4): 278-283.

[15] Le Berre et al. Concomitant acute aortic thrombosis and pulmonary embolism complicating COVID-19 pneumonia.Diagn Interv Imaging.2020; 101; 321-322.

[16] La Vignera et al. Sex-Specific SARS-CoV-2 Mortality: Among Hormone-Modulated ACE2 Expression, Risk of Venous Thromboembolism and Hypovitaminosis D. Int. J. Mol. Sci. 2020; 21: 2948.

[17] Zhu et al. Cardiovascular Complications in Patients with COVID-19: Consequences of Viral Toxicities and Host Immune Response. Curr Cardiol Rep.2020;22:32

[18] Celina M, Oliva G. Acute pulmonary embolism in a patient with COVID-19 pneumonia.Diagn Interv Imaging.2020.

[19] Gonzallez-Jamarilo N, Low N, Franco OH. The double burden of disease of COVID-19 in cardiovascular patients: overlapping conditions could lead to overlapping treatments. Eur. J. Epidemiol. 2020; 35:335-333.

[20] Gao et al. Prognostic value of NT-proBNP in patients with severe COVID-19. Respir Res. 2020; 21:83.

[21] Rico-Mesa JS, White A, Anderson AS. Outcomes in Patients with COVID-19 Infection Taking ACEI/ARB.Curr Cardiol Rep. 2020; 22:31.

[22] Wang Z, Xu X. scRNA-seq Profiling of Human Testes Reveals the Presence of the ACE2 Receptor, A Target for SARS-CoV-2 Infection in Spermatogonia, Leydig and Sertoli Cells.Cells 2020; 9: 920.

[23] Rizzo et al. COVID-19 in the heart and the lungs: could we "Notch" the inflammatory storm?Basic Research in Cardiology 2020; 115:31

[24] Schiffrin et al. Hypertension and COVID-19. Am. J. Hypertens.2020;1-2.

[25] Tan W, Aboulhousn J. The cardiovascular burden of coronavirus disease 2019 (COVID-19) with a focus on congenital heart disease.Int. J. Cardiol. 2020; 309: 70-77

[26] Gupta R, Misra A. Contentious issues and evolving concepts in the clinical presentation and management of patients with COVID-19 infectionwith reference to use of therapeutic and other drugs used in Co-morbid diseases (Hypertension, diabetes etc). Diabetes Metab Syndr.2020;14: 251-254.

[27] Gackowski et al. Echocardiography during the coronavirus disease 2019 (COVID-19) pandemic: expert opinion of the Working Group on Echocardiography of the Polish Cardiac Society. Kardiologia Polska 2020; 78 (4):357-363.

[28] Guo et al. Coronavirus Disease 2019 (COVID-19) and Cardiovascular Disease: A Viewpoint on the Potential Influence of Angiotensin-Converting Enzyme Inhibitors/Angiotensin Receptor Blockers on Onset and Severity of Severe Acute Respiratory Syndrome Coronavirus 2 Infection. J Am Heart Assoc. 2020b;9:e016219.

[29] Sommerstein et al. Coronavirus Disease 2019 (COVID-19): Do Angiotensin-Converting Enzyme Inhibitors/Angiotensin Receptor Blockers Have a Biphasic Effect?J Am Heart Assoc. 2020;9:e016509

[30] Vanduganathan et al. Renin–Angiotensin–Aldosterone System Inhibitors in Patients with Covid-19. N Eng J Med. 2020; 1-7. DOI: 101056/NEJMsr2005160

[31] Chen et al. The ACE2 expression in human heart indicates new potential mechanismof heart injury among patients infected with SARS-CoV-2. Cardiovasc Res, 2020:1-4.

[32] Chen C, Zhou Y,Wen Wang D. SARS-CoV-2: a potential novel etiology of fulminant myocarditis.Herz volume 2020; 45:230-232

[33] Hulot J-S. COVID-19 in patients with cardiovascular diseases. Arch. Cardiovasc. Dis. 2020; 113: 225—226.

[34] South AM, Diz DI, Chappell MC. COVID-19, ACE2, and the cardiovascular consequences. Am J Physiol Heart Circ Physiol 2020; 318: H1084–H1090.

[35] Abassi et al. Angiotensin-converting enzyme 2: an ally or a Trojan horse? Implications to SARS-CoV-2-related

cardiovascular complications. Am J Physiol Heart Circ Physiol. 2020; 318: H1080–H1083.

[36] Gori T, Lelieveld J, Münzel T. Perspective: cardiovascular disease and the Covid-19 pandemic. Basic Res Cardiol. 2020; 115:32.

[37] Zhang H, Penninger JM, Li Y, Zhong N and Slutsky AS. Angiotensin-converting enzyme 2 (ACE2) as a SARS-CoV-2 receptor: molecular mechanisms and potential therapeutic target. *Intensive Care Med*. March 3, 2020. doi: 10.1007/s00134-020-05985-9.

Chapter 10

Post COVID-19 Conditions and the Cardiovascular System

Iana Simova, Denislava Hristova, Hristina Tzanovska, Denis Nikolov, Diliana Iakova, Anyuta Ivanova, Maria-Magdalena Pintova, Pavlin Pavlov, Ognyan Matkov, Todor Samardjiev, Vladimir Kornovski, Jordan Krasnaliev, Todor Kundurzhiev, Nikolay Dimitrov and Toni Vekov

Abstract

One out of four patients affected by COVID-19 will experience persistent (>3-4 weeks) signs and symptoms (Post COVID-19 conditions or Post-Acute Sequelae of SARS-CoV-2 – PASC) and this fact will have a major significance for the healthcare and economic systems in the upcoming years. The cardiovascular system is one of the key targets for the Post COVID-19 syndrome, given the pathogenesis of the virus and prevalence of ACE-2 receptors. According to our initial personal experience via the campaign "Life after COVID" of the Bulgarian Cardiac Institute, a substantial proportion of patients having suffered from COVID-19 develop long-term cardiovascular consequences. They could range from rhythm disorder and blood pressure variation, through impairment of myocardial mechanics and heart failure, and to acute vascular manifestations of Post COVID-19 conditions, such as acute coronary syndrome, acute pulmonary embolism, and acute limb ischemia. These cardiovascular complications require special and dedicated medical attention, and we could share our personal experience on the matter.

Keywords: post COVID-19 conditions, cardio-vascular system, acute coronary syndrome, acute pulmonary embolism

1. Introduction

1.1 Definition

According to its definition, post COVID-19 conditions comprise all signs and symptoms of COVID-19 that persist after the acute phase (3 to 4 weeks), without an upper limit of duration (as for the present state of knowledge). Another term for these conditions, introduced by Antoni Fauci, is "Post-Acute Consequences of SARS-CoV-2 Infection" (PASC) [1].

1.2 Time frame

The acute phase of the disease usually lasts about 3-4 weeks from the onset of symptoms, after which replication competent SARS-CoV-2 has not been isolated in the nasopharynx [1].

Accumulated data show that the consequences for the body can be just as serious and continue for an unusually long time after the initial encounter with the virus. It is the long persistence of complaints of varying degrees and manifestations after the infection that are known as post COVID-19 conditions. There is no precise scientific definition for the reason, duration, and prognosis of PASC [2].

The acute phase of the disease does not determine the onset of Post COVID-19 syndrome, because even patients with mild or asymptomatic infection may report PASC. There is no age limit for the manifestation of post Covid-19 conditions, but the reported frequency is higher in the elderly population [3, 4].

According to the latest data from the World Health Organization, the consequences of an infectious disease can last for two to three years [5].

1.3 Pathogenetic considerations

There are several pathogenetic hypotheses for PASC. The first is direct cell damage by binding of SARC-CoV-2 to ACE 2, initiating a violent immune response leading to increased cytokine production and triggering of procoagulant states [6].

It was later found that the reason for prolonged viral replication is the fact that SARS-CoV-2 can be transmitted by a different route from the respiratory tract, namely through the gastrointestinal tract, which could be considered a second hypothesis. The gastrointestinal tract is a major immunological organ in the human body and disruption of its microbiome leads to severe dysbacteriosis. Intestinal inflammation exacerbates the expression of ACE2, and the virus stays in the gut for much longer, which in turn can modulate immune responses and cause prolonged symptoms [6, 7]. This has been demonstrated by an intestinal biopsy, which detects the presence of the virus for months [7].

COVID-19 has also been shown to provoke autoimmune reactions, leading to a more severe course of the disease and the development of post COVID-19 conditions [7].

The suboptimal immune response leads to a higher viral load associated with decreased balance in interferon production. It was found that in severe disease the body lacks IFN-beta and the level of IFN-alpha and lambda is reduced [7, 8].

Lymphopenia and unregulated inflammation have been observed in patients with severe COVID-19 and prolonged persistence of the infection as a result of decreased production of granular lymphocytes (NK cells), CD16 + monocytes, plasmacytoid dendritic cells, which are responsible for innate immunity [8].

1.4 Symptoms

The severity of symptoms can range from mild to inability to perform normal daily duties. Every system could be involved, with a typical fluctuation and changing of symptoms over time. As the pathogenesis has shown, prolonged exposure to viral load can cause multisystem inflammatory syndrome (MIS) or trigger autoimmune conditions. The involvement in PASC is multi-organ, with the most common being complaints from the nervous system [2, 9]. Post COVID-19 conditions are more common among people with chronic diseases such as hypertension, diabetes, kidney disease, obesity. Genetic pre-exposure to the disease has not yet been specified.

The main systems that are affected are the nervous, cardiovascular, pulmonary, and excretory systems, musculoskeletal system, skin (**Table 1**).

System	Symptoms	Sign
Neuropsychiatric	fatigue, dizziness, headache, dysautonomia and cognitive impairment (brain fog), anxiety, depression, sleep disturbances	Direct damage to nerve tissue by the virus in patients with severe disease. [2] Psycho-emotional changes may include a wide range of symptomatic complexes characteristic of severe patients who are being treated in intensive care, known as "Post Intensive Care Syndrome"
Pulmonary	dyspnea, decreased exercise capacity and hypoxia	Reduced difusion capacity, restrictive pulmonary physiology, destruction of the alveolar-capillary membrane, secondary bacterial infections, pulmonary fibrosis," ground-glass opacity" [2, 3]
Cardiovascular	palpitations, dyspnea and chest pain, high blood pressure, fatigue, swelling of the lower extremities, acute pain and discoloration of the arm or leg due to ischemia	Thromboembolic events. It is already known that many patients re-admitted to the hospital with chest pain and positive cardiac enzymes (Troponin, CK, CK-MB,) and high levels of D-dimer. Pulmonary embolism is very common. In patients at high cardiovascular risk or underlying ischemic heart disease, acute thrombotic occlusion of the coronary artery are diagnosed. Non-obstructive coronary heart disease has been verified in many patients: myocardial infarction with non-obstructive coronary arteries (MINOCA), endothelial dysfunction, and microcirculation of arterial vascular disease [9, 10]. Acute limb ischemia may be observed. Some patients have pericardial effusion or the development of dilated cardiomyopathy of viral origin, after myocarditis [10]
Gastrointestinal	loss of appetite, weight loss, nausea, vomiting, diarrhea, abdominal pain	increased transaminases dysbiosis in the intestinal microflora (disturbed microbiome) with, increase in pathogenic bacteria and decrease in the normal microflora in the gut [7]
Endocrine	• new or worsening control of existing diabetes mellitus • bone demineralization • subacute thyroiditis	• Hyperglycaemia is due to a stress response of the body as a result of the disease as well as due to treatment with corticosteroids. • lack of vitamin D and / or immobilization • autoimmune conditions [2, 3]
Excretory and urogenital system	impaired renal function decreased urine output, pain in the kidneys	elevated levels of waste products (urea and creatinine), requiring hemodialysis [2]
Reproductive system	Impaired spermatogenesis	The male sex is more affected in reproductive system, and one of the hypotheses for this is the higher amount of ACE 2 in the male gonads compared to the uterus [11, 12]
Musculoskeletal system	occurrence of long-lasting arthralgia/myalgia	Due to immobilization, they can lead to cachexia due to loss of muscle mass. Sarcopenia - impaired muscle function due to loss of muscle tissue [2, 13]
Ear Nose Throat	pain and "noise" in the ears, throat irritation, loss of taste and smell(anosmia)	Nasal congestion, pharyngeal erythema [14]

System	Symptoms	Sign
Dermatology	hair loss, skin rash, urticaria, dry skin	disturbed cycle in hair growth, (telogen effuvium); stress after infection "COVID toes" syndrome - reddish-purple discoloration on the toes; In children, a rare condition similar to Kawasaki disease or Multisystem inflammatory syndrome in children (MIS-C) [2, 15, 16]

Table 1.
Affecting the basic systems in post COVID-19 conditions.

1.5 Duration

Many global medical centers are opening specialized clinics to provide care for people who have persistent symptoms or related illnesses after COVID-19. It is important to know that most people who have COVID-19 recover. The scientific community should focus on that part of the people in whom the effects of the disease leave lasting traces and change their lives. It is still unknown how long PASC can last. In 30% of COVID-19 survivors, symptoms may persist indefinitely. Data show that 76% of patients reported persistence of at least one of the symptoms of PASC for at least six months after the acute phase [17]. Many COVID-19 survivors cannot return to their normal lifestyle. At this stage, there is no accurate scientific data on whether these long symptoms can lead to a chronicity of the condition.

1.6 Sequelae

Understanding the pathogenesis of PASC may provide answers to additional questions to guide the medical community to the right management of the condition.

The loss of human lives, the disability of the population, the increase in the costs of health care and services burden the health systems. Persistence of post COVID-19 conditions affects various levels of medical and social life, and the negative effects on healthcare and the economy may be fully appreciated in years to come.

The psychological and social consequences of ongoing Covid19 should be considered as part of clinical care models [17].

2. COVID-19 and the cardiovascular system

The primary target for SARS-CoV-2 is the respiratory tract, but the cardiovascular system can be involved too [18, 19].

As well as the mild flu-like symptoms, COVID-19 often causes serious damage to the cardiovascular system - pulmonary vascular endothelialitis, microangiopathy, diffuse thrombosis, cardiac arrhythmias, heart failure, myocarditis, pericarditis and acute coronary syndromes [19].

Once in the nasopharynx, the SARS-CoV-2 enters the body by binding through its S-binding protein to angiotensin I-converting enzyme 2 (ACE2) receptors, found mainly in the lungs, cardiac myocytes, and endothelial cells in the vessel wall [20].

ACE2 is known to have protective effects by counteracting angiotensin II and over activating renin-angiotensin-aldosterone system (RAAS), which occurs in conditions of cardiovascular disease (CVD) such as hypertension, congestive heart failure and atherosclerosis [19, 21].

Entering through endocytosis, this RNA virus begins to replicate, causing widespread infection. Since ACE2 converts angiotensin I and II to cardioprotective peptides - angiotensin 1-9 and angiotensin 1-7, its loss on cell surface may potentiate cardiac damage, resulting in endothelial dysfunction, inflammation and thrombosis [21, 22].

ACE2 activity is known to be reduced in vessels with established atherosclerotic plaques and diabetes, while it is increased in women and young people due to the action of estrogens [21].

Decreased ACE2 activity may potentiate the so-called cytokine storm. This is an overreaction of the immune system caused by dysregulating RAAS and activating ACE2/bradykinin axis. The overproduction of cytokines and hyperinflammation leads to exacerbation of underlying cardiovascular diseases or triggering new ones.

According to the latest epidemiological data, about 80% of patients with COVID 19 have mild symptoms, about 45% have symptoms requiring hospitalization, while 5% of patients need mechanical ventilation [21–25]. The difference in course is related to the degree of viral load, host immune response, age of the patient and the presence of concomitant diseases such as hypertension, diabetes and coagulation abnormalities.

Aging is associated with slowing of body functions, increased oxidative stress, reduced role of endogenous defense mechanisms. With age, reduced efficiency of thrombolysis, lower protection afforded by physical exercise against myocardial ischemia and more frequent manifestations of heart failure are more often observed [21, 22].

It has not yet been established whether the patient's older age or greater immune response to the virus or both are responsible for myocardial damage with subsequent complications [21–24].

2.1 Cardiovascular complications in COVID-19

Direct viral infection, cytokine dysregulation and direct myocyte involvement can lead to acute myocardial injury in patients with COVID-19. Thus except for the high levels of CRP (C-reactive protein), elevated troponin levels suggest acute myocardial injury. It can be a result of myocarditis, ischemic injury, Takotsubo's cardiomyopathy, septic cardiomyopathy, acute cor pulmonale (as a result of acute pulmonary embolism) [7, 26, 27].

Acute coronary syndromes can be a manifestation of imbalance between myocardial supply and demand as a result of systemic changes – hypoxemia, tachycardia, hypotension, vasoconstriction; or acute thrombosis in the coronary arteries. Often, when the right coronary artery is affected a complete atrioventricular heart block can be seen. Other location of the coronary lesion may lead to severe ischemic cardiomyopathy, left ventricular aneurysm formation with apical thrombosis [28, 29].

The most frequent arrhythmia seen in COVID-19 patients is atrial fibrillation, which is a result of the acute respiratory failure. Electrolyte imbalance – hypokalemia and hypomagnesaemia can also lead to arrhythmic states [30].

Some of the medications used in the treatment of COVID-19 have proarrhythmogenic effects and should be used with caution, as they can provoke long QT interval, ventricular tachycardia and sudden cardiac death [30, 31].

A hypercoagulable state and thrombotic events, that are related to markedly elevated D-dimer and fibrin degradation products, are thought to be secondary to systemic inflammatory response [32, 33].

Takotsubo cardiomyopathy, predominantly seen in women, is mainly a result of increased sympathetic stimulation, which is usually observed in patients with COVID-19. It can be due to physical and psychological stress. This state can mimic acute coronary syndrome, which can develop within severe sepsis, hypoxemia, or metabolic acidosis [34–36].

Acute myocarditis due to myocardial inflammation can lead to ventricular dysfunction as a result of focal or global myocarditis or necrosis [37]. Life- threatening arrhythmias can be a consequence of myocarditis. When linked with pericardial effusion, further deteriorating of the hemodynamics might lead to acute heart failure (HF) and cardiogenic shock [38, 39].

The pathogenic mechanisms and clinical manifestations of cardiovascular complications of COVID-19 are presented in **Table 2**.

Cardiovascular disease	**Pathogenic mechanism**	**Clinical manifestation**
Acute coronary syndrome with or without ST elevation	Cytokine storm, hypercoagulability, plaque instability, imbalance between cardiac supply and demand	Typical chest pain or atypical pain and/or dyspnea, elevated levels of troponin, ECG changes (ST elevation or depression) and LV WMAs associated with specific region of distribution of a coronary artery
Myocarditis	Cytokine storm, direct cellular damage (possible)	Chest pain (possible), dyspnea (possible), elevated levels of troponin, ECG changes (possible), diffuse LV WMAs not related to specific coronary artery territory distribution
Pericarditis	Cytokine storm, direct cellular damage (possible)	Chest pain, dyspnea (possible), elevated troponin, ECG changes, impaired LV diastolic function and/or pericardial effusion
TTS	Emotional stress, microvascular and endothelial dysfunction, sepsis, acidosis, hypoxemia	Chest pain and/or dyspnea, elevated troponin, ECG changes, LV WMAs not related to specific coronary artery territory distribution (circumferential pattern, apical ballooning most frequently)
PE	Hypercoagulability	Chest pain and/or dyspnea, perioral cyanosis, elevated troponin (possible), ECG changes - S1Q3T3 pattern (possible), RV enlargement and dysfunction (McConnell sign, 60/60 sign)
Decompensated chronic HF	Hypoxia, elevated metabolic demand	Dyspnea, fatique, orthopea, tachydyspnea, hepatomegalia, anasarca, elevated levels of troponin (possible), LV WMAs without de novo abnormalities
Acute myocardial injury	Cytokine storm, direct cellular damage (possible), microvascular and endothelial dysfunction, hypoxia	Chest pain and/or dyspnea (possible), elevated levels of troponin, ECG changes (possible), LV WMAs (possible) not associated with specific coronary artery territory distribution (if absence of coexistent CAD)
Arrhytmias	Electrolyte abnormalities and medications for treatment of COVID 19 that have proarrhythmic effects	Dyspnea and chest pain (possible), ECG changes

ACS, acute coronary syndrome; CAD, coronary artery disease; CMR, cardiac magnetic resonance; CT, computed tomography; ECG, electrocardiogram; HF, heart failure; ICA, invasive coronary angiography; LV, left ventricular; PE, pulmonary embolism; RV, right ventricular; TTE, transthoracic echocardiography; TTS, Takotsubo syndrome, WMAs, wall motion abnormalities. Modified from Ref. [40].

Table 2.
Pathogenetic mechanisms and clinical presentations of cardiovascular complications seen in patients with COVID-19.

2.2 Imaging of cardiovascular complications

As COVID 19 is an infectious disease clinicians should use methods of imaging, minimizing the risk of spreading infection. Most suitable are transthoracic echocardiography and point of care ultrasound. They are the first-line cardiac imaging techniques in this clinical setting, due to its portability, bedside feasibility in emergency settings and low cost [41].

The ultrasound is a diagnostic method for imaging the heart structures, valve lesions and kinetics. According to the European Association of Cardiovascular Imaging it is recommended performing echocardiography in patients with abnormally high levels of cardiac biomarkers and/or ECG signs of myocardial damage, while acknowledging that other imaging diagnostic tests are not routinely used in the emergency context of the COVID-19 pandemic [42, 43].

Findings in echocardiography could be normal heart or uchanged from prior exams, global left ventricular dysfunction and strain, regional left ventricular dysfunction, right ventricuar dilatation, pylmonary hypertention and pericardial effusion.

CT scan and MRI can also be used for distinguising cardiovascular implication, but they have higher cost and lower availability [44].

2.3 Treatment of cardiovascular complications during acute COVID-19

Every hospital in the world should develop appropriate protocols for rapid diagnosis, triage, isolation, and management of patients with COVID-19 and concomitant cardiovascular complications. These protocols should be well-rehearsed for proper use of health services and to minimize the exposure of the medical staff [45].

Most of the patients with COVID-19 have hypertension, treated with ACE inhibitors or (ACEi) or angiotensin II receptor blockers (ARBs). The amount of cardiac ACE2 mRNA could be increased significantly by the use of ACEi and ARBs [46, 47]. However, major cardiology scientific associations, have recommended continuation of renin-angiotensin system inhibitors (RASi) in patients who have been prescribed them [47–49].

Statin therapy is important for patients with diabetes, history of stroke or chronic heart disease, and familial hypercholesterolemia. However, in cases with COVID-19 there is still not an approved opinion whether it is risky or beneficial [50, 51].

As various anti-retroviral drugs might interact with cardiac drugs, a dose modification should be performed as well as careful monitoring [52]. Even though chloroquine or hydroxychloroquine could interfere with cellular endocytosis of the virus, prolongation of the QT interval might be observed. Therefore ECG monitoring is crucial and should be done [52, 53].

Colchicine is a drug that has been shown to restrict the production of pro-inflammatory cytokines (tumor necrosis factor [TNF]-α, interleukin [IL]-1 and IL-6) and chemokines (IL-8), usually observed in patients with severe COVID-19 [54, 55].

As patients with COVID-19 may have elevated levels of D-dimer and higher platelet counts, it is suggested that coagulopathy is a major clinical feature in severe cases. This makes the use of anticoagulant and/or antiplatelet therapy very reasonable [56, 57].

2.4 Long-term cardiovascular consequences as a part of the post COVID-19 conditions

Most people recover completely from COVID-19, but some of them have persisting symptoms after their initial recovery. This is the group of “long haulers” and the condition is called post-COVID-19 syndrome/conditions. [57, 58] The most common signs are fatigue, shortness of breath, cough, joint paint, chest pain. Every system could be affected, and the cardiovascular system is one of the frequent targets. Imaging tests taken months after recovery have shown lasting damage to the heart muscle [58–60]. This may increase the risk of heart failure or other complications such as arrhythmias and micropulmonary embolism. Careful follow-up of patients recovering from COVID-19 would be of great importance to understand the long-term impact of this illness [37, 61, 62].

3. "Life after COVID" campaign of the Bulgarian Cardiac Institute

Bulgarian Cardiac Institute is a leading organization for cardiovascular diagnosis and treatment in South-eastern Europe. The institute manages the largest and fastest growing medical group in Bulgaria. The medical establishments cover 2/3 of the patient flow and ¾ from the territory of the country. The Bulgarian Cardiac Institute is unique in the development of modern scientific, educational and medical activities in the field of cardiology, cardiac surgery, neurology, neurosurgery, vascular surgery, oncology, surgery, orthopedics, genetics, immunology, radiation therapy and radiosurgery.

Despite the growing population of patients surviving COVID-19, the long-term consequences remain a clinical challenge. Currently, just under 1% of studies focus on Post COVID-19 conditions. That is why the Bulgarian Cardiac Institute has launched a large-scale, free-of-charge, voluntary and indefinite screening campaign "Life after COVID-19". It aims to establish the effects of the infection on the cardiovascular system, diagnosis, treatment, long-term follow-up and adequate actions to improve the quality of life by providing specialized medical care.

The campaign covers citizens who have suffered from COVID-19. Those who wish to participate answer a survey with questions related to their health. When they answer in the affirmative to at least one of the questions (yes, i.e.there is a problem), we offer a free medical examination. It is held in one of the seven high-tech hospitals, with the highest third level of competence, according to national medical standards or in one of the 15 medical centers in the country, by leading specialists in the field of cardiology. The initial examination includes a detailed history, complete examination, blood pressure measurement and electrocardiogram, on the basis of which we determine whether the patient needs additional instrumental or laboratory tests and treatment. According to the results and the leading symptoms, patients are consulted with trained in Europe and USA specialists in the field of cardiac surgery, neurology, neurosurgery, vascular surgery and others. If necessary and with persistence of symptoms, despite treatment, citizens are hospitalized.

As the population of recovering from COVID-19 grows, it is crucial to identify the health problems that surround them. The campaign creates round-the-clock access to high-quality and specialized medical care at European level, based on a multidisciplinary approach and dedicated medical care.

4. Initial results of the campaign "Life after COVID"

More than 1,500 citizens took part in the survey - 77% of them were treated at home, 23% were hospitalized, of which 2% in intensive care units. Of all respondents, 80% answered in the affirmative (Yes, i.e.there is a problem) to at least one of the initial survey questions. Signs and symptoms such as fatigue (67%), palpitations (41%), shortness of breath (31%), chest pain (30%), joint pain (27%), headache (22%), impaired concentration (17%), persistent cough (16%), dizziness (15%) were among the most frequently reported in the questionnaire responses (**Figure 1**). A significant proportion of patients had more than two symptoms.

Medical examination was offered to citizens with persistent symptoms. We analyzed data from 808 patients (57% women and 43% men). The most common pathological changes we found were destabilization of blood pressure control (51%) - hypertension (92%), hypotension (5%) or fluctuation in blood pressure (3%). Heart rhythm disorders are the next most common finding (29%), expressed in tachycardia (97%) or bradycardia (3%). Manifestations of heart failure were found in 15% of cases.

According to the anamnesis and the objective condition, additional examinations had to be performed in 65% of the examined. These examinations included:

- Instrumental methods: echocardiography (41%), holter ECG (3%), radiography (3%)
- Laboratory diagnostics (9.4%): complete blood count, NT-proBNP, D-dimer, blood glucose test
- consultations with specialists (10%): neurologist (28%), pulmonologist (22%), endocrinologist (12%), vascular surgeon (5%), rheumatologist (4%) and other

At the end of the examination, a change in therapy was required for 62% of those followed.

At the time of the secondary examination, new studies were performed in 5% and a change in therapy in 2.6%. Despite all interventions, in 6% of the cases, due to the persistence of the symptoms, the citizens were hospitalized.

Our experience shows that the care of patients with COVID-19 should not stop at the end of the acute illness. From the responders to our survey, 4/5 reported persistent signs and symptoms months later. The most common complaints were: fatigue, palpitations, shortness of breath, chest pain. Other reported symptoms included joint pain, headache, and impaired concentration. High values of blood pressure, tachycardia, and manifestations of heart failure were the leading objective changes. Our study showed that in more than half of the cases of COVID-19,

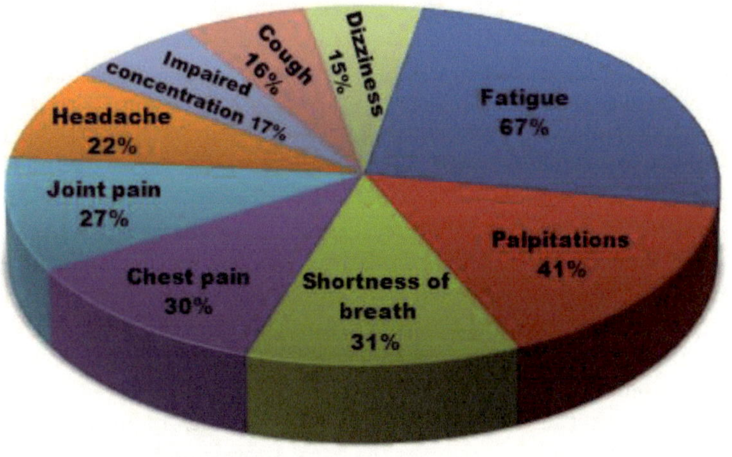

Figure 1.
The most common signs and symptoms persisting after COVID-19.

additional tests and changes in treatment were required. The range of symptoms required the inclusion of doctors with different specialties in the overall follow-up. Despite the measures taken, the symptoms may be so severe and difficult to control that re-hospitalization may be necessary.

People suffering from post COVID-19 conditions constitute already a significant part of the world's population, and their numbers will continue to grow. This necessitates a long-term commitment of human and material resources and will test the health and economic system of the countries. Regardless of the obstacles we face, dedication and professionalism, good organization and a holistic approach are the main prerequisites for good results. By tracking and caring for these patients, we will not only contribute to increasing humanity's knowledge of this new, dangerous pathogen, but we will also make progress in the process of diagnosis and treatment guidelines.

5. Imaging of myocardial involvement in post COVID-19 conditions

COVID-19 is a multiorgan systemic inflammatory disease caused by SARS-CoV-2 virus. Patients with COVID-19 often exhibit cardiac dysfunction and myocardial injury [63], which we can recognize with laboratory parameters and imaging methods. The most used imaging method is transthoraic echocardiography (TTE), which gives us information about the heart function. Global longitudinal strain (GLS) by speckle tracking echocardiography is an important additive method for evaluation of LV function at global and regional level. It is more sensitive method for detecting myocardial dysfunction, compared with Left ventricular ejection fraction (LVEF) [64]. Another very informative method is MRI, however it is not used that often, due to higher expenses and need of contrast material. According to studies, almost all patients with severe COVID-19 and most of the patients with moderate illness, had a certain degree of cardiac dysfunction [63].

Conventional echocardiography usually does not show significant changes in the LVEF and LV sizes in patients with mild or moderate COVID- 19. According to one trial in China, however, in 78.3% from the patients with mild infection and 98% of the patients who were in critical condition, some echocardiographic parameters showed deviations. For example, the motion of the LV walls was abnormal and the wall thickness was slightly thickened, particularly for the septum [63]. But in patients who were with critical conditions, lower LVEF could be found [65]. These changes are in correlation with elevated serum levels of cardiac biomarkers, such as cardiac troponin I (cTnI) and N-terminal pro-B-type natriuretic peptide (NT-proBNP), pulse oxygen saturation (SpO2) and inflammatory markers, such as C-reactive protein and cytokines [63].

Although abnormalities in conventional echocardiography are found mostly in patients with severe COVID- 19, global longitudinal strain (GLS) can identify subclinical myocardial dysfunction. Moreover, measuring GLS gives us the opportunity for earlier diagnosis of myocardial injury, even before a reduction in the LVEF occurs. Studies showed that reduced LV-GLS is more frequent, occurring in 80% of the patients, while LV function parameters such as reduced EF and wall motion abnormalities were less frequent findings [66].

2D- speckle tracking echocardiography is a method, which evaluates myocardial function at global and regional level. It shows the percentage of deformation between two points in the myocardium. Studies in COVID-19 patients show that the abnormal GLS predominantly involves the basal-septal and basal-lateral segments of the LV. This pattern reminded of a "reverse tako-tsubo" morphology, and is not typical for other viral myocarditis [67]. Another interesting finding is that the reduction of the LV-GLS is usually reversible, with normalization of the findings for one to three months [66].

Cardiac magnetic resonance (CMR) is the current gold standard to evaluate cardiac morphology and function. It has higher sensitivity for detecting occult cardiac dysfunction than hs-cTnI. With its mapping techniques, such as T1, T2, extracellular volume (ECV) and Late Gadolinium Enhancement (GLE), this method can assess quantitatively diffuse or local myocardial fibrosis and edema [68]. One study in Frankfurt with 100 patients recently recovered from COVID-19, showed that 78% of them had abnormal CMR findings, namely lower left ventricular ejection fraction, higher left ventricle volumes, raised signals in native T1 and T2 mapping, which illustrate edema and changes in LGE, showing myocardial fibrosis. Endomyocardial biopsy was performed in patients with severe findings and revealed active lymphocytic inflammation [37].

Our experience in "Life after COVID" campaign (unpublished data) shows that about two-thirds of PASC patients referred for echocardiography have the typical post COVID-19 GLS impairment, involving predominantly the basal segments. We observe such findings in severe as well as non-severe COVID-19 cases. Our management strategy in these cases includes prolongation of antiaggregant therapy, initiation of cardioprotective therapy (could include some or all of the following: beta-blocker, trimetazidine, molsidomine), antiviral therapy (hydroxychloroquine) and advice to refrain from vigorous physical activity, although maintaining moderate physical activity or inclusion in a rehabilitation program. Our initial experience with 3-month follow-up of these patients shows a resolution of the abnormality in about 80% of the cases in this time period.

From our experience, we think that global longitudinal strain is very sensitive for recognizing subclinical myocardial dysfunction and a valuable imaging method for prognosis, management, sport activity resumption advice, and long-term following of the patients recovered from COVID-19.

6. Acute coronary syndrome as part of the post COVID-19 conditions

Apart from the direct lung damage, the virus infection is associated with multiple organ damage, including the heart, causing conditions such as congestive heart failure, myocarditis, conduction abnormalities, arrhythmias, and acute coronary syndromes [69, 70]. The SARS-CoV-2 infection can frequently induce coagulation abnormalities that are associated with cardiopulmonary damage in all patients, despite presence or absence of concomitant risk factors and diseases.

The range of clinical responses to COVID-19 is extremely broad. Endothelial injury is an underlying mechanism that links the inflammation and consequent thrombosis [71, 72]. It is currently hypothesized that ACE-2 receptor is the entry gate for the virus to invade and infect tissues [73]. The vascular endothelium appears to be targeted directly by the virus as ACE-2 is expressed widely in the blood vessels and the heart. The result is exocytosis of endothelial granules containing VWF (von Willebrand factor), P-selectin, and other proinflammatory cytokines, which mediate platelets adhesion, aggregation, and leukocyte adherence to the vessel wall, with a final result of intravascular thrombosis [74].

In addition, many patients with severe COVID-19 undergo thromboembolic events, due to this particular coagulopathy [75, 76]. One of the most and life-threatening types of this coagulation abnormality is the one involving the coronary blood flow, thus causing a heart attack. In this scenario many additional problems arise – for example: access to a Cath lab, exposure of additional medical personnel, more complications and increased mortality for the patients. Invasive coronary angiography for COVID-19 patients is a logistic challenge and, in some cases, there is not a need for intervention since the main problem is the thrombosis and the dysfunction of the microcirculation. For this reason, we evaluated in detail a case series of ten patients referred for primary percutaneous coronary intervention (pPCI) for MI in our catheterization laboratory during the course of COVID-19 infection. The goal was to evaluate if there are any factors or parameters that could predict the presence of an interventional target – infarct related artery (IRA), prior to catheterization, and to determine their sensitivity and specificity.

During November and December 2020, 214 patients were treated in our COVID-19 department. Ten of them were referred to the Cath lab with MI defined by the fourth universal definition [77]. Most of the patients in our study were sent to our hospital due to acute coronary syndrome, while others developed ACS during their stay in the COVID-19 department.

After coronary angiography, we found that 7 patients (70%) had an IRA, and they underwent pPCI. The other 3 (30%) did not have an IRA, they did not require pPCI, and the diagnosis of myocardial infarction with no obstructive coronary arteries (MINOCA) was made, most probably due to myocarditis or microvascular dysfunction.

Comparing the patients with IRA to those without we found that the subjects who required pPCI had significantly higher high-sensitivity troponin I(hsTRI) values, had typical chest pain, and had more often ST elevation. The other studied variables did not differ significantly between the groups with or without IRA. Regarding hsTrI concentrations, all but one patient with IRA and pPCI had hsTrI>7.5 times URL, and all patients without IRA and pPCI had hsTrI ≤7.5 times URLN. Therefore, for hsTrI>1.5 ng/ml (>7.5 times URL) to predict the presence of IRA and the need for pPCI the sensitivity is 86%, the specificity is 100%, positive predictive value (PPV) is 100%, while the negative predictive value (NPV) is 10%.

Even though our analysis is on a small number of patients, similar incidence of arterial (coronary and cerebral) thrombosis (4%) has been described by other authors. In this study, however, the authors have not provided a guide to the right moment of interventional treatment. According to our published data search, we were not able to find another study, analyzing the predictors for the presence of IRA and the need for pPCI in COVID-19 MI patients.

So in conclusion, myocardial infarction, could complicate up to 5% of COVID-19 cases. In our study group, most of the patients (30%) with MI did not have an IRA and, did not need a coronary intervention. Patients with MI and IRA had significantly higher hsTrI values and exclusively typical chest pain compared to patients with MI but without an IRA, whose hsTrI values were lower and chest pain was atypical or non-stenocardic. ECG changes had only a minor statistical significance for distinguishing between MI patients with or without IRA. Our results suggest that using a higher cut-off value for hsTrI increases the specificity for diagnosing a MI and therefore - interventional treatment.

7. Pulmonary thromboembolism in patients after COVID-19 - predictive indicators for correct diagnosis

Infection caused by SARS-CoV-2 has been shown to lead to significant procoagulant events, in some cases involving life-threatening pulmonary thromboembolism (PE) [78]. A number of abnormalities have been described in coagulation parameters, which are a predictor of poor prognosis in patients with COVID-19 and PE [79]. Due to the lack of large prospective studies, little is known about the pathogenesis underlying PE, caused by COVID-19 [80]. Additional conditions complicating the diagnosis are the presence of risk factors for PE in almost all patients with COVID-19, as well as the overlap of the clinical presentation between PE and COVID-19.

We, therefore designed a study to find the indicators that predict the presence of PE in patients with acute or Post-acute COVID-19 conditions. It was a single-center study, conducted at the Heart and Brain Hospital, Pleven in the period December 2020-February 2021. It included 27 consecutively hospitalized patients with recent pneumonia caused by Covid-19 and clinical presentation referring to PE. The cohort was divided into two groups - without and with a definitive diagnosis of PE, proven by CT pulmoangiography. During treatment with COVID-19, all patients received a prophylactic dose of anticoagulant and antiplatelet drug.

Our results showed that eight patients from the group had PE, and 19 had not evidence of PE. The mean age of the group was 65 years and 18 of the patients were women. The two groups did not differ significantly in age and distribution between the sexes. Statistically significant differences in electrocardiographic findings were observed in the two groups. In patients without PE, 18 (94.7%) had no evidence of S-wave greater than 1.5 mm in I, aVL. On the other hand, in the group diagnosed with PE in 3 (37.5%) this ECG criteria was not present, and in 5 (62.5%) it was present ($p = 0.004$). Similar ratios were found in terms of the presence of Q-wave in III, aVF. In patients without PE, 18 (94.7%) did not have this ECG sign, while it was present in half of the patients with PE($p = 0.017$).

In patients without PE, the median value of oxygen saturation was 92.0% (69-97), and in those with proven - 88.5% (83-95) ($p < 0.001$). Statistically significant differences between the two groups were observed in regard to the indicator - the ratio RV/LV diameters ≥1.0 ($p = 0.001$). In patients without PE there was none with an increase in the ratio ≥ 1 in favor of the right ventricle, while in the group of patients with massive form 5 (62.5%) had the ratio RV/ LV diameters ≥1.0, and 3 (37, 5%) did not have it. The same results were demonstrated for the indicator right ventricular dysfunction ($p = 0.001$). The RV/LV diameter ratios ≥1.0 as well as right ventricular dysfunction showed sensitivity 62.5%, specificity 100%, positive predictive value 100% and negative such 86.4% to verify the PE diagnosis.

D-dimer values differed significantly in the two groups. In patients without PE, the mean D-dimer value was 1546 ng/ml (109-8840), while in those with PE - 6489.75 ng/ml (570-17051) ($p = 0.021$). For our laboratory, the upper limit of the normal range is 500 ng/ml. As a result of the ROC analysis we found that the D-dimer cut-off value of 1032 ng/ml (2,064 times higher above the upper limit of the normal range) had an optimal sensitivity (Se) of 87.5%, specificity (Sp) 57.9%, positive predictive value (PPV) 46.7% and negative predictive value (NPV) of 91.7% for the diagnosis of PE ($p = 0.021$) (**Figure 2**).

Regarding D-dimer as a binary variable (cut-off 1032 ng/ml), we found that in the group without PE, in 11 (57.9%) of patients the D-dimer was ≤1032 ng/ml, while in 8 (42.1%) it was >1032 ng/ml. Of the patients with massive PE, only 1 (12.5%) had a D-dimer ≤1032 ng/ml, and the remaining 7 (87.5%) were > 1032 ng/ml (Fisher's exact tests, $p = 0.043$).

When performing binary logistic regression, part of the ECG criteria - S-wave over 1.5 mm in I lead and aVL ($p = 0.007$), Q-wave in III and aVF ($p = 0.020$), as well as the D-dimer as quantitative variable ($p = 0.025$) proved to be independent predictors of PE.

Our results show that against the background of acute and Post-acute COVID-19 conditions ECG and EchoCG criteria remain predictive of PE. As for the D-dimer values, we found that a cut-off concentration with optimal Se, Sp, PPV and NPV for diagnosis of PE, is two times higher than the upper limit of normal, with high Se and

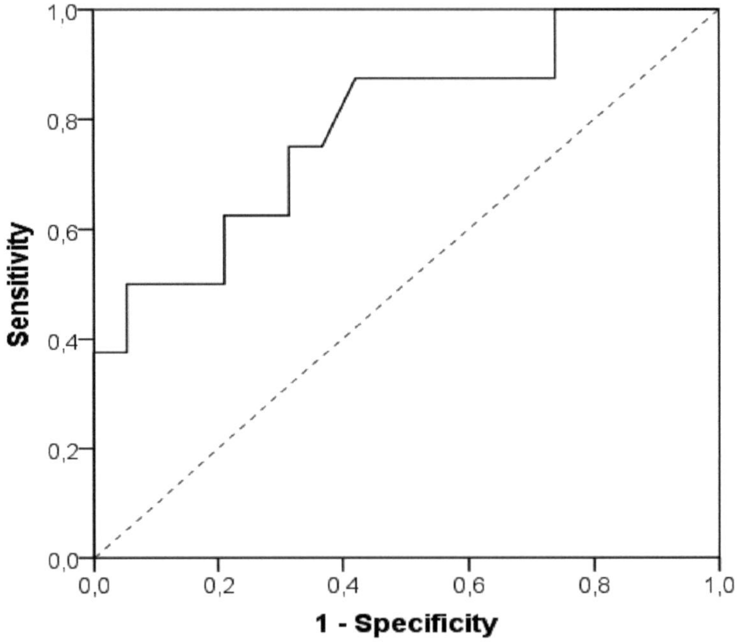

Figure 2.
ROC analysis for D-dimer values and the probability of PE.

NPV. We suggest that a higher D-dimer cut-off value should be applied in COVID-19 and post-COVID-19 patients in order to confirm/dismiss the diagnosis PE.

8. Acute limb ischemia as part of the post COVID-19 conditions

The vascular bed, being rich in ACE2 receptors, is not devoid of complications during the acute or post-acute COVID-19 conditions. Our analysis is to report our experience in the Department of Vascular Surgery of Heart and Brain Center of Clinical Excellence, Pleven, Bulgaria, focusing on management of COVID-19 patients who developed severe acute ischemia with impending lower and upper limb loss.

We carried out a retrospective data collection of COVID-19 patients with severe acute ischemia of the lower or upper limbs between December 2020, and April 2021. We included only those COVID-19 patients suffering from acute lower limb ischemia. Primary outcomes of the analysis were early reoperations, amputation and postoperative mortality.

Admitted to our department were 16 patients (13 male, 3 female) with acute ischemia of the lower limbs and 2 patients (both male) with acute ischemia of the upper limbs. The median age was 70 years (range 50–85 years). All patients tested positive for COVID-19 and all had general clinical symptoms. In all patients, the limb was at risk, and the only alternative was a major amputation. Seven of the cases had previous claudication symptoms and peripheral artery disease (PAD). Computed tomography-angiography (CT-A) showed acute thrombosis over atherosclerotic occlusive disease. The rest of the patients [11] had no clinical evidence of PAD. The occlusion was related to acute thrombosis of the arteries or distal embolization and confirmed by (CT-A).

Generally, based on the patient's overall stability, degree of ischemia, and limb viability, a determination needs to be made whether intervention is appropriate,

	All procedures	Generally good condition	Mortality
All patients	18	11 (61.1%)	7 (38.9%)
Open surgery	15	8 (53.3%)	7 (46.7%)
PTA/Stent	3	3 (100%)	0 (0%)
Re-operation	4	3 (75%)	1 (25%)
Amputation	6	3 (50%)	3 (50%)

Table 3.
Operative vascular procedures at the Vascular Surgery Department of Heart and Brain Center of Clinical Excellence, Pleven, Bulgaria

and if so, whether an endovascular or open approach should be used. It is crucial to consider the severity of systemic illness when considering intervention. Because of the severe pulmonary complications associated with COVID-19, critically ill patients may not be candidates for revascularization. Similar to damage control in trauma patients, the principle of "life over limb" is justified.

Laboratory parameters in our group showed increased levels of serum D-Dimer, C-reactive protein (CRP), and a decreased platelet count. All 18 patients underwent urgent revascularization, (embolectomy, open surgery procedures, percutaneous transluminal angioplasty with catheter balloon and stenting or primary amputation). Postoperatively, all patients received heparin therapy with low molecular weight heparin, combined with clopidogrel 75 mg and, in some cases, acetylsalicylic acid 100 mg.

Ten of the patients suffered from early (1st or 2nd day) postoperative re-thrombosis. All of them underwent reoperation (embolectomy), but 6 of them suffered from re-re-thrombosis and eventually required above-the-knee amputation and one patient required above-the-elbow amputation. Unfortunately, 7 patient died from multiple organ failure (MOF). 11 patients left the hospital in generally good condition. One patient with femoral-popliteal thrombosis left with symptoms of claudication but without critical limb ischemia. After one month this patient underwent endovascular revascularization with percutaneous transluminal angioplasty (PTA) and stent implantation (**Table 3**).

9. Conclusions

In our experience, the incidence of acute limb ischemia increased significantly during the COVID-19 pandemic in Bulgaria. Successful revascularization and survival was lower than expected, which we believed was due to a virus-related hypercoagulable state. The use of prolonged systemic heparin might improve surgical treatment efficacy, limb salvage, and overall survival.

10. Cardiac surgery during the COVID-19 pandemic

The COVID-19 pandemic posed serious challenges not only to modern cardiac surgery, but to medicine in general. As a result of the epidemic situation, the planned admission to hospitals and elective operations were stopped, and some of the health facilities were transformed into COVID-19 centers. Our hospital has developed a special algorithm for admission of patients in need of urgent or emergent cardiac surgery.

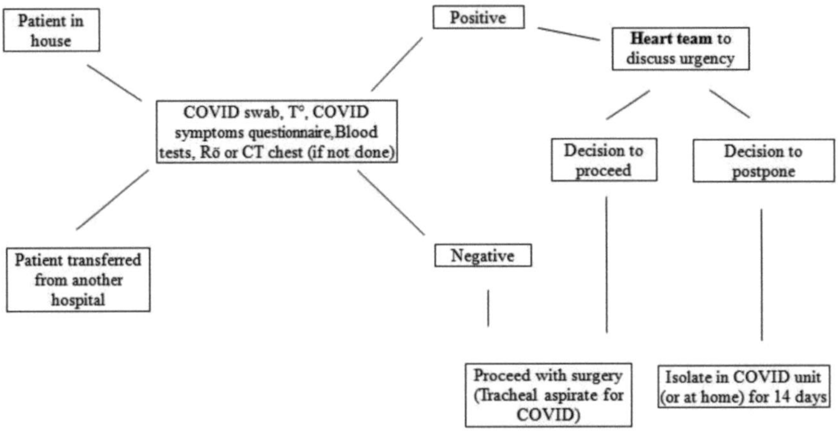

The epidemic situation has led to a reduction in hospital admissions. One of the reasons is certainly the fear of intra-hospital infection and transmission of COVID-19. The other reason is the postponement of elective operations. According to statistics, the number of hospitalized patients with acute coronary syndrome has decreased by 30%. If we consider that the mortality from COVID-19 is about 3% and the mortality from untreated STEMI reaches 30%, then the fear seems unjustified [81]. Important in this case, from a cardiac surgery point of view, is the definition of the concepts of elective and emergency admission and treatment, as well as treatment in accelerated and urgent order, as well as the nosological units to the respective groups:

- True elective (isolated MR, isolated AS)
- Accelerated elective (AS combined with CAD)
- Urgent (CAD withLM disease or LM equivalent)
- Emergent (Infective endocarditis, Acute myocardial infarction)
- Salvage life saving (Aortic dissection Stanford type A, mechanical complications after AMI)

While the first two groups may remain on the waiting list, for the next three the waiting time is shortened according to the disease (24 hours, 6 hours and as soon as possible in case of urgent, emergency and life-saving surgery, respectively). The functioning of such a system requires particularly good communication and collaboration between GPs, specialized outpatient and inpatient care, proper categorization of patients and optimal timing of treatment.

Unfortunately, there is still no formal international protocol or guidelines for optimal timing of cardiac surgery in patients with active COVID-19 infection. Since the beginning of the pandemic, 18 patients with identified COVID-19 infection pre- or postoperatively have undergone cardiac surgery (4.9% of all operated patients). The results of the operative treatment are excellent, as the intraoperative and early (up to 7th day) postoperative mortality is zero. Late postoperative mortality was 44%, with no patients dying from cardiovascular disease. It is noteworthy, contrary to expectations, that it is not the complexity of surgical treatment that is the leading risk factor for the complicated postoperative period in patients with proven COVID-19, but the development of viral pneumonia. Interstitial changes typical of COVID-19 pneumonia (ground-glass opacities, vascular enlargement, bilateral abnormalities, lower lobe involvement, and posterior predilection) have been demonstrated by CT scan in 75% of the deaths, with respiratory failure being the leading cause of death.

The question how long after recovery from a COVID-19 infection can a patient be transferred to surgery also remains open. Several studies on the subject are currently conducted. The data collected so far from 116 countries on 140,231 patients may finally show some resolve [82]. 2.2% of the patients included in the study were diagnosed preoperatively with COVID-19 infection. Mortality is highest in the first 7 weeks after the illness.

Thus, with surgical treatment 0-2 weeks, 3-4 weeks, and 5-6 weeks after COVID-19, the 30-day mortality was 4.1%, 3.9% and 3.6%, respectively. In surgical treatment after the seventh week, the results were the same as in patients without COVID-19 infection (1.5%). The estimated 30-day postoperative mortality in patients without COVID-19 infection was 1.5%. It should be borne in mind, however, that these are not specific studies in the field of cardiac surgery, but concern surgery in general. Probably the specific risk for cardiac surgery patients would be higher if we consider the complicated procedure of cardiac surgery, the aging of the population and the polymorbidity of the Bulgarian population. The role of the Heart team is crucial and the preparation of precise general hospital protocols and individual approach to each patient are extremely important for achieving good results.

Author details

Iana Simova[1,2,3*], Denislava Hristova[1], Hristina Tzanovska[1], Denis Nikolov[1], Diliana Iakova[1,3], Anyuta Ivanova[1], Maria-Magdalena Pintova[1], Pavlin Pavlov[1], Ognyan Matkov[1], Todor Samardjiev[1], Vladimir Kornovski[4], Jordan Krasnaliev[1], Todor Kundurzhiev[5], Nikolay Dimitrov[1,3,4] and Toni Vekov[2,3]

1 Heart and Brain Centre of Excellence, Pleven, Bulgaria

2 Bulgarian Cardiac Institute, Sofia, Bulgaria

3 Medical University, Pleven, Bulgaria

4 Heart and Brain Centre of Excellence, Burgas, Bulgaria

5 Medical University, Sofia, Bulgaria

*Address all correspondence to: ianasimova@gmail.com

References

[1] COVID-19 rapid guideline: managing the long-term effects of COVID-19. NICE guideline [NG188]. Published date: 18 December 2020 https://www.nice.org.uk/guidance/ng188

[2] Nalbandian, A., Sehgal, K., Gupta, A. et al. Post-acute COVID-19 syndrome. Nat Med 27, 601-615 (2021).https://doi.org/10.1038/s41591-021-01283-z

[3] Logue JK, Franko NM, McCulloch DJ, et al. Sequelae in Adults at 6 Months After COVID-19 Infection. *JAMA Netw Open.* 2021;4(2):e210830. doi:10.1001/jamanetworkopen.2021.0830

[4] Damian McNamara. Infectious COVID-19 Can Persist in Gut for Weeks, September 11, 2020, MedScape

[5] World Health Organization (WHO). COVID-19 Clinical management Living guidance 25 January 2021 ,

[6] Robert J. Mason. Pathogenesis of COVID-19 from a cell biology perspective. European Respiratory Journal 2020 55: 2000607; DOI: 10.1183/13993003.00607-2020

[7] Yeoh YK, Zuo T, Lui GC, et al Gut microbiota composition reflects disease severity and dysfunctional immune responses in patients with COVID-19 Gut 2021;70:698-706

[8] Srinivas Murthy, Todd C Lee. IL-6 blockade for COVID-19: a global scientific call to arms. Lancet Respir Med 2021 Published Online March 4, 2021 https://doi.org/10.1016/S2213-2600(21)00127-2

[9] Chaolin Huang, Lixue Huang , Yeming Wang. 6-month consequences of COVID-19 in patients discharged from hospital: a cohort study, The Lancet , Published:January 08, 2021 doi:https://doi.org/10.1016/S0140-6736(20)326568

[10] Bert R. Everaert , Jan Muylle , Theodorus Bartholomeus Twickler. Emerging cardiological issues during the COVID-19 pandemic https://doi.org/10.1111/eci.13270

[11] Morelli F, Meirelles LEF, de Souza MVF, Mari NL, Mesquita CSS, Dartibale CB, Damke GMZF, Damke E, da Silva VRS, Souza RP, Consolaro MEL. COVID-19 Infection in the Human Reproductive Tract of Men and Nonpregnant Women. Am J Trop Med Hyg. 2021 Jan 18;104(3):814-25. doi: 10.4269/ajtmh.20-1098. Epub ahead of print. PMID: 33534765; PMCID: PMC7941816

[12] Li H, Xiao X, Zhang J, Zafar MI, Wu C, Long Y, Lu W, Pan F, Meng T, Zhao K, Zhou L, Shen S, Liu L, Liu Q, Xiong C. Impaired spermatogenesis in COVID-19 patients. EClinicalMedicine. 2020 Nov;28:100604. doi: 10.1016/j.eclinm.2020.100604. Epub 2020 Oct 23. PMID: 33134901; PMCID: PMC7584442

[13] William S. Effects of covid-19 on the human musculoskeletal system, Young scientists journal, 14, 2020

[14] El-Anwar MW, Elzayat S, Fouad YA. ENT manifestation in COVID-19 patients. Auris Nasus Larynx. 2020;47(4):559-564. doi:10.1016/j.anl.2020.06.003

[15] Alexis E. and Stephanie E. COVID-19 rashes: How your skin can be a sign of the virus, 23 July 2020

[16] Alexis E. Carrington et.al. Dermatology experts tell all about how COVID-19 can affect the skin

[17] Post-COVID Conditions, Centers for Disease Control and prevention, Apr. 8, 2021 https://www.cdc.gov/

[18] Manish Bansal, Cardiovascular disease and COVID-19

[19] Claudio Napoli, Isabella Tritto, Giuditta Benincasa, Gelsomina Mansueto and Giuseppe Ambrosioc, Cardiovascular involvement during COVID-19 and clinical implications in elderly patients. A review AnnMedSurg (Lond). 2020 Sep; 57: 236-243. Published online 2020 Aug 5. doi: 10.1016/j.amsu.2020.07.054

[20] Hoffmann M., Kleine-Weber H., Schroeder S., Krüger N., Herrler T., Erichsen S. SARS-CoV-2 cell entry depends on ACE2 and TMPRSS2 and Is blocked by a clinically proven protease inhibitor. Cell. 2020;181(271-80):e8

[21] YasarSattar, Waqas Ullah, Hiba Rauf, Hafeez ul Hassan Virk,d Sunita Yadav, Medhat Chowdhury, Michael Connerney,a Sahil Mamtani,e Mohit Pahuja, Raj D. Patel, Tanveer Mir, Talal Almas, Homam Moussa Pacha, and M. ChadiAlraiesg. COVID-19 cardiovascular epidemiology, cellular pathogenesis, clinical manifestations and management Int J CardiolHeartVasc. 2020 Aug; 29: 100589. Published online 2020 Jul14. doi: 10.1016/j.ijcha.2020.100589

[22] Ksiazek TG, Erdman D, Goldsmith CS, et al. A novel coronavirus associated with severe acute respiratory syndrome. N Engl J Med 2003; 348: 1953-1966.

[23] Wang D., Hu B., Hu C., Zhu F., Liu X., Zhang J., Wang B., Xiang H., Cheng Z., Xiong Y., Zhao Y., Li Y., Wang X., Peng Z. Clinical characteristics of 138 hospitalized patients with 2019 novel coronavirus-infected pneumonia in Wuhan, China. J. Am. Med. Assoc. 2020;323:1061-1069. doi: 10.1001/jama.2020.1585.

[24] Huang C., Wang Y., Li X. Clinical features of patients infected with 2019 novel coronavirus in Wuhan, China. Lancet. 2020;395:497-506.doi: 10.1016/S0140-6736(20)30183-5

[25] Chen N., Zhou M., Dong X., Qu J., Gong F., Han Y., Qiu Y., Wang J., Liu Y., Wei Y., Xia J., Yu T., Zhang X., Zhang L. Epidemiological and clinical characteristics of 99 cases of 2019 novel coronavirus pneumonia in Wuhan, China: a descriptive study. Lancet. 2020;395:507-513. doi: 10.1016/S0140-6736(20)30211-7

[26] Li B., Yang J., Zhao F. Prevalence and impact of cardiovascular metabolic diseases on COVID-19 in China. Clin Res Cardiol. 2020

[27] Zhou F., Yu T., Du R. Clinical course and risk factors for mortality of adult inpatients with COVID-19 in Wuhan, China: a retrospective cohort study. Lancet. 2020

[28] Mihatov N, Januzzi JL, Gaggin HK. Type 2 myocardial infarction due to supply-demand mismatch. Trends Cardiovasc Med. 2017 Aug;27(6):408-417

[29] Asrress KN, Williams R, Lockie T, Khawaja MZ, De Silva K, Lumley M, Patterson T, Arri S, Ihsan S, Ellis H, Guilcher A, Clapp B, Chowienczyk PJ, Plein S, Perera D, Marber MS, Redwood SR. Physiology of Angina and Its Alleviation With Nitroglycerin: Insights From Invasive Catheter Laboratory Measurements During Exercise. Circulation. 2017 Jul 04;136(1):24-34

[30] Chen D., Li X., song q, Hu C., Su F., Dai J. Hypokalemia and clinical implications in patients with coronavirus disease 2019 (COVID-19) medRxiv. 2020 doi:10.1101/2020.02.27.20028530

[31] Xiong T.Y., Redwood S., Prendergast B., Chen M. Coronaviruses and the cardiovascular system: acute and long-term implications. Eur Heart J. 2020

[32] JuanEstebanGómez-Mesa, MD, FSIAC, Stephania Galindo-Coral, MD,

Maria Claudia Montes, MD, and Andrés J. Muñoz Martin, MD, PhD Thrombosis and Coagulopathy in COVID-19 CurrProbl Cardiol.2021 Mar; 46(3): 100742. Published online 2020 Nov 2. doi: 10.1016/j.cpcardiol. 2020.100742

[33] Tang N, Li D, Wang X, Sun Z. Abnormal coagulation parameters are associated with poor prognosis in patients with novel coronavirus pneumonia. J Thromb Haemostasis: JTH. 2020;18(4):844-847

[34] Knight DS, Kotecha T, Razvi Y, Chacko L, Brown JT, Jeetley PS. COVID-19: Myocardial injury in survivors. Circulation. 2020

[35] Guo T, Fan Y, Chen M, Wu X, Zhang L, He T. Cardiovascular implications of fatal outcomes of patients with coronavirus disease 2019 (COVID-19) JAMA Cardiol. 2020

[36] Sala S, Peretto G, Gramegna M, Palmisano A, Villatore A, Vignale D. Acute myocarditis presenting as a reverse Tako-Tsubo syndrome in a patient with SARS-CoV-2 respiratory infection. Eur Heart J. 2020;41(19):1861-1862.

[37] Puntmann VO, Carerj ML, Wieters I, Fahim M, Arendt C, Hoffmann J. Outcomes of Cardiovascular Magnetic Resonance Imaging in Patients Recently Recovered From Coronavirus Disease 2019 (COVID-19) JAMA Cardiol. 2020

[38] Hua A, O'Gallagher K, Sado D, Byrne J. Life-threatening cardiac tamponade complicating myo-pericarditis in COVID-19. Eur Heart J. 2020;41(22):2130.

[39] Manka R, Karolyi M, Polacin M, Holy EW, Nemeth J, Steiger P. Myocardial edema in COVID-19 on cardiac MRI. J Heart Lung Transplant. 2020;39(7):730-732.

[40] Rodolfo Citro,Gianluca Pontone, Michele Bellino,Angelo Silverio, Giuseppe Iuliano, Andrea Baggiano, Robert Manka, Severino Iesu, Carmine Vecchione, Federico Miguel Asch, Jelena Rima Ghadri and Christian Templinf. Role of multimodality imaging in evaluation of cardiovascular involvement in COVID-19 Trends Cardiovasc Med. 2021 Jan; 31(1): 8-16. Published online 2020 Oct 13. doi: 10.1016/j.tcm.2020.10.001

[41] Zhang L, Wang B, Zhou J, Kirkpatrick J, Xie M, Johri AM. Bedside focused cardiac ultrasound in COVID-19 from the Wuhan Epicenter: the role of cardiac point-of-care ultrasound, limited transthoracic echocardiography, and critical care echocardiography. J Am Soc Echocardiogr: Off Publ Am Soc Echocardiogr. 2020;33(6):676-682.

[42] Skulstad H, Cosyns B, Popescu BA, Galderisi M, Salvo GD, Donal E. COVID-19 pandemic and cardiac imaging: EACVI recommendations on precautions, indications, prioritization, and protection for patients and healthcare personnel. Eur Heart J Cardiovasc Imaging. 2020;21(6):592-598.

[43] Cosyns B, Lochy S, Luchian ML, Gimelli A, Pontone G, Allard SD. The role of cardiovascular imaging for myocardial injury in hospitalized COVID-19 patients. Eur Heart J Cardiovasc Imaging. 2020;21(7):709-714.

[44] Motwani M, Kidambi A, Greenwood JP, Plein S. Advances in cardiovascular magnetic resonance in ischaemic heart disease and non-ischaemic cardiomyopathies. Heart (British Cardiac Society) 2014;100(21):1722-1733

[45] Tam C.F., Cheung K.S., Lam S. Impact of coronavirus disease 2019 (COVID-19) outbreak on ST-segment-elevation myocardial infarction care in

Hong Kong, China. Circ Cardiovasc Qual Outcomes. 2020 CIRCOUTCOMES120006631.

[46] Ferrario C.M., Jessup J., Chappell M.C. Effect of angiotensin-converting enzyme inhibition and angiotensin II receptor blockers on cardiac angiotensin-converting enzyme 2. Circulation. 2005;111:2605-2610. 31.

[47] HFSA/ACC/AHA statement addresses concerns Re: using RAAS antagonists in COVID-19. https://www.acc.org/latest-in-cardiology/articles/2020/03/17/08/59/hfsa-acc-aha-statement-addresses-concerns-re-using-raas-antagonists-in-covid-19

[48] Position statement of the ESC council on hypertension on ACE-inhibitors and angiotensin receptor blockers. https://www.escardio.org/Councils/Council-on-Hypertension-(CHT)/News/position-statement-of-the-esc-council-on-hypertension-on-ace-inhibitors-and-ang

[49] Information for clinicians on therapeutic options for COVID-19 patients. https://www.cd.gov/coronavirus/2019-ncov/hcp/therapeutic-options.html

[50] Su, Yen-Boa,b; Kuo, Ming-Jena,b; Lin, Ting-Yua,b; Chien, Chian-Shiuc; Yang, Yi-Pingc; Chou, Shih-Jiec; Leu, Hsin-Banga,b,d,*Cardiovascular manifestation and treatment in COVID-19 Journal of the Chinese Medical Association: August 2020 - Volume 83 - Issue 8 - p 704-709

[51] Vandermeer ML, Thomas AR, Kamimoto L, Reingold A, Gershman K, Meek J, et al. Association between use of statins and mortality among patients hospitalized with laboratory-confirmed influenza virus infections: a multistate study. J Infect Dis 2012;205:13-9.

[52] Chauvin B, Drouot S, Barrail-Tran A, Taburet AM. Drug-drug interactions between HMG-CoA reductase inhibitors (statins) and antiviral protease inhibitors. Clin Pharmacokinet 2013;52:815-31.

[53] Ayman F, Ping W, Mahmoud A, Hesham S. Identification of FDA approved drugs targeting COVID-19 virus by structure-based drug repositioning. ChemRxiv 2020Doi:10.26434/chemrxiv.12003930.

[54] Kawaguchi M, Takahashi M, Hata T, Kashima Y, Usui F, Morimoto H, et al. Inflammasome activation of cardiac fibroblasts is essential for myocardial ischemia/reperfusion injury. Circulation 2011;123:594-604.

[55] Demidowich AP, Davis AI, Dedhia N, Yanovski JA. Colchicine to decrease NLRP3-activated inflammation and improve obesity-related metabolic dysregulation. Med Hypotheses 2016;92:67-73.

[56] Zhou X, Li Y, Yang Q. Antiplatelet therapy following percutaneous coronary intervention in patients complicated by COVID-19: implications from clinical features to pathological findings. Circulation 2020;141:1736-8.

[57] Thachil J, Tang N, Gando S, Falanga A, Cattaneo M, Levi M, et al. ISTH interim guidance on recognition and management of coagulopathy in COVID-19. J Thromb Haemost 2020;18:1023-6.

[58] Mayo Clinic COVID-19 (coronavirus): Long-term effects https://www.mayoclinic.org/diseases-conditions/coronavirus/in-depth/coronavirus-long-term-effects/art-20490351

[59] Lambert NJ, et al. COVID-19 "long hauler" symptoms survey report. Survivor Corps. https://www.survivorcorps.com/reports. Accessed Nov. 13, 2020.

[60] McIntosh K. Coronavirus disease 2019 (COVID-19): Clinical features. https://www.uptodate.com/contents/search. Accessed July 23, 2020.

[61] Yancy CW, et al. Coronavirus disease 2019 (COVID-19) and the heart — Is heart failure the next chapter? JAMA Cardiology. 2020; doi:10.1001/jamacardio.2020.3575.

[62] Mitrani RD, et al. COVID-19 cardiac injury: Implications for long-term surveillance and outcomes in survivors. Heart Rhythm. 2020; doi:10.1016/j.hrthm.2020.06.026.

[63] Rui Li, Hong Wang, Fei Ma, et al. Widespread myocardial dysfunction in COVID-19 patients detected by myocardial strain imaging using 2-D speckle-tracking echocardiography. ActaPharmacologicaSinica (2021). 0:1-8.

[64] Sigve Karlsen, Thomas Dahlslett, Bjørnar Grenne, Benthe Sjøli , Otto Smiseth, Thor Edvardsen and Harald Brunvand Karlsen et al. Global longitudinal strain is a more reproducible measure of left ventricular function than ejection fraction regardless of echocardiographic training. Cardiovascular Ultrasound (2019) 17:18

[65] Li SS, Cheng CW, Fu CL, et al. Left ventricular performance in patients with severe acute respiratory syndrome: a 30-day echocardiographic follow-up study. Circulation. 2003 Oct 14; 108(15):1798-803.

[66] Shmueli H., Shah M., Ebinger J., et al. Left ventricular global longitudinal strain in identifying subclinical myocardial dysfunction among patients hospitalized with COVID-19. Int J Cardiol Heart Vasc. 2021 Feb; 32: 100719.

[67] Stöbe St., Richter S., Seige M. Echocardiographic characteristics of patients with SARS-CoV-2 infection. ClinicalResearchinCardiology. 2020. Vol.109, 1549-1566.

[68] Huang L, Zhao P, Tang D, et al. Cardiac involvement in recovered COVID-19 patients identified by magnetic resonance imaging. JACC Cardiovasc Imaging. Published online May 12, 2020. doi:10.1016/j.jcmg.2020.05.004

[69] Rattka M, Dreyhaupt J, Winsauer C, et al. Effect of the COVID-19 pandemic on mortality of patients with STEMI: a systematic review and meta-analysis. Heart 2021;107:482-487.

[70] Samidurai A, Das A. Cardiovascular Complications Associated with COVID-19 and Potential Therapeutic~Strategies. Int J Mol Sci. 2020;21(18):6790. Published 2020 Sep 16. doi:10.3390/ijms21186790

[71] ZsuzsannaVarga, Andreas J Flammer, Peter Steiger, Martina Haberecker, Rea Andermatt, Annelies S, Zinkernagel et al. Endothelial cell infection and endotheliitis in COVID-19. Lancet. 2020 May 2;395(10234): 1417-1418. doi: 10.1016/S0140-6736(20)30937-5. Epub 2020 Apr 21.

[72] Charles J. Lowenstein, Scott D. Solomon. Severe COVID-19 Is a Microvascular Disease. Circulation. 2020;142:1609-1611

[73] Kasal DA, De Lorenzo A, Tibiriçá E. COVID-19 and Microvascular Disease: Pathophysiology of SARS-CoV-2 Infection With Focus on the Renin-Angiotensin System. Heart Lung Circ. 2020;29(11):1596-1602. doi:10.1016/j.hlc.2020.08.010

[74] James D. McFadyen, Hannah Stevens, Karlheinz Peter. The Emerging Threat of (Micro)Thrombosis in COVID-19 and Its Therapeutic Implications. Circulation Research. 2020;127:571-587. https://doi.org/10.1161/CIRCRESAHA.120.317447

[75] Asakura, H., Ogawa, H. COVID-19-associated coagulopathy and disseminated intravascular coagulation. Int J Hematol 113, 45-57 (2021). https://doi.org/10.1007/s12185-020-03029-y

[76] Schiavone M, Gobbi C, Biondi-Zoccai G, et al. Acute Coronary Syndromes and Covid-19: Exploring the Uncertainties. J Clin Med. 2020;9(6):1683. Published 2020 Jun 2. doi:10.3390/jcm9061683

[77] Kristian Thygesen, Joseph S Alpert, Allan S Jaffe, Bernard R Chaitman, Jeroen J Bax, David A Morrow, Harvey D White, ESC Scientific Document Group, Fourth universal definition of myocardial infarction (2018), *European Heart Journal*, Volume 40, Issue 3, 14 January 2019, Pages 237-269. https://doi.org/10.1093/eurheartj/ehy462

[78] Sakr Y., Giovini M., Leone M., et al. Pulmonary embolism in patients with coronavirus disease-2019 (COVID-19) pneumonia: a narrative review. AnnIntensive Care. 2020; 10: 124

[79] Rouhezamin, M. R., & Haseli, S. Diagnosing Pulmonary Thromboembolism in COVID-19: A Stepwise Clinical and Imaging Approach. Academic Radiology. 2020

[80] Helms, J., Tacquard, C., Severac, F. et al. High risk of thrombosis in patients with severe SARS-CoV-2 infection: a multicenter prospective cohort study. Intensive Care Medicine. 2020

[81] De Filippo et al. Reduced Rate of Hospital Admissions for ACS during Covid-19 Outbreak in Northern Italy NEJM 2020; doi; 10. 1056/NEJMc2009166

[82] https://associationofanaesthetists-publications.onlinelibrary.wiley.com/doi/10.1111/anae.15458

Chapter 11

COVID-19 and Type 2 Diabetes Mellitus

Ritwika Mallik and Mohammed S.B. Huda

Abstract

COVID-19 pandemic caused by SARS-COV-2 virus has evolved into a global crisis and is a major concern especially for the diabetes community. People with diabetes mellitus have increased morbidity and mortality associated with COVID-19 infection. Conversely, COVID-19 infection and treatment may predispose to hyperglycemia. Potentially modifiable risk factors have been discussed and urgent need to mitigate the risks is warranted. In this book chapter we summarize the available evidence on COVID-19 and type 2 diabetes mellitus including link between COVID-19 and type 2 diabetes, pathophysiology, clinical manifestations, management and complications.

Keywords: COVID-19, SARS-COV-2, diabetes mellitus, hyperglycaemia, type 2 diabetes

1. Introduction

From the offset of Coronavirus disease (COVID-19), groups that are more vulnerable to COVID-19 were identified. Presence of diabetes mellitus (DM), both type 1 (T1DM) and type 2 (T2DM) independently increases the adverse effects of COVID-19 [1]. A meta-analysis found that the proportion of diabetes in COVID-19 patients was 9.7% and that having cardiac disease and diabetes increased the risk of death by twice as much as the other risk factors [2]. The purpose of this chapter is to discuss in detail the current evidence available regarding type 2 diabetes mellitus and COVID-19.

2. Pathophysiology of T2D and COVID-19

There has been some insight into the pathophysiological mechanisms of COVID-19 infection and diabetes, but much remains to be investigated. The SARS-CoV2 utilizes angiotensin converting enzyme 2 (ACE2) to gain entry into infected cells and reduces expression of ACE2, and over activation of renin angiotensin aldosterone system (RAAS) is proposed to contribute to adverse effects in patients with diabetes (PWD) and COVID-19 infection [3].

Mechanisms accentuated in PWD include increased inflammatory cytokines, increased lipopolysaccharides, and increased RAAS (angiotensin 2) which results in vascular endothelial damage, increased ROS and IL-6 in increased insulin resistance (due to exaggerated angiotensin 2 activity) which results in hyperglycaemia [4]. There is increased blood viscosity due to increased fibrinogen and d-dimer [4].

The S1 spike protein of SARS-Cov2 is predicted to bind to DPP4 which may facilitate epithelial infection [1, 5].

It has been noted that infection with SARS-Cov-2 virus results in damage to pancreatic beta-cells [6]. Apart from COVID-19 related impaired insulin production [7], COVID-19 can cause insulin resistance due to activation of integrated stress response (ISR) initiating serine/threonine kinases which can induce IRS-1 serine phosphorylation. Hence, patients with COVID-19 infection can present with hyperglycaemia for the first time and may require insulin for insulin naïve patients or the one on insulin may have increased requirements [8].

Patients with type 2 diabetes (T2D) have a dysregulated immune response with higher ratio of lymphopenia, and increased levels of neutrophils, CRP and IL-6 have been noted in PWD with COVID-19 infections. T2D is associated with activation of the RAAS in different tissues [3]. In PWD pulmonary dysfunction has been reported involving changes in lung volume, lung diffusing capacity, ventilation, bronchomotor tone and neuroadrenergic bronchial innervation [3].

Increased metabolic rate, dysregulation of glucose metabolism, aggravation of inflammation and immune modulation result in increased oxidative stress, cytokine production, endothelial damage, increased glucotoxicity which ultimately can result in increased severity of COVID-19 and rapid progression of cardiorespiratory failure [4].

3. Clinical manifestations

The most common symptoms of COVID-19 infection are fever, cough [9], fatigue and shortness of breath [10]. Other symptoms such as sore throat, rhinorrhoea, ageusia, anosmia, vomiting and diarrhea have also been reported [11]. An observational study noted that male patients were more vulnerable than female patients to COVID-19 infection [9]. Common comorbidities include diabetes mellitus, hypertension obesity and cardiovascular disease [10].

Multiple comorbidities are associated with more severe disease and higher mortality [9]. Patients with T2D are more likely to develop severe COVID-19 infection as compared with patients without diabetes [12]. An increased prevalence of chronic obstructive pulmonary disease (COPD) and chronic kidney disease (CKD) has been noted in patients with T2D and COVID-19 infection [11]. COVID-19 infection may result in severe insulin resistance and insulin deficiency precipitating diabetic ketoacidosis (DKA) in patients with T1DM and not commonly but still possible in T2DM, result in new onset diabetes, or in PWD result in new or increased insulin therapy at times with very high dose requirements. Dexamethasone therapy which has been found to be beneficial in COVID-19 infection, can result in further hyperglycaemia and has the potential of precipitating Hyperosmolar hyperglycaemic state (HHS) and DKA [7]. Regular monitoring of capillary blood glucose (CBGs) is warranted for inpatients. As hyperglycaemia with ketosis may occur in COVID-19 infection, ketones should be checked in all patients with diabetes initially or if CBG > 12 mmol/L [13].

Laboratory findings include lymphopenia, thrombocytopenia, raised CRP, raised ALT and other markers of inflammation such as ferritin [10]. Compared with patients without diabetes, patients with T2DM were found to have a higher ESR, CRP, IL-6, TNF-α and procalcitonin but lower lymphocyte and T lymphocyte subsets [12]. HbA1C, IL-6 and lymphocyte count have been proposed as risk factors for the severity of COVID-19 infection and T2DM [12]. CT scan changes are common and include ground glass abnormalities, lung lesions and enlargement of lymph nodes [10].

4. Management of type 2 diabetes and COVID-19 infection

Diabetes UK, a British-based patient, healthcare professional and research charity, has provided advice for healthcare professionals on COVID-19 and inpatient diabetes care on their website and topics include front door guidance, managing inpatient hyperglycaemia, dexamethasone therapy and safe discharge endorsed by the Joint British Diabetes Society (JBDS) and Association of British Clinical Diabetologists (ABCD) [14].

Front door guidance is available for inpatients [13]. An ABCDE (Airway, breathing, circulation, disability and exposure) approach is warranted initially if patient is unwell, CBG> 12 mmol/L or known diabetes. Aim is rule out DKA, HHS and watch out for new presentation of diabetes, sepsis, steroid use, uncontrolled diabetes or delayed and missed treatment of diabetes [13]. Be aware of the possibility of euglycaemic DKA. Stop Metformin and SGLT2 inhibitors on admission. Fluid requirements may differ in patients with COVID-19 infection and have to be tailored individually due to ARDS, cardiac involvement or AKI. Contact the diabetes specialist team and early involvement of critical care team where appropriate.

Target glucose levels are 6–10 mmol/L, and up to 12 mmol/L is acceptable. The guidance for managing inpatient hyperglycaemia should be used if glucose levels are >12 mmol/L and a corrective dose is appropriate and the patient is not in DKA or HHS [14]. It provides information for patients on insulin and insulin naïve patients too, regarding insulin dose adjustment as while recovering from COVID-19 related insulin resistance, doses may require rapid reduction to avoid hyperglycemia [14]. Initiation of IV insulin with monitoring of blood glucose, electrolytes, pH and ketones should be done as appropriate. Blood ketones <0.6 mmol/L is safe, blood ketones 1.5–2.9 mmol/L signifies increased risk of DKA [13], and if 3 mmol/L or greater, then check pH and bicarbonate for possibility of DKA [13].

If patients unable to manage insulin pump start on variable rate intravenous insulin infusion (VRII) or subcutaneous (S/C) insulin. For S/C insulin find out the total daily insulin dose and if not available can be calculated as 0.5 units multiplied by weight. Half this dose is given as basal and remaining half as bolus dose divided by 3 to give the meal time dose [13]. If patient is placed in prone position, feeding may be affected and that needs to be taken into account while dosing insulin.

Continuous glucose monitors (CGMs) and flash glucose monitoring (FGM) can be left on but capillary blood glucose monitoring must still continue. For magnetic imaging such as MRIs, these devices including pumps should be removed [13]. Always check the feet on admission to look for foot infection and rule out critical limb ischaemia.

4.1 Medications used in diabetes

As it was not feasible to conduct RCTs initially, expert opinion and observational studies regarding treatment with medication for T2D suggest the following [15]:

Regular monitoring blood glucose of patients on insulin should be encouraged [15]. A retrospective study in patients in China found that patients with T2D required more medical interventions and had a significantly higher mortality and multiple organ injury than the non-diabetic individuals [3]. Within PWD they found that well controlled BG (CBG 3.9–10 mmol/L) was associated with reduction in adverse outcomes including lower mortality as compared with poorly controlled BG while in hospital. Hence correlation of improved glycaemic control with better outcomes was made and aggressive blood glucose lowering treatment with tablets and insulin was advocated.

4.1.1 Insulin

Insulin therapy is the mainstay in acute unwell PWD admitted to hospital where oral tablets have been stopped or not enough to control the hyperglycaemia. However, there is some evidence that insulin treatment is associated with adverse clinical outcomes in patients with T2D and COVID-19, including increased mortality. Use of insulin was associated with enhanced inflammation (increased IL-1β-dependent CRP and IL-6) and injury of vital organs (acute cardiac injury and acute kidney injury) during the progression of COVID-19 in patients with T2D [16]. Hypoglycaemia was higher in patients on insulin and may have contributed to the increased mortality although a sub-group without hypoglycaemia still had increased mortality. Insulin has been the mainstay in ill PWD and if hyperglycaemia and insulin result in adverse outcomes, there is a difficult dilemma for clinicians [17]. A UK study of 2.85 million PWD, a higher risk of COVID-19 related mortality was seen in patients on insulin, but the higher risk was thought to be due to residual confounding factors rather than direct drug effects [18]. Currently guidelines continue to endorse insulin in unwell PWD. Caution and close monitoring is to be exerted while using insulin treatment in PWD and COVID-19.

4.1.2 Metformin

Metformin, a lipophilic biguanide, has been associated with reduced mortality in women with obesity or T2D admitted to hospital with COVID-19 infection [19]. Several explanations have been provided including decreased inflammatory factors. Retrospective studies evaluating use of Metformin in T2D and COVID-19 infection have mainly suggested some benefit or no harm or benefit whereas a single study has suggested some harm, but overall use of Metformin is considered to be safe [20]. The CORONADO study which was a prospective study noted that Metformin was associated with a lower risk of death in PWD hospitalized with COVID-19 infection [21]. Dehydration with Covid-19 may increase the risk of lactic acidosis in patients taking metformin, hence temporary cessation of the drug along with usual sick day rules should be followed. Renal function should be monitored closely [15]. As metformin may reduce progression to severe COVID-19 infection, after initial cessation and review of clinical parameters including hypoxic state, lactate and renal parameters, metformin may be re-introduced if appropriate [13]. The MET-Covid Trial is an RCT designed to evaluate use of Metformin versus placebo for outpatient treatment and post exposure prophylaxis of COVID-19 infection [22].

4.1.3 Sodium glucose co-transporter 2 inhibitors

Sodium glucose co-transporter 2 inhibitors (SGLT2i) primarily act on the proximal tubule to block sodium and glucose absorption. Given that the mechanisms that are attributed to the protective effects of SGLT2i overlap with the mechanisms that are activated in COVID-19 infection, SGLT2i seem to have the potential to protect against end organ damage through cardio-renal protection [23]. Initiation of this medication should not be done during any likely infection, and for patients with T2D with COVID-19 infection, on SGLT2I, risk of dehydration and euglycemic DKA remains and should temporarily stop this medication and follow sick day rules. Renal function should be monitored closely [15]. A retrospective study to evaluate SGLT2i and COVID19 infection in a large UK based primary care dataset concluded that as compared to DPP4i, SGLT2i did not confer an increased risk of COVID-19 infection [24]. They deemed that clinicians can safely use SGLT2i the everyday care of PWD during COVID-19. DARE-19, is the first randomized controlled multi-centre trial investigating the use of Dapagliflozin, and the goals are to prevent COVID-19 related organ dysfunction or mortality and to improve clinical recovery [23].

4.1.4 Glucagon like peptide receptor agonists

Glucagon like peptide receptor agonist (GLP-1 RA) in animal studies has shown to activate ACE-2 expression and there have been speculations if this accelerated virus entrance into host cells but also if this expression neutralizes the virus limiting infection [25]. There is support for the hypothesis that GLP-1 RA may mitigate a more adverse clinical course in PWD and COVID-19 infection [26]. GLP-1 RA also are beneficial with weight loss. There are a few studies on GLP1RA and COVID-19 infection and even the final report of the CORONADO study did not find any benefit or harm with its use [27]. Dehydration is likely to lead to serious illness so patients on GLP1RA with COVID-19 should be monitored [15]. Regular meals and adequate hydration should be encouraged [15].

4.1.5 Dipeptidyl peptidase-4 inhibitors

It has been proposed that SARS Cov-2 binds to Dipeptidyl peptidase-4 inhibitors (DPP4), but the clinical implications are not known. Dipeptidyl peptidase-4 inhibitors (DPP4i) are well tolerated in COVID-19 infection [15]. The majority of studies have shown either benefit with DPP4i in PWD and COVID-19, or no harm or benefit [20], Although DPP4 inhibitors appear to be safe in T2D and COVID-19 infection [4], in an observational study of 717 patients, in the diabetes sub-group, patients on DPP4I were at a higher risk of ICU admission [5]. As study that compared GLP-1 RA or DPP4i with SGLT2i did not note associated improved outcomes in patients with COVID-19 infection [28]. As DPP4 upregulation may be an indicator for severity of COVID-19 infection, there is interest regarding the use of DPP4i in COVID-19 infection and available information may form the path to discovering novel therapies [29]. RCTs involving Linagliptin versus placebo and Sitagliptin versus placebo have been registered [30, 31].

4.1.6 Sulphonylureas

The use of sulphonylureas with regard to COVID-19 infection has not shown any harm or benefit according to some retrospective studies [20]. If there is a risk of hypoglycaemia, they may be stopped. Sulphonylureas are not recommended in the context of dexamethasone induced hyperglycaemia as beta cell function maybe impaired with COVID-19 infection and there is insulin resistance too [7].

4.1.7 Thiazolidinediones

Several studies have shown a reduction in proinflammatory cytokines with pioglitazone, but no studies have reported outcomes in pioglitazone users with COVID-19 infection, and due to small numbers of users meaningful data is unlikely to be available soon [20].

4.1.8 Steroid induced hyperglycaemia

Dexamethasone has been proven to reduce mortality in patients dependent on oxygen therapy and ventilation. However, recommended dose of 6 mg orally or intravenously are bound to affect glucose metabolism and guidance for glucocorticoid therapy in patients with and without diabetes is provided by DUK [14].

4.2 Hypertension

Treatment with angiotensin-converting enzyme inhibitors (ACEI) and angiotensin receptor blockers (ARBs) could increase the expression of ACE2 and accelerate entry of the virus into the cells. However, in COVID-19 infection, impairment of the ACE2/Mas receptor pathway and increase in angiotensin-2 activity could occur, and RAAS blockade may protect against this serious lung injury. Thus it is recommended that ACEI and ARBs should continue [15].

4.3 Lipid medications

Reduction on ACE2 by hyperlipidemia is restored by statins. It is believed that statins should not be discontinued in patients with COVID-19 infection due to it pleiotropic effects and potential for a cytokine storm due to rebound increase in interleukins [15].

4.4 Renal transplant recipients

Potential effect of COVID-19 on pancreatic function of patients with solid organ transplants is not known. Monitoring is required for patients with PTDM and without diabetes at risk of PTDM [15].

4.5 Fatty liver disease

Should be considered at an increased risk of cytokine storm and should be considered at risk of severe disease. Hence patients at risk of a cytokine storm and are to be considered at an increased risk of severe disease. There may be some benefit of screening and monitoring tests for hyperinflammation [15].

4.6 Discharge

Advice regarding safe and supported discharge is available [14]. Patients using insulin pumps or wearable diabetes technology should have them returned to the patient if not being used and ensure enough consumables are available at home. If a patient has had DKA, SGLT2i should not be used. Metformin can be re-started once the patient is well, eGFR>30 ml/min and lactate is normal. Sulphonylureas may have been withheld due to risk of hypoglycaemia, and assessment should be made if re-starting it is appropriate.

4.7 Outpatient management

It is suggested that patients with diabetes (PWD) not yet infected with the SARS-CoV-2 virus should intensify their treatment to prevent COVID-19 infection including glycaemic control, management of hypertension and raised cholesterol. Tele medicine and virtual appointments should continue to ensure adequate follow up [15]. The priority was to contain spread of COVID-19 but health care services need to ensure that the needs of PWD are met is imperative which includes continuous supply of medications and available healthcare services in the primary care [32].

4.8 Prevention

Patients with COVID-19 infection without diabetes should be monitored for new onset diabetes especially if on steroids. PWD and COVID-19 infection should have good glycaemic control [15].

4.9 Lifestyle management

While lockdown was the best armamentarium we had while the vaccination program was established and rolled out, it lead to potential for more sedentary activity, unhealthy diet, mental health related issues and possible delay in seeking care due to fear of contracting COVID-19 especially for patients with chronic conditions. Maintaining a healthy lifestyle is important now more than ever [32]. Adoption of dietary advice and restriction of dietary carbohydrates has been proposed for people with metabolic syndrome [33]. Smoking was associated with a higher mortality rate in hospitalized patients and advice regarding smoking cessation should be given [9].

4.10 Prediabetes

Prediabetes is associated with increased CRP and IL-6, and hospitalized patients with moderate to severe COVID-19 infection have been noted to have prediabetes, hence it has been proposed that pre-diabetes be treated as a comorbidity for COVID-19 infection [34]. Whether screening of all COVID-19 infected patients for prediabetes to improve patient care is feasible or beneficial remains to be seen as there is currently no therapeutic drug approved for prediabetes.

5. Complications

Apart from the known pulmonary complications, extra pulmonary complications from COVID-19 include neurological, cardiovascular, gastro-intestinal, renal, endocrine and dermatological complications are being reported [35]. Due to COVID-19 infection, there have been increased risk of hyperglycaemia, euglycaemic ketosis and diabetic ketoacidosis (DKA) [35]. With COVID-19 infection, there is a risk of atypical presentations of complications such as DKA or mixed hyperosmolar states with associated increased mortality. A retrospective case series confirmed that PWD are at a risk of combined DKA and HHs with COVID-19 infection [36]. Data from our own centre has shown that DKA in T2DM is increased significantly and that the frequency of HHS increased seven fold during the first Covid pandemic in the UK [37]. Fluid management is a challenge in such patients especially in case of renal impairment and ARDS should be avoided. Guidelines for management of DKA is available on the Diabetes UK website and it is worth remembering that euglycaemic DKA can occur in patients taking SGLT2i or in pregnancy [14]. In a whole population study assessing risks of in-hospital death in England, people with T1DM were found to be three-and-a-half times more at risk of dying from COVID-19 infection, while people with T2D are at twice the risk of dying than people without diabetes [38]. Hence, continued measures to mitigate the risks of people with diabetes of becoming seriously ill or dying due to COVID-19 infection is warranted.

6. Conclusion

COVID-19 infection and diabetes mellitus have important and clinically relevant interactions. It is important for all physicians to be aware of these, particularly in view of likely further COVID-19 pandemics.

Author details

Ritwika Mallik and Mohammed S.B. Huda*
Department of Diabetes and Metabolism, St. Bartholomew's and Royal London Hospital, Barts Health Trust, London, United Kingdom

*Address all correspondence to: bobby.huda1@nhs.net

References

[1] Gregory JM, Slaughter JC, Duffus SH, Smith TJ, LeStourgeon LM, Jaser SS, McCoy AB, Luther JM, Giovannetti ER, Boeder S, Pettus JH, Moore DJ. COVID-19 severity is tripled in the diabetes community: A prospective analysis of the pandemic's impact in type 1 and type 2 diabetes. Diabetes Care. 2021 Feb;44(2):526-532. DOI:10.2337/dc20-2260. Epub 2020 Dec 2.

[2] Li B, Yang J, Zhao F, Zhi L, Wang X, Liu L, Bi Z, Zhao Y. Prevalence and impact of cardiovascular metabolic diseases on COVID-19 in China. Clin Res Cardiol. 2020 May;109(5):531-538. DOI:10.1007/s00392-020-01626-9.

[3] Zhu L, She ZG, Cheng X, Qin JJ, Zhang XJ, Cai J, Lei F, Wang H, Xie J, Wang W, Li H, Zhang P, Song X, Chen X, Xiang M, Zhang C, Bai L, Xiang D, Chen MM, Liu Y, Yan Y, Liu M, Mao W, Zou J, Liu L, Chen G, Luo P, Xiao B, Zhang C, Zhang Z, Lu Z, Wang J, Lu H, Xia X, Wang D, Liao X, Peng G, Ye P, Yang J, Yuan Y, Huang X, Guo J, Zhang BH, Li H. Association of blood glucose control and outcomes in patients with COVID-19 and pre-existing type 2 diabetes. Cell Metab. 2020 Jun 2;31(6):1068-1077.e3. DOI:10.1016/j.cmet.2020.04.021.

[4] Lim S, Bae JH, Kwon HS, Nauck MA. COVID-19 and diabetes mellitus: From pathophysiology to clinical management. Nat Rev Endocrinol. 2021 Jan;17(1):11-30. DOI:10.1038/s41574-020-00435-4.

[5] Dalan R, Ang LW, Tan WYT, Fong SW, Tay WC, Chan YH, Renia L, Ng LFP, Lye DC, Chew DEK, Young BE. The association of hypertension and diabetes pharmacotherapy with COVID-19 severity and immune signatures: An observational study. Eur Heart J Cardiovasc Pharmacother. 2021 May 23;7(3):e48-e51. DOI:10.1093/ehjcvp/pvaa098.

[6] Govender N, Khaliq OP, Moodley J, Naicker T. Insulin resistance in COVID-19 and diabetes. Prim Care Diabetes. 2021 Apr 8;15(4):629-634. DOI:10.1016/j.pcd.2021.04.004.

[7] Rayman G, Lumb AN, Kennon B, Cottrell C, Nagi D, Page E, Voigt D, Courtney HC, Atkins H, Higgins K, Platts J, Dhatariya K, Patel M, Newland-Jones P, Narendran P, Kar P, Burr O, Thomas S, Stewart R. Dexamethasone therapy in COVID-19 patients: Implications and guidance for the management of blood glucose in people with and without diabetes. Diabet Med. 2021 Jan;38(1):e14378. DOI:10.1111/dme.14378.

[8] Santos A, Magro DO, Evangelista-Poderoso R, Saad MJA. Diabetes, obesity, and insulin resistance in COVID-19: Molecular interrelationship and therapeutic implications. Diabetol Metab Syndr. 2021 Mar 1;13(1):23. DOI:10.1186/s13098-021-00639-2.

[9] Abbas HM, Nassir KF, Al Khames Aga QA, Al-Gharawi AA, Rasheed JI, Al-Obaidy MW, Al Jubouri AM, Jaber AS, Al Khames Aga LA. Presenting the characteristics, smoking versus diabetes, and outcome among patients hospitalized with COVID-19. J Med Virol. 2021 Mar;93(3):1556-1567. DOI:10.1002/jmv.26487.

[10] Israfil SMH, Sarker MMR, Rashid PT, Talukder AA, Kawsar KA, Khan F, Akhter S, Poh CL, Mohamed IN, Ming LC. Clinical characteristics and diagnostic challenges of COVID-19: An update from the global perspective. Front Public Health. 2021 Jan 11;8:567395. DOI:10.3389/fpubh.2020.567395.

[11] Maddaloni E, D'Onofrio L, Alessandri F, Mignogna C, Leto G, Coraggio L, Sterpetti S, Pascarella G, Mezzaroma I, Lichtner M, Pozzilli P,

Agrò FE, Rocco M, Pugliese F, Mastroianni CM, Buzzetti R; CoViDiab study group. Clinical features of patients with type 2 diabetes with and without Covid-19: A case control study (CoViDiab I). Diabetes Res Clin Pract. 2020 Nov;169:108454. DOI:10.1016/j.diabres.2020.108454.

[12] Cheng Y, Yue L, Wang Z, Zhang J, Xiang G. Hyperglycemia associated with lymphopenia and disease severity of COVID-19 in type 2 diabetes mellitus. J Diabetes Complications. 2021 Feb;35(2):107809. DOI:10.1016/j.jdiacomp.2020.107809.

[13] Guidance for inpatient diabetes care. Concise advice on Inpatient Diabetes (COVID:Diabetes) – Front Door Guidance Available from: https://www.diabetes.org.uk/professionals/resources/coronavirus-clinical-guidance/inpatient-guidance [Accessed on 2021-06-28].

[14] Guidance for inpatient diabetes care. Advice for healthcare professionals on coronavirus (covid-19) and inpatient diabetes care. https://www.diabetes.org.uk/professionals/resources/coronavirus-clinical-guidance/inpatient-guidance [Accessed 2020-06-28]

[15] Bornstein SR, Rubino F, Khunti K, Mingrone G, Hopkins D, Birkenfeld AL, Boehm B, Amiel S, Holt RI, Skyler JS, DeVries JH, Renard E, Eckel RH, Zimmet P, Alberti KG, Vidal J, Geloneze B, Chan JC, Ji L, Ludwig B. Practical recommendations for the management of diabetes in patients with COVID-19. Lancet Diabetes Endocrinol. 2020 Jun;8(6):546-550. DOI:10.1016/S2213-8587(20)30152-2.

[16] Yu B, Li C, Sun Y, Wang DW. Insulin treatment is associated with increased mortality in patients with COVID-19 and type 2 diabetes. Cell Metab. 2021 Jan 5;33(1):65-77.e2. DOI:10.1016/j.cmet.2020.11.014.

[17] Donath MY. Glucose or insulin, which is the culprit in patients with COVID-19 and diabetes? Cell Metab. 2021 Jan 5;33(1):2-4. DOI:10.1016/j.cmet.2020.11.015.

[18] Khunti K, Knighton P, Zaccardi F, Bakhai C, Barron E, Holman N, Kar P, Meace C, Sattar N, Sharp S, Wareham NJ, Weaver A, Woch E, Young B, Valabhji J. Prescription of glucose-lowering therapies and risk of COVID-19 mortality in people with type 2 diabetes: A nationwide observational study in England. Lancet Diabetes Endocrinol. 2021 May;9(5):293-303. DOI:10.1016/S2213-8587(21)00050-4.

[19] Bramante CT, Ingraham NE, Murray TA, Marmor S, Hovertsen S, Gronski J, McNeil C, Feng R, Guzman G, Abdelwahab N, King S, Tamariz L, Meehan T, Pendleton KM, Benson B, Vojta D, Tignanelli CJ. Metformin and risk of mortality in patients hospitalised with COVID-19: A retrospective cohort analysis. Lancet Healthy Longev. 2021 Jan;2(1):e34-e41. DOI:10.1016/S2666-7568(20)30033-7.

[20] Singh AK, Singh R, Saboo B, Misra A. Non-insulin anti-diabetic agents in patients with type 2 diabetes and COVID-19: A critical appraisal of literature. Diabetes Metab Syndr. 2021 Jan-Feb;15(1):159-167. DOI:10.1016/j.dsx.2020.12.026.

[21] Lalau JD, Al-Salameh A, Hadjadj S, Goronflot T, Wiernsperger N, Pichelin M, Allix I, Amadou C, Bourron O, Duriez T, Gautier JF, Dutour A, Gonfroy C, Gouet D, Joubert M, Julier I, Larger E, Marchand L, Marre M, Meyer L, Olivier F, Prevost G, Quiniou P, Raffaitin-Cardin C, Roussel R, Saulnier PJ, Seret-Begue D, Thivolet C, Vatier C, Desailloud R, Wargny M, Gourdy P, Cariou B; CORONADO investigators. Metformin use is associated with a reduced risk of mortality in patients with diabetes

hospitalised for COVID-19. Diabetes Metab. 2020 Dec 10;47(5):101216. DOI:10.1016/j.diabet.2020.101216.

[22] Met-Covid: Outpatient Metformin Use for Covid 19 [Internet]. Available from: https://clinicaltrials.gov/ct2/show/NCT045110194 [Accessed on 2021-06-28].

[23] Kosiborod M, Berwanger O, Koch GG, Martinez F, Mukhtar O, Verma S, Chopra V, Javaheri A, Ambery P, Gasparyan SB, Buenconsejo J, Sjöström CD, Langkilde AM, Oscarsson J, Esterline R. Effects of dapagliflozin on prevention of major clinical events and recovery in patients with respiratory failure because of COVID-19: Design and rationale for the DARE-19 study. Diabetes Obes Metab. 2021 Apr;23(4):886-896. DOI:10.1111/dom.14296.

[24] Sainsbury C, Wang J, Gokhale K, Acosta-Mena D, Dhalla S, Byne N, Chandan JS, Anand A, Cooper J, Okoth K, Subramanian A, Bangash MN, Taverner T, Hanif W, Ghosh S, Narendran P, Cheng KK, Marshall T, Gkoutos G, Toulis K, Thomas N, Tahrani A, Adderley NJ, Haroon S, Nirantharakumar K. Sodium-glucose co-transporter-2 inhibitors and susceptibility to COVID-19: A population-based retrospective cohort study. Diabetes Obes Metab. 2021 Jan;23(1):263-269. DOI:10.1111/dom.14203.

[25] Pang J, Liu M, Ling W, Jin T. Friend or foe? ACE2 inhibitors and GLP-1R agonists in COVID-19 treatment. Obes Med. 2021 Mar;22:100312. DOI:10.1016/j.obmed.2020.100312.

[26] Monda VM, Porcellati F, Strollo F, Gentile S. ACE2 and SARS-CoV-2 infection: Might GLP-1 receptor agonists play a role? Diabetes Ther. 2020 Sep;11(9):1909-1914. DOI:10.1007/s13300-020-00898-8.

[27] Wargny M, Potier L, Gourdy P, Pichelin M, Amadou C, Benhamou PY, Bonnet JB, Bordier L, Bourron O, Chaumeil C, Chevalier N, Darmon P, Delenne B, Demarsy D, Dumas M, Dupuy O, Flaus-Furmaniuk A, Gautier JF, Guedj AM, Jeandidier N, Larger E, Le Berre JP, Lungo M, Montanier N, Moulin P, Plat F, Rigalleau V, Robert R, Seret-Bégué D, Sérusclat P, Smati S, Thébaut JF, Tramunt B, Vatier C, Velayoudom FL, Vergès B, Winiszewski P, Zabulon A, Gourraud PA, Roussel R, Cariou B, Hadjadj S; CORONADO investigators. Predictors of hospital discharge and mortality in patients with diabetes and COVID-19: updated results from the nationwide CORONADO study. Diabetologia. 2021 Apr;64(4):778-794. DOI:10.1007/s00125-020-05351-w.

[28] Israelsen SB, Pottegård A, Sandholdt H, Madsbad S, Thomsen RW, Benfield T. Comparable COVID-19 outcomes with current use of GLP-1 receptor agonists, DPP-4 inhibitors or SGLT-2 inhibitors among patients with diabetes who tested positive for SARS-CoV-2. Diabetes Obes Metab. 2021 Jun;23(6):1397-1401. DOI:10.1111/dom.14329.

[29] Bassendine MF, Bridge SH, McCaughan GW, Gorrell MD. COVID-19 and comorbidities: A role for dipeptidyl peptidase 4 (DPP4) in disease severity? J Diabetes. 2020 Sep;12(9):649-658. DOI:10.1111/1753-0407.13052.

[30] Effects of DPP4 Inhibition on COVID-19 [Internet]. Available from: https://clinicaltrials.gov/ct2/show/NCT04341935 [Accessed on 2021-06-28].

[31] The effect of sitagliptin treatment in COVID-19 positive diabetic patients (SIDIACO). Available from: https://clinicaltrials.gov/ct2/show/NCT04365517 [Accessed on 2021-06-28].

[32] Beran D, Aebischer Perone S, Castellsague Perolini M, Chappuis F, Chopard P, Haller DM, Jacquerioz Bausch F, Maisonneuve H, Perone N, Gastaldi G. Beyond the virus: Ensuring continuity of care for people with diabetes during COVID-19. Prim Care Diabetes. 2021 Feb;15(1):16-17. DOI:10.1016/j.pcd.2020.05.014.

[33] Demasi M. COVID-19 and metabolic syndrome: Could diet be the key? BMJ Evid Based Med. 2021 Feb;26(1):1-2. DOI:10.1136/bmjebm-2020-111451.

[34] Sosibo AM, Khathi A. Pre-diabetes and COVID-19, could we be missing the silent killer? Exp Biol Med (Maywood). 2021 Feb;246(4):369-370. DOI:10.1177/1535370220973451.

[35] Tsai PH, Lai WY, Lin YY, Luo YH, Lin YT, Chen HK, Chen YM, Lai YC, Kuo LC, Chen SD, Chang KJ, Liu CH, Chang SC, Wang FD, Yang YP. Clinical manifestation and disease progression in COVID-19 infection. J Chin Med Assoc. 2021 Jan 1;84(1):3-8. DOI:10.1097/JCMA.0000000000000463.

[36] Chan KH, Thimmareddygari D, Ramahi A, Atallah L, Baranetsky NG, Slim J. Clinical characteristics and outcome in patients with combined diabetic ketoacidosis and hyperosmolar hyperglycemic state associated with COVID-19: A retrospective, hospital-based observational case series. Diabetes Res Clin Pract. 2020 Aug;166:108279. DOI:10.1016/j.diabres.2020.108279.

[37] Huda MSB, Shaho S, Trivedi B, Fraterrigo G, Chandrarajan L, Zolfaghari P, Dovey TM, Garrett CG, Chowdhury TA. Diabetic emergencies during the COVID-19 pandemic: A case-control study. Diabet Med. 2021 Jan;38(1):e14416. DOI:10.1111/dme.14416.

[38] Holman N, Knighton P, Kar P, O'Keefe J, Curley M, Weaver A, Barron E, Bakhai C, Khunti K, Wareham NJ, Sattar N, Young B, Valabhji J. Risk factors for COVID-19-related mortality in people with type 1 and type 2 diabetes in England: A population-based cohort study. Lancet Diabetes Endocrinol. 2020 Oct;8(10):823-833. DOI:10.1016/S2213-8587(20)30271-0.

Chapter 12

Pregnancy and COVID-19

Sushruti Kaushal and Harpreet Kaur

Abstract

Pregnancy is a physiological state that alters the body's response to infections. COVID-19 has been found to cause severe disease in pregnancy with morbidity and mortality that is higher than in non-pregnant adults. There is risk of transmission of SARS-CoV2 infection to fetus during ante-natal period, intra-partum and post-delivery from an infected mother. It is necessary to provide an un-interrupted ante-natal care and delivery services to pregnant women during the pandemic. Tele-consultation is important modality to reduce the physical exposure of pregnant women to the hospital environment and should be utilised. Screening, isolation, testing and treatment for SARS-CoV2 infection in pregnant women should follow the local guidelines and remain essentially the same as in non-pregnant adults. Admission, if required, should be in a facility that can provide obstetric maternal and fetal monitoring in addition to care for COVID-19 illness. Use of nitrous oxide and inhalational oxygen for fetal indication should be avoided during labor. Second stage of labor is considered an aerosol generating procedure and should be managed with adequate precautions. Mode of delivery should be as per obstetric indications. Regional anaesthesia should be preferred during caesarean. COVID-19 is not a contra-indication to breast feeding. For antenatal women, COVID-19 vaccination can be considered after shared decision making.

Keywords: Pregnancy, COVID-19, vaccine, labor, delivery

1. Introduction

Pregnancy is a physiological state that alters the body's immune system and response to viral infections. Pregnant women have been found to have higher risk of complications during the previous corona virus outbreaks, namely Severe Acute Respiratory Syndrome (SARS) in 2002–2004 and Middle East Respiratory Syndrome (MERS) in 2012. The risk of maternal morbidity and mortality was high with these infections. With Covid-19, though initially there were different opinions but currently there is sufficient evidence to suggest that pregnant women are at increased risk for complications of COVID19. Additionally, there is evidence to support risk of transmission of infection to fetus intra- or postpartum and concerns about obstetrical outcome.

2. Physiological changes in pregnancy and SARS-CoV2 infection

Pregnancy induces changes in all organ systems of body, notable one being a state of altered immunity and body's response to various infections. This results in increased severity of illnesses during pregnancy as evidenced in previous respiratory disease outbreaks.

Changes in pregnancy that alter the response to illness are:

2.1 Immune system

a. Shift in population of CD4+ T Cells population towards Th2 phenotype promoting humoral immunity in place of cellular immunity [1].

b. Decrease in the population of natural killer cells, possibly altering viral clearance [2].

c. Phagocytic dendritic cells are decreased and so, interferon response to viruses is altered [3]

d. Hormonal changes in the form of increased progesterone, oestrogen and androgens alter the body's immune system because of immunomodulatory properties [4]. Whether these hormones predispose to severe disease or have protective effect is yet to be known.

2.2 Respiratory system

a. Elevation of diaphragm due to gravid uterus leading to reduction in lung volume and total lung capacity.

b. Increase in tidal volume (30–40%)

c. Decrease in functional residual capacity, residual volume and end expiratory volumes

d. Decreased clearance of secretions

These changes make pregnant women more susceptible to severe disease [5].

2.3 Coagulation pathway

Pregnancy is a hypercoagulable state with:

a. increase in thrombin and other coagulation factors

b. increased fibrinolytic factors such as plasmin

Covid 19 is associated with high rate of thromboembolic complications which is compounded by changes of pregnancy.

2.4 Vascular system

Pregnancy increases maternal blood volume, heart rate and cardiac output while systemic resistance decreases. There is an increase in intravascular inflammation [6]. These vascular changes have the potential to impact endothelial function which is a major factor in development of Acute Respiratory Distress Syndrome (ARDS) with Covid19.

Preeclampsia is an important complication of pregnancy associated with endothelial cell dysfunction and higher rates of preeclampsia have been noted in pregnancies complicated with Covid19 [7].

3. Physiology of placenta and placental transmission of COVID-19

Placenta acts as a barrier for transmission of pathogens by various mechanisms. Placental decidua contains large number of NK cells, macrophages and T cells. Decidual macrophages perform antimicrobial functions while CD8+ T cells protect the fetus from viral infections [8]. Additional protection is provided by syncytiotrophoblast and cytotrophoblast mediated by toll-like receptors. Placenta also has antimicrobial peptides which prevent fetal transmission of various pathogens [9].

The first prerequisite for transmission of any virus through placenta is viremia, which, in case of SARS-CoV2, may be present for a relatively short duration. Although earlier studies documented viremia in only 1–15% of patients infected with SARS-CoV2 virus, recent study using WHO RT-qPCR protocol demonstrated viremia in up to 80% patients, although mostly with low levels of viral load [10].

The second element necessary for fetal transmission is placental tropism or the ability of the virus to infect placental cells. In lungs, SARS-CoV2 uses ACE-2 receptor to enter cells and a serine protease named TMPRSS2 to cleave the spike glycoprotein, facilitating fusion. Although ACE-2 and TMPRSS2 have not been shown to be co-expressed in placental cells, they have been demonstrated in trophoblast, blastocyst and hypoblast. It has been suggested that SARS-CoV2 could enter placenta using other proteases like DPP4, CD147 or trypsin [11].

Another route for this virus to enter the placenta could be through infected blood cells like lymphocytes and macrophages but this has not been proven yet for SARS-CoV2. Transcytosis of free virus particles can infect the fetus, as in case of HIV but this method is thought be less important with maternal SARS-CoV2 infections because of low viremia.

Infection may also cross over to fetus through cervico-vaginal secretions which would raise concerns for the mode of delivery of the fetus. The evidence we have till now does not favour this mode of transmission as one study on ten infected women did not find viral RNA in vaginal secretions in any patient [12].

There is convincing evidence that placental transmission of the virus causing COVID-19 is possible, though rarely. Presence of SARS-CoV2 viral RNA in placenta and SARS-CoV2 virions in syncytiotrophoblast has been reported in multiple cases. IgM antibodies directed against SARS-CoV2 virus have been documented in neonates born to mothers with SARS-CoV2 infection, making a strong case for in-utero transmission of this virus [13].

Placental histology in parturient women who contracted SARS-CoV2 infection during the ante-natal period shows vascular malperfusion, chronic villitis, placental infarcts and fibrin deposition [14].

It has been estimated that maternal to fetal transmission occurs in 3.2% of pregnant women infected with SARS-CoV2 virus. Viral positivity rate for placental and cord samples and fetal serology fall in the same range, supporting the transmission rate of 3.2% [13].

4. Effects of SARS-CoV 2 infection on pregnant women

Pregnancy is an immuno-deficient state and high morbidity has been reported during previous corona virus outbreaks, both MERS and SARS. Earlier studies done in China showed key outcomes in pregnant women infected with SARS-CoV2 virus to be similar to those in non-pregnant adults [15, 16]. These studies were limited by small sample sizes and a retrospective design. A national analysis of all Covid related ICU admissions in Sweden was one of the first studies to report increased morbidity during pregnancy [17]. Studies later done in France and the USA supported these findings. The largest study addressing this topic was the review of all laboratory confirmed cases of Covid19 from January to June 2020 in the USA. They found increased risk of hospitalisation, ICU admission and mechanical ventilation but not mortality [18]. This data was recently updated through October 2020 to report increased risk of hospitalisation, ICU admission, mechanical ventilation, extracorporeal membranous oxygenation (ECMO) and death [19]. Though risk appears to be increased when compared with non-pregnant adults, absolute risk remains low.

Clinical course of COVID-19 is believed to be mild in majority (86%) of pregnant females, severe in 9% and critical in 5% [20]. This is similar to incidences reported in non-pregnant Covid19 patients.

In data reported from the UK, most women with more severe illness were in third trimester of pregnancy or postpartum [21]. Risk factors associated with hospital admission in pregnant women include Black, Asian or minority ethnicity, pre-existing co-morbidity (e.g. diabetes, hypertension, asthma), obesity/overweight and maternal age more than 35 years. It has been postulated that this risk is due to genetic differences, socio-economic disparity or difference in response to infection. Vitamin D deficiency has been associated with respiratory infections and ARDS, a common complication of Covid19. South Asian population has been documented to be deficient in Vitamin D and this could be a factor in increased morbidity in this population [21].

COVID-19 increases the risk of thromboembolic complications and pregnancy is itself associated with increased risk of thrombo-embolism. Royal College of Obstetricians and Gynaecologists (RCOG) has emphasised the risk of thromboembolism in COVID-19 with pregnancy and recommends appropriate use of thromboprophylaxis.

5. Risks to the fetus

Many studies have shown increased chances of preterm delivery in SARS-CoV2 infected women. Most of these preterm births have been seen to be iatrogenic. Most of the preterm babies have been delivered by caesarean section due to intrauterine foetal distress. Symptomatic women have been found to have increased risk of preterm delivery compared to asymptomatic SARS-CoV2 infected women. Some studies have shown a decrease in mean gestational age at the time of delivery in women who were diagnosed with COVID-19 within 14 days before delivery. One study also reported increased chances of stillbirth in foetuses born to SARS-CoV2 positive mothers [22].

Till date no association has been found with first trimester losses or teratogenicity and COVID-19 infection is not an indication for medical termination of pregnancy. Though this is ever changing situation and we may get more information in future as the evidence is pooled in. Amniocentesis to diagnose fetal infection is also not recommended at present [23].

6. Diagnostic testing for SARS-CoV2 infection in pregnancy

The criteria for testing pregnant women for SARS-CoV 2 infection remain the same as for general population. Local testing guidelines as per the local, state and regional governments should be followed. Basically, it includes testing symptomatic women, contacts of SARS-CoV2 positive people and those with history of travel.

Nasopharyngeal swab is the recommended sample for testing, oropharyngeal swab is also acceptable. Lower respiratory samples are recommended in intubated patients and in those with severe illness and negative nasopharyngeal swabs.

RT-PCR is the most commonly used test in pregnancy. Nucleic Acid Amplification Tests (NAAT) can be used as per availability and regional guidelines.

Rapid antigen tests and serological tests can all be used in pregnancy as per regional protocols and there are no specific considerations for diagnostic testing in pregnancy [24].

7. Ante-natal care during COVID-19 pandemic

Providing adequate antenatal care during the COVID-19 pandemic is a priority and a minimum number of antenatal visits should be ensured. Federation International of Gynaecology and Obstetrics (FIGO) suggests a minimum of six in-person antenatal visits i.e. at 12 weeks, 20 weeks, 28 weeks, 32 weeks, 36 weeks and at 37–41 weeks. Telemedicine can be used for any additional advice and facilities should be made available for tele-consultation.

Appointments should be taken before consultation and screening for any symptoms for COVID-19 should either be done telephonically or before entering the antenatal area [25]. Screening should include symptoms suggestive of COVID-19 illness, any history of recent travel, history of exposure to infected person and any history of immune-suppression [25].

FIGO recommends that any pregnant women testing positive on screening should have a minimum waiting period, should be tested for severity of symptoms, and evaluated as per local guidelines [25]. Screen-positive women should be isolated and not allowed near other pregnant women.

Screen-positive woman who contacts telephonically should be advised to defer the visit for 14 days unless there is an urgent need.

During antenatal visits, pregnant woman should be counselled about the general measures to prevent spread of infection like social distancing, use of face masks and respiratory hygiene. They should be educated about the symptoms of SARS-CoV2 infection and that even if they become infected, they are likely to have mild disease in most cases. They should be told that if they develop severe symptoms or recovery is delayed, they should seek care [25].

Pregnant women should be allowed only one accompanying person and he/she should also be screened at entrance to hospital.

They should also be counselled about the possible modifications in her antenatal plan in view of the ongoing pandemic. She should be told about dedicated COVID facilities in her neighbourhood and facilities where SARS-Cov2 positive women can deliver.

She should be advised to keep taking her routine health supplements e.g. folic acid during pregnancy.

There should a mechanism in place to track antenatal women who miss scheduled visits and they should be contacted telephonically.

Clinicians should be aware of the increased risk of psychological problems and domestic abuse during the pandemic and appropriate steps should be taken to address these issues including looking for signs, counselling and referral if needed. Particular concern has been raised about the increased need of psychological counselling and support services to the antenatal women during this time of pandemic when face to face consultation is not possible [25].

8. Antenatal care for women with suspected/confirmed covid-19

Care of symptomatic pregnant women suffering from Covid-19 should be a multidisciplinary team approach.

American College of Obstetricians & Gynaecologists (ACOG) has developed an algorithm for management of outpatient pregnant women with suspected or confirmed COVID-19. If a woman has no symptoms to suggest infection with SARS-CoV2, she should receive routine prenatal care. If she has symptoms, severity of symptoms should be assessed. Assessment of severity of illness should include any shortness of breath, coughing up blood, dizziness, chest pain, not being able to keep down fluids and any history of confusion. If any of these are present, pregnant woman is at elevated risk and should be asked to seek care in an emergency department in a centre that has facilities for antenatal and obstetric care. If the woman has symptoms but those are not severe, she should be screened for any co-morbidities and any obstetric complications. If any co-morbidities or obstetric complications are present, she is categorised as having moderate risk and should be evaluated in ambulatory setting as soon as possible and should be investigated for severity of illness. CT Scan with abdominal shielding should be done if clinically indicated. If the woman does not have any high risk factors, she should be sent for symptomatic care at home, including hydration and rest and evaluated repeatedly for development of any of the above symptoms [26].

Indian Council of Medical Research (ICMR) recommends that symptomatic women with fever >38°C and respiratory symptoms should be hospitalised in a tertiary care centre with facilities for maternal and fetal monitoring. Seriousness of maternal situation is assessed by quick SOFA score, parameters of severity being systolic blood pressure < 100 mmHg, respiratory rate > 22, and Glasgow consciousness scale <15. Any pregnant woman with more than one of these factors should be admitted in Intensive Care Unit (ICU) [27].

FIGO recommends anomaly scan at 18–23 weeks in women with confirmed SARS-CoV2 infection and monthly scan after that for fetal growth. ICMR (Indian Council for Medical Research) recommends a growth scan 14 days after recovery from acute illness [25].

9. Management during labor

9.1 Preparation before admission

Admission for labor and delivery represents a unique scenario in that admission, though planned, cannot be delayed. The basic principles remain the same as those for outpatient visits, i.e., to avoid unnecessary hospital visits, maintain social distancing and other measures to prevent spread of SARS-CoV2. Women should be advised to quarantine themselves or work from home at least 14 days before planned admission for delivery or caesarean. This should start in most women by 37 weeks of gestation. Woman and her birthing partner should be screened for symptoms of COVID-19 telephonically one day before admission [28].

9.2 Screening on arrival

All women arriving for admission for delivery should be screened verbally for fever, cough and respiratory symptoms. Birthing partner should be similarly screened. Those testing positive should be sent for testing and care by Obstetric care provider. Some women would already be diagnosed with SARS-CoV2 infection and they should directly be delegated to area dedicated for infected patients.

Case can be made for testing all women at the time of admission to labor and delivery unit because of high number of asymptomatic infections [20]. Local guidelines could also mandate testing at the time of admission.

After screening at the time of admission, women will be categorised into one of the three categories: infected, suspect and non-infected. Under ideal circumstances, all health care facilities caring for pregnant women should have well demarcated zones with separate passageways for all of these categories. These zones should include separate wards, intensive care areas and operation theatres. If not possible, all care should be taken to avoid infected and non-infected people coming in proximity of each other.

9.3 General precautions during admission

All women and their birthing partners should wear triple layer surgical masks throughout admission. All healthcare providers should wear triple layer surgical mask for each patient contact. Hands should be sanitised with alcohol based hand-rub after every patient contact. Droplet precautions should be used when caring for women with respiratory symptoms. This requires the use of gloves, gown, surgical mask and face shield. Gown, gloves, face shield and N95 mask should be used for any woman with suspected COVID and during any aerosol generating procedure including second stage of labour [28]. Disinfection of rooms should be done between patients.

Women should be allowed to have one birthing partner who should stay throughout admission. Other support persons should be given option to provide support through video. Visitors should not be allowed in person, although visitation may be considered in end of life situations.

Shifting of woman from one area to other should be avoided and all efforts should be made to provide services at women's bedside.

All preoperative investigations needed for caesarean should also be done on the day of admission to decrease the number of pre-admission hospital visits.

9.4 Intrapartum care

Management of first stage of labour remains essentially the same as in a woman not infected with Covid-19. Women with mild disease require management of fluid-electrolyte balance during labor, in addition to symptomatic management and close monitoring of maternal well-being. Woman should be encouraged to take oral fluids to maintain hydration. Intravenous fluids should be used with caution because of association of Covid-19 with Acute Respiratory Distress Syndrome (ARDS) [25]. Early use of oxytocin for slow and dysfunctional labour is recommended to avoid the stress and complications of a prolonged labor. Use of Nitrous Oxide during labour should be avoided because of insufficient data about cleaning, filtering and potential aerosolization of nitrous oxide systems [28].

Oxygen is used intrapartum for fetal benefit, to increase fetal oxygenation. A recent meta-analysis has shown that it does not provide fetal benefit and may even be harmful [29, 30]. ACOG recommends against the use of oxygen therapy for fetal resuscitation during labour [28].

Second stage of labour is considered an aerosol generating procedure and should be managed with appropriate precautions. Obstetric management remains the same as before the pandemic.

Blood resources have become scarce during the pandemic because of inability to conduct donation drives. Maintaining pre-delivery haemoglobin is the most efficient way to decrease the use of blood during labour and delivery admissions. Utmost importance should be given to aggressively treat anaemia detected during pregnancy. Blood transfusion should only be used when absolutely necessary and in minimum quantity.

Misoprostol and tranexamic acid should be used prophylactically in third stage of labor to decrease blood loss after delivery.

10. Management of pregnant woman with COVID-19

A pregnant woman with SARS-CoV2 infection should be counselled about the risk of serious infection and the methods to protect family members from infection. Next step is to assess systemic status of woman for severity of infection and need of hospitalisation.

Management of infection should be same as management of non-pregnant patients with COVID-19. If the patient needs hospitalisation, she should be admitted in a facility where maternal as well as fetal monitoring can be done [31]. The facility should be able to provide fetal and uterine contraction monitoring, individualised delivery planning and team based approach including obstetrician, paediatrician, anaesthetist and respiratory medicine specialist. The basic principles and medications remain the same as in non-pregnant patients. Potentially effective treatment for COVID-19 should not be withheld from pregnant women due to theoretical concerns regarding safety. Decisions regarding treatment options should be made keeping in mind safety of the medication, the severity of maternal disease and in shared decision-making with the patient [31].

A very important limitation is exclusion of pregnant women from most clinical trials involving new treatment modalities and the safety data remains scarce.

In most cases, timing of delivery should not be altered by maternal COVID-19 infection [32]. Patients who get infected in early pregnancy and subsequently recover do not require any change in the timing of delivery. For patients who contract SARS-CoV2 infection in the third trimester of pregnancy, attempt should be made to postpone delivery till negative SARS-CoV2 report or lifting of quarantine status to decrease the risk of perinatal transmission. Maternal COVID-19 infection is not an indication for caesarean section, which should be done for obstetric indication or on maternal request [32]. Because the risk of transmission from umbilical cord blood is low, delayed cord clamping should be continued as pre-pandemic. Similarly, umbilical cord blood banking can be done if the parents desire.

11. Lactation and COVID-19

Several studies have detected SARS-CoV2 nucleic acid in breast milk. However, infectious virus particles have not been detected in breast milk [33]. Also, antibodies specific to SARS-CoV2 have also been detected in breast milk, which could potentially protect the neonate. Therefore, it is recommended to continue breastfeeding in mothers with SARS-CoV2 infection, with precautions. These precautions include hand hygiene before breast feeding and wearing a face mask. Breast milk may be expressed after hand-hygiene and fed to infant by uninfected care-provider after disinfection (pasteurisation) [33].

12. Pregnancy and COVID-19 vaccines

Clinical trials to determine safety and efficacy of SARS-CoV2 vaccines have excluded pregnant women and so data on safety of vaccines in pregnancy is sparse. However, the vaccines that are not live attenuated are generally considered safe in pregnancy. Also, the animal studies done for safety and efficacy of the current vaccines for SARS-CoV2 have not shown any evidence of teratogenicity. RCOG recommends that SARS-CoV2 vaccine should be offered to pregnant women at the same time as general population [34]. ACOG recommends that mRNA vaccines for SARS-CoV2 should not be withheld from pregnant women and should be offered to lactating women [35]. It would be prudent to make the decision regarding use of SARS-CoV2 vaccines in pregnancy keeping in mind the activity of virus in community, risks and potential severity of illness in woman, efficacy of vaccine and risks to mother and fetus due to vaccination [35].

Author details

Sushruti Kaushal and Harpreet Kaur*
Obstetrics and Gynecology, All India Institute of Medical Sciences (AIIMS), Bilaspur, Himachal Pradesh, India

*Address all correspondence to: drharpreetsidhu7@gmail.com

References

[1] Piccinni MP, Romagnani S. Regulation of fetal allograft survival by a hormone-controlled Th1- and Th2 type type cytokines. Immunol Res. 1996;15:141-150.

[2] Veenstra van Nieuwenhoven AL, Heineman MJ, Faas MM. The immunology of successfulm pregnancy. Hum Reprod Update. 2003;9:347-357.

[3] Reizis B. Plasmacytoid dendritic cells: development, regulation and function. Immunity. 2019;37-50.

[4] Drukmann R, Drokmann MA. Progesterone and the immunology of pregnancy. J Steroid Biochem Mol Biol. 2005;97:389-396.

[5] Goodnight WH. Pneumonia in pregnancy. Crit Care Med. 2005;33:S390–S397.

[6] Di Renzo GC, Giardina I. Coronavirus disease 2019 in pregnancy: consider thromboembolic disorders and thromboprophylaxis. Am J Obstet Gynecol. :135.

[7] Di Mascio D, Khalil A, Saccone G et al. Outcome of coronavirus spectrum infections (SARS, MERS, COVID-19) during pregnancy: a systematic review and meta-analysis. Am J Obstet Gynecol MFM2. 2020;100-107.

[8] . van Egmond A, van der Keur C, Swings GM et al. The possible role of virus-specific CD8(+) memory T cells in decidual tissue. J Reprod Immunol. 2016;1-8.

[9] Groß R, Bauer R, Krüger F, et al. A Placenta Derived C-Terminal Fragment of βHemoglobin With Combined Antibacterial and Antiviral Activity. Front Microbiol. 2020;508.

[10] Hadjadj Jerome, Yatim Nader, Barnabei Laura, Corneau Aurelien, Boussier Jeremy, Pere Helene, Charbit Bruno. Impaired type I interferon activity and exacerbated inflammatory responses in severe Covid-19 patients. edRxiv. 2020;

[11] WASTNEDGE ET AL. Pregnancy and Covid19. Physiol Rev. 2020;101:303-318.

[12] Qiu Lin, Liu Xia, Xiao Meng, Xie Jing, Cao Wei, Liu Zhengyin, Morse Abraham, Xie Yuhua, Li Taisheng, Lan Zhu. SARS-CoV-2 is not detectable in the vaginal fluid of women with severe COVID-19 infection. Clin Infect Dis. 2020;

[13] Alexander M Kotlyar et al. Vertical transmission of coronavirus disease 2019: a systematic review and metaanalysis. Am J Obstet Gynecol. :35-53.

[14] Shanes ED, Mithal LB, Otero S, Azad HA,, Miller ES, Goldstein JA. Placental pathology in COVID-19. Am J Clin Pathol 202015423-32. 2020;23-32.

[15] Wang Z, Wang Z, Xiong G. Clinical characteristics and laboratory results of pregnant women with COVID-19 in Wuhan, China. Int J Gynecol Obstet. 2020;150:312-317.

[16] Liu F, Liu H, Hou L, Li J, Zheng H, Chi R, et al. Clinico-radiological features and outcomes in pregnant women with COVID-19 pneumonia compared with age-matched nonpregnant women. Infect Drug Resist 2020;13:2845-54. Infect Drug Resist. 2020;2845-54.

[17] Collin J, Bystr€om E, Carnahan AS, Ahrne M. Public Health Agency of Sweden's brief report: pregnant and postpartum women with severe acute respiratory syndrome coronavirus 2 infection in intensive care in Sweden. Acta Obstet Gynecol Scand. 2020; 819-822.

[18] Ellington S, Strid P, Tong VT, Woodworth K, Galang RR, Zambrano LD, et al. Characteristics of women of reproductive age with laboratory-confirmed SARS-CoV-2 infection by pregnancy status—United States, January 22–June 7, 2020. MMWR Morb Mortal Wkly Rep. 2020;769-775.

[19] Zambrano LD, Ellington SR, Strid P, Galang RR, Oduyebo T, Tong VT, et al. Characteristics of women of reproductive age with laboratory-confirmed SARS-CoV-2 infection by pregnancy status—United States,January 22– October 3, 2020. MMWR Morb Mortal Wkly Rep. 2020;1641-1647.

[20] Breslin N, Baptiste C, Gyamfi-Bannerman C, et al. Coronavirus disease 2019, infection among asymptomatic and symptomatic pregnant women: two weeks of confirmed presentations to an affiliated pair of New York City hospitals. Am J Obstet Gynecol MFM. 2020;2:100-18.

[21] Royal College of Obstetricians and Gynaecologists. Coronavirus (COVID-19) infection in pregnancy. London: RCOG; 2020.

[22] Naima T. Joseph, M.D., M.P.H.,a Sonja A. Rasmussen, M.D., M.S.,b and Denise J. Jamieson, M.D., M.P.H.a. The effects of COVID-19 on pregnancy and implications for reproductive medicine. Fertil Steril. 2021;115:824-30.

[23] Singh, et al. Managing pregnancy in COVID-19 pandemic: A review article. J Fam Med Prim Care 202095468-73. 2020;9:5468-73.

[24] Information on COVID-19 Treatment, Prevention and Research [Internet]. COVID-19 Treat. Guidel. [cited 2021 Apr 9]. Available from: https://www.covid19treatmentguidelines.nih.gov/

[25] Khoiwal K, Kapur D, Gaurav A, Chaturvedi J. Management of Pregnant Women in Times of Covid-19: A Review of Current Literature. J Obstet Gynecol Ind. 70:262-268.

[26] Novel Coronavirus 2019 (COVID-19) [Internet]. [cited 2021 Apr 9]. Available from: https://www.acog.org/en/clinical/clinical-guidance/practice-advisory/articles/2020/03/novel-coronavirus-2019

[27] Guidance for Management of Pregnant Women in COVID-19 Pandemic. :17.

[28] Rupsa C. Boelig, MD, MS; Tracy Manuck, MD; Emily A. Oliver, MD; Daniele Di Mascio, MD; Gabriele Saccone, MD;, Federica Bellussi, MD; Vincenzo Berghella, MD. Labor and delivery guidance for COVID-19. Am J Obstet Gynecol MFM. May2020;1-10.

[29] Raghuraman N, Wan L, Temming LA,, et al. Effect of oxygen vs room air on intrauterine fetal resuscitation: a randomized noninferiority clinical trial. JAMA Pediatr 2018;172:818-23. JAMA Pediatr. 172:818-23.

[30] Hamel MS, Anderson BL, Rouse DJ. Oxygen for intrauterine resuscitation: of unproved benefit and potentially harmful. Am J Obstet Gynecol. Am J Obstet Gynecol. 2014;124-127.

[31] Pregnancy [Internet]. COVID-19 Treat. Guidel. [cited 2021 Apr 16]. Available from: https://www.covid19treatmentguidelines.nih.gov/special-populations/pregnancy/

[32] COVID-19 FAQs for Obstetrician-Gynecologists, Obstetrics [Internet]. [cited 2021 Apr 16]. Available from: https://www.acog.org/en/clinical-information/physician-faqs/covid-19-faqs-for-ob-gyns-obstetrics

[33] FAQs: Management of Infants Born to Mothers with Suspected or Confirmed COVID-19 [Internet].

[cited 2021 Apr 19]. Available from: http://services.aap.org/en/pages/2019-novel-coronavirus-covid-19-infections/clinical-guidance/faqs-management-of-infants-born-to-covid-19-mothers/

[34] COVID-19 vaccines, pregnancy and breastfeeding [Internet]. R. Coll. Obstet. Amp Gynaecol. [cited 2021 Apr 20]. Available from: https://www.rcog.org.uk/en/guidelines-research-services/coronavirus-covid-19-pregnancy-and-womens-health/covid-19-vaccines-and-pregnancy/covid-19-vaccines-pregnancy-and-breastfeeding/

[35] Vaccinating Pregnant and Lactating Patients Against COVID-19 [Internet]. [cited 2021 Apr 20]. Available from: https://www.acog.org/en/clinical/clinical-guidance/practice-advisory/articles/2020/12/vaccinating-pregnant-and-lactating-patients-against-covid-19

Chapter 13

Neurological Involvement in COVID-19

Valentina Opancina, Kristijan Krstic, Predrag Sazdanovic, Nebojsa Zdravkovic, Ruzica Radojevic Marjanovic and Radisa Vojinovic

Abstract

The respiratory system is the most common target of COVID-19, however, various experimental studies and case reports have shown its affinity for neural tissues. In this chapter, we described pathogenesis and propagation of SARS-CoV-2 virus in the nervous system, potential routes of the SARS-CoV-2 invasion in the brain, as well as indirect effects of COVID-19 on multiorgan disorders. We have also presented all of the reported neurological manifestations in COVID-19 with an explanation of possible underlying pathways. Among patients who tested positive on SARS-CoV-2, various neurological irregularities have been described, affecting both the central and peripheral nervous systems. In general, neurological complications in COVID-19 patients occur within 1 and 14 days, in most cases on average on the 5th day of the incubation period. We have demonstrated all of the reported neurological findings, whereas the most commonly reported were headache, dizziness, myalgia, hypogeusia, hyposmia, and impaired consciousness. More serious neurological conditions in COVID-19 included meningitis, encephalitis, and ischemic or hemorrhagic stroke.

Keywords: SARS-CoV-2, neurologic manifestations, pathogenesis, COVID-19, coronavirus

1. Introduction

The infection of coronavirus (SARS-CoV-2) severe acute respiratory syndrome coronavirus 2 (SARS-CoV-2) was declared a pandemic by the World Health Organization (WHO) on March 11, 2020 [1]. Regarding its structure and infection mechanism, SARS-CoV-2 is mostly similar to familiar coronaviruses such as the SARS-CoV-1 and Middle East respiratory syndrome (MERS) [2, 3]. Identified in Wuhan, China, it has abruptly spread all over the world with more than 164.513.450 reported cases to date [4]. The respiratory system is the most common target of infection however, various experimental studies and case reports have shown an affinity for neural tissues. Considering observational studies, SARS-CoV-2 patients were registered with complaints of headache, nausea, vomiting, dizziness, myalgia, hypogeusia, hyposmia, and impaired consciousness, all symptoms that indicate involvement of the nervous system [5]. Even though, the exact mechanism which SARS-CoV-2 penetrates the central nervous system has not yet been determined, prior experimental models have shown that other coronaviruses can compromise the nervous system and respiratory drive by directly targeting neurons located in cardiorespiratory centers [6], due to the preliminary observation of cases concerning the COVID-19 pandemic, suggesting a higher affinity of SARS-CoV-2 virus for CNS targets.

The aim of this chapter is to present all of the reported neurological manifestations in COVID-19 with the explanation of possible underlying pathways.

2. COVID-19 and nervous system

In the previous months, reports of meningitis, encephalitis, myelitis, or peripheral nerve affection in regard to COVID-19 infection were presented, implying that SARS-CoV-2 can directly infect the nervous system.

2.1 Pathogenesis

The SARS-CoV-2 spike protein (S) can bind to the host cellular angiotensin-converting enzyme 2 (ACE-2) receptor because of its high binding affinity, which is of importance to cell tropism [7]. Preparing and processing of the S protein by the transmembrane protease serine 2 (TMPRSS2) have been demonstrated to be crucial for the synthesis of viral and host cellular membranes, furthermore entrance of SARS-CoV-2 [8]. The increased expression of the ACE-2 receptor has been found on neurons and glial cells of several brain structures including the cerebral cortex, the striatum, the posterior hypothalamic area, the substantia nigra, and brain stem. ACE-2 is strongly expressed in the ventrolateral medulla and the nucleus of tractus solitarius, both areas involved in the regulation of the respiratory cycle [9].

Arguably, several mechanisms could be taken into account as possible viral access routes, such as axonal transport and trans-synaptic transfer, and hematogenous or potentially lymphatic system routes. The infiltration of the CNS through the transcribial system describes an infection of the olfactory epithelium continuing transmission through the cribriform plate to the subarachnoid space. On the other side, the axonal and trans-synaptic transport would combine numerous peripheral nerve terminals which leads to contamination by spreading onward neurons (olfactory bulb, the trigeminal nerve, the vagus nerve, etc.) [10].

Another way of CNS infiltration could be through the circulatory system or on the other hand, the lymphatic system routes. Transfer over the brain endothelium could be accomplished through abluminal virus release into the CNS parenchyma, by direct infection of brain microvascular endothelial cells (BMEC), or via endocytosis, through virally affected leukocytes or disrupted tight junctions on BMEC-s [11].

However, direct contamination of cells is not the only way of virus transmission. Indirect neurotoxicity may be caused by immune system disorders, coagulation disorders, cardiovascular comorbidities, disorders of glucose and lipid metabolism, hypoxic encephalopathy, and/or gastrointestinal disorders.

Other than ACE-2, SARS-CoV-2 may utilize extracellular matrix metalloproteinase inducer also known as basigin (BSG; CD147) and transmembrane glycoprotein neuropilin-1 (NRP1) as receptors. Some enzymes that catalyze proteolysis such as TMPRSS11A/B, cathepsin B and L, and furin (FURIN), have been presented to promote viral cell entry and replication [12].

2.2 Propagation of SARS-CoV-2 virus in the nervous system

Dissemination of SARS-CoV-2, in which the virus has an effect on peripheral neurons via active transport, synaptic terminals, and retrograde transport to the neuronal body of the cell, has been hypothesized [13]. Studies have been conducted, explaining the mechanism of trans-synaptic transfer involving the hemagglutinating encephalomyelitis virus strain 67 N (HEV-67 N), which represents the first SARS-CoV-2 strain that was found to infect the porcine cerebrum [14]. Data from human single nuclei RNA-seq databases suggest that vascular endothelial cells may express ACE-2 in the human cerebrum at low levels, however non-canonical SARS-CoV-2 receptors (e.g., BSG/CD147) are displayed in several different brain cell types, making them exposed to the virus [15].

2.3 Potential routes of SARS-CoV-2 invasion in brain

Provided by other viruses of the family Coronaviridae, certain possible routes of entry for SARS-CoV-2 have been established [16].

2.3.1 Olfactory route

The olfactory nerve (CN I) is the first and shortest cranial nerve. It is a special visceral afferent nerve, which transmits information relating to smell. The sense of smell is distinguished by olfactory receptors situated within the nasal epithelium. Their axons amass into small bundles of olfactory nerves, which infiltrate small foramina in the cribriform plate of the ethmoid bone and enter the cranial cavity. The absence of the sense of smell is defined as anosmia. A temporary loss of smell can be caused by infection or by local disorders, in contrast, a permanent loss of smell may be caused by head injury or tumors. Infection of the olfactory system is consistent with the observation that loss of smell is a frequent neurological manifestation in COVID-19. Some evidence, demonstrate increased MRI signal in the olfactory cortex during the acute phase of SARS-CoV-2 infection [17]. As represented in the case of other coronaviruses, the virus could be disguised in nerve terminals by endocytic mechanisms, transported retrogradely, and spread trans-synaptically to other regions of the cerebrum [18]. As described before, ACE-2 and TMPRSS2 have been identified in the nasal mucosa, epithelial cells (sustentacular cells), but not olfactory neurons [19]. However, there are some evidences of neuronal involvement.

2.3.2 Blood: brain route

The blood–brain barrier (BBB) acts as an additional boundary between circulating blood and the extracellular space of the brain. The barrier is highly selective, protecting the brain from toxins, pathogens and even circulating neurotransmitters (e.g. glutamate) that can be potentially damaging to neurons. The BBB is a typical route of entry of blood-borne viruses into the brain. In SARS-CoV-2 infection, dissemination of the virus into the blood has been reported, even though frequencies are extensively ranging (1–41%) [16]. Immunoreactivity of ACE-2 was described in brain vessels of a patient with multiple ischemic infarcts. However, the cellular localization was not resolved. Other receptors, such as NRP1 and BSG, could be another possibility of infection due to their more widely expression in the cerebral vasculature [20]. Nonetheless, SARS-CoV-2 associated cytokines – interleukins (IL-6, IL-1b, IL-17) and tumor necrosis factor (TNF) can potentially damage the BBB, which is another way of virus invasion [21]. In several autopsy studies, a lack of florid cerebrovascular inflammation has been described [22]. Comorbidities, as have oftentimes been seen in COVID-19, such as cardiovascular risk factor or pre-existing neurological diseases, in combinations with activation of cytokines, increase the permeability of BBB [21].

2.3.3 Infiltration of infected immune cells

Infected immune cells (monocytes, neutrophils, and T cells) can cause brain infestation through the vasculature, the meninges, and choroid plexus [16]. In a study conducted by Chen et al., 2020, SARS-CoV-2 nucleocapsid protein (NP) immunoreactivity was observed in CD68+ cells in lymphoid organs, while single-cell RNA seq data showed viral RNA in macrophages of COVID-19 patients [23]. However, data about virus proliferation in macrophages are limited due to the unknown mechanisms of virus propagation (phagocytic uptake of virus-infected cells or extracellular virions) [24].

3. COVID-19 and nervous system: indirect effects of systemic factors

Indirect effects of systemic factors of SARS-CoV-2 can lead to acute and chronic consequences, such as respiratory failure, systemic inflammation, hypercoagulable state and, lethal systemic organ failure.

3.1 Respiratory failure

SARS-CoV-2 has been predominantly detected in pneumocytes and epithelial progenitors, which can lead to potential lung damage, causing massive alveolar damage, inflammatory cell infiltration, edema, microvascular thrombosis, and hemorrhage resulting in severe hypoxia and acute respiratory distress syndrome (ARDS) [25, 26]. The most sensitive brain regions to hypoxia, such as the neocortex, hippocampus, and cerebellum have shown neuronal impairment [27].

3.2 Systemic inflammation

The correlation between immunosuppression and disease severity has been established. Most COVID-19 patients have higher circulating levels of IL-6, IL-1b, and TNF, but also additionally IL-2, IL-8, IL-17, G-CSF, GM-CSF, IP10, MCP1, and MIP1a2, and serum levels of IL-6 and TNF leading to cytokine release syndrome [28–30]. After brain entry through the damaged BBB, certain molecules such as the nuclear protein high mobility group box 1 (HMGB1), could act as pathogen-associated molecular patterns (PAMPs) and damage-associated molecular patterns (DAMPs) [31]. This process activates an immune response in pericytes, brain macrophages, and microglia, which express toll-like receptors (TLR) which act as mediators for pro-inflammatory effects of SARS-CoV-2 spike protein on human macrophages through nuclear factor-kB (NF-kB) [32]. In this way, immune response boosts the level of cytokine production which results in impairment of brain function [33].

3.3 Hypercoagulable state

Another vital element of COVID-19 is significant coagulopathy. The multicenter study has been conducted, suggesting that 88% of patients displayed evidence of a hypercoagulable state. The prothrombin time (PT), activated partial thromboplastin time (aPTT), and complete blood count (CBC) are in the reference range. However, fibrinogen level, and fibrin breakdown products indicative of intravascular thrombosis (D-dimer), are both increased. Coagulopathy may start in the lungs causing endothelial damage, complement activation, activation of the procoagulant effect of IL-6, and neutrophil release of extracellular traps (NETs) that leads to the formation of a clot, resulting in intravascular thrombosis [34].

3.4 Systemic organ failure

There are many metabolic and pathological evidence of systematic impairment in different organs (heart, liver, gastrointestinal tract, and endocrine system) [35]. Hypoperfusion of the cerebrum could be impacted by a compromised function of the heart [36]. Many neurological symptoms, for instance, headache, confusion, agitation, can be correlated to systemic metabolic changes including electrolyte disbalance, hormonal dysfunction and accumulation of toxic metabolites [37, 38].

4. COVID-19 and nervous system: neurological manifestations

Although, SARS-CoV-2 is primarily causing the insufficient function of the respiratory system, there are overwhelming amounts of evidence implying that neurological complications appear as a serious problem in the ongoing COVID-19 pandemic. In the long-term, COVID-19 could negatively affect the nervous system [39].

Among patients who tested positive on SARS-CoV-2, various neurological irregularities have been described, affecting both the central and peripheral nervous system. Clinical condition and symptoms may vary from mild to severe, regardless of patient clinical status (severe form or asymptomatic infection). According to Helms et al., neurological abnormalities have been displayed in 30% of hospitalized patients, 45% of those with severe respiratory problems, and 85% of those who developed ARDS [40]. Patients with mild or asymptomatic infection were more likely to develop nonspecific neurological irregularity including headache, dizziness, malaise, and loss of sense of smell and taste.

In the review by Leonardi M, Padovani A, McArthur JC (2020) [41], authors have classified the reported neurological findings, into three distinctive categories:

a. Central (headache, dizziness, impaired consciousness, acute cerebrovascular disease, seizures, and meningitis/encephalitis)

b. Peripheral (hypogeusia, hyposmia)

c. Musculoskeletal (ischemic or hemorrhagic stroke)

In general, neurological complications in COVID-19 patients occur within 1 and 14 days, in most cases on average on the 5th day of the incubation period [42].

4.1 Headache and dizziness: central neurological findings

Headache is one of the most commonly reported neurological symptoms of a systemic viral infection. Although direct mechanisms of this symptom are yet to be discovered, there are some possible causes. High body temperature directly causes activation of several immunoinflammatory mediators (cytokines, glutamate, cyclooxygenase-2/prostaglandin E2 system, and nitric oxide system) and activation of substances that are capable of inducing interleukins (exogenous and endogenous pyrogens). Some of the indirect causes are dehydration, electrolyte disbalance, hypoxia, systemic inflammation, and cytokine release syndrome (CRS).

One of the possibilities for developing this symptom could also be direct infection of the nervous system via ACE-2 receptors [43].

Vertigo or dizziness has been described as the most common neurological manifestation of COVID-19. Neurotropism of SARS-CoV-2 causes the virus to invade neural tissue from circulation through capillary endothelium (ACE-2 receptors). Aside from this mechanism, direct invasion, hypoxia, and systemic inflammation play the part in causing this symptom. Approximately 7.0% (2.5% to 21.4%) of the COVID-19 patients were reported to have this symptom.

Combined manifestation of dizziness and headache occurred in 12.1% as has been reported in eight studies, with a total of n=654 patients [44].

4.2 Impaired consciousness: central neurological findings

As anticipated, severe or critical patients tend to develop impaired consciousness (11.9%) due to hypoxia and cerebrum impairment. In patients with mild or asymptomatic clinical manifestations, the prevalence of this symptom is considerably lower (3.2%). The number of studies taken into account was nine, including n=2890 patients with impaired consciousness [45].

4.3 Acute cerebrovascular complications: central neurological findings

The most common display of cerebrovascular disease is an acute stroke with rapidly evolving symptoms which may include weakness of one side of the face or body, numbness, motor or sensory aphasia, ataxia, visual impairment. Those symptoms could be manifested due to compromised blood supply to the brain and which symptom will develop depends on the compromised area of the cerebrum. Regarding this clinical problem, two cohort studies were conducted. The first study by Mao et al. noted that among 214 hospitalized patients, 6 patients developed acute cerebrovascular manifestation (2.8%) [46]. The second study by Li et al. reported 11 patients with acute ischemic stroke (including a total of 221 COVID-19 patients). It has been shown that developing acute cerebrovascular events is highly correlated with the age of the patients (71.6 ± 15.7 years/52.1 ± 15.3 years) [47].

4.4 Seizures: central neurological findings

An epileptic seizure is a "transient occurrence of signs and/or symptoms due to abnormal excessive or synchronous neuronal activity in the brain" [48]. There are few reports of acute seizures in SARS-CoV-2 positive patients. The first study regarding this clinical manifestation was noted in a COVID-19 patient, a 24-year-old male with generalized seizures, from Japan [49]. The second publication reported a COVID-19 patient, a 30-year-old female with generalized tonic–clonic seizures, from Iran. In both cases, there was no evidence of previous seizures, prior to hospitalization [50]. Even though these and similar reports may suggest that correlation between seizures and COVID-19 infection exist, there are a relatively low number of reported cases so far, therefore a seizure risk is caused by nonspecific mechanisms (hypoxia, cerebrovascular events, cytokine proliferation, etc.).

4.5 Meningitis/encephalitis: central neurological findings

By definition, meningitis is inflammation of the meninges, in almost all cases identified by an abnormal number of leukocytes in the cerebrospinal fluid and specific symptoms. The etiology may be noninfectious and associated with a systemic disease, medication, or other pathologic factors. However, most cases of aseptic meningitis are caused by viruses. There have been interpreted few single-case reports, regarding meningitis/encephalitis in correlation with COVID-19. Anyhow, only a few of reported cases tested positive for SARS-CoV-2. The first described case was reported from China, but the amount of clinical evidence was underwhelming [51]. Another case was reported in a SARS-CoV-2 positive patient from Japan, manifested as generalized seizure and pathological cerebral MRI (right lateral ventriculitis and encephalitis mainly on the right mesial temporal lobe and hippocampus) [52]. In other reported cases, patients tested negative for SARS-CoV-2, or even were not tested at all [53].

4.6 Hypogeusia/hyposmia: peripheral neurological findings

The presence of taste and smell alterations seems to be a usual clinical manifestation going from 19.4–88% of patients [54]. The specific pathogenesis of these issues has not yet been explained. ACE-2 has been distinguished as the cell receptor for SARS-CoV-2. These receptors are expressed diffusely on the mucous membrane of the entire oral cavity, especially on the tongue and furthermore on the nasal mucosa where it takes part in respiratory inflammatory infections by regulating the level of inflammatory peptides, for example, bradykinin. There have been many reports regarding alteration of the senses of smell and taste. The one particular larger study, including a total of 417 patients with mild to moderate SARS-CoV-2 infection, described smell impairment in 85.6% and taste impairment in 88.8% [55].

4.7 Stroke: musculoskeletal neurological findings

Stroke is commonly defined as sudden neurological deficit as a result of infarction or hemorrhage in the central nervous system [56]. This is a traditional definition, which has been updated over time with the fact that the neurological symptoms need to last more than 24 hours or CT and MRI confirmed focal infarction or hemorrhage compatible with the symptoms [57]. The typical subdivision of stroke includes ischemic stroke (infarction of brain, retina, or spinal infarction) and hemorrhagic stroke (intracerebral or subarachnoid hemorrhage) [58]. The cause of ischemic stroke is thromboembolism from the small vessel, larger artery, or the heart [59]. Classification of the hemorrhagic stroke depends on the anatomical location, whereas the most common are supratentorial hemorrhages [60].

There are numerous studies that report acute stroke complicating COVID-19 [61, 62]. The reported incidence of acute stroke in COVID-19 varies from 0.4% to 8.1%, due to the different ethnic and geographical variations: Asia (3.1%), Europe (1.2%) and, North America (1.1%) [63]. The reported incidence of stroke in COVID-19 patients treated in the intensive care units (ICU) is 1–3% [64–68]. Given the extent of the COVID-19 pandemic, this reported incidence is very high. Hemorrhagic stroke has been described from 21.7% to 25.7% COVID-19 patients with stroke, while the rest were ischemic strokes [69].

It has been stated that male COVID-19 patients, the median age of 63 years, are more likely to experience a stroke than women, but it is also known that the majority of ICU COVID-19 patients are older men as well [67]. Other reported risk factors include hypertension, diabetes mellitus [66, 70]. Race/ethnicity is also an important risk factor and it was observed that the black race had shown the highest prevalence (47%) [71]. A severe type of COVID-19 infection was observed as one of the most important risk factors for stroke in these patients [72–76]. There is a causal relationship between COVID-19 and stroke since the infection itself is more likely to induce thrombotic vascular events [63].

Described mechanisms of stroke in COVID-19 patients are diverse and multifactorial, considering that COVID-19 could be a trigger to typical stroke mechanisms, or alternatively, there are specific pathophysiological mechanisms [63]. The mechanisms for ischemic stroke in COVID-19 include sepsis-induced coagulopathy, presence of antiphospholipid antibodies, and thromboembolism, which show activated coagulation pathway in patients with COVID-19 who ordinarily already have elevated D-dimer and fibrinogen [77–81]. It is well known that COVID-19 uses the ACE-2 receptor to enter the cells, which leads to increased sympathetic activity, loss of blood pressure auto-regulation, and subsequent cerebral hypoperfusion [82]. Cytokine storm has also been suggested as one of the mechanisms in stroke development in COVID-19, due to its impact on atherosclerosis and thrombosis [83]. Finally, hypoxemia in COVID-19 patients may cause cerebral hypoperfusion and increase the risk of ischemia, together with previously explained thromboembolic mechanisms [84, 85].

Hemorrhagic strokes are less prevalent than ischemic strokes, but it has been implicated that some mechanism which plays a role in ischemic stroke, could lead to intracerebral hemorrhage in COVID-19 [86]. The proposed mechanisms include viral damage of vessel wall, downregulation of RAS and hypertension, cytokine destruction of blood–brain barrier, consumption coagulopathy caused by COVID-19 and cerebral hypoxia which induces micro-hemorrhages and microbleeds [87, 88]. It has been reported that COVID-19 patients who develop stroke are distinctly susceptible to large vessel occlusion, multi-territorial involvement and engagement of else ways infrequently affected vessels such as pericallosal artery [66, 68, 89].

Neuroimaging of stroke in COVID-19 patients standardly includes CT, MRI, and CT angiography (CTA). Small vessel occlusion in acute ischemic stroke was reported in 9% of cases, while large vessel infarctions were seen in almost 65% of cases [67, 68, 71, 90]. More frequent were ischemic strokes in posterior circulation [91]. It has been demonstrated that CTA verified occlusion in anterior or medial cerebral arteries with the co-development of floating thrombi in aorta and carotid arteries in patients with high D-dimer values, which confirms the influence of hypercoagulable state [71, 92]. Apart from standardly seen ischemic lesions, a small number of the patients (two of them were children) with acute stroke had: vasculitis or wall enhancement on MRI in the arterial wall [93]. Imaging findings of the hemorrhagic stroke include extensive hemispheric hematomas or multiple hematomas [94–97]. Hemorrhages may develop in severely ill patients, especially due to the failure of multiple organs or as a transformation of ischemic stroke, aneurysm rupture, or thrombosis of central venous sinus [66, 97, 98]. Some authors report a possible correlation between COVID-19 and arterial dissection, seen in the carotid artery, cervical vertebral artery or in posterior inferior cerebellar artery [99, 100].

A very small samples of patients were presented with acute stroke confirmed on neuroimaging and PCR confirmed COVID-19 [101]. Described atypical neuroimaging findings are seen in small number of COVID-19 patients with stroke and consist of: brain perfusion abnormalities, leptomeningeal enhancement [eight patients], focal cortico-pial enhancement in one patient, posterior reversible encephalopathy syndrome, microbleeds or leuco-encephalopathy [66, 102, 103]. Atypical findings express latent thrombotic angiopathy, vascular disruption and impairment of vascular autoregulation of the brain which happens in COVID-19 patients with stroke [103, 104].

5. Conclusions

Even though the COVID-19 virus is primarily a respiratory infection, new reported cases of neurological involvement have been presented daily all over the world [105]. In this chapter, we portrayed the neurological manifestations and possible pathophysiological mechanisms of SARS-CoV-2 on nervous system [105]. Given the extent of the COVID-19 pandemic, it is important to monitor COVID-19 patients for potential neurological complications to provide them with timely diagnostics and treatment.

Conflict of interest

The authors declare no conflict of interest.

Author details

Valentina Opancina[1*], Kristijan Krstic[2], Predrag Sazdanovic[3], Nebojsa Zdravkovic[4], Ruzica Radojevic Marjanovic[5] and Radisa Vojinovic[1]

1 Department of Radiology, Faculty of Medical Sciences, University of Kragujevac, Serbia

2 Department of Physical Medicine and Rehabilitation, Faculty of Medical Sciences, University of Kragujevac, Serbia

3 Department of Anatomy, Faculty of Medical Sciences, University of Kragujevac, Serbia

4 Department of Medical Statistics and Informatics, Faculty of Medical Sciences, University of Kragujevac, Serbia

5 Clinic for Infectious Diseases, University Clinical Centre Kragujevac, Serbia

*Address all correspondence to: valentina.opancina@gmail.com

References

[1] Cucinotta M. Vanelli, WHO declares COVID-19 a pandemic, Acta Biomed. 91 (1) (2020) 157-160

[2] YC Li, EZ Bai, T Hashikawa. The neuroinvasive potential of SARS-CoV2 may play a role in the respiratory failure of COVID-19 patients, J. Med. Virol. DOI:10.1002/jmv.25728

[3] D. Wang, et al., Clinical Characteristics of 138 Hospitalized Patients with 2019 Novel Coronavirus-Infected Pneumonia in Wuhan, China, JAMA 2020. DOI:10.1001/jama.2020.1585

[4] E Dong, H Du, L. Gardner. An interactive web-based dashboard to track COVID-19 in real time, Lancet Infect. Dis. 2020. DOI:10.1016/S1473-3099(20)30120-1

[5] L. Mao, et al., Neurologic Manifestations of Hospitalized Patients with Coronavirus Disease 2019 in Wuhan, China, JAMA Neurol. 2020. DOI:10.1001/jamaneurol.2020.1127

[6] J Netland, et al., Severe acute respiratory syndrome coronavirus infection causesneuronal death in the absence of encephalitis in mice transgenic for human ACE2, J. Virol. 82 (15). 2008. 7264-7275. DOI:10.1128/JVI.00737-08

[7] Hoffmann M, Kleine-Weber H, Schroeder S, Kruger N, Herrler T, Erichsen S, Schiergens TS, Herrler G, Wu NH, Nitsche A, et al. SARSCoV-2 Cell Entry Depends on ACE2 and TMPRSS2 and Is Blocked by a Clinically Proven Protease Inhibitor. Cell 181, 271-280. DOI:10.1016/j.cell.2020.02.052

[8] Hamming I, Timens W, Bulthuis MLC, Lely AT, Navis G, and van Goor H. (2004). Tissue distribution of ACE2 protein, the functional receptor for SARS coronavirus. A first step in understanding SARS pathogenesis. J Pathol. 203, 631-637. DOI:10.1002/path.1570

[9] Li Y, Zhou W, Yang L, You R. Physiological and pathological regulation of ACE2, the SARS-CoV-2 receptor. Pharmacol Rec. 2020. 157:104833. DOI:10.1016/j.phrs.2020.104833.

[10] Baig AM (2017) Emerging insights for better delivery of chemicals and stem cells to the brain. ACS Chem Neurosci 8:1119-1121

[11] Desforges M, Le Coupanec A, Dubeau P et al. (2019) Human coronaviruses and other respiratory viruses: Underestimated opportunistic pathogens of the central nervous system? Viruses 12:14. DOI:10.3390/v12010014

[12] Cantuti-Castelvetri L, Ojha R, Pedro LD, Djannatian M, Franz J, Kuivanen, S, Kallio K, Kaya T, Anastasina M, Smura T, et al. (2020). Neuropilin-1 facilitates SARS-CoV-2 cell entry and provides a possible pathway into the central nervous system. bioRxiv. DOI:10.1101/science.abd2985

[13] AM Baig, et al., Evidence of the COVID-19 virus targeting the CNS: Tissue distribution, host-virus interaction, and proposed neurotropic mechanisms, ACS Chem. Neurosci. 11 (7) (2020) 995-998. DOI:10.1021/aschemneuro.0c00122

[14] YC Li, EZ Bai, T Hashikawa, The neuroinvasive potential of SARS-CoV2 may play a role in the respiratory failure of COVID-19 patients, J. Med. Virol. (2020). DOI:10.1002/jmv.25728

[15] Wang K, Chen W, Zhou YS, Lian JQ, Zhang Z, Du P, Gong L, Zhang Y, Cui HY, Geng JJ, et al. (2020b). SARS-CoV-2 invades host cells via a novel

route: CD147-spike protein. bioRxiv. DOI:10.1002/jmv.25728

[16] Bergmann CC, Lane TE, and Stohlman SA (2006). Coronavirus infection of the central nervous system: Host-virus stand-off. Nat. Rev. Microbiol. 4, 121-132. DOI:10.1038/nrmicro1343

[17] Politi LS, Salsano E, and Grimaldi M. (2020). Magnetic resonance imaging alteration of the brain in a patient with coronavirus disease 2019 (COVID-19) and anosmia. JAMA Neurol. Published online may 29, 2020. DOI:10.1001/jamaneurol.2020.2125

[18] Dube´ M, Le Coupanec A, Wong AHM, Rini JM, Desforges M, and Talbot PJ. (2018). Axonal transport enables neuron-to-neuron propagation of human coronavirus OC43. J. Virol. 92, e00404-e00418. DOI:10.1128/JVI.00404-18

[19] Sauve, F, Ternier G, Fernandois D, Coelho C, Imbernon M, Deligia E, Perbet R, Florent V, Baroncini M, et al. (2020). The hypothalamus as a hub for SARS-CoV-2 brain infection and pathogenesis. bioRxiv. DOI:10.1101/2020.06.08.139329.

[20] Cantuti-Castelvetri L, Ojha R, Pedro LD, Djannatian M, Franz J, Kuivanen S, Kallio K, Kaya T, Anastasina M, Smura T, et al. (2020). Neuropilin-1 facilitates SARS-CoV-2 cell entry and provides a possible pathway into the central nervous system. bioRxiv. DOI:10.1101/2020.06.07.137802

[21] Erickson MA, and Banks WA. (2018). Neuroimmune axes of the blood-brain barriers and blood-brain interfaces: Bases for physiological regulation, disease states, and pharmacological interventions. Pharmacol. Rev. 70, 278-314. DOI:10.1124/pr.117.014647

[22] Teuwen LA, Geldhof V, Pasut A, and Carmeliet P. (2020). COVID-19: The vasculature unleashed. Nat. Rev. Immunol. 20, 389-391. DOI:10.1038/s41577-020-0343-0

[23] Chen Y, Feng Z, Diao B, Wang R, Wang G, Wang C, Tang Y, Liu L, Wang C, Liu Y, et al. (2020). The novel severe acute respiratory syndrome coronavirus 2 (SARS-CoV-2) directly decimates human spleens and lymph nodes. MedRxiv. DOI:10.1101/2020.03.27.20045427

[24] Merad M, and Martin JC (2020). Pathological inflammation in patients with COVID-19: A key role for monocytes and macrophages. Nat. Rev. Immunol. 20, 355-362. DOI:10.1038/s41577-020-0331-4

[25] Carsana L, Sonzogni A, Nasr A, Rossi RS, Pellegrinelli A, Zerbi P, Rech R, Colombo R, Antinori S, Corbellino M, et al. (2020). Pulmonary post-mortem findings in a series of COVID-19 cases from northern Italy: A two-Centre descriptive study. Lancet Infect. Dis. 2020. DOI:10.1016/S1473-3099(20)30434-5

[26] Qin C, Zhou L, Hu Z, Zhang S, Yang S, Tao Y, Xie C, Ma K, Shang K, Wang W, and Tian DS (2020). Dysregulation of immune response in patients with coronavirus 2019 (COVID-19) in Wuhan, China. Clin. Infect. Dis. 71, 762-768. DOI:10.1093/cid/ciaa248

[27] Kantonen J, Mahzabin S, Ma MI, Tynninen O, Paetau A, Andersson N, Sajantila A, Vapalahti O, Carpe´ n, O, Keka E, et al. (2020). Neuropathologic features of four autopsied COVID-19 patients. Brain Pathol. 2020. DOI:10.1111/bpa.12889

[28] Diao B, Wang C, Tan Y, Chen X, Liu Y, Ning L, Chen L, Li M, Liu Y, Wang G, et al. (2020). Reduction and functional exhaustion of T cells in

patients with coronavirus disease 2019 (COVID-19). Front. Immunol. 11, 827. DOI:10.3389/fimmu.2020.00827

[29] Qin C, Zhou L, Hu Z, Zhang S, Yang S, Tao Y, Xie C, Ma K, Shang K, Wang W, and Tian DS. (2020). Dysregulation of immune response in patients with coronavirus 2019 (COVID-19) in Wuhan, China. Clin. Infect. Dis. 71, 762-768. DOI:10.1093/cid/ciaa248

[30] Vabret N, Britton GJ, Gruber C, Hegde S, Kim J, Kuksin M, Levantovsky R, Malle L, Moreira A, Park MD, et al.; Sinai Immunology Review Project (2020). Immunology of COVID-19: Current state of the science. Immunity 52, 910-941. DOI:10.1016/j.immuni.2020.05.002

[31] Chen L, Long X, Xu Q, Tan J, Wang G, Cao Y, Wei J, Luo H, Zhu H, Huang L, et al. (2020b). Elevated serum levels of S100A8/A9 and HMGB1 at hospital admission are correlated with inferior clinical outcomes in COVID-19 patients. Cell. Mol. Immunol. 368, 1-3. DOI:10.1038/s41423-020-0492-x

[32] Dosch SF, Mahajan SD, and Collins AR. (2009). SARS coronavirus spike protein-induced innate immune response occurs via activation of the NF-kappaB pathway in human monocyte macrophages in vitro. Virus Res. 142, 19-27. DOI:10.1016/j.virusres.2009.01.005

[33] Dantzer R. (2018). Neuroimmune interactions: From the brain to the immune system and vice versa. Physiol. Rev. 98, 477-504. DOI:10.1152/physrev.00039.2016.

[34] Helms J, Tacquard C, Severac F, Leonard-Lorant, I, Ohana M, Delabranche X, Merdji H, Clere-Jehl R, Schenck M, Fagot Gandet F, et al.; CRICS TRIGGERSEP Group (Clinical Research in Intensive Care and Sepsis Trial Group for Global Evaluation and Research in Sepsis) (2020b). High risk of thrombosis in patients with severe SARS-CoV-2 infection: A multicenter prospective cohort study. Intensive Care Med. 46, 1089-1098. DOI:10.1007/s00134-020-06062-x

[35] Goyal P, Choi JJ, Pinheiro LC, Schenck EJ, Chen R, Jabri A, Satlin MJ, Campion TR, Jr Nahid M, Ringel JB, et al. (2020). Clinical characteristics of Covid-19 in new York City. N. Engl. J. Med. 382, 2372-2374. DOI:10.1056/NEJMc2010419

[36] Inciardi RM, Adamo M, Lupi L, Cani DS, Di Pasquale M, Tomasoni D, Italia L, Zaccone G, Tedino C, Fabbricatore D, et al. (2020). Characteristics and outcomes of patients hospitalized for COVID-19 and cardiac disease in northern Italy. Eur. Heart J. 41, 1821-1829. DOI:10.1093/eurheartj/ehaa388

[37] Pan L, Mu M, Yang P, Sun Y, Wang R, Yan J, Li P, Hu B, Wang J, Hu C, et al. (2020). Clinical characteristics of COVID-19 patients with digestive symptoms in Hubei, China: A descriptive, cross-sectional, Multicenter study. Am. J. Gastroenterol. 115, 766-773. DOI:10.14309/ajg.000000 0000000620

[38] Su H, Yang M, Wan C, Yi LX, Tang F, Zhu HY, Yi F, Yang HC, Fogo AB, Nie X, and Zhang C. (2020). Renal histopathological analysis of 26 postmortem findings of patients with COVID-19 in China. Kidney Int. 98, 219-227. DOI:10.1016/j.kint.2020.04.003

[39] Lau KK, Yu WC, Chu CM, Lau ST, Sheng B, Yuen KY (2004). Possible central nervous system infection by SARS coronavirus. Emerg Infect Dis 10:342-344. DOI:10.1016/j.kint.2020.04.003

[40] Helms J, Kremer S, Merdji H, Clere-Jehl R, Schenck M, Kummerlen C, Collange O, Boulay C, Fafi-Kremer S,

Ohana M, et al. (2020a). Neurologic features in severe SARS-CoV-2 infection. N. Engl. J. Med. 382, 2268-2270. DOI:10.1056/NEJMc2008597

[41] Leonardi M, Padovani A, McArthur JC (2020) Neurological manifestations associated with COVID-19: A review and a call for action. J Neurol 267:1573-1576. DOI:10.1007/s00415-020-09896-z

[42] Li Q, Guan X, Wu P, Wang X, Zhou L, Tong Y, Ren R, Leung KSM, Lau EHY, Wong JY, Xing X, Xiang N, WuY, Li C, Chen Q, Li D, Liu T, Zhao J, Liu M, TuW, Chen C, Jin L, Yang R, Wang Q, Zhou S, Wang R, Liu H, Luo Y, Liu Y, Shao G, Li H, Tao Z, Yang Y, Deng Z, Liu B, Ma Z, Zhang Y, Shi G, Lam TTY, Wu JT, Gao GF, Cowling BJ, Yang B, Leung GM, Feng Z (2020) Early transmission dynamics in Wuhan, China, of novel coronavirus-infected pneumonia. NEngl J Med 382:1199-1207. DOI:10.1007/s00415-020-09896-z

[43] Mao L, Jin H, Wang M, Hu Y, Chen S, He Q, et al. Neurologic manifestations of hospitalized patients with coronavirus disease 2019 in Wuhan, China. JAMA neurology. 2020. Headache classification Committee of the International Headache Society (IHS). The international classification of headache disorders (beta version). Cephalalgia. 2013;33(9), 629-808. DOI:10.1177/0333102413485658

[44] Shi H, Han X, Jiang N et al (2020) Radiological findings from 81 patients with COVID-19 pneumonia in Wuhan, China: A descriptive study. Lancet Infect Dis 20:425-434.

[45] Guan W, Liang W, Zhao Y et al (2020) Comorbidity and its impact on 1,590 patients with COVID-19 in China: A nationwide analysis. Eur Respir J 55:2000547

[46] Mao L, Jin H, Wang M et al (2020) Neurologic manifestations of hospitalized patients with coronavirus disease 2019 in Wuhan, China. JAMA Neurol 77:1-9. DOI:10.1001/jamaneurol.2020.1127

[47] Li Y, Li M, Wang M et al (2020) Acute cerebrovascular disease following COVID-19: A single center, retrospective, observational study. Stroke Vascul Neurol. DOI:10.1136/svn-2020-000431

[48] Fisher RS, van Emde Boas W, Blume W, et al. Epileptic seizures and epilepsy: Definitions proposed by the international league against epilepsy (ILAE) and the International Bureau for Epilepsy (IBE). Epilepsia 2005;46(4):470-472. DOI:10.1111/j.0013-9580.2005.66104.x

[49] Moriguchi T, Harii N, Goto J et al (2020) A first case of meningitis/encephalitis associated with SARS-Coronavirus-2. Int J Infect. Dis 94:55-58. DOI:10.1016/j.ijid.2020.03.062

[50] Duong L, Xu P, Liu A (2020) Meningoencephalitis without respiratory failure in a young female patient with COVID-19 infection in downtown Los Angeles, early April 2020. Brain Behav Immun 87:33. DOI:10.1016/j.bbi.2020.04.024

[51] SARS-CoV-2 patients: a cross-sectional study. Clin Infect Dis. (in press). Epub 2020. DOI:10.1093/cid/ciaa330

[52] Lahiri D, Ardila A. COVID-19 pandemic: A neurological perspective. Curteus. 2020: 12(4): e7889. DOI:10.7759/cureus.7889

[53] Pilotto A, Si O, Masciocchi S et al (2020) Steroid-responsive severe encephalopathy in SARS-CoV-2 infection. Ann Neurol. DOI:10.1002/ana.25783

[54] Vaira L, Salzano G, Deiana G, De Riu G. Ageusia and anosmia: common findings in COVID-19 patients.

Laryngoscope. (in press). Epub 2020. DOI:10.1002/lary.28698.

[55] Lechien JR, Chiesa-Estomba CM, De Siati DR et al (2020) Olfactory and gustatory dysfunctions as a clinical presentation of mild-to-moderate forms of the coronavirus disease (COVID-19): A multicenter European study. Eur Arch Otorhinolaryngol. DOI:10.1007/s00405-020-05965-1

[56] Sacco RL, Kasner SE, Broderick JP, Caplan LR, Connors JJ, Culebras A, Elkind MS, George MG, Hamdan AD, Higashida RT, Hoh BL, Janis LS, Kase CS, Kleindorfer DO, Lee JM, Moseley ME, Peterson ED, Turan TN, Valderrama AL, Vinters HV; American Heart Association Stroke Council, Council on Cardiovascular Surgery and Anesthesia; Council on Cardiovascular Radiology and Intervention; Council on Cardiovascular and Stroke Nursing; Council on Epidemiology and Prevention; Council on Peripheral Vascular Disease; Council on Nutrition, Physical Activity and Metabolism. An updated definition of stroke for the 21st century: a statement for healthcare professionals from the American Heart Association/American Stroke Association. Stroke. 2013;44(7):2064-89. DOI:10.1161/STR.0b013e318296aeca

[57] Hankey GJ. Stroke. Lancet. 2017;389(10069):641-654. DOI:10.1016/S0140-6736(16)30962-X

[58] Smith EE, Saposnik G, Biessels GJ, Doubal FN, Fornage M, Gorelick PB, Greenberg SM, Higashida RT, Kasner SE, Seshadri S; American Heart Association Stroke Council; Council on Cardiovascular Radiology and Intervention; Council on Functional Genomics and Translational Biology; and Council on Hypertension. Prevention of Stroke in Patients With Silent Cerebrovascular Disease: A Scientific Statement for Healthcare Professionals From the American Heart Association/American Stroke Association. Stroke. 2017;48(2):e44-e71. DOI:10.1161/STR.0000000000000116

[59] Hart RG, Diener HC, Coutts SB, Easton JD, Granger CB, O'Donnell MJ, Sacco RL, Connolly SJ; cryptogenic stroke/ESUS international working group. Embolic strokes of undetermined source: The case for a new clinical construct. Lancet Neurol. 2014;13(4):429-438. DOI:10.1016/S1474-4422(13)70310-7

[60] Rannikmäe K, Woodfield R, Anderson CS, Charidimou A, Chiewvit P, Greenberg SM, Jeng JS, Meretoja A, Palm F, Putaala J, Rinkel GJ, Rosand J, Rost NS, Strbian D, Tatlisumak T, Tsai CF, Wermer MJ, Werring D, Yeh SJ, Al-Shahi Salman R, Sudlow CL. Reliability of intracerebral hemorrhage classification systems: A systematic review. Int J Stroke. 2016;11(6):626-636. DOI:10.1177/1747493016641962

[61] Beyrouti R, Adams ME, Benjamin L, Cohen H, Farmer SF, Goh YY, Humphries F, Jäger HR, Losseff NA, Perry RJ, Shah S, Simister RJ, Turner D, Chandratheva A, Werring DJ. Characteristics of ischaemic stroke associated with COVID-19. J Neurol Neurosurg Psychiatry. 2020;91(8):889-891. DOI:10.1136/jnnp-2020-323586

[62] Dogra S, Jain R, Cao M, Bilaloglu S, Zagzag D, Hochman S, Lewis A, Melmed K, Hochman K, Horwitz L, Galetta S, Berger J. Hemorrhagic stroke and anticoagulation in COVID-19. J Stroke Cerebrovasc Dis. 2020;29(8):104984. DOI:10.1016/j.jstrokecerebrovasdis.2020.104984

[63] Nannoni S, de Groot R, Bell S, Markus HS. Stroke in COVID-19: A systematic review and meta-analysis. Int J Stroke. 2021;16(2):137-149. DOI:10.1177/1747493020972922

[64] Iadecola C, Anrather J, Kamel H. Effects of COVID-19 on the Nervous

System. Cell. 2020;183(1):16-27.e1. DOI:10.1016/j.cell.2020.08.028

[65] Ellul MA, Benjamin L, Singh B, Lant S, Michael BD, Easton A, Kneen R, Defres S, Sejvar J, Solomon T. Neurological associations of COVID-19. Lancet Neurol. 2020;19(9):767-783. DOI:10.1016/S1474-4422(20)30221-0

[66] Li Y, Li M, Wang M, Zhou Y, Chang J, Xian Y, Wang D, Mao L, Jin H, Hu B. Acute cerebrovascular disease following COVID-19: A single center, retrospective, observational study. Stroke Vasc Neurol. 2020;5(3):279-284. DOI:10.1136/svn-2020-000431

[67] Tan YK, Goh C, Leow AST, Tambyah PA, Ang A, Yap ES, Tu TM, Sharma VK, Yeo LLL, Chan BPL, Tan BYQ. COVID-19 and ischemic stroke: A systematic review and meta-summary of the literature. J Thromb Thrombolysis. 2020;50(3):587-595. DOI:10.1007/s11239-020-02228-y

[68] Siegler JE, Cardona P, Arenillas JF, Talavera B, Guillen AN, Chavarría-Miranda A, de Lera M, Khandelwal P, Bach I, Patel P, Singla A, Requena M, Ribo M, Jillella DV, Rangaraju S, Nogueira RG, Haussen DC, Vazquez AR, Urra X, Chamorro Á, Román LS, Thon JM, Then R, Sanborn E, de la Ossa NP, Millàn M, Ruiz IN, Mansour OY, Megahed M, Tiu C, Terecoasa EO, Radu RA, Nguyen TN, Curiale G, Kaliaev A, Czap AL, Sebaugh J, Zha AM, Liebeskind DS, Ortega-Gutierrez S, Farooqui M, Hassan AE, Preston L, Patterson MS, Bushnaq S, Zaidat O, Jovin TG. Cerebrovascular events and outcomes in hospitalized patients with COVID-19: The SVIN COVID-19 Multinational Registry. Int J Stroke. 2020 Sep 30:1747493020959216. DOI:10.1177/1747493020959216

[69] Vogrig A, Gigli GL, Bnà C, Morassi M. Stroke in patients with COVID-19: Clinical and neuroimaging characteristics. Neurosci Lett. 2021;743:135564. DOI:10.1016/j.neulet.2020.135564

[70] Morassi M, Bagatto D, Cobelli M, D'Agostini S, Gigli GL, Bnà C, Vogrig A. Stroke in patients with SARS-CoV-2 infection: Case series. J Neurol. 2020;267(8):2185-2192. DOI:10.1007/s00415-020-09885-2

[71] Oxley TJ, Mocco J, Majidi S, Kellner CP, Shoirah H, Singh IP, De Leacy RA, Shigematsu T, Ladner TR, Yaeger KA, Skliut M, Weinberger J, Dangayach NS, Bederson JB, Tuhrim S, Fifi JT. Large-vessel stroke as a presenting feature of Covid-19 in the Young. N Engl J Med. 2020;382(20):e60. DOI:10.1056/NEJMc2009787

[72] Li Y, Li M, Wang M, Zhou Y, Chang J, Xian Y, Wang D, Mao L, Jin H, Hu B. Acute cerebrovascular disease following COVID-19: A single center, retrospective, observational study. Stroke Vasc Neurol. 2020;5(3):279-284. DOI:10.1136/svn-2020-000431

[73] Klok FA, Kruip MJHA, van der Meer NJM, Arbous MS, Gommers D, Kant KM, Kaptein FHJ, van Paassen J, Stals MAM, Huisman MV, Endeman H. Confirmation of the high cumulative incidence of thrombotic complications in critically ill ICU patients with COVID-19: An updated analysis. Thromb Res. 2020;191:148-150. DOI:10.1016/j.thromres.2020.04.041

[74] Pinna P, Grewal P, Hall JP, Tavarez T, Dafer RM, Garg R, Osteraas ND, Pellack DR, Asthana A, Fegan K, Patel V, Conners JJ, John S, Silva ID. Neurological manifestations and COVID-19: Experiences from a tertiary care center at the frontline. J Neurol Sci. 2020;415:116969. DOI:10.1016/j.jns.2020.116969

[75] Mao L, Jin H, Wang M, Hu Y, Chen S, He Q, Chang J, Hong C, Zhou Y, Wang D, Miao X, Li Y, Hu B. Neurologic

manifestations of hospitalized patients with coronavirus disease 2019 in Wuhan, China. JAMA Neurol. 2020;77(6):683-690. DOI:10.1001/jamaneurol.2020.1127

[76] Karadaş Ö, Öztürk B, Sonkaya AR. A prospective clinical study of detailed neurological manifestations in patients with COVID-19. Neurol Sci. 2020;41(8):1991-1995. DOI:10.1007/s10072-020-04547-7

[77] Fan S, Xiao M, Han F, Xia P, Bai X, Chen H, Zhang H, Ding X, Zhao H, Zhao J, Sun X, Jiang W, Wang C, Cao W, Guo F, Tian R, Gao P, Wu W, Ma J, Wu D, Liu Z, Zhou X, Wang J, Guan T, Qin Y, Li T, Xu Y, Zhang D, Chen Y, Xie J, Li Y, Yan X, Zhu Y, Peng B, Cui L, Zhang S, Guan H. Neurological manifestations in critically ill patients with COVID-19: A retrospective study. Front Neurol. 2020;11:806. DOI:10.3389/fneur.2020.00806

[78] Spence JD, de Freitas GR, Pettigrew LC, Ay H, Liebeskind DS, Kase CS, Del Brutto OH, Hankey GJ, Venketasubramanian N. Mechanisms of stroke in COVID-19. Cerebrovasc Dis. 2020;49(4):451-458. DOI:10.1159/000509581

[79] Hess DC, Eldahshan W, Rutkowski E. COVID-19-related stroke. Transl Stroke Res. 2020;11(3):322-325. DOI:10.1007/s12975-020-00818-9

[80] Iba T, Levy JH, Warkentin TE, Thachil J, van der Poll T, Levi M; scientific and standardization committee on DIC, and the scientific and standardization committee on perioperative and critical Care of the International Society on thrombosis and haemostasis. Diagnosis and management of sepsis-induced coagulopathy and disseminated intravascular coagulation. J Thromb Haemost. 2019;17(11):1989-1994. DOI:10.1111/jth.14578

[81] Zhang Y, Xiao M, Zhang S, Xia P, Cao W, Jiang W, Chen H, Ding X, Zhao H, Zhang H, Wang C, Zhao J, Sun X, Tian R, Wu W, Wu D, Ma J, Chen Y, Zhang D, Xie J, Yan X, Zhou X, Liu Z, Wang J, Du B, Qin Y, Gao P, Qin X, Xu Y, Zhang W, Li T, Zhang F, Zhao Y, Li Y, Zhang S. Coagulopathy and Antiphospholipid antibodies in patients with Covid-19. N Engl J Med. 2020;382(17):e38. DOI:10.1056/NEJMc2007575

[82] Zhou P, Yang XL, Wang XG, Hu B, Zhang L, Zhang W, Si HR, Zhu Y, Li B, Huang CL, Chen HD, Chen J, Luo Y, Guo H, Jiang RD, Liu MQ, Chen Y, Shen XR, Wang X, Zheng XS, Zhao K, Chen QJ, Deng F, Liu LL, Yan B, Zhan FX, Wang YY, Xiao GF, Shi ZL. A pneumonia outbreak associated with a new coronavirus of probable bat origin. Nature. 2020;579(7798):270-273. DOI:10.1038/s41586-020-2012-7

[83] Marchandot B, Sattler L, Jesel L, Matsushita K, Schini-Kerth V, Grunebaum L, Morel O. COVID-19 related coagulopathy: A distinct entity? J Clin Med. 2020;9(6):1651. DOI:10.3390/jcm9061651

[84] Helms J, Kremer S, Merdji H, Clere-Jehl R, Schenck M, Kummerlen C, Collange O, Boulay C, Fafi-Kremer S, Ohana M, Anheim M, Meziani F. Neurologic features in severe SARS-CoV-2 infection. N Engl J Med. 2020;382(23):2268-2270. DOI:10.1056/NEJMc2008597

[85] Williams OH, Mohideen S, Sen A, Martinovic O, Hart J, Brex PA, Sztriha LK. Multiple internal border zone infarcts in a patient with COVID-19 and CADASIL. J Neurol Sci. 2020;416:116980. DOI:10.1016/j.jns.2020.116980

[86] Sharifi-Razavi A, Karimi N, Rouhani N. COVID-19 and intracerebral haemorrhage: Causative or coincidental? New Microbes New Infect.

2020;35:100669. DOI:10.1016/j.nmni.2020.100669

[87] Valderrama EV, Humbert K, Lord A, Frontera J, Yaghi S. Severe acute respiratory syndrome coronavirus 2 infection and ischemic stroke. Stroke. 2020;51(7):e124-e127. DOI:10.1161/STROKEAHA.120.030153

[88] Conklin J, Frosch MP, Mukerji S, Rapalino O, Maher M, Schaefer PW, Lev MH, Gonzalez RG, Das S, Champion SN, Magdamo C, Sen P, Harrold GK, Alabsi H, Normandin E, Shaw B, Lemieux J, Sabeti P, Branda JA, Brown EN, Westover MB, Huang SY, Edlow BL. Cerebral Microvascular Injury in Severe COVID-19. medRxiv [Preprint]. 2020:2020.07.21.20159376. DOI:10.1101/2020.07.21.20159376. Update in: J Neurol Sci. 2021;421:117308

[89] John S, Kesav P, Mifsud VA, Piechowski-Jozwiak B, Dibu J, Bayrlee A, Elkambergy H, Roser F, Elhammady MS, Zahra K, Hussain SI. Characteristics of large-vessel occlusion associated with COVID-19 and ischemic stroke. AJNR Am J Neuroradiol. 2020;41(12):2263-2268. DOI:10.3174/ajnr.A6799

[90] Goyal P, Choi JJ, Pinheiro LC, Schenck EJ, Chen R, Jabri A, Satlin MJ, Campion TR Jr, Nahid M, Ringel JB, Hoffman KL, Alshak MN, Li HA, Wehmeyer GT, Rajan M, Reshetnyak E, Hupert N, Horn EM, Martinez FJ, Gulick RM, Safford MM. Clinical characteristics of Covid-19 in new York City. N Engl J Med. 2020;382(24):2372-2374. DOI:10.1056/NEJMc2010419

[91] Hernández-Fernández F, Sandoval Valencia H, Barbella-Aponte RA, Collado-Jiménez R, Ayo-Martín Ó, Barrena C, Molina-Nuevo JD, García-García J, Lozano-Setién E, Alcahut-Rodriguez C, Martínez-Martín Á, Sánchez-López A, Segura T. Cerebrovascular disease in patients with COVID-19: Neuroimaging, histological and clinical description. Brain. 2020;143(10):3089-3103. DOI:10.1093/brain/awaa239

[92] Viguier A, Delamarre L, Duplantier J, Olivot JM, Bonneville F. Acute ischemic stroke complicating common carotid artery thrombosis during a severe COVID-19 infection. J Neuroradiol. 2020;47(5):393-394. DOI:10.1016/j.neurad.2020.04.003

[93] Dixon L, Coughlan C, Karunaratne K, Gorgoraptis N, Varley J, Husselbee J, Mallon D, Carroll R, Jones B, Boynton C, Pritchard J, Youngstein T, Mason J, Gabriel C. Immunosuppression for intracranial vasculitis associated with SARS-CoV-2: therapeutic implications for COVID-19 cerebrovascular pathology. J Neurol Neurosurg Psychiatry. 2020:jnnp-2020-324291. DOI:10.1136/jnnp-2020-324291

[94] Jain R, Young M, Dogra S, Kennedy H, Nguyen V, Jones S, Bilaloglu S, Hochman K, Raz E, Galetta S, Horwtiz L. COVID-19 related neuroimaging findings: A signal of thromboembolic complications and a strong prognostic marker of poor patient outcome. J Neurol Sci. 2020;414:116923. DOI:10.1016/j.jns.2020.116923

[95] Sharifi-Razavi A, Karimi N, Rouhani N. COVID-19 and intracerebral haemorrhage: Causative or coincidental? New Microbes New Infect. 2020;35:100669. DOI:10.1016/j.nmni.2020.100669

[96] Giorgianni A, Vinacci G, Agosti E, Mercuri A, Baruzzi F. Neuroradiological features in COVID-19 patients: First evidence in a complex scenario. J Neuroradiol. 2020;47(6):474-476. DOI:10.1016/j.neurad.2020.05.005

[97] Gonçalves B, Righy C, Kurtz P. Thrombotic and Hemorrhagic neurological complications in critically ill COVID-19 patients. Neurocrit Care.

2020;33(2):587-590. DOI:10.1007/s12028-020-01078-z

[98] Poillon G, Obadia M, Perrin M, Savatovsky J, Lecler A. Cerebral venous thrombosis associated with COVID-19 infection: Causality or coincidence? J Neuroradiol. 2021;48(2):121-124. DOI:10.1016/j.neurad.2020.05.003

[99] Morassi M, Bigni B, Cobelli M, Giudice L, Bnà C, Vogrig A. Bilateral carotid artery dissection in a SARS-CoV-2 infected patient: Causality or coincidence? J Neurol. 2020;267(10): 2812-2814. DOI:10.1007/s00415-020-09984-0

[100] Dakay K, Kaur G, Gulko E, Santarelli J, Bowers C, Mayer SA, Gandhi CD, Al-Mufti F. Reversible cerebral vasoconstriction syndrome and dissection in the setting of COVID-19 infection. J Stroke Cerebrovasc Dis. 2020;29(9):105011. DOI:10.1016/j.jstrokecerebrovasdis.2020.105011

[101] Garcia S, Dehghani P, Grines C, Davidson L, Nayak KR, Saw J, Waksman R, Blair J, Akshay B, Garberich R, Schmidt C, Ly HQ, Sharkey S, Mercado N, Alfonso CE, Misumida N, Acharya D, Madan M, Hafiz AM, Javed N, Shavadia J, Stone J, Alraies MC, Htun W, Downey W, Bergmark BA, Ebinger J, Alyousef T, Khalili H, Hwang CW, Purow J, Llanos A, McGrath B, Tannenbaum M, Resar J, Bagur R, Cox-Alomar P, Stefanescu Schmidt AC, Cilia LA, Jaffer FA, Gharacholou M, Salinger M, Case B, Kabour A, Dai X, Elkhateeb O, Kobayashi T, Kim HH, Roumia M, Aguirre FV, Rade J, Chong AY, Hall HM, Amlani S, Bagherli A, Patel RAG, Wood DA, Welt FG, Giri J, Mahmud E, Henry TD; Society for Cardiac Angiography and Interventions, the Canadian Association of Interventional Cardiology, and the American College of Cardiology Interventional Council. Initial Findings From the North American COVID-19 Myocardial Infarction Registry. J Am Coll Cardiol. 2021;77(16):1994-2003. DOI:10.1016/j.jacc.2021.02.055

[102] Helms J, Kremer S, Merdji H, Clere-Jehl R, Schenck M, Kummerlen C, Collange O, Boulay C, Fafi-Kremer S, Ohana M, Anheim M, Meziani F. Neurologic features in severe SARS-CoV-2 infection. N Engl J Med. 2020;382(23):2268-2270. DOI:10.1056/NEJMc2008597

[103] Sachs JR, Gibbs KW, Swor DE, Sweeney AP, Williams DW, Burdette JH, West TG, Geer CP. COVID-19-associated Leukoencephalopathy. Radiology. 2020;296(3):E184-E185. DOI:10.1148/radiol.2020201753

[104] Levinson R, Elbaz M, Ben-Ami R et al (2020) Anosmia and dysgeusia in patients with mild SARS-CoV-2 infection. Infect Dis. DOI:10.1016/S1473-3099(20)30086-4

[105] Helms J, Kremer S, Merdji H et al (2020) Neurologic features in severe SARS-CoV-2 infection. N Engl J Med 382:2268-2270. DOI:10.1056/NEJMc2008597

Chapter 14

"Neurocovid": An Analysis of the Impact of Covid-19 on the Older Adults. Evolving Psychological and Neuropsychological Understanding

Sara Palermo

Abstract

When SARS-CoV-2 began to spread, older adults experienced disproportionately greater adverse effects from the pandemic, including exacerbation of pre-existing physical and cognitive frailty conditions. More severe complications, higher mortality, and concerns about disruptions to their daily routines and access to care. Knowledge about the impact of COVID-19 on the brain is rapidly accumulating and this is reflected in the increasing use of the term "*neurocovid*". Co-involvement of the central and peripheral nervous system had already been observed in SARS patients, but COVID-19 seems to invade it with greater affinity than other coronaviruses. This chapter provides an overview of the expanding understanding of the multiple ways in which COVID-19 affects the human brain, discuss the likelihood of long-term sequelae of neurocovid, and their implications for cognitive functions and behaviors in the elderly.

Keywords: COVID-19; SARS-CoV-2, neurocovid, long term pandemic fatigue, mechanisms of brain damage, brain dysfunction, neurology, neuropsychology, neuropsychiatry, cognitive dysfunctions, mood changes, anxiety, depression, social isolation, frailty, elderly, older adults

1. Introduction

Europe is a country that is getting older every day. An increasingly significant number of people find themselves in a condition of vulnerability and are at greater risk of suffering a functional loss and/or loss of autonomy [1, 2]. These conditions have been accentuated during the health emergency due to the current pandemic situation [3].

The elderly population has been burdened with a higher incidence and mortality of infection: the older adults have been shown to contract the infection in a more severe clinical form and this is especially true in Europe which, having, after Japan, the highest percentage of elderly people, has paid a very high toll in terms of mortality [3]. More than 95 per cent of the deaths involved people over the age of 60, and 50 per cent of all deaths were aged ≥80 [4].

IntechOpen

The disease did not strike indiscriminately; it was mainly the elderly with serious concomitant chronic diseases (cardiovascular diseases, respiratory diseases, diabetes, neurodegenerative diseases, oncological diseases, etc.) who paid the highest price in terms of mortality [3, 4]. A particular incidence of fatal events has occurred among people living in social and health care residences throughout Europe [3, 4]. It is reasonable to assume that the virus has affected residential care facilities because of the community life that takes place there, affecting people already suffering from frailty and polypathology, so that the damage caused by the virus has been superimposed on that caused by coexisting diseases.

Considering the above, social distancing measures severely penalized the elderly, since they needed to be isolated as they could act as healthy carriers for the community and, if they became ill, would produce extraordinary pressure on intensive care [4].

The Covid-19 pandemic has also brought to light the concept that it is above all the frail elderly who are at high risk of functional, cognitive and psycho-social disabilities that make it difficult for the elderly to return to their pre-infection condition: this is the key to interpreting the relationship between the elderly and the coronavirus infection.

This inference is derived from what is observed about the global population. It seems increasingly likely that the majority of all those infected wills experience chronic sequelae of the disease, resulting in disability or diminished quality of life, a phenomenon now described as "*long-covid*" [5, 6]. Indeed, COVID-19 survivors can suffer from persistent symptoms after recovering [5], especially related to organ damage, post viral syndrome, and post-critical care syndrome [6]. Long-covid is characterized by breathlessness, chest tightness, cough, fatigue, myalgia, palpitations, sleep disorders and difficulty to focus [5, 6]. Anxiety and depression were also reported [5].

The SARS-CoV-2 pandemic has rekindled attention on the possible neurovirulence of this virus and the possible involvement of the central nervous system and peripheral nervous system [7, 8]. The spectrum of central and peripheral nervous systems disease in COVID-19 patients is much broader than previously thought. Some form of "*neurocovid*" appears to occur in up to 30% of positive patients. It is therefore a phenomenon that deserves to be carefully investigated and evaluated when screening and monitoring short- and long-term patients, especially the elderly.

2. Aging, frailty, and COVID-19

Aging is a natural phenomenon involving a progressive physiological transformation of the human body and of neuropsychological and behavioral functions [1, 2]. The aging phenomenon, in addition to the growing quantitative data on the total population, is characterized by the different attributes that qualitatively characterize this process and transition. In fact, elderly life is structured by different levels of independence and dependence of individuals with respect to both primary family networks and secondary networks of assistance and care [1, 2].

The conceptualization of frailty is presented as an attempt to define this heterogeneity of conditions. Frailty is a condition of marked vulnerability to adverse events caused by a reduction in the functional reserves of multiple systems of the body due to the aging process and chronic polypathology. It is a condition that represents a risk factor for disability, hospitalization, institutionalization, and death [1–3]. At first, frailty appeared in the literature with a distinctly bio-medical or clinical meaning [9], but in the last decade it has acquired bio-psycho-social connotations as well as medical ones. Starting from the works of Gobbens et al. [10] and Van Campen [11], it is preferred to define frailty as a condition of vulnerability at a bio-psycho-social level. Today we prefer to speak of frailty in the plural. There are functional, cognitive, psycho-social, clinical, and - finally - economic frailty. These different dimensions interact together in moments of greatest difficulty. The definition of "frail elderly" therefore refers to a person who, faced with a stressful event -such as the SARS-CoV-2 pandemic - is unable to respond adequately, and therefore succumbs, with an increased risk of adverse events: mortality, disability and worsening of his/her general condition.

An increasingly significant number of older people are in a frail state, making this a hot topic. Physical and cognitive frailty have proved more useful than ever in understanding the impact of the SARS-CoV-2 pandemic on the elderly population and in guiding the principles of vaccine clinical trials [3]. Indeed, not only frail older people are particularly vulnerable to serious or life-threatening infections, but the age-related dysregulation of the immune system (due to immunosenescence and inflammaging) results in poorer responses to vaccination [3].

3. Neurological presentations of COVID-19: the polyform entity of neurocovid

Psychiatric and neurological complications were reported during the SARS epidemic in 2003 [11].

Apart from depression, anxiety disorders and suicidal ideations, fear for survival, and fear of infecting others; across all timeframes, stigmatization, reduced quality of life, psychological distress, and posttraumatic stress symptoms were reported [11]. Moreover, cases of organic hallucinosis (visual and auditory hallucinations), deliriums of persecution, temporo-spatial disorientation and hypomanic disorder were reported. In some cases, these manifestations have been classified as secondary to steroid therapy. Isolated cases of fatal Coronavirus OC43 encephalomyelitis in the face of little pulmonary involvement [12] and generalized tonic–clonic convulsion in patients with infection and cerebrospinal fluid positivity for SARS-CoV [13] have also been described.

Recent data suggesting that the COVID-19 virus also reaches the central nervous system [7, 8, 14]. It has been shown that (like SARS-CoV) COVID-19 virus exploits the receptor for the angiotensin converting enzyme 2 (ACE2) to enter cells. This discovery made it possible to investigate the expression of ACE2 in the neurological tissue and to determine the possible contribution of neurological tissue damage to morbidity and mortality caused by COVID-19 [7, 14].

The neuroinvasiveness, neurotropism and neurovirulence of the COVID-19 has been demonstrated [7]. Pathological studies suggest a direct route of neuroinvasion via haematogenous diffusion and retrograde transport by the olfactory nerve. Retrograde transport via the vagus and olfactory nerves remains hypothetical [7].

In most cases, COVID-19 would not make a direct attack on vulnerable structures. This would explain why various manifestations of the nervous system are favorable to immune suppression or immune modulation [8].

Direct affection of the central nervous system is uncommon and may result in meningitis/encephalitis [8, 15, 16], manifesting as headache, seizures, confusion, ataxia, pyramidal signs, or impaired consciousness. Direct affection of the peripheral nervous system includes hyposmia or hypogeusia [8].

Neurological disease due to the immune reaction against the COVID-19 embraces acute disseminated encephalomyelitis; acute, haemorrhagic, myoclonus; necrotizing encephalopathy [17, 18]; cytokine release syndrome (a new nosographic entity characterized by aphasia, behavioral alterations, central hypothyroidism, cerebellar ataxia, coma, confusion, cranial nerve palsy, dysautonomia, pyramidal signs, and tremor) and mononeuritis [19]; myositis [20]; cerebral vasculitis; delirium; psychosis; transverse myelitis [21]; cranial nerve palsy; Guillain-Barre syndrome [22]. Neurological long-term complications may be also secondary to affection of the heart or the kidneys [8]. Cardiac involvement may be responsible for cardioembolic, ischemic stroke, or ischemic stroke due to hypotension [8].

The COVID-19 pandemic continues to affect millions of people globally, with increasing reports of neurological manifestations but limited data on their incidence and associations with outcome. Two recent papers report the presence of neurological symptoms in 36.2% [23] and 80% [24] of patients hospitalized with COVID-19. Neurocovid is a polymorphic entity [25]. More than seventy different symptom combinations have been reported in the literature. Symptoms of a general nature seem to be present in almost all patients, often with abnormal laboratory tests [25]. The timing of symptoms varies from early states (anosmia, headache, myalgia) to later stages (altered mental status, neuromuscular disorders, seizures, stroke) [25]. Some neurological symptoms may persist (such as anosmia or headache), while others may cause persistent disability (such as stroke or polyneuropathy) [25].

4. Brain imaging findings and new classification system

The existence of alterations in brain structure as a result of SARS-CoV-2 infection appears to be well established [26, 27], even in subjects whose only symptom was anosmia [28]. Post-mortem structural MRI examinations revealed brain parenchymal abnormalities, subcortical micro and macro hemorrhages, cortico-subcortical oedema, non-specific deep white matter changes and asymmetrical olfactory bulbs [29]. Similar evidence is also found in hospitalized patients [30–33]. The most common neuroimaging findings include cortical signal abnormalities on fluid-attenuated inversion recovery images, associated with leptomeningeal enhancement or cortical diffusion restriction [26], which may reflect autoimmune or infectious encephalitis, hypoglycaemia, hypoxia, or seizures [34]. Acute demyelinating lesions have also been depicted [35–38].

Starting from the observation that different neurobiological processes and mechanisms may lie behind the onset of neurocovid, a three-stage MRI classification system to categorize patients has been recently proposed [39]:

- *Neurocovid Stage 1*: Viral damage is limited to epithelial cells of the nose and mouth with temporary loss of smell and taste.

- *Neurocovid Stage 2*: Inflammation floods from the lungs through the blood stream, leading to blood clots that prompt small and large strokes.

- *Neurocovid Stage 3*: The inflammation damages the blood–brain barrier. Inflammatory markers and viral particles infiltrate the brain, causing confusion, coma, encephalopathy, and seizures.

5. Aging, COVID-19, and neurocovid

Frailty elderly are more prone to cognitive impairment and SAR-CoV-2 infection [3]. Preexisting comorbidities (i.e., cerebrovascular, and cardiovascular diseases, diabetes, hypertension, obesity, malignancy, and respiratory diseases) seem to be predictor of disease severity and neurological complications [40]. Moreover, elderly individuals with pre-existing neurological diseases are susceptible to more severe forms of COVID-19 infection and higher mortality rates [40, 41]. Indeed, it is now established that older people with Alzheimer's and Parkinson's diseases exhibit independent association with the rate of change in both physical frailty and cognitive impairment [42], placing these individuals at higher risk of COVID-19 disease severity [40]. Specifically, patients with Parkinson's disease are vulnerable to infection due to advanced age, bulbar symptoms, respiratory dysfunction, frailty and cognitive impairment. Similarly, patients with Alzheimer's disease and major neurocognitive disorder are at increased risk of infection and adverse events [43].

Elderly patients aged 65 years or older are known to have higher rates of neurological complications [40]. Commonly reported neurological dysfunctions include dizziness, confusion, fatigue, and headache. They may experience also atypical presentations such as falling or postural instability. Other neurological complications include cerebrovascular disease, cognitive impairment and neuropsychiatric disease [40]. Altered mental status and epilepsy have been also reported [25].

Older patients are particularly vulnerable to the psychological burden of COVID-19 [40]. Disturbed sleep, moderate to severe depression and anxiety have been reported [44]. Loneliness related to quarantine and social isolation has had a significant impact on mental health outcomes in the elderly [45], especially for those with chronic neurological diseases and neurocognitive disorder [46]. Quarantine comes to induce a rapid increase in behavioral and psychological symptoms in ~60% of patients and stress-related symptoms in two-thirds of caregivers [46]. The most common symptoms included agitation, anxiety, apathy, irritability, and sleep disturbances [46]. Similarly, a worsening of symptoms was observed in 67.5% of Parkinson's patients during the quarantine period [47].

6. Implications for neurocognitive and neuropsychiatric disorders

COVID-19 causes high levels of acute respiratory distress, hypoxia, and proinflammatory cytokines - all of which contribute to the onset of cognitive decline in the elderly [26]. It therefore seems reasonable that cardiovascular and cerebrovascular disease secondary to infection may contribute to an increased long-term risk of cognitive decline and major neurocognitive disorders in recovered individuals [26, 48, 49].

After the SARS pandemics, one in five infected individuals reported memory problems [50]. Likewise, the current pandemic situation appears to have resulted in a dysexecutive syndrome in one in three individuals who have been hospitalized [50]. Poor memory, attention and speed of information processing impairments have commonly been reported with COVID-19 [39, 51].

This could lead to a vicious circle whereby impaired cognitive abilities may cause poor occupational and functional outcomes for individuals recovered from COVID-19 that precipitate or exacerbate mental health concerns, and poor mental health may likewise contribute to cognitive dysfunction [52].

Abnormalities in the mental status (defined as a severe change in personality, behavior, cognition, or consciousness) have been reported [39, 53], in line with what happened previously with the SARS pandemic [26]. COVID-19 patients experienced a high level of post-traumatic stress symptoms and a significantly higher level of depressive symptoms [39, 54]. In the post-illness phase, the point prevalence of post-traumatic stress disorder seems to be around 32%, depression and anxiety disorder both around 15% [50]. Patients with pre-existing psychiatric disorders reported a worsening of their symptomatology [54].

Viral infections of the brain may have an impact on the risk of AD or Parkinson's disease [26]. Olfactory deficits (hyposmia/anosmia) are among the sentinel symptoms of COVID-19 infection [55] and are characteristic of neurodegenerative disorders [56–58]. Indeed, anosmia is associated with high levels of interleukin-6, an inflammatory mediator causally implicated in brain disorders and which action is blocked by tocilizumab as part of COVID-19 treatment [59].

To date, the mechanisms by which neurological abnormalities result from SARS-CoV-2 infection have yet to be fully established. Nevertheless, the contribution resulting from direct effects of SARS-CoV-2 on neuronal function and survival or glial reactivity, exaggerated cytokine responses or anti-neuronal antibodies are all likely, as are sequelae of cerebrovascular accidents [26]. The data available to date suggest an increase in neuropsychiatric and neuropsychological long-term sequelae, including cognitive decline, motor impairment, and affective and psychotic disorders [26].

7. Management and treatment of neurocovid in elderly patients

Treatment of neurocovid is currently based on existing evidence-based treatment for specific neurologic conditions in conjunction with systemic treatment of COVID-19 infection (i.e., antivirals, corticosteroids, and immunomodulators) [25, 40].

The contagion is associated with neuropsychiatric symptoms [60] and it is recommended to set up a baseline mental status examination for all hospitalized COVID-19 old patients [61].

Delirium management has long been a priority in the care of older adults [25]. Every hospitalized older person should be considered at high risk for developing delirium, and prevention should be optimized [58]. Non-pharmacologic interventions include patient-centered care with adequate hydration and sleep, optimization of hearing and vision, early mobilization, frequent re-orientation, reduction of social isolation and regular visits, connecting patients with their families, and minimization of unnecessary lines, tubes, polypharmacy, and precipitating medications [61, 62]. Low-potency neuroleptics and alpha-2 adrenergic agents may be useful [60].

Neurologists, geriatricians and neuropsychologists must be involved at an early stage and be prepared to handle the peculiarities of neurocovid. It is advisable to have patients undergo neuropsychological assessment even 6–8 months after their discharge from hospital, especially if cognitive problems, slowness in processing information or poor attention persist [39].

Patients with below cut-off test scores should be evaluated for rehabilitation and cognitive enhancement interventions. This would reduce the risk of facilitating an earlier/rapid age-related cognitive decline [3, 39].

8. Conclusions

The high probability of long-term neurological and neuropsychological consequences of COVID-19 indicates the importance of continuous surveillance for neuroimmune and neurodegenerative disorders in infected individuals, especially the elderly [7]. Until an effective treatment is discovered, or the expected global population-wide vaccination coverage is achieved, clinicians need to be alert to neurocovid [25].

Researchers have postulated several explanations for the severity with which COVID-19 occurs in the elderly and the increased mortality rate in this population group. Age-related epigenetic changes, inflammasome activity, covalent modifications of human and viral proteins, etc. are all possibilities currently being explored by scientists [63]. Future research will lead to a full understanding of the key factors leading to the vulnerability of the elderly population, especially about the intersection of aging, vulnerability to infection and alterations in cognitive-behavioral patterns. A neurocognitive approach could prove extremely useful for this purpose. It seems particularly appropriate to deepen our knowledge of the deleterious effects of SARS-CoV-2 and COVID-19 infection on the central and peripheral nervous system (in both structural and functional terms), and to assess through predictive medicine how these effects may contribute to the chronic burden of disease in the coming years. Notably, key questions need to be answered about the impact of the risk of cognitive decline in old age, Alzheimer's disorder, Parkinson's disorder and other neurodegenerations. In addition, a change of pace in the observation of the various conditions of elderly life can make it possible to construct complementary health and welfare interventions that have the characteristic of elasticity and immediacy to be placed alongside the traditional ones - above all in response to phenomena such as neurocovid.

Acknowledgements

No funding was available to the author.

Conflict of interest

The authors declare that the manuscript was written in the absence of any commercial or financial relationships that could be construed as a potential conflict of interest.

Author details

Sara Palermo[1,2]

1 European Innovation Partnership on Active and Healthy Ageing, Brussels, Belgium

2 Diagnostic and Technology Department, Neuroradiology Unit, Neurological Institute "Carlo Besta" IRCCS Foundation, Milan, Italy

*Address all correspondence to: sara.palermo@istituto-besta.it

References

[1] Morese R, Palermo S, Defedele M, Nervo J, Borraccino A. Vulnerability and Social Exclusion: Risk in Adolescence and Old Age. In: Morese R, Palermo S, editors. The New Forms of Social Exclusion. London: IntechOpen Limited; 2019. p. 1-16. DOI: 10.5772/intechopen.85463

[2] Palermo S. Frailty, Vulnerability, and Plasticity: Towards a New Medicine of Complexity. In: Palermo S, editor. Frailty in the Elderly - Understanding and Managing Complexity. London: IntechOpen Limited; 2021. p. 1-11. DOI: 10.5772/intechopen.96244.

[3] Palermo S. Covid-19 pandemic: Maximising future vaccination treatments considering ageing and frailty. Front. Med. 2020; 7:558835. DOI: 10.3389/fmed.2020.558835

[4] AA.VV. A timeline of WHO's response to COVID-19 in the WHO European Region: a living document (version 2.0 from 31 December 2019 to 31 December 2020). Copenhagen: WHO Regional Office for Europe; 2021. Licence: CC BY-NC-SA3.0 IGO.

[5] Iwu CJ, Iwu CD, Wiysonge CS. The occurrence of long COVID: a rapid review. Pan Afr Med J 2021; 38:65. DOI: 10.11604/pamj.2021.38.65.27366.

[6] Raveendran AV, Jayadevan R, Sashidharan S. Long COVID: An overview. Diabetes Metab Syndr. 2021; 15(3):869-875. DOI: 10.1016/j.dsx.2021.04.007.

[7] Zhang L, Wei L, Wang ZX, Huang YN, Schwarz G, Wheelock V. COVID-19: Neuro invasiveness, Neurotropism and Neurovirulence. J Neurol Exp Neurosci. 2020; 6(S1): S24-S31. DOI: 10.17756/jnen.2020-S1-006

[8] Finsterer J, Scorza FA. Clinical and Pathophysiologic Spectrum of Neuro-COVID. Mol Neurobiol. 2021; 8:1-5. DOI: 10.1007/s12035-021-02383-0.

[9] Fried LP, Tangen CM, Walston J, Newman AB, Hirsch C, Gottdiener J, Seeman T, Tracy R, Kop WJ, Burke G, McBurnie MA; Cardiovascular Health Study Collaborative Research Group. Frailty in older adults: evidence for a phenotype. J Gerontol A Biol Sci Med Sci. 2001; 56(3):M146-M156. DOI: 10.1093/gerona/56.3.m146.

[10] Gobbens RJ, van Assen MA, Luijkx KG, Wijnen-Sponselee MT, Schols JM. Determinants of frailty. J Am Med Dir Assoc. 2010; 11(5):356-364. DOI: 10.1016/j.jamda.2009.11.008.

[11] Gardner PJ and Moallef P. Psychological impact on SARS survivors: Critical review of the English language literature. Canadian Psychology/Psychologie Canadienne 2015; 56(1):123-135. DOI: 10.1037/a0037973.

[12] Morfopoulou S, Brown JR, Davies EG, Anderson G, Virasami A, Qasim W, Chong WK, Hubank M, Plagnol V, Desforges M, Jacques TS, Talbot PJ, Breuer J. Human Coronavirus OC43 Associated with Fatal Encephalitis. N Engl J Med. 2016; 375(5):497-498. doi: 10.1056/NEJMc1509458.

[13] Lau KK, Yu WC, Chu CM, Lau ST, Sheng B, Yuen KY. Possible central nervous system infection by SARS coronavirus. Emerg Infect Dis. 2004; 10(2):342-344. DOI: 10.3201/eid1002.030638.

[14] Baig AM, Khaleeq A, Ali U, Syeda H. Evidence of the COVID-19 Virus Targeting the CNS: Tissue Distribution, Host-Virus Interaction, and Proposed

Neurotropic Mechanisms. ACS Chem Neurosci. 2020; 11(7):995-998. doi: 10.1021/acschemneuro.0c00122.

[15] Schweitzer F, Kleineberg NN, Göreci Y, Onur OA, Franke C, Warnke C. Neuro-COVID-19 is more than anosmia: clinical presentation, neurodiagnostics, therapies, and prognosis. Curr Opin Neurol. 2021. DOI: 10.1097/WCO.0000000000000930.

[16] Gallacher SD, Seaton A. Meningococcal meningitis and COVID-19 co-infection. BMJ Case Rep. 2020; 13(8):e237366. doi: 10.1136/bcr-2020-237366.

[17] Delamarre L, Gollion C, Grouteau G, Rousset D, Jimena G, Roustan J, Gaussiat F, Aldigé E, Gaffard C, Duplantier J, Martin C, Fourcade O, Bost C, Fortenfant F, Delobel P, Martin-Blondel G, Pariente J, Bonneville F, Geeraerts T; NeuroICU Research Group. COVID-19-associated acute necrotising encephalopathy successfully treated with steroids and polyvalent immunoglobulin with unusual IgG targeting the cerebral fibre network. J Neurol Neurosurg Psychiatry. 2020; 91(9):1004-1006. DOI: 10.1136/jnnp-2020-323678.

[18] Ghosh R, Dubey S, Finsterer J, Chatterjee S, Ray BK. SARS-CoV-2-Associated Acute Hemorrhagic, Necrotizing Encephalitis (AHNE) Presenting with Cognitive Impairment in a 44-Year-Old Woman without Comorbidities: A Case Report. Am J Case Rep. 2020; 21:e925641. DOI: 10.12659/AJCR.925641.

[19] Perrin P, Collongues N, Baloglu S, Bedo D, Bassand X, Lavaux T, Gautier-Vargas G, Keller N, Kremer S, Fafi-Kremer S, Moulin B, Benotmane I, Caillard S. Cytokine release syndrome-associated encephalopathy in patients with COVID-19. Eur J Neurol. 2021; 28(1):248-258. DOI: 10.1111/ene.14491.

[20] Zhang H, Charmchi Z, Seidman RJ, Anziska Y, Velayudhan V, Perk J. COVID-19-associated myositis with severe proximal and bulbar weakness. Muscle Nerve. 2020; 62(3):E57-E60. DOI: 10.1002/mus.27003.

[21] Kaur H, Mason JA, Bajracharya M, McGee J, Gunderson MD, Hart BL, Dehority W, Link N, Moore B, Phillips JP, Rogers D. Transverse Myelitis in a Child With COVID-19. Pediatr Neurol. 2020; 112:5-6. DOI: 10.1016/j.pediatrneurol.2020.07.017.

[22] Finsterer J, Scorza FA, Fiorini AC. SARS-CoV-2-associated Guillain-Barre syndrome in 62 patients. Eur J Neurol. 2021;28(1):e10-e12. DOI: 10.1111/ene.14544.

[23] Oliveira V, Seabra M, Rodrigues R, Carvalho V, Mendes M, Pereira D, Caldeiras C, Martins B, Silva R, Azevedo A, Lima MJ, Monteiro C, Varela R, Malheiro S, Abreu M, Azevedo E, Leal Loureiro J, Tedim Cruz V, Silva MR, Magalhães R, Silva C, Maia LF, Correia M. Neuro-COVID frequency and short-term outcome in the Northern Portuguese population. Eur J Neurol. 2021; 10.1111/ene.14874. DOI: 10.1111/ene.14874. Epub ahead of print.

[24] Chou SH, Beghi E, Helbok R, et al. Global Incidence of Neurological Manifestations Among Patients Hospitalized With COVID-19—A Report for the GCS-NeuroCOVID Consortium and the ENERGY Consortium. JAMA Netw Open. 2021;4(5):e2112131. DOI:10.1001/jamanetworkopen.2021.12131

[25] García-Azorín D, Abildúa MJA, Aguirre MEE, Fernández SF, Moncó JCG, Guijarro-Castro C, Platas MG, Delgado FR, Andrés JML, Ezpeleta D; Spanish neuroCOVID registry group. Neurological presentations of COVID-19: Findings

from the Spanish Society of Neurology neuroCOVID-19 registry. J Neurol Sci. 2021; 423:117283. DOI: 10.1016/j.jns.2020.117283.

[26] de Erausquin GA, Snyder H, Carrillo M, Hosseini AA, Brugha TS, Seshadri S; CNS SARS-CoV-2 Consortium. The chronic neuropsychiatric sequelae of COVID-19: The need for a prospective study of viral impact on brain functioning. Alzheimers Dement. 2021. DOI: 10.1002/alz.12255.

[27] Mankad K, Perry MD, Mirsky DM, Rossi A. COVID-19: A primer for Neuroradiologists. Neuroradiology. 2020; 62(6):647-648. DOI: 10.1007/s00234-020-02437-5.

[28] Politi LS, Salsano E, Grimaldi M. Magnetic Resonance Imaging Alteration of the Brain in a Patient With Coronavirus Disease 2019 (COVID-19) and Anosmia. JAMA Neurol. 2020; 77(8):1028-1029. DOI: 10.1001/jamaneurol.2020.2125.

[29] Coolen T, Lolli V, Sadeghi N, Rovai A, Trotta N, Taccone FS, Creteur J, Henrard S, Goffard JC, Dewitte O, Naeije G, Goldman S, De Tiège X. Early postmortem brain MRI findings in COVID-19 non-survivors. Neurology. 2020; 95(14):e2016-e2027. DOI: 10.1212/WNL.0000000000010116.

[30] Radmanesh A, Raz E, Zan E, Derman A, Kaminetzky M. Brain Imaging Use and Findings in COVID-19: A Single Academic Center Experience in the Epicenter of Disease in the United States. AJNR Am J Neuroradiol. 2020; 41(7):1179-1183. DOI: 10.3174/ajnr.A6610.

[31] Jain R, Young M, Dogra S, Kennedy H, Nguyen V, Jones S, Bilaloglu S, Hochman K, Raz E, Galetta S, Horwtiz L. COVID-19 related neuroimaging findings: A signal of thromboembolic complications and a strong prognostic marker of poor patient outcome. J Neurol Sci. 2020; 414:116923. DOI: 10.1016/j.jns.2020.116923.

[32] Katal S, Balakrishnan S, Gholamrezanezhad A. Neuroimaging and neurologic findings in COVID-19 and other coronavirus infections: A systematic review in 116 patients. J Neuroradiol. 2021; 48(1):43-50. DOI: 10.1016/j.neurad.2020.06.007.

[33] Md Noh MSF. Brain imaging findings in COVID-19: What do we know so far? J Neuroradiol. 2020; 47(5):329-330. DOI: 10.1016/j.neurad.2020.05.004.

[34] Kandemirli SG, Dogan L, Sarikaya ZT, Kara S, Akinci C, Kaya D, Kaya Y, Yildirim D, Tuzuner F, Yildirim MS, Ozluk E, Gucyetmez B, Karaarslan E, Koyluoglu I, Demirel Kaya HS, Mammadov O, Kisa Ozdemir I, Afsar N, Citci Yalcinkaya B, Rasimoglu S, Guduk DE, Kedir Jima A, Ilksoz A, Ersoz V, Yonca Eren M, Celtik N, Arslan S, Korkmazer B, Dincer SS, Gulek E, Dikmen I, Yazici M, Unsal S, Ljama T, Demirel I, Ayyildiz A, Kesimci I, Bolsoy Deveci S, Tutuncu M, Kizilkilic O, Telci L, Zengin R, Dincer A, Akinci IO, Kocer N. Brain MRI Findings in Patients in the Intensive Care Unit with COVID-19 Infection. Radiology. 2020; 297(1):E232-E235. DOI: 10.1148/radiol.2020201697.

[35] Zanin L, Saraceno G, Panciani PP, Renisi G, Signorini L, Migliorati K, Fontanella MM. SARS-CoV-2 can induce brain and spine demyelinating lesions. Acta Neurochir (Wien). 2020; 162(7):1491-1494. DOI: 10.1007/s00701-020-04374-x..

[36] Brun G, Hak JF, Coze S, Kaphan E, Carvelli J, Girard N, Stellmann JP. COVID-19-White matter and globus pallidum lesions: Demyelination or small-vessel vasculitis? Neurol

Neuroimmunol Neuroinflamm. 2020; 7(4):e777. DOI: 10.1212/ NXI.0000000000000777.

[37] Novi G, Rossi T, Pedemonte E, Saitta L, Rolla C, Roccatagliata L, Inglese M, Farinini D. Acute disseminated encephalomyelitis after SARS-CoV-2 infection. Neurol Neuroimmunol Neuroinflamm. 2020; 7(5):e797. DOI: 10.1212/ NXI.0000000000000797. Erratum in: Neurol Neuroimmunol Neuroinflamm. 2020;8(1).

[38] Abdi S, Ghorbani A, Fatehi F. The association of SARS-CoV-2 infection and acute disseminated encephalomyelitis without prominent clinical pulmonary symptoms. J Neurol Sci. 2020; 416:117001. DOI: 10.1016/j. jns.2020.117001.

[39] Fotuhi M, Mian A, Meysami S, Raji CA. Neurobiology of COVID-19. J Alzheimers Dis. 2020; 76(1):3-19. DOI: 10.3233/JAD-200581.

[40] Mainali S, Darsie ME. Neurologic and Neuroscientific Evidence in Aged COVID-19 Patients. Front Aging Neurosci. 2021; 13:648662. DOI: 10.3389/fnagi.2021.648662.

[41] García-Azorín D, Martínez-Pías E, Trigo J, Hernández-Pérez I, Valle-Peñacoba G, Talavera B, Simón-Campo P, de Lera M, Chavarría-Miranda A, López-Sanz C, Gutiérrez-Sánchez M, Martínez-Velasco E, Pedraza M, Sierra Á, Gómez-Vicente B, Guerrero Á, Ezpeleta D, Peñarrubia MJ, Gómez-Herreras JI, Bustamante-Munguira E, Abad-Molina C, Orduña-Domingo A, Ruiz-Martin G, Jiménez-Cuenca MI, Juarros S, Del Pozo-Vegas C, Dueñas-Gutierrez C, de Paula JMP, Cantón-Álvarez B, Vicente JM, Arenillas JF. Neurological Comorbidity Is a Predictor of Death in Covid-19 Disease: A Cohort Study on 576 Patients. Front Neurol. 2020; 11:781. DOI: 10.3389/fneur.2020.00781.

[42] Buchman AS, Yu L, Wilson RS, Boyle PA, Schneider JA, Bennett DA. Brain pathology contributes to simultaneous change in physical frailty and cognition in old age. J Gerontol A Biol Sci Med Sci. 2014; 69(12):1536-1544. DOI: 10.1093/gerona/glu117.

[43] Brown EE, Kumar S, Rajji TK, Pollock BG, Mulsant BH. Anticipating and Mitigating the Impact of the COVID-19 Pandemic on Alzheimer's Disease and Related Dementias. Am J Geriatr Psychiatry. 2020; 28(7):712-721. DOI: 10.1016/j.jagp.2020.04.010.

[44] Parlapani E, Holeva V, Nikopoulou VA, Sereslis K, Athanasiadou M, Godosidis A, Stephanou T, Diakogiannis I. Intolerance of Uncertainty and Loneliness in Older Adults During the COVID-19 Pandemic. Front Psychiatry. 2020; 11:842. DOI: 10.3389/fpsyt.2020.00842.

[45] Okruszek Ł, Aniszewska-Stańczuk A, Piejka A, Wiśniewska M, Żurek K. Safe but Lonely? Loneliness, Anxiety, and Depression Symptoms and COVID-19. Front Psychol. 2020; 11:579181. DOI: 10.3389/ fpsyg.2020.579181.

[46] Cagnin A, Di Lorenzo R, Marra C, Bonanni L, Cupidi C, Laganà V, Rubino E, Vacca A, Provero P, Isella V, Vanacore N, Agosta F, Appollonio I, Caffarra P, Pettenuzzo I, Sambati R, Quaranta D, Guglielmi V, Logroscino G, Filippi M, Tedeschi G, Ferrarese C, Rainero I, Bruni AC; SINdem COVID-19 Study Group. Behavioral and Psychological Effects of Coronavirus Disease-19 Quarantine in Patients With Dementia. Front Psychiatry. 2020; 11:578015. DOI: 10.3389/fpsyt. 2020.578015.

[47] Santos-García D, Oreiro M, Pérez P, Fanjul G, Paz González JM, Feal

Painceiras MJ, Cores Bartolomé C, Valdés Aymerich L, García Sancho C, Castellanos Rodrigo MDM. Impact of Coronavirus Disease 2019 Pandemic on Parkinson's Disease: A Cross-Sectional Survey of 568 Spanish Patients. Mov Disord. 2020; 35(10):1712-1716. DOI: 10.1002/mds.28261.

[48] Heneka MT, Golenbock D, Latz E, Morgan D, Brown R. Immediate and long-term consequences of COVID-19 infections for the development of neurological disease. Alzheimers Res Ther. 2020; 12(1):69. DOI: 10.1186/s13195-020-00640-3

[49] Vallamkondu J, John A, Wani WY, Ramadevi SP, Jella KK, Reddy PH, Kandimalla R. SARS-CoV-2 pathophysiology and assessment of coronaviruses in CNS diseases with a focus on therapeutic targets. Biochim Biophys Acta Mol Basis Dis. 2020; 1866(10):165889. DOI: 10.1016/j.bbadis.2020.165889.

[50] Rogers JP, Chesney E, Oliver D, Pollak TA, McGuire P, Fusar-Poli P, Zandi MS, Lewis G, David AS. Psychiatric and neuropsychiatric presentations associated with severe coronavirus infections: a systematic review and meta-analysis with comparison to the COVID-19 pandemic. Lancet Psychiatry. 2020; 7(7):611-627. DOI: 10.1016/S2215-0366(20)30203-0.

[51] Kumar S, Veldhuis A, Malhotra T. Neuropsychiatric and Cognitive Sequelae of COVID-19. Front Psychol. 2021; 12:577529. DOI: 10.3389/fpsyg.2021.577529.

[52] Cothran TP, Kellman S, Singh S, Beck JS, Powell KJ, Bolton CJ, Tam JW. A brewing storm: The neuropsychological sequelae of hyperinflammation due to COVID-19. Brain Behav Immun. 2020; 88:957-958. DOI: 10.1016/j.bbi.2020.06.008.

[53] Varatharaj A, Thomas N, Ellul MA, Davies NWS, Pollak TA, Tenorio EL, Sultan M, Easton A, Breen G, Zandi M, Coles JP, Manji H, Al-Shahi Salman R, Menon DK, Nicholson TR, Benjamin LA, Carson A, Smith C, Turner MR, Solomon T, Kneen R, Pett SL, Galea I, Thomas RH, Michael BD; CoroNerve Study Group. Neurological and neuropsychiatric complications of COVID-19 in 153 patients: a UK-wide surveillance study. Lancet Psychiatry. 2020; 7(10):875-882. DOI: 10.1016/S2215-0366(20)30287-X.

[54] Vindegaard N, Benros ME. COVID-19 pandemic and mental health consequences: Systematic review of the current evidence. Brain Behav Immun. 2020; 89:531-542. DOI: 10.1016/j.bbi.2020.05.048.

[55] Han AY, Mukdad L, Long JL, Lopez IA. Anosmia in COVID-19: Mechanisms and Significance. Chem Senses. 2020; 17:bjaa040. DOI: 10.1093/chemse/bjaa040.

[56] Dibattista M, Pifferi S, Menini A, Reisert J. Alzheimer's Disease: What Can We Learn From the Peripheral Olfactory System? Front Neurosci. 2020; 14:440. DOI: 10.3389/fnins.2020.00440.

[57] Hustad E, Aasly JO. Clinical and Imaging Markers of Prodromal Parkinson's Disease. Front Neurol. 2020; 11:395. DOI: 10.3389/fneur.2020.00395.

[58] Van Regemorter V, Hummel T, Rosenzweig F, Mouraux A, Rombaux P, Huart C. Mechanisms Linking Olfactory Impairment and Risk of Mortality. Front Neurosci. 2020; 14:140. DOI: 10.3389/fnins.2020.00140.

[59] Gialluisi A, de Gaetano G, Iacoviello L. New challenges from Covid-19 pandemic: an unexpected opportunity to enlighten the link between viral infections and brain disorders? Neurol Sci. 2020; 41(6):1349-1350. DOI: 10.1007/s10072-020-04444-z.

[60] Baller EB, Hogan CS, Fusunyan MA, Ivkovic A, Luccarelli JW, Madva E, Nisavic M, Praschan N, Quijije NV, Beach SR, Smith FA. Neurocovid: Pharmacological Recommendations for Delirium Associated With COVID-19. Psychosomatics. 2020; 61(6):585-596. DOI: 10.1016/j.psym.2020.05.013.

[61] Oh ES, Fong TG, Hshieh TT, Inouye SK. Delirium in Older Persons: Advances in Diagnosis and Treatment. JAMA. 2017; 318(12):1161-1174. DOI: 10.1001/jama.2017.12067.

[62] Kotfis K, Williams Roberson S, Wilson JE, Dabrowski W, Pun BT, Ely EW. COVID-19: ICU delirium management during SARS-CoV-2 pandemic. Crit Care. 2020; 24(1):176. DOI: 10.1186/s13054-020-02882-x.

[63] Mueller AL, McNamara MS, Sinclair DA. Why does COVID-19 disproportionately affect older people? Aging (Albany NY). 2020; 12(10):9959-9981. DOI: 10.18632/aging.103344.

Chapter 15

Consequences of the SARS-CoV-2 Pandemic on Mental Health: Integrative Review

Jucier Gonçalves Júnior, Gislene Farias de Oliviera and Modesto Leite Rolim-Neto

Abstract

The lack of specific treatment and knowledge about the exact pathophysiology of the 2019 Coronavirus disease (COVID-19) and its vaccines makes the organic aspects of the pandemic a concern and puts the psychiatric consequences and psychological effects of SARS-CoV-2, COVID-19, in second place. Hence, the psychiatric impacts of the COVID-19 pandemic have not been well established yet. We have performed an integrative literature review in three electronic databases: Medline, PsycINFO, and Published International Literature on Traumatic Stress (PILOTS). The findings were then divided into five subcategories: impacts of COVID-19 on the mental health of psychiatric patients; use of technology as an ally in combating impacts on mental health in the context of the COVID-19 pandemic; mental health promotion measures in the context of the COVID-19 pandemic for the population; mental health promotion measures in the context of the COVID-19 pandemic for health professionals; and mental health in specific groups in the context of the COVID-19 pandemic. This study has showed that the situation and measures proposed to fight the COVID-19 pandemic cause stress, anxiety, fear, and uncertainty in the population. Psychiatric patients, the elderly, refugees, and migrant workers are more vulnerable due to the stigmatization and lack of specialized support in health services and reduced access to medications. Therefore, they require care from governments and health authorities. In addition, measures to promote hospital health for health professionals seem to be essential to improve care and reduce the psychologic/psychiatric impacts on professionals. Thus, technology is a valuable ally in this process.

Keywords: Mental Health, Coronavirus infections, Pandemic, Stress, Affective Disorders

1. Introduction

A pandemic creates its own objective reality as a backdrop for all forms of psychopathology. There are economic downturns, job layoffs, prolonged school and business closings, and threatened supply chain disruptions during such period [1–5]. It also compromises the care and mental health of individuals who already have diseases.

According to the WHO [6], 792 million (10.7%) people in the global population have a mental disorder – 264 million (3.4%) with depression, 284 million (3.8%) with anxiety disorders, and 46 million (0.6%) with bipolar disorders. However, the lack of a specific treatment, knowledge about the exact pathophysiology of the disease and its vaccines makes the organic aspects of the pandemic a concern and puts the psychiatric consequences and psychological effects of COVID-19 in second place [7–9]. Thus, the psychiatry impacts by COVID-19 pandemic have not been well established yet.

We aimed to carry out an integrative literature review based on the following guiding question: What practical contributions does the current scientific literature may provide regarding the impact of COVID-19 on mental health? This review highlighted that not only previous mental illnesses are exacerbated during a pandemic, but also negative feelings. In addition, pandemic prevention and control measures can be triggers for causing the population's sickness.

2. Method

2.1 Literature review

We have performed an integrative literature review in three electronic databases: Medline, PsycINFO, and Published International Literature on Traumatic Stress (PILOTS). The electronic searches used variants of the following research terms with a syntax adjusted to each database: #1 "COVID-19" OR "Coronavirus Infections" (Medical Subject Headings – [MeSH term] AND #2 ("Health Personnel" OR "Health Care Provider" [MeSH] term); and "Mental Health" [keyword].

2.2 Data collection

Manuscripts were selected primarily through the analysis of their titles and abstracts. Two researchers collected data individually in order to ensure trustworthiness of the findings, and divergences were solved by a third senior researcher. Each sample article was thoroughly read, and the information was inserted in a spreadsheet (**Table 1**) that included the author, publishing year, journal, and main findings.

2.3 Eligibility criteria

Papers were analyzed based on the following eligibility criteria: at least one combination of the terms described in the search strategy in the title; written in English, Portuguese or Spanish; addressing the psychiatric impact of COVID-19 pandemic; original articles with the full text available through the Journal Portal of the Brazilian Coordination of Personal Improvement of Higher Level (CAPES), which is a virtual library created by the Brazilian Department of Health where content is restricted to authorized users. Monographs, dissertations, and thesis were excluded.

Manuscripts repeated in more than one of the databases were counted only once. Some papers were excluded because they approached other viruses/pandemics.

2.4 Ethical issue

Considering this is an integrative literature review, Resolution 510/16 of the Brazilian National Health Council (CNS, acronym in Portuguese) ensures the dismissal of submission to an Ethics Committee on Research (Human Beings).

Rolim-Neto et al. [10]	Psychiatry Res.	Importance of recognizing how to combat stress, anxiety, and negative symptoms such as depression in the face of death figures as a mental health strategy for healthcare workers.
Xiang et al. [11]	Int. J. Biol. Sci.	In China, the lack of psychiatrists' training in the management of infectious diseases in pandemics is a major challenge to mental health and an impasse to health promotion in the pandemic.
Mental health in specific groups in the COVID-19 pandemic context		
Zhai and Du [12]	Lancet	Exchange students may have their mental health affected due to stigmatization, bullying and mistreatment in the countries where they are studying because they could be classified as potential transmitters of the virus.
Bao et al. [13]	Lancet	Triggering of mental disorders, post-traumatic stress disorder, depression, and anxiety in healthcare workers.
Perlis [14]	JAMA	Chronic shess of COVID-19 pandemic can cause anxiety and major depression in healthcare workers.
Jawaid [15]	Science	Encouraging the spread of news with mental health benefits; mental health supports with hotline; and maintaining regular phone contact are possible measures to deal with the mental health consequences of elderly people with COVID-19.
Brasil [16]	—	List of a series of measures to promote childreifs mental health in the COYID-19 pandemic context.
Liem et al. [17]	Lancet	Impasses of the communities of intemational mi grant workers, since their pre-exposure condition is more fragile, and they are more exposed to psychiatric diseases in pandemics than the general population.
Yang et al. [18]	Lancet Psych.	The outbreak of COVID-19 has raised great challenges regarding mental health semces for older adults in the community. There seems to be insufficient and inadequate attention paid to this vulnerable population in the recently established crisis of psychological services in China.
Gonçalves Júnior et al. [19]	Psychiatry Res.	Populations as refugees have a much greater risk of developing mental disorders compared to the general population due to the precarious hygienic-sanitary conditions, nutrition, housing and access to information that they have.
Source: *Authors.*		

Table 1.
Main Findings.

3. Results

The findings were then divided into five subcategories: impacts of COVID-19 on the mental health of psychiatric patients; use of technology as an ally in combating mental health impacts in the context of COVID-19 pandemic; mental health promotion measures in the context of the COVID-19 pandemic for the population; mental health promotion measures in the context of the COVID-19 pandemic for health professionals; and mental health in specific groups in the context of the COVID-19 pandemic (**Table 1**).

4. Discussion

4.1 Impacts of COVID-19 on the mental health of psychiatric patients

Patients with confirmed or suspected COVID-19 may experience fear of the consequences of being infected by a potentially harmful virus, and those in quarantine might experience boredom, loneliness, and anger [20]. In a Chinese study with 263 participants, the majority (53.3%) of individuals did not feel helpless due to the COVID-19 pandemic. However, 52.1% of the participants felt horrified and apprehensive due to the pandemic. Additionally, most participants (57.8 to 77.9%) received more support from friends and family members, more shared feeling and caring with family [21].

Indeed, a pandemic causes profound changes in social dynamics. One example is supermarkets, which were clear of essential items and faced a rationing procedure at the beginning of the pandemic. Schools and other educational institutions have been affected, with compulsory examinations postponed and most children remaining at home. The financial implications are profound, even though governments have implemented various supportive measures [22]. This situation causes stress, anxiety, depressive symptoms, insomnia, denial, anger, and fear [23].

Moreover, such feelings may especially arise due to fake news and conspiracy theories that circulate as a result of social media "infodemic", particularly in areas with low social capital and public trust [24]. According to Gao et al. [25], the prevalence of depression, anxiety, and a combination of depression and anxiety in 4,872 participants from 31 provinces and autonomous regions in China was 48.3% (95%CI: 46.9–49.7%), 22.6% (95%CI: 21.4–23.8%) and 19.4% (95%CI: 18.3–20.6%), respectively, during COVID-19. More than 80% (95%CI: 80.9–83.1%) of the participants reported frequent exposure to social media.

This impact is more dangerous and worrying in psychiatric patients. Schizophrenia, bipolar, depression and anxiety disorders or autism have an increased risk for infection due to immunogenetic vulnerability. The elderly psychiatric patients are the most vulnerable group, and there is a high exacerbation risk of psychic disorders and an aggravation of existing psychiatric symptoms, cognitive disorders, and loss of autonomy. The elderly may have difficulties adopting "barrier measures" (behavioral measures to protect oneself and others from the virus) and complying with confinement instructions. Severe social isolation, precarious housing, restricted solidarity networks for the informal monitoring of these patients' health condition complicate this population's situation [26].

Furthermore, people with mental disorders can be exposed to more barriers in accessing timely health services due to discrimination associated with patients who have mental illness in health care settings. The elderly could be more substantially influenced by emotional responses brought on by the COVID-19 pandemic, resulting in relapses or worsening of an already existing mental health condition due to high susceptibility to stress compared with the general population. The treatment for mental disease could make that of COVID-19 more challenging [27].

4.2 Use of technology as an ally in combating impacts on mental health in the COVID-19 pandemic context

Health services around the world have been mobilized and reinvented in an attempt to meet the population's mental health demands during the COVID-19 pandemic. The literature states that technology to reduce risk is a way out of proper pandemic management [28].

In France [29], there has been a 90% shift in outpatient activity with the use of telepsychiatry. There is a hotline for psychiatry teleconsultation, and meetings with more than five people became virtual. In addition, psychiatrists alternately present themselves in the department or teleworking. According to Starace and Serrara [30], during phone check-ins, the professional provides information of open hours, changes in access to services, and public health recommendations about limiting social contacts.

In Siena, Italy, more than 90% of the outpatient consultations were transformed into telemedicine consultations, which also made use of cell phones. Hence, health workers may benefit from social contact provided via the Internet, in a group setting, at the end of a working day, from their houses, without wearing the protective garments they wore all day long. They believe that offering a space to talk electronically, to share experiences, and to provide comfort to each other can be helpful, especially for those who live alone [31].

In Croatia, the use of digital technologies in post-traumatic stress disorder (PTSD) mitigation was the main topic of the researches carried out by Cosic et al. [32]. According to the authors, based on their experience, the development of computer tools and methods for emotion elicitation, estimation and regulation, cognitive-behavioral therapy, stress inoculation/resilience training, prevention of stress-related disorders and soldiers' ability strength to cope with highly stressful situations, as well as assessments of individual and group stress resilience features, created the NATO research and development project "Multidisciplinary Metrics for Soldier Resilience Prediction and Training" with researches from Turkey, Croatia, and Austria. It can use these expertise's origin strategies to face the COVID-19 psychology and psychiatric impact.

Increasing the communication with friends, family members and loved ones, even if from a distance, from video-chats or group calls with family members, may help to reduce loneliness and precariousness. In case of insufficient social network, professional helplines are particularly useful, if managed by qualified trained professionals [33].

Mainstream media, such as television and radio, may play an important role by including content that promotes quality information and safety for the population [15]. They should get ahead and educate people about the importance and existence of not only physical health issues, but also mental health ones during a pandemic, along with medical and mental health professionals in order to sustain scientific- and fact-based presentation and suggestions while addressing the importance of COVID-19 control practices [34].

In Singapore, the government have kept the public abreast on the progress of the outbreak with regular broadcasts of news and announcements on social media. These include daily updates, such as the number of new and current infections, patients who are at critical condition or have been discharged, and preventive measures. Social media channels have also been set up by the state to curb the spread of false information and "fake news." Regular dialog with Cabinet Ministers and infectious diseases physicians is aired to clear questions [35].

4.3 Mental health promotion measures in the COVID-19 pandemic context for the population

A significant distress decrease has been associated with the nationwide quarantine, medical supports and resources from all over the country, public education, individual protection strength, medical isolation, population mobility control, reduction of gatherings to stop the virus spread, and social and spiritual support. These are very important elements of community resilience and anti-fragility during COVID-19 crisis periods [3, 36].

During the COVID-19 pandemic, the National Institutes of Health in the USA and other funders must provide administrative supplements and notifications that encourage researchers to go fully remote; assess the mental health impact of COVID-19; prioritize repurposing of psychiatric human and pharmacologic resources for COVID-19 research efforts; and continue working, leveraging the unique clinical research resources in psychiatry to help as many people as possible through the crisis [28].

China created 26 protocols and guidelines regarding mental health promotion between January and February in 2020 [37]. In these protocols, psychological crisis interventions have included three key points: understanding the mental health condition in different populations influenced by the COVID-19 outbreak, identifying people that are at high risk of suicide and aggression, and providing appropriate psychological interventions for those in need [37].

Based on Fiorillo and Gorwood [33] in Italy, some measures to face the mental impacts of the pandemic are: limiting the sources of stress, *i.e.* decrease of access to unofficial channels and uncontrolled sources; breaking isolation, by increasing communication of family and friends via social media; maintaining the usual routine rhythm; focusing on the isolation benefits and asking for professional help when needed. According to Ho, Che and Ho [35], the integration of hospital and community resources, more support for frontline health workers, accurate dissemination of health and related information to the public, identification of high-risk groups, improved screening of psychiatric morbidities, mode and content of psychological intervention encourage the use of a psychodynamic approach as a way to improve the population's adherence to preventive measures [38]. A Chinese study that evaluated 1,304 people showed that cognitive therapy can provide information or evidence to enhance confidence in the doctor's ability to diagnose COVID-19 [39].

Measures for a better health promotion and for combating the COVID-19 include the use of personal protective equipment, mainly of fluid-resistant surgical masks, telemedicine, avoiding crowds/visits, offering individual educational sessions to patients admitted at the unit, providing printed materials, and encouraging hand hygiene [30].

4.4 Mental health promotion measures in the COVID-19 pandemic context for health professionals

As if exposure to the COVID-19 during the global pandemic was not enough, healthcare workers face another risk: burnout due to overstress in an increasingly overloaded healthcare system [10]. Thus, health care professionals have accepted an overwhelming responsibility. They are coping with the psychological distress of losing patients, as well as lack of clarity and unpredictability within their work environments, while trying to protect their own health [22], particularly in countries with limited resources [24]. Health professionals have been dealing with high risk of infection and inadequate protection against contamination, overwork, frustration, discrimination, isolation, patients with negative emotions, lack of family contact, and exhaustion [23].

A study with 1,287 workers in hospitals equipped with fever clinics or wards for patients with COVID-19 in Wuhan and other regions in China reported that health workers have been experiencing psychological burden (depression, anxiety, insomnia, and distress), especially female nurses [40]. After surveying more than 1,200 nurses and physicians in 34 hospitals in the Wuhan region and across mainland China, approximately 14% of the physicians and nearly 16% of the nurses described moderate or severe depressive symptoms. There were also reports of insomnia and anxiety [14].

Some strategies for dealing with COVID-19 impacts include: routine support processes (such as peer support programs) available to the healthcare staff with a briefing on moral injuries, as well as awareness on other causes of mental ill health and what to look out for [10, 41]; training on psychological skills to deal with patients' anxiety, panic and other emotional problems, and, if possible, for mental health staff to be on hand to directly help these patients [42]; formation of psychological intervention teams and intra hospital support for professionals [43] in public policies that aim to articulate these joint efforts in a centralized and strategic way [11, 13].

4.5 Mental health in specific groups in the COVID-19 pandemic context

During the COVID-19 pandemic, individuals at age extremes (children and the elderly) also suffer an impact on their mental health. Social isolation by COVID-19 pandemic in elderly people has been associated with increased depression and suicidality, as well as to increased pro-inflammatory and decreased anti-viral immune responses. Virtual solutions may be less comfortable for children and the elderly [15], who may also have limited access to internet services and smartphones to enter in mental health services online. Also, the current mass quarantines and restrictions to public transport make it more difficult for them to acquire medicine from previous psychiatric pathologies, which is common in this age range [18].

Some suggestions for managing mental health in institutionalized elderly people include establishing a contingency plan and strategies to deal with more serious psychiatric symptoms; maintaining transparency and trust with employees that prioritize equity and well-being with adequate training and personal protective equipment; ensuring care for the mental health of family members; reassuring them about feelings of fear, sadness and anxiety; and promoting a healthy climate of communication and empathy [44].

In the case of children, stressful and potentially traumatic situations, such as illness and hospitalization, can trigger the emergence of unusual behaviors, such as sucking finger, enuresis, or desire to sleep with parents. Therefore, encouraging the maintenance of routine and creative activities, such as painting, drawing or playing with family members, is essential to reduce psychological impacts. In the event of hospitalization, children should be maintained with constant contact and communication with the family and belongings that fulfill the function of emotional connection. No one should lie about their diagnosis and treatment, making it clear that the child is not to blame for being sick, providing an open communication channel for them [16].

As for young people in universities, the Chinese, mainly, were denied entry in many countries. They face discrimination and isolation in some countries due to being deemed as potential COVID-19 carriers, consequently, such students are at risk of hate crimes, especially when individuals consider them contagious. This situation can lead to mental health problems, such as denial, stress, anxiety, and fear [12].

Refugees and international migrant workers have a higher burden of common mental disorders (*e.g.* depression) and a lower quality of life than local populations. Many domestic workers cannot obtain masks from pharmacies because they must stay with employers and adhere to government-recommended self-quarantine [17]. Severe risk factors for COVID-19 are common for mental disorders in this population: overcrowding, disruption of sewage disposal, poor standards of hygiene, poor nutrition, negligible sanitation, and lack of access to shelter, health care, public services and safety [19, 45–48].

5. Conclusions

This study has showed that the situation and measures proposed to fight the COVID-19 pandemic cause stress, anxiety, fear, and uncertainty in the population. Psychiatric patients, the elderly, refugees, and migrant workers are more vulnerable groups due to stigmatization and lack of specialized support in health services and reduced access to medications. Therefore, they require care from governments and health authorities. In addition, measures to promote hospital health for health professionals seem to be essential to improve care and reduce the psychologic/psychiatric impacts on professionals, and thus technology is a valuable ally in this process. Finally, the weakness of this study is the absence of more robust studies to compose the sample.

Author details

Jucier Gonçalves Júnior[1*], Gislene Farias de Oliviera[2] and Modesto Leite Rolim-Neto[2]

1 Department of Rheumatology, Faculty of Medicine - University of São Paulo (FMUSP), São Paulo, Brazil

2 School of Medicine, Federal University of Cariri, Barbalha, Ceará, Brazil

*Address all correspondence to: juciergjunior@hotmail.com

References

[1] Guo YR, Cao QD, Hong ZS, Tan YY, Chen SD, Jin HJ, et al. The origin, transmission, and clinical therapies on coronavirus disease 2019 (COVID-19) outbreak – an update on the status. Mil. Med. Res. 2020; 13: 1-11 [PMID: 32169119 DOI: 10.1186/s40779-020-00240-0].

[2] Li Q, Guan X, Wu P, Wang X, Zhou L, Tong Y, et al. Early transmission dynamics in Wuhan, China, of novel coronavirus-infected pneumonia. N. Engl. J. Med. 2020; 382: 1199-1207 [PMID: 31995857 DOI: 10.1056/NEJMoa2001316].

[3] World Health Organization – WHO. Coronavirus disease (COVID-19) outbreak situation. 2020a. Available at: https://www.who.int/emergencies/diseases/novel-coronavirus-2019 (accessed 25 March 2020).

[4] Anzai A, Kobayashi T, Linton NM, Kinoshita R, Hayashi K, Suzuki A, et al. Assessing the impact of reduced travel on exportation dynamics of novel coronavirus infection (COVID-19). J Clin Med. 2020; 9: 601 [PMID: 32102279 DOI: 10.3390/jcm9020601].

[5] Goldberg JF. Psychiatry's Niche Role in the COVID-19 Pandemic. J. Clin. Psychiatry. 2020; 81, 20com13363 [DOI: 10.4088/JCP.20com13363].

[6] World Health Organization – WHO. Mental disorders. 2020b. Available at: https://ourworldindata.org/mental-health (accessed 25 March 2020).

[7] Shigemura J, Ursano RJ, Morganstein JC, Kurosawa M, Benedek DM. Public responses to the novel 2019 coronavirus (2019-nCoV) in Japan: Mental health consequences and target populations. Psychiatry Clin. Neurosci. 2020; 74: 281-282 [PMID: 32034840 DOI: 10.1111/pcn.12988].

[8] Brooks SK, Webster RK, Smith LE, Woodland L, Wessely S, Greenberg N, et al. The psychological impact of quarantine and how to reduce it: rapid review of the evidence. Lancet. 2020; 395: 912-920 [DOI: 10.1016/S0140-6736(20)30460-8].

[9] Ahmad A, Muller C, Konstantinos T. Covid-19 pandemic: a public and global mental health opportunity for social transformation? BMJ. 2020; 369: m1383 [DOI: 10.1136/bmj.m1383].

[10] Rolim-Neto M, Almeida HG, Esmeraldo JD, Nobre CB, Pinheiro WR, de Oliveira CR, et al. When health professionals look death in the eye: the mental health of professionals who deal daily with the 2019 coronavirus outbreak. Psychiatry Res. 2020; 288: 112972 [PMID: 32302817 DOI: 10.1016/j.psychres.2020.112972].

[11] Xiang YT, Zhao YJ, Liu ZH, Li XH, Zhao N, Cheung T, et al. The COVID-19 outbreak and psychiatric hospitals in China: managing challenges through mental health service reform. Int. J. Biol. Sci. 2020b; 16: 1741-1744 [PMID: 32226293 DOI: 10.7150/ijbs.45072].

[12] Zhai Y, Du X. Mental health care for international Chinese students affected by the COVID-19 outbreak. Lancet Psychiatr. 2020; 7: e22 [PMID: 32199511 DOI: 10.1016/S2215-0366(20)30089-4].

[13] Bao Y, Sun Y, Meng S, Shi J, Lu L. 2019-nCoV epidemic: address mental health care to empower society. Lancet. 2020; 295: e37-e38 [PMID: 32043982 DOI: 10.1016/S0140-6736(20)30309-3].

[14] Perlis RH. Exercising heart and head in managing coronavirus disease 2019 in Wuha. JAMA Netw Open. 2020; 3: e204006. [PMID: 32202641 DOI: 10.1001/jamanetworkopen.2020.4006].

[15] Jawaid A. Protecting older adults during social distancing. Science. 2020; 368, 145 [PMID: 32273460 DOI: 10.1126/science.abb7885].

[16] Brasil. Ministério da Saúde. Recomendações para Cuidado das Crianças em Isolamento Hospitalar. Brasília, DF: Fundação Oswaldo Cruz; 2020. p.7.

[17] Liem A, Wang C, Wariyanti Y, Latkin CA, Hall BJ. The neglected health of international migrant workers in the COVID-19 epidemic. Lancet Psychiatr. 2020; 7: e20 [PMID: 32085842 DOI: 10.1016/S2215-0366(20)30076-6].

[18] Yang Y, Li W, Zhang Q, Zhang L, Cheung T, Xiang Y-T. Mental health services for older adults in China during the COVID-19 outbreak. Lancet Psychiat. 2020; 7: e19 [PMID: 32085843 DOI: 10.1016/S2215-0366(20)30079-1].

[19] Gonçalves Júnior J, de Sales JP, Moreira MM, Pinheiro WR, Woneska R, Lima CK, et al. A crisis within the crisis: the mental health situation of refugees in the world during the 2019 coronavirus (2019-nCoV) outbreak. Psychiatry Res. 2020; 288: 113000 [DOI: 10.1016/j.psychres.2020.113000].

[20] Xiang Y-T, Yang Y, Li W, Zhang L, Zhang Q, Cheung T, et al. Timely mental health care for the 2019 novel coronavirus outbreak is urgently needed. Lancet Psychiatr. 2020a; 7: 228-229 [PMID: 32032543 DOI: 10.1016/S2215-0366(20)30046-8].

[21] Zhang Y, Ma ZF. Impact of the COVID-19 pandemic on mental health and quality of life among local residents in Liaoning Province, China: a cross-sectional study. Int. J. Environ. Res. Public Health. 2020; 17: 2381 [PMID: 32244498 DOI: 10.3390/ijerph17072381].

[22] Yahya AY, Khawaja S, Chukwuma SJ. The impact of COVID-19 in Psychiatry. Prim. Care Companion CNS Disord. 2020; 22: 20l02627 [PMID: 32302070 DOI: 10.4088/PCC.20l02627].

[23] Torales J, O'Higgins M, Castaldelli-Maia JM, Ventriglio A. The outbreak of COVID-19 coronavirus and its impact on global mental health. Int. J. Soc. Psychiatry. 2020; 66: 317-320 [PMID: 32233719 DOI: 10.1177/0020764020915212].

[24] Assari S, Habibzadeh P. The COVID-19 emergency response should include a mental health component. Arch Iran Med. 2020; 23: 281-282 [DOI: 10.34172/aim.2020.12].

[25] Gao J, Zheng P, Jia Y, Chen H, Mao Y, Chen S, et al. Mental health problems and social media exposure during COVID-19 outbreak. PLoS ONE. 2020; 15, e0231924 [DOI: 10.1371/journal.pone.0231924].

[26] Chevance A, Gourion D, Hoertel N, Llorca PM, Thomas P, Bocher R, et al. Ensuring mental health care during the SARS-CoV-2 epidemic in France: a narrative review. Encephale. 2020; 46: 193-201 [PMID: 32370982 DOI: 10.1016/j.encep.2020.04.005].

[27] Yao H, Chen J-H, Xu Y-F. Patients with mental health disorders in the COVID-19 epidemic. Lancet Psychiat. 2020; 7: e21 [PMID: 32199510 DOI: 10.1016/S2215-0366(20)30090-0].

[28] Nicol GE, Karp JF, Reiersen AM, Zorumski CF, Lenze EJ. "What were you before the war?" repurposing psychiatry during the COVID-19 pandemic. J. Clin. Psychiatry. 2020; 81: 20com13373 [PMID: 32271506 DOI: 10.4088/JCP.20com13373].

[29] Corrouble E. A viewpoint from Paris on the COVID-19 pandemic: a necessary turn to telepsychiatry. J. Clin. Psychiatry. 2020; 81, 20com13361 [PMID: 32237302 DOI: 10.4088/JCP.20com13361].

[30] Starace F, Ferrara M. COVID-19 disease emergency operational instructions for Mental Health Departments issued by the Italian Society of Epidemiological Psychiatry. Epidemiol Psychiatr Sci. 2020; 29: e116 [PMID: 32228737 doi: 10.1017/S2045796020000372].

[31] Fagiolini A, Cuomo A, Frank E. COVID-19 diary from a Psychiatry department in Italy. J. Clin. Psychiatry. 2020; 81, 20com13357 [PMID: 32237301 DOI: 10.4088/JCP.20com13357].

[32] Cosic K, Popovic S, Sarlija M, Kesedzic I. Impact of human disasters and covid-19 pandemic on mental health: potential of digital psychiatry. Psychiatr. Danub. 2020; 32: 25-31 [PMID: 32303026 DOI: 10.24869/psyd.2020.25].

[33] Fiorillo A, Gorwood P. The consequences of the COVID-19 pandemic on mental health and implications for clinical practice. Eur Psychiatry. 2020; 63: e32 [PMID: 32234102 DOI: 10.1192/j.eurpsy.2020.35].

[34] Shuja KH, Aqeel M, Jaffar A, Ahmed A. COVID-19 pandemic and impending global mental health implications. Psychiatr Danub. 2020; 32: 32-35 [PMID: 32303027 DOI: 10.24869/psyd.2020.32].

[35] Ho C, Che CY, Ho RCM. Mental Health Strategies to Combat the Psychological Impact of Coronavirus Disease 2019 (COVID-19) Beyond Paranoia and Panic. Ann Acad Med Singap. 2020; 49: 155-160 [PMID: 32200399].

[36] Jakovljevic M, Bjedov S, Jaksic N, Jakovljevic I. COVID-19 pandemia and public and global mental health from the perspective of global health security. Psychiatr Danub. 2020; 32, 6-14 [PMID: 32303023 DOI: 10.24869/psyd.2020.6].

[37] Li W, Yang Y, Liu Z-H, Zhao Y-J, Zhang Q, Zhang L, et al. Progression of mental health services during the COVID-19 outbreak in China. Int. J. Biol. Sci. 2020; 16: 1732-1738 [PMID: 32226291 DOI: 10.7150/ijbs.45120].

[38] Marčinko D, Jakovljevic M, Jaksic N, Bjedov S, Drakulic AM. The importance of psychodynamic approach during COVID-19 pandemic Psychiatr Danub. 2020; 32: 15-21 [PMID: 32303024 DOI: 10.24869/psyd.2020.15].

[39] Wang C, Pan R, Wan X, Tan Y, Xu L, Ho CS, et al. Immediate psychological responses and associated factors during the initial stage of the 2019 coronavirus disease (COVID-19) epidemic among the general population in China. Int. J. Environ. Res. Public Health. 2020; 17: 1729 [PMID: 32155789 DOI: 10.3390/ijerph17051729].

[40] Lai J, Ma S, Wang Y, Cai Z, Hu J, Wei N, et al. Factors associated with mental health outcomes among health care workers exposed to coronavirus disease 2019. JAMA Netw Open. 2020; 3: e203976 [PMID: 32202646 DOI: 10.1001/jamanetworkopen.2020.3976].

[41] Greenberg N, Docherty M, Gnanapragasam S, Wessely S. Managing mental health challenges faced by healthcare workers during covid-19 pandemic. BMJ. 2020; 368: m1211 [PMID: 32217624 DOI: 10.1136/bmj.m1211].

[42] Chen Q, Liang M, Li Y, Guo J, Fei D, Wang L, et al. Mental health care for medical staff in China during the COVID-19 outbreak. Lancet Psychiatry. 2020; 7: e15–e16 [PMCID: PMC7129426 DOI: 10.1016/S2215-0366(20)30078-X].

[43] Kang L, Li Y, Hu S, Chen M, Yang C, Yang BX, et al. The mental health of medical workers in Wuhan, China dealing with the 2019 novel coronavirus. Lancet Psychiatr. 2020;

7: e14 [PMID: 32035030 DOI: 10.1016/S2215-0366(20)30047-X].

[44] Ornell F, Schuch JB, Sordi AO, Kessler FH. Pandemic fear and COVID-19: mental health burden and strategies. Braz J Psychiat. 2020; 42: 232-235 [PMID: 32267343 DOI: 10.1590/1516-4446-2020-0008].

[45] Duan L, Zhun G. Psychological interventions for people affected by the COVID-19 epidemic. Lancet Psych. 2020; 7: 300-302 [PMID: 32085840 DOI: 10.1016/S2215-0366(20)30073-0].

[46] Li S, Wang Y, Xue J, Zhao N, Zhu T. The Impact of COVID-19 Epidemic Declaration on Psychological Consequences: A Study on Active Weibo Users. Int. J. Environ. Res. Public Health 2020; 17 (6): 2032 [PMID: 32204411 DOI: 10.3390/ijerph17062032].

[47] Liu S, Yang L, Zhang C, Xiang Y-T, Liu Z, Hu S, et al. Online mental health services in China during the COVID-19 outbreak. Lancet Psychiatry. 2020; 7: e17-e18 [PMID: 32085841 DOI: 10.1016/S2215-0366(20)30077-8].

[48] Word Health Organization – WHO. Infection prevention and control guidance for Long-Term Care Facilities in the context of COVID-19. 2020c. Available at: https://apps.who.int/iris/handle/10665/331508 (accessed 24 April 2020).

Chapter 16

COVID-19 in India: Problems, Challenges and Strategies (Psychological Aspects)

Sarika Jain and Manish Yadav

Abstract

The pandemic COVID-19 is a global challenge which has infected and killed people worldwide. Some people do not show any symptom while some have fever, cough, sore throat, general weakness and fatigue and muscular pain and in most severe cases, severe pneumonia, acute respiratory distress syndrome, sepsis and septic shock all leading to death. It has adversely affected the economy and social integrity of countries. There is rising concern about the mental health challenges of the general population (children, adults, or elderly), along with health workers and family of infected people. This study aims to determine effect of COVID-19 on mental health of people in India. It also focuses on the stigma and discriminating factors in our society and ways to cope with such conditions. A structured survey was conducted with 250 participants of different age groups. Our analysis focuses on the factors affecting mental health of any person, changes in behavior and daily routine due to stress, anxiety or fear of transmission of virus in their family and friends, some are worried for their lifestyle and career. There is a need to understand that pandemic is affecting everyone, either physically or mentally. There must be increase in the study of the aspects of mental health during the pandemic and methods to cope with issues like discrimination for better mental health during pandemic period.

Keywords: adaptive coping, COVID-19, pandemic, resilience, stigma

1. Introduction

Along with great increase in mortality and morbidity due to this pandemic in India, COVID-19 has caused mental health issues among general population, children, adults, elderly, migrant workers, healthcare workers and their families. As per a study performed to assess the youth mental health after COVID-19 in China, it is observed that mental health problems are majorly found in youth group. This study indicates that low education level, post-traumatic stress disorder (PTSD) and negative coping styles were the influence factors of youth mental health [1].

A recent study indicates that structured websites and toll free helpline numbers may be launched for alleviating psychological distress among the general public regarding this ongoing pandemic. Social media is to be used in good sense so that people can get education regarding transmission dynamics and symptoms of disease. To protect social media from devaluations, strict government laws and legislation regarding fake news, social media rumors, disinformation and misinformation are to be implemented [2].

It is important to understand different reasons of mental health issues, ways in which they are affecting our society and resilience of people and the ways they try to cope up with such situations. Therefore, the current study will aim to show impact of COVID-19 on mental health of people in India.

Human beings are social species which require most satisfying environment with social relationship and physical well beings. The pandemic has affected lifestyle, education, career, development and economy in few months as there has been sudden increase in number of patients. Isolation, contact restrictions and economic shutdown impose a complete change to the psycho-social environment. These measures have the potential to threaten the mental health of children, adolescent and elders significantly.

2. Mental health issues during COVID-19

During COVID-19 pandemic, people were bound to stay at home and maintain social distancing. This sudden change in their lifestyle along with fear of COVID-19 created discomfort in their life. Long term anxiousness and fear leads to negative psychological effects including post-traumatic stress symptoms, confusion and anger. Personality disorders and Alzheimer's disease, irritability, restlessness, difficulty in concentration, fatigue, dizziness are also some psychological disorders.

As pandemic was spreading rapidly, complete lockdown had been implemented at most of the places and due to non-availability of transport system people were not able to move around. People from various age groups are reporting loneliness as they were away from their family members. A study revealed that depression, anxiety, and stress play an important role in enhancing the fear of COVID-19.

The general population can experience the fear and anxiety of dying, helplessness, blame the people who are already affected and precipitate the mental breakdown. Let us briefly discuss the impact of COVID-19 on different age groups.

2.1 Children

Unaware of everything happening young children are enjoying the company of their family members with no efforts of going school. As children were not permitted to play outside home they feel irritated sometimes sitting at home. They are also curious to know the reason of drastic change in lifestyle as they cannot judge the actual reasons. Some youngsters are happy to stay home, especially those who are family focused. According to a study done over children and adolescents in the age groups of 9 years to 18 years during COVID-19 outbreak in India. Children and adolescents who were under quarantine had faced more psychological problems than those who were not quarantined. Fear ($p < 0.0001$), nervousness ($p < 0.0001$) and annoyance ($p < 0.001$) were most significantly seen in the quarantined group. Anxiety related insomnia, isolation, boredom (not statistically significant) and sadness was also more common in the quarantine group [3].

Teenagers caring most about their privacy, peers and independence are under depression living with their family while younger kids are happy to get much attention. The notion of social distancing becomes difficult for youngsters who think of themselves not getting ill and takes it as restriction. So primarily being unhappy they start being cutoff from other family members, which results their aggressive behaviors. Having healthy conversation can make them understand and they can be given their personal space at home, even can be allowed to play video games and stay connected to their friends through internet.

Children are also worried about their future. Some self motivated kids have set their goals to achieve something during this period. They are busy with video of their interest and some tutorial, but have become physically less active and have much screen time, irregular sleep pattern and less favorable diets resulting in weight gain and loss of cardio-respiratory fitness.

2.2 Adults

During the pandemic, this age group are afraid of losing their jobs as few companies were not able to survive and few were still operating offline. This age group decided not to go to office and choose work from home as they were concerned about the spread of virus. In this case, the fear of losing jobs increases. Some are getting depressed and feeling alone as maintaining distance. According to Italian study, during the second week of mandatory lockdown, Italian adults paid much attention to information about COVID-19, they perceived it as very severe, and they were particularly worried about infecting their relatives [4]. Loneliness is recognized as a contributing and maintaining factor in the development of Alcohol abuse. Alcohol does affect the user's ability to perceive, integrate and process information. This distortion in the user's thinking does not cause violence but may increase the risk that the user will misinterpret his partner or other's behavior [5]. Consumption of alcohol make a person emotionally weak and might give rise to domestic violence. Which affects the whole family and cause loss of concentration of each family member and make emotionally weak. Some poor labor just focused to reach their home, lost their life due to psychiatric disorders.

Women have started taking measure to protect their family from virus, each item bought to home is sanitized and then used. This increases burden on women due to which they feel tensed, depressed and facing psychiatric disorders like mood extremes. The disruption of social and protective networks, loss of income and decreased access to services, all can exacerbate the risk of violence for women [6]. Women are ones who are more affected by nosophobia of COVID-19 as allergy or climate change may also result some illness. They are more worried about family members.

2.3 Elder and special population

Person with pre-existing mental illness have been inevitably affected by the pandemic. In patients, especially aged and those who require long term hospitalization in closed wards are under great risk [7]. Elderly people were at a higher risk of spreading and catching virus so other family members started keeping themselves away from them. Neither elders are having proper conversations with family nor getting absolute care. Even they are not taken to hospital for any other disease as they can come in the contact of some corona infected person. Watching news related to COVID-19 whole day is depressing them as it seems to be the end of human life (**Figure 1**).

3. Survey

To clearly understand the pandemic impact on different age group a survey on 250 people has been done by preparing a questionnaire. Each questionnaire was divided into four sections. The questionnaire included scaled questions that have

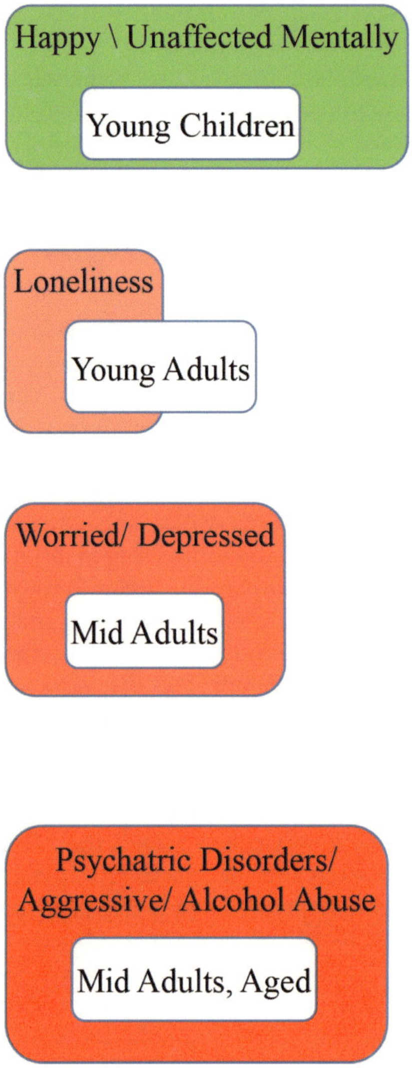

Figure 1.
Impact on mental health of different age groups due to COVID-19 (green is least, and red is most affected).

already been used worldwide in the previous studies and we are using same type of questionnaire for India [8]. In the first section, questions were framed to gather data on the personal profile of the respondents. The second section consisted of questions on personal awareness and attitude. The third and fourth sections of the questionnaire comprised attitude towards family and country. Questions asked the respondents to inform their choices (i) (not at all), (ii) (many times), (iii) (mostly), (iv) (every time) about various factors that affect their awareness, attitude, behavior and methods they follow to keep themselves fit.

3.1 Participants

We used a snowball sampling approach to distribute questionnaire online. The questionnaire was shared on different platforms, when a participant completed it, they forwarded it to their group of friends to expand the size. Out of total 250 respondents, 138 are males that is 55.2% and 112 are females that is 44.8%. Based on the distribution of age, majority of respondents belonged to the age group of 25–44

(50.8%). Whereas 34.8% of the respondents belonged to the age group of 18–24 years and 9.6% were in the age group of 45–above years and 4.8% of the respondents were of the age group of 1–17 years of age (**Table 1**).

Occupation of the respondents has been assessed using 7 categories including medical/security/defense (4.4%), full time employed (31.6%), part time employed (2.8%), unemployed (2.8%), homemaker (0.8%) and majority of respondents lie in category student (41.6%) and others (16%).

The work from home permission of the respondents indicates that most of the respondents as (47.2%) lies in yes and (28.8%) lies in the category of no and there were 8% respondents who were partially allowed to work from home while 16% falls in category of not applicable.

3.2 Awareness

People awareness plays an instrumental role in determining their behavior. This section describes the effectiveness of the awareness for people in the pandemic. The people awareness has been measured with indicators (0 to 4) which include the level of awareness as (0) do not know anything, (1) know very less things, (2) know few things, (3) know many things, (4) know everything (**Table 2**).

The above table describes the study respondents awareness about COVID-19 divided in age groups which are 1–17, 18–24, 25–44 and 44–above. In category Age

Characteristics	Count	Percentage
Gender		
Male	138	55.2%
Female	112	44.8%
Age		
4–17	12	4.8%
18–24	87	34.8%
25–44	127	50.8%
45 and above	24	9.6%
Occupation		
Health worker/security	11	4.4%
Full time employed (except above)	79	31.6%
Part time employed (except above)	7	2.8%
Unemployed	7	2.8%
Homemaker	2	0.8%
Student	104	41.6%
Others	40	16%
Work from home		
Yes	118	47.2%
No	72	28.8%
Partially (at least once in week)	20	8%
Not applicable	40	16%

Table 1.
Descriptive profile of the respondents.

How much they know about corona-virus?		
Scale	**Count**	**Percentage**
Age group (4–17)		
0	2	16.67%
1	1	8.33%
2	3	25%
3	3	25%
4	3	25%
Age group (18–24)		
0	3	3.4%
1	3	3.4%
2	13	14.9%
3	35	40.2%
4	33	37.9%
Age group (25–44)		
0	3	2.4%
1	2	1.6%
2	19	15%
3	57	44.9%
4	46	36.2%
Age group (45–above)		
0	0	0%
1	1	4.16%
2	4	16.67%
3	9	37.5%
4	10	41.67%

Table 2.
Awareness about COVID-19 in respondents.

group (4–17) maximum results come in favor of 2, 3, 4, In age group (18–24) and (25–44) maximum results come in favor of 3 while in age group (44–above) maximum respondents lie in category of 4. This implies that most of the people were aware about the pandemic situation (**Figure 2**).

3.3 Attitude

In age group of 18–24 and 25–44 approximately 35% people were worried more about their health while 10.5% are worried every time with ~33% of 18–24 and ~28% of 25–44 do not worry at all (**Figure 3**).

In age group of 18–24 there are ~32% people worrying about nation or world everytime and in 25–44 age group there ~21% people worrying about nation or world everytime. While ~34% of 18–24 years and 37% of 25–44 years worrying most of the time. While only 8% and 11% of 18–24 and 25–44 resp. do not worry at all (**Figure 4**).

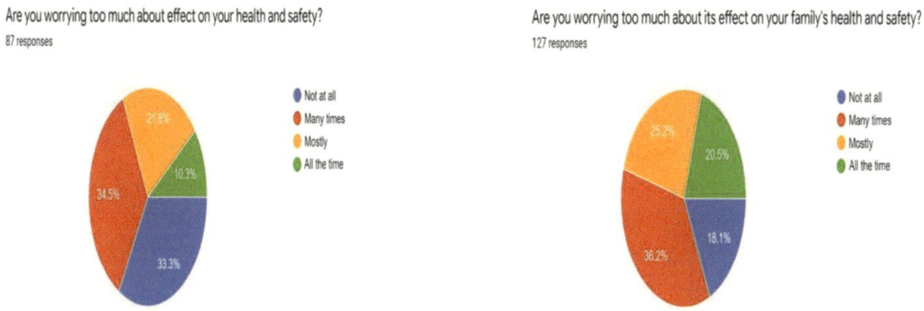

Figure 2.
Percentage of different age group people worrying about their health and safety during pandemic.

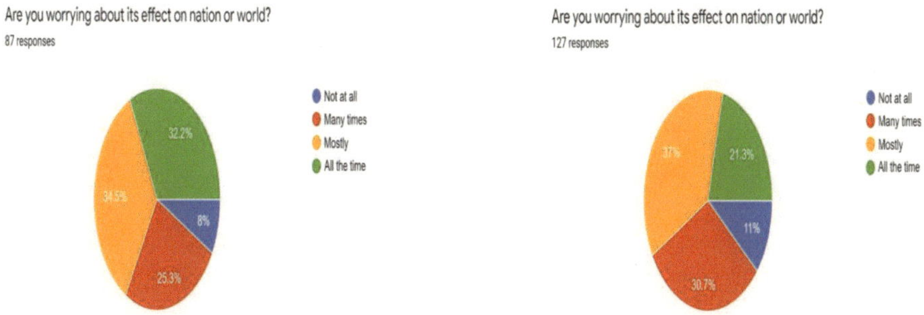

Figure 3.
Percentage of different age group people worrying about effect on nation and world during pandemic.

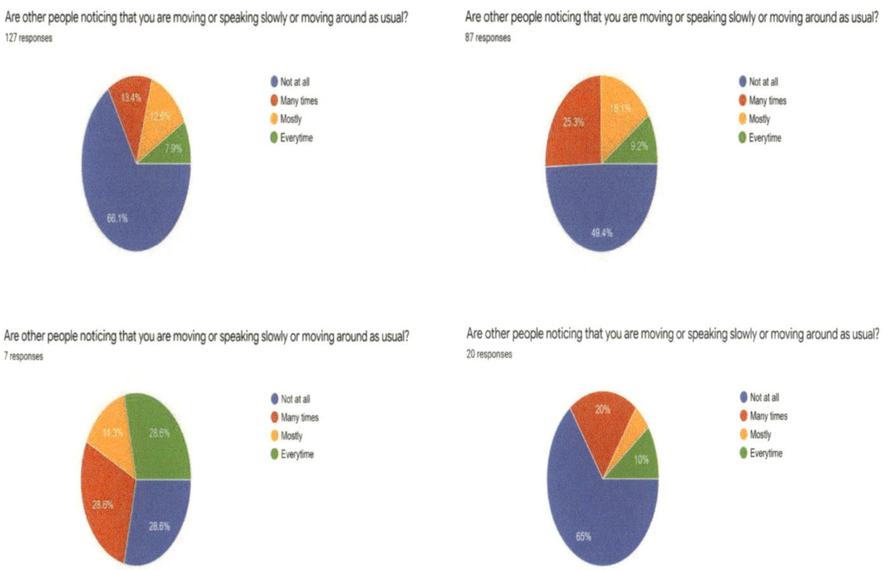

Figure 4.
Percentage of different age group people change in their behavior life speaking slowly or moving around usually during pandemic.

3.4 Behavior

According to Survey, ~28% of teenagers, ~9% of 18–24 age group people, ~8% of 25–44 age group people and 10% of 44+ have been every time noticed moving or

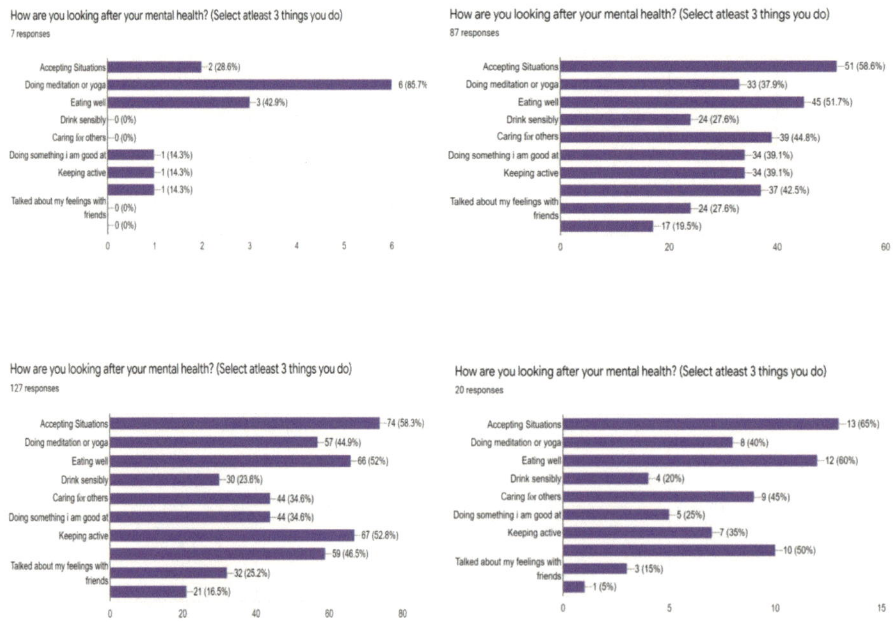

Figure 5.
Percentage of different age group people taking care of mental health by caring others, eating well, accepting situation, taking about their feelings etc. during pandemic.

speaking slowly. Approx 14% and 28% of children are mostly and many times seen moving slowly while ~28% are not at all effected. In case of 18–24 age group 16% and 24% have been noticed mostly and many times moving slowly than usual (**Figure 5**).

Most people have accepted the situation to look after of their mental health, 86% of 13–17 years, ~38% of people of 18–24 years, ~45% of people of 25–44 years and 40% of people of 45+ age group have engaged themselves in doing meditation or yoga. People of 18–24 years opted to eat well (~52%), care others (~45%) and talk to someone they have not talked for long (~42%) for their better mental health. In 25–44 age group, opted to keep themselves active (~53%), eat well (52%), to do things they are good at and care others are (~35%). While in 44+ people tried to be active (35%), contact people they have not contacted so long (50%), care others (45%) and drink sensibly (20%).

Similarly, this questionnaire gives us more details about people's anxiousness, tiredness and concentration problem being faced. Survey shows that most of the people have only one hour of news watching time a day, some are irritated and facing arguments resulting into fights. Few families are also facing Domestic violence during period of pandemic and lockdown.

4. Resilience and adaptive coping

Resilience helps to protect one from mental illness by using the available resources. Resilience is a protective factor against development of mental disorder and a risk factor for a number of clinical conditions, e.g. suicide [9]. On one side, the nation as a whole focuses on controlling the pandemic by adapting different strategies like isolation and quarantined period, other side some organizations are paying attention towards mental health during COVID-19. Lack of social interactions and staying home for longer time effects mental wellness. One should not be over exposed to media coverage, should maintain happy relationship, get in touch

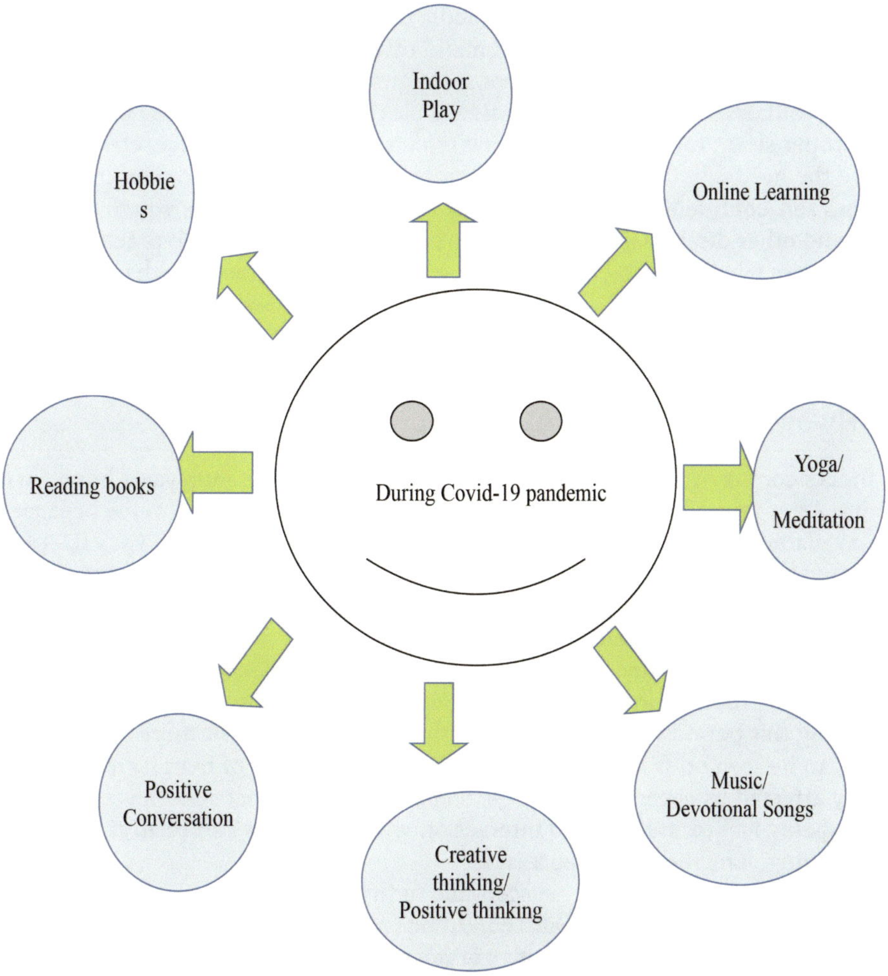

Figure 6.
People can adopt following various lifestyles to resilient/cope with mental health challenges.

Do's	Don't s
1) Positive thinking	1) Excessive Crying/ Negative Thinking
2) Get plenty of sleep	2) Use of alcohol/Drugs
3) Balanced exercise and balanced diet	3) Consuming fast food/ Aerated drinks
4) Talk with your child about Covid-19	4) Partying/Travelling
5) Exercise/Yoga/Meditation	5) Excessive Media Exposure
6) Connect with your favourite ones through social media.	6) Spreading/ Believing Fake News

Figure 7.
Points for good mental health during COVID-19 pandemic.

of friends and relatives through social media to whom you have not been contacting since too long. Reaching out to children and others is good for everyone as feeling close to others reduces anxiety and boost the immune system. For coping with mental health issues people should follow a particular routine such as regular exercise, proper sleep, follow a strict routine which helps us to be active, efficient, reduce the need of will power, reduces procrastination, builds momentum and a person's self-confident by reducing stress, staying calm also helps you to overcome stress and other diseases such as hypertension diseases, one should practice breathing exercises which maintains the proper blood flow in the body with calmness in mind (**Figures 6** and 7).

5. Adjustment problems

India's coronavirus forced many citizens to return their countryside homes with family. After few days of pandemic, daily wagers were in a great trouble because of non-availability of work so their survival become very difficult. The COVID-19 lockdown has the most daunting impact on such people whereby most of them must fight for survival on a daily basis. Many agencies are trying to support daily wage workers, but the entire cycle of revenue has been greatly troubled in few weeks.

During this time of uncertainty, employers may experience changes in productivity. When productivity drops, it has direct impact on jobs. One cannot get new job during this period and siting home in this situation makes it more difficult and effect can be seen on faces of family members too. Millions of lives have been heavily affected by several psychological changes such as increased levels of loneliness as being locked in home, no interaction with neighbors and relatives result in overthinking, loneliness and depression.

Aged people are particularly susceptible to the risk of infection from COVID-19, especially those with chronic health conditions such as hypertension, cardiovascular diseases, and diabetes. Older persons are not just struggling with great health risks but are also less capable of keeping themselves in isolation. Although social distancing is necessary to reduce the spread of diseases, but some families are understanding that elders also require proper care and interaction. Mostly getting locked in a room alone irritates them, and inability to use technology and differentiate between real and fake news also makes them worried and unable to adjust with family. Pandemic and lockdown increased the burden of household work for all families. Children are off school, no service provider (dhobi, cook, driver, gardener, etc.) and regardless to whether they hold job or not. Women are taking care of cleanliness and disinfecting everything and everyone coming in house other than daily works.

6. COVID-19 related stigma among people

Social stigma in the context of health is the negative factor between a person or group of people sharing certain characteristics or symptoms of specific disease. During this outbreak, individuals are branded, treated badly, discriminated, and suffer status loss due to merging with infected people. Such treatment impacts adversely to those with symptoms as well as their caregivers, family, friends and communities. People who do not have the disease but share other characteristics with this group may also suffer from stigma [10].

The level of stigma associated with COVID-19 is based on three main factor:

1. It is a disease that is new and for which there are still many unknowns;

2. We are usually afraid of the unidentified; and

3. It is easy to associate that fear with 'others' there is confusion and anxiety among the public.

Unfortunately, these factors are also fueling harmful stereotypes.

Effects that stigma can cause: Drive people to hide illness to void discrimination, prevent people from seeking health care immediately and discourage them from adopting healthy behaviors. To understand the ways in which this can incite violence and push public in harm, one needs to look at a case of Himachal Pradesh, where Mohammad Dilshad, a 37 year old resident of Una district, hung himself after being continuously taunted and harassed by community despite he tested corona negative (**Figure 8**) [11].

In the COVID-19 emergency, medical workers and security services were at high risk of infection. They were facing overwork, frustration, discrimination, isolation, patients with negative emotions, a lack of contact with their families and exhaustion. This situation causes mental health problems such as stress, anxiety, depressive symptoms insomnia, denial, anger and fear. These mental health problems not only affect attention, understanding and decision-making capacity of medical workers, which could hinder the fight against COVID-19 but they could also have a lasting effect on their overall well being. Stigmatized groups may often be deprived of the resources they need to take care of themselves and their families. Stigma can present major barriers against healthcare seeking, social marginalization, distrust in health authorities and distortion of public perception of risk, resulting in massive panic among citizen.

Groups experiencing stigma related to COVID-19 are mostly the health workers and emergency respondents, people returning from travel, people with the disease, their family and friends and people released from quarantine. The stigmatized people may be excluded or shunned in social situations, denied some kind of opportunity, may be denied access to adequate housing and health caregiver and they might be targets of verbal, emotional and physical abuse.

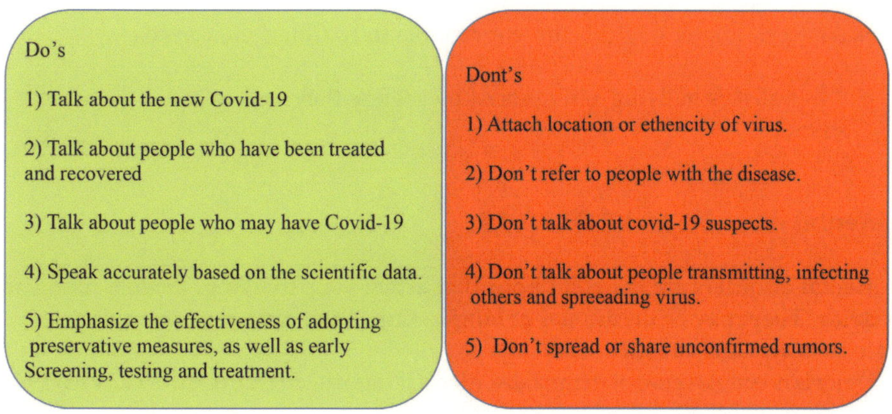

Figure 8.
There are some do's and dont's on language when talking.

7. Stigma and discrimination with corona positive people

The threat of getting infected can change our responses to ordinary interactions, leading us to behave in unexpected ways. Publishing the personal data of people infected with COVID-19 or data of those who are suspicious of having the virus, jeopardizes their safety and well being. This way people themselves are exposed to public lynching, and declared dangerous to public health, the blame for the infection is sought on them and they are marked as irresponsible, reckless, and dangerous citizen. The WHO has also issued specific psycho-social considerations for abating the growing stigma of COVID-19 [12].

People who tested positive often become fearful of seeking help or even discussing symptoms. They put themselves and society into risk and increase the rate of transmission. We are all fed by fear, internalized racism and misinformation. And this will increase with increase of no. of cases, rising mortality rate and limited testing facilities.

How are corona positive been discriminated?

1. Food is thrown through a passage in a quarantine center.

2. Society does not allow their family members to enter their society.

3. They are not allowed to go in public even after treatment and recovery.

4. They are teased as they got infection by their own mistake.

Effects of stigma and discrimination with corona positive:

1. Family members of COVID-19 positive patients who have been tested COVID-19 negative will also face trouble in society and will be considered as guilty which in result will affect them mentally.

2. A treated patient will also feel insecure in the society as everyone will look at him as a risk for society.

3. Family members even after getting symptoms similar to COVID-19 will neglect the test in fear of social discrimination.

4. Affected family might be having trouble in fulfilling their needs.

5. After all this bullying and ignored by society they may take a step towards suicide.

8. Mental disorder and COVID-19

Mental disorders are the conditions that affect your thinking, feeling, mood and behavior. They may be occasional or long lasting. They can affect our ability to relate to others and function each day.

There is no single cause of mental disorder, factors causing it in case of COVID-19 are:

1. having few friends and feeling lonely.

2. having a serious medical condition.

3. life experience as person having symptoms like COVID-19 is started to be discriminated.

4. use of alcohol and recreational drugs.

Some common type of disorders being faced during COVID-19 pandemic:

1. Eating disorders: these are serious mental health disorders. They involve severe problem with your thought about food and your eating behavior, you may eat less or more than you need. They affect ability of our body to get proper nutrition. Causes of eating in this case are psychological and social factors. In long term it can result in some problems like: Muscle weakness, low blood pressure, brain damage, multi-organ failure, feeling tired all time and infertility [13].

2. Depression: depression is serious medical illness. it's more than just a feeling of being sad. Symptoms may include: loss of interest in favorite things, overeating, feeling hopeless, irritated, digestive problems and thoughts of death or suicide. Depression is a disorder of brain which can be caused at any stage of life but it begins often in teens and adults. It can be treated by being socially active or going to psychiatrist [14].

3. Obsessive compulsive disorders: it is a disorder in which we have thoughts of something again and again, but one cannot control them. Obsession are repeated thoughts such as fear of infection in case of COVID-19, fear of losing and misplacing something as one might have fear of losing their parents of family member during this pandemic. Compulsions are the behaviors that you feel like you need to do repeatedly to try to reduce or stop your obsession thoughts. Some compulsions include: excessive cleaning hands and items, ordering and arranging things in a particular way [15].

9. India vs. global situation

This pandemic not only impacted India, but its impact can be seen worldwide. In terms of mental health, the situation globally was also similar. Children, adults, and aged people were facing same type of problems. The pandemic impact can be seen both on developed and developing countries. Initially mortality rate was very high in both developed and developing countries. But due to high population and less resources, India faced more challenges during this situation. The medical facilities were also not as good in India as they are in other developed countries.

10. Conclusion

COVID-19 causes strong mental health issues, as number of deaths, death of family members and friends and lockdown are factors affecting the thought of a person. During the pandemic people facing the problem with inadequate supplies, inadequate information, financial loss, stigma and infection fear. According to our survey children are having lesser knowledge about pandemic while they are curious to know but are not able to understand scientific complexities. Children are little bit irritated locked at home but mostly happy with their families and do not have any anxiety or fear of death. While teenagers are not much happy and worried for their family and friends' health. They were eagerly waiting to meet their friends as being unsocial makes them lonely, irritated and anxious which motivates them to fight with other family members. Adults are most mentally affected, as they have load on their shoulder and see whole life been affected due to corona virus. This group has people mostly worried about its effect on studies/jobs/financial condition. They are not very easily irritated and annoyed but hard to sit still. Most people in this age group are accepting situation, eating well and keeping themselves active. Aged are mostly facing loneliness, anxious and irritated due to being separated from other family members. They watch news channels for atleast one hour a day and afraid that something awful might happen. The number of person infected and died were increasing every day. Even isolation, lockdown and physical distancing are prolonged. Opportunities are decreasing and as a result financial problem are increasing. This leads to increase of mental health issues exponentially. There is stigma related to COVID-19 among people which might be initiating factor of mental health issues. To avoid stigma one can believe that not all who are having symptoms like cough and sneeze have COVID-19, despite precautions if anybody catches COVID-19 its not their fault, one should face fear and anxiety with facts not discrimination, stay positive and remember COVID-19 will heal but stigma and mental trauma left behind will not. In India there is lack of clear and effective communication and a knowledge-based stigma reduction strategy that can translate into public education, community engagement and trust in the health care system. Firstly, we should have knowledge that virus will not be going away any time soon. Any long term strategy must be introduced, broad based and transparent with key public figures who can help the state to communicate on this daily. Secondly, we must move from language of fear and paranoia to one of empathy. We can stop using terms such as "infected" "carrier" and switch to "affected" and "acquired." This reminds people that patients and those at risk are people like us. A public awareness campaign around breaking stereotypes that harm social cohesion and empathy is the need of the hour. We have already seen sections of mainstream media demolishing certain communities and ethnicity. This is not just unethical, but also has an impact on disease control and people lives. There is need to understand the side of mental health during the pandemic, increase the number of researches and find the actions to cope with issues for their effective management.

A. Appendix

A.1 Questionnaire

Dear Sir/Madam,

I request you to please take a few minutes of your precious time to complete the questionnaire of study on "COVID-19 IN INDIA: PROBLEMS, CHALLENGES AND STRATEGIES, PSYCHOLOGICAL ASPECTS". Hence, your participation in the survey will be highly appreciated. I ensure the anonymity of all the participants and complete confidentiality of responses collected. The responses will only be used for my research and not for any other commercial purposes. The study aims at surveying the Mental health of people during COVID-19 pandemic.

Please put a tick mark against the most appropriate choice.
Section A: Demographic Profile

1. Name:

2. Age (in years):

    a. 1–17

    b. 18–24

    c. 25–44

    d. 45 or above

3. Gender:

    a. Male

    b. Female

4. Occupation?

    a. Medical staff/security/police

    b. Full time employed (except above)

    c. Part time employed (except above)

    d. Unemployed

    e. Homemaker

    f. Student

    g. Others

5. Does anyone in your home belongs to medical staff/security/police?

    a. Yes

    b. No

6. Do you have option to work from home?

    a. Yes

    b. No

    c. Partially (need to go at least once a week)

    d. Not applicable

Section B: Inferential Analysis
Awareness:

7. How much you know about Coronavirus?

   a. 0

   b. 1

   c. 2

   d. 3

   e. 4

Attitude:

8. Are you feeling nervous, anxious on edge?

   a. Not at all

   b. Many times

   c. Mostly

   d. Everytime

9. Are you worrying too much about affect on your health and safety?

   a. Not at all

   b. Many times

   c. Mostly

   d. Everytime

10. Are you worrying too much about its affect on your family's health and safety?

    a. Not at all

    b. Many times

    c. Mostly

    d. Everytime

11. Are you worrying too much about its effect on studies/jobs/financial conditions?

    a. Not at all

b. Many times

c. Mostly

d. Everytime

12. Are you worrying about its affect on nation or world?

a. Not at all

b. Many times

c. Mostly

d. Everytime

13. Are you afraid as if something awful might happen?

a. Not at all

b. Many times

c. Mostly

d. Everytime

14. Are you feeling bad for not being able to help yourself, your family or the community in difficult time?

a. Not at all

b. Many times

c. Mostly

d. Everytime

15. Are you feeling helpless or annoyed?

a. Not at all

b. Many times

c. Mostly

d. Everytime

People Behavior:

16. Are You restless that it is hard to sit still?

a. Not at all

b. Many times

c. Mostly

d. Everytime

17. Are you easily irritated or annoyed?

a. Not at all

b. Many times

c. Mostly

d. Everytime

18. How often you fight with family members?

a. Not even once in last month

b. Once in a week

c. Often

d. Daily once

e. More than once in a day

19. Was there any type of domestic violence in your home?

a. Yes

b. No

20. Are you loosing interest in doing things?

a. Not at all

b. Many times

c. Mostly

d. Everytime

21. Are you facing trouble in falling asleep or stay asleep or sleeping too much?

a. Not at all

b. Many times

c. Mostly

d. Everytime

22. Are you feeling tired or having little energy?

    a. Not at all

    b. Many times

    c. Mostly

    d. Everytime

23. Are you over eating or experiencing poor appetite?

    a. Not at all

    b. Many times

    c. Mostly

    d. Everytime

24. Are you having trouble in concentrating on things such as reading books or newspaper or playing games?

    a. Not at all

    b. Many times

    c. Mostly

    d. Everytime

25. Are other people noticing that you are moving or speaking slowly or moving around usually?

    a. Not at all

    b. Many times

    c. Mostly

    d. Everytime

26. Do you miss someone or want to meet?

    a. Not at all

    b. Yes but can wait to meet

    c. Cannot wait anymore

    d. Missing badly

27. Number of hours you watch news?

    a. Not at all

    b. one hour a day

    c. More than one hour a day

    d. most of the time

28. How are you looking after your mental health? (Select atleast 3 things you do)

    a. Accepting situations

    b. Doing meditation or yoga

    c. Eating well

    d. Drink sensibly

    e. Caring others

    f. Doing Something I am good at

    g. Keeping active

    h. Being in touch with family and friends

    i. Talked about my feelings with friends

    j. Contacted person you have not been talking earlier

29. Any comment or suggestions: ....

Author details

Sarika Jain* and Manish Yadav
Department of Mathematics, Amity School of Applied Sciences, Amity University Haryana, Gurugram, India

*Address all correspondence to: sarika33jain@gmail.com

References

[1] Liang, L., Ren, H., Cao, R., et al. (2020). The Effect of COVID-19 on Youth Mental Health. Springer Publication. https://link.springer.com/content/pdf/10.1007/s11126-020-09744-3.pdf

[2] Dubey, S., Biswas, P., Ghosh, R., Chatterjee, S., et al. (2020). Psychological Impact of COVID-19. PMC US National Institute of Medicine National Institute of Health. https://www.ncbi.nlm.nih.gov/pmc/articles/PMC7255207/#bib16

[3] Saurabh, K., and Ranjan, S. (2020). Compliance and Psychological Impact of Quarantine in Children and Adolescents due to COVID-19 Pandemic. Springer Publication. https://link.springer.com/content/pdf/10.1007/s12098-020-03347-3.pdf

[4] Germani, E., Buratta, L., Delvecchio, E., and Mazzeschi, C. (2020). Emerging Adults and COVID-19: The Role of Individualism-Collectivism on Perceived Risks and Psychological Maladjustment. International Journal of Environmental Research and Public Health. https://www.mdpi.com/1660-4601/17/10/3497/htm

[5] Alcohol and Domestic Violence. http://hrlibrary.umn.edu/svaw/domestic/link/alcohol.htm

[6] COVID-19 and Violence Against Women (2020). What the Health Sector/System Can Do. World Health Organisation: Human Reproduction Programme. https://www.who.int/reproductivehealth/publications/emergencies/COVID-19-VAW-full-text.pdf

[7] Kluge, H. H. (2020). Older people are at highest risk from COVID-19, but all must act to prevent community spread. Copenhagen. World Health Organization: Regional Office for Europe. https://www.euro.who.int/en/health-topics/health-emergencies/coronavirus-covid-19/statements/statement-older-people-are-at-highest-risk-from-covid-19,-but-all-must-act-to-prevent-community-spread

[8] Chukwu, E. (2020). https://docs.google.com/forms/d/e/1FAIpQLSfed7oMpx4yx5u8cKfpeT7p942-50L3YO4TJwbBFeKFME79qg/viewform

[9] Shrivastava, A., and Desousa, A. (2016). Resilience: A psychobiological construct for psychiatric disorders. Indian Journal of Psychiatry. https://www.ncbi.nlm.nih.gov/pmc/articles/PMC4776579/

[10] WHO UNICEF (2020). Social Stigma Associated With COVID-19. https://www.who.int/publications/m/item/a-guide-to-preventing-and-addressing-social-stigma-associated-with-covid-19?gclid=CjwKCAjw88v3BRBFEiwApwLevVKu723YGq9eyhGgBaFNtGtEFo2NCVIJw42cujFBmBuAnEOeyO4naBoCAFUQAvD_BwE

[11] Himachal Pradesh Man Accused of Spreading Virus Kills Self (2020). The Tribune India. https://www.tribuneindia.com/news/himachal/himachal-pradesh-man-accused-of-spreading-virus-kills-self-66217

[12] Mental Health and Psychosocial Considerations During the COVID-19 Outbreak (2020). World Health Organization. https://www.who.int/docs/default-source/coronaviruse/mental-health-considerations.pdf

[13] Brennan, P. F. (2020). Eating Disorder. National Institute of Health, US National Library of Medicine. https://medlineplus.gov/eatingdisorders.html

[14] Brennan, P. F. (2020). Depression. National Institute of Health, US National Library of Medicine. https://medlineplus.gov/depression.html

[15] Brennan, P. F. (2020). Compulsive Disorder. National Institute of Health, US National Library of Medicine. https://medlineplus.gov/obsessive compulsivedisorder.html

Chapter 17

COVID-19 and Multiorgan Dysfunction Syndrome

Jitendra D. Lakhani, Sajni Kapadia, Rohit Choradiya, Roop Preet Gill and Som J. Lakhani

Abstract

Severe acute respiratory syndrome (SARS) is the leading cause of death in COVID-19 infection, however, multi-organ dysfunction due to COVID-19 and/or because of co-morbidities is a usual accompaniment causing unfavorable outcome. Early detection of organ failure and giving appropriate organ support may improve the chances of survival. Arterial Blood Gas (ABG) analysis; electrolytes coupled with clinical picture and with organ related laboratory investigations may help in diagnosis of MODS and sepsis in COVID-19 SEVERE SYNDROME. Acute kidney injury (AKI), myocarditis, thromboembolism, acute liver de-compensation, hospital acquired infections, cardiac arrest, glycemic variability, thyroid dysfunction and other organ failure may lead to MODS. As patients having multiple organ syndrome requires ICU admission and interventions like intubation, hemodialysis and other extracorporeal treatment support knowing holistically about "COVID-19 MODS" is important for treating physicians.

Keywords: COVID-19, SARS-CoV-2, Multi-organ dysfunction, cytokine storm, sepsis

1. Introduction

Corona viruses (CoVs) are a group of spherical/pleomorphic, enveloped, single stranded RNA viruses having club shaped glycoprotein projections, having four genera: alpha, beta, gamma and delta. Alpha and beta corona viruses infect many mammalian species ranging from bats to humans. Gamma and Delta Corona viruses affecting mainly birds known as Avian corona viruses [1]. First corona virus was isolated in chick embryo in 1937 and is known as Avian infectious bronchitis virus. The virus affects various organs as it is replicating in epithelial tissues of respiratory, genitourinary and enteric tracts of birds [1, 2]. Evolution of corona virus as etiological agent of avian bronchitis to present COVID-19 pandemic is known to cause involvement of various organs like lung, intestine, liver and brain of animals and humans [2].

SARS-CoV-1, human beta-corona virus was first identified in 2003 as a causative agent of Severe Acute Respiratory Syndrome (SARS) outbreak of China which spread to four other countries [3, 4]. Number of corona viruses were identified then after which included Middle East Respiratory Syndrome (MERS) named MERS-CoV-2 which had features of acute respiratory distress with acute renal failure which was reported in large number of severe MERS cases [5, 6].

Corona Virus	Genera	Year of isolation	Organ involved/syndrome manifested
Avian infectious bronchitis virus	Gamma and Delta Corona viruses	1937	Chick Embryo / infectious bronchitis
Further evolution of Avian corona virus	Gamma and Delta Corona viruses	Poultry outbreaks	Epithelial tissues of respiratory, genito-urinary and enteric tracts of birds.
SARS-CoV-1	Beta	2003	Severe Acute respiratory syndrome (SARS)
MERS	Beta	2012	SARS with Kidney involvement
SARS-CoV-2	Beta	2019	SARS/Multi-organ involvement
SARS-CoV-2Variants: B.1.1.7, B.1.351P.1,B.1.427 B.1.429,B.1.617(delta Variant)	Beta	2020-2021	Variants of concern(VOC) having increased transmissibility, more severe disease

Table 1.
Evolution of corona viruses and their relation to organ involvement [1–10].

In December 2019, cases of pneumonia of unknown etiology were reported from Wuhan, China, which was identified to be caused by virus referred as "novel corona virus (NCV)-2019"/"2019-nCoV"and lung manifestation as "novel corona virus pneumonia (NCP)". WHO declared disease caused by new corona virus as COVID-19 (Corona Virus Disease) which appeared in 2019 [7]. As main manifestations of COVID-19 causing virus is Severe Acute Respiratory Syndrome, SARS-CoV-2 was the accepted name of the virus causing COVID-19. This new corona virus, had genetic and phylogenetic similarity to SARS-CoV-1 and MERS-CoV. All these three new corona viruses; SARS-CoV-1, MERS-CoV and SARS-CoV-2 are Beta corona virus causing human disease have some similarity and also having some dissimilarities, which is important to be noted as to understand pathogenicity and manifestations [8].

Though severe respiratory distress is an important feature of COVID-19 infection, it also causes acute kidney injury (AKI) like MERS virus and leads to multi-organ dysfunction syndrome (MODS). Multiple organ dysfunction in SARS-CoV-2 can be designated as MODS-CoV-2 which can represent multi-organ involvement of COVID-19 infection [9]. Like other viruses, genomic sequence of SARS-CoV-2 (COVID-19 virus) is changing over time and such variants are of concern (VOC); as it may cause rapid transmission, more severe disease and insufficient host response (**Table 1**) [10].

2. Pathogenesis and profile of various organ involvement in COVID-19

COVID-19 disease affects all organs of the body, predominantly lung, manifesting in form of severe acute respiratory syndrome (SARS) [11–14]. Multiple organ dysfunction is reported in severe manifestation of COVID-19 infection and is considered as late manifestation, while loss of sense of smell and of taste; a neurological manifestation, is reported as an early sign [11]. Mechanisms of COVID-19 induced multi-organ dysfunction is multi factorial.

Angiotensin-converting enzyme-2 (ACE 2) receptors, inflammatory mediators, rouge antibodies (autoantibodies), and dysregulated host response play important role in pathogenesis of COVID-19 organ involvement [12]. COVID-19 can also regarded as autoimmune disorder in which auto-antibodies formation leads to organ dysfunction and severe disease and are called Rouge antibodies". They are auto- antibodies which is non-protective and may play part in targeted longer term organ demage [12].

SARS-CoV-2 virus enters human respiratory epithelial cells through attachment of its spike (S) protein to the human angiotensin converting enzyme-2(h-ACE2). Angiotensin-converting enzyme 2 (ACE2) is a key player in pathogenesis of lung involvement leading to SARS. ACE-2 also works as a receptor site and entry point of virus to host cells. Disruption of ACE/ACE2 balance and RAAS activation is responsible for COVID-19 progression which can lead to severe disease and result in multi organ dysfunction especially in patients having co-morbidities like diabetes mellitus, hypertension, and cardiovascular disease [13]. Massive cytokine release, immune depression, cytopathic effect of virus are other mechanisms by which severe COVID-19 disease develops which can result in multi-organ dysfunction [14].

3. Various organ involvement in COVID-19

Various organ and systems are involved in COVID-19 infection. Lung can be entry site, can cause atypical pneumonia and may results in ARDS. Liver, Kidney, Blood, Heart, Brain, Endocrine glands, Gastro-intestinal tract, and Skin are involved which is discussed in sections 4 to 11 of this chapter. **Table 2** summarizes manifestations of various organ involvement and their surrogate markers.

4. Hepatobiliary involvement

The hepatic injury has been found in increasing number in COVID-19 patients [15–18]. It has been evident from altered liver enzymes and total bilirubin. It ranges from mild to severe hepato-cellular damage. It was observed and reported by American college of gastroenterology News Team, that 20-30% individuals with COVID-19 infection had raised transaminases on admission [15]. Liver injury can be attributed to multi-organ dysfunction or the disease process itself causing viral induced hepatitis. The mechanism underlying the liver injury is yet not clear, but few theories might explain the patho-physiology. Firstly, critical illness and immune mediated injury and secondly ACE2 mediated direct hepatocyte injury by the virus itself [16]. The role of ACE2 receptor in infecting the cells by COVID-19 virus has been well established and these receptors are highly expressed in gastrointestinal epithelial cells which can infect cholangiocytes as well [17]. With severe COVID-19 infection, severe hepatic injury has been observed [18]. In severe infection, liver failure can occur due to hypotension and immune mediated mechanisms. Liver dysfunction is heightened in COVID-19 infection due to cytokine storm. Patients who already have underlying chronic liver disease like hepatitis B infection, alcohol induced hepatitis, primary biliary cholangitis may get decompensated during COVID-19 infection. As these patients are at increased risk of acquiring infection due to their immuno-compromised status, liver enzymes should be carefully monitored [18].

5. Renal system involvement and electrolyte imbalance in COVID-19 infection

COVID-19 infection and kidney injury has been well observed and reported. In one study by Chen et al., in 710 patients, 15.5% had raised creatinine on admission and 44% had hematuria and proteinuria [19–24]. It implies that kidney involvement

	Organ.	Clinical manifestations	Clinical marker	Investigatory marker	Evidence of organ involvement	Possible Management/ intervention
1.	Lung	Cough, Fever, Shortness of breath, chest pain, dyspnea and fatigue	ARDS	Nasal and throat swab, Chest X-Ray, HRCT Thorax, Arterial Blood Gas (ABG) analysis	Pneumonia, Atelectasis, Peripheral ground glass opacities, consolidative pulmonary opacities, crazy paving pattern on HRCT Thorax. Hypoxemia with acute respiratory alkalosis on ABG	Oxygenation, hemodynamic resuscitation and awake prone positioning. Steroids in patients who need supplemental oxygen. Non-invasive ventilation like BiPap/CPAP and mechanical ventilation.
2.	GIT	Nausea, Vomiting, Diarrhea, Abdominal pain and loss of appetite	Low Volume pulse, Hypotension, Tenderness on palpation of abdomen	Stool samples	Detection of SARS-CoV-2 RNA in stool samples of infected patients,suggest that ACE2 receptors are highly expressed in the GI tract.	Intravenous fluids, proton pump inhibitors, anti-emetics, anti-spasmodic and other supportive treatment.
3.	Kidney	Hematuria, and proteinuria	AKI, Sepsis, multi-organ failure, shock	Renal function test, Urine routine and microscopy, ABG analysis	Albuminuria, Proteinuria, hematuria, raised levels of serum creatinine and blood urea nitrogen, and eGFR<60ml/min in per 1.73 m^2, Metabolic acidosis on ABG.	Renal Replacement Therapy
4.	Hematopoietic system	Thrombosis and bleeding	Clots, pulmonary embolism, DVT and hemorrhage	Complete blood picture, PT INR, APTT, D-Dimer levels, ferritin, Procalcitonin, Serum LDH, ESR.	Lymphopenia, Leukopenia, thrombocytopenia, raised neutrophil/lymphocyte and platelet/ lymphocyte ratios and raised PT INR, APTT, D-Dimer, Serum LDH, Ferritin Procalcitonin and ESR.	LMWH or Unfractionated Heparin

	Organ.	Clinical manifestations	Clinical marker	Investigatory marker	Evidence of organ involvement	Possible Management/ intervention
5.	Immune System	Unremitting fever along with other cardinal features, ARDS, ACS	Hyperthermia, Hyper inflammatory state, shock	Complete Blood Picture, ESR, CRP, Serum Ferritin, IL-6 levels	Hyperferriteinemia, cytopenia, surge in inflammatory biomarkers and IL-6 levels can lead to cytokine storm resulting in ARDS, MODS and other severe syndromes, and even death.	Corticosteroids, Hydroxychloroquine, chloroquine and Tocilizumab.
6.	Cardio-Vascular System	Palpitations, dyspnea, chest tightness	Sinus tachycardia, DVT, thromboembolic complications	ECG, 2D-Echo, Troponin and creatine kinase levels, TTE, and Cardiac MRI	Acute cardiac injury, Reduced ejection fraction, increased levels of troponin and creatine kinase. Acute myocarditis, myocardial infarction and chronic DCMP.	Continuation of ACE inhibitors and ARBs. Statins, and antiplatelets.
7.	Nervous system	Loss of smell (Anosmia) and taste (dysgeusia), headache, dizziness, myalgia, neuralgia, fatigue, delirium, seizures.	Impaired consciousness, acute flaccid paralysis, seizure, ataxia	CT SCAN, MRI, ABG	Hypoxemia on ABG can detect hypoxic ischemic encephalopathy, CT SCAN can detect symmetric hypoattenuation of bilateral medial thalami and hemorrhagic rim lesions of bilateral thalami and medial temporal lobes can be evident on MRI.	Oxygenation, anticoagulation for stroke, mechanical ventilation in view of poor outcomes.
8.	Liver	Abdominal pain, loss of appetite, vomiting	Icterus (Acute Viral Hepatitis)	Liver function tests, GGT, Alkaline phosphatase, Serum LDH, USG Abdomen and pelvis, CT Abdomen and pelvis	Elevated levels of LDH, Bilirubin and ALT and AST, GGT and ALP levels suggestive of acute liver injury. USG may suggest fatty liver and portal venous gas on CT SCAN. Can be drug induced.	Avoidance of Hepato toxic drugs

	Organ.	Clinical manifestations	Clinical marker	Investigatory marker	Evidence of organ involvement	Possible Management/ intervention
9.	Pancreas	Acute pancreatitis	Pancreatic injury, Prolonged hyperglycemia	Serum amylase and lipase levels, USG abdomen and pelvis.	Elevated levels of serum amylase and lipase	Use of high doses of insulin
10.	Thyroid	Palpitations, subacute thyroiditis, thyrotoxicosis	Swelling of thyroid gland	Thyroid function test	Low T3 levels with normal or low TSH	Continuation of thyroid medications.
11.	Skin.	Pseudo-chilblains (COVID-19 toes), Vesicular and maculo-papular eruptions, urticaria	COVID-19 heel	Clinical and local examination	Urticarial rash, confluent erythematous/ maculopapular/morbilliform rash, papulovesicular exanthema, chilblain-like acral pattern, livedoreticularis/racemose-like pattern, purpuric "vasculitic" pattern.	

Table 2.
Manifestations and markers of organ involvement

can be direct; perhaps in the form of glomerulonephritis that can be immune complex mediated or secondary to hypotension and multi organ dysfunction. The mechanism of injury can be multi-factorial. The presence of co-morbidities also play role in pathogenesis, as underlying renal injury in patients with diabetic nephropathy can get exacerbated due to decreased renal perfusion owing to shock. It has been found that this virus can have direct cytopathic effect on renal cells, as ACE2 is highly expressed in kidneys as well [20]. As cytokine storm can affect other organs due to increased pro-inflammatory markers like IL10, IL7, TNF alpha etc., which can result in injury to kidneys [21].

The electrolyte imbalances have also been found in form of hyponatremia and hypokalemia. In patients requiring ICU care, the strong association of electrolyte imbalance with severity of illness has been found [22]. In one multicenter case-control study in adult patients presenting in emergency department conducted in France, they found that 20.4% patients with infection had hyponatremia whereas it was found only in 12.3% controls [23]. Again, the possible role of ACE2, which is an important enzyme of RAS system can be postulated. As many patients have co-morbid conditions like hypertension and heart failure and are on diuretics, their water excretion is already disturbed and above that the severe COVID-19 infection with severe acute respiratory illness requiring ventilatory support renders these patients more dehydrated with fluid and electrolyte imbalance. In above mentioned French study, they found that hyponatremia was associated with most severe presentation of the disease and that it can be linked to increased ADH secretion in response to dehydration and volume depletion. Also, the syndrome of inappropriate ADH secretion occurs secondary to ARDS in such patients. The urinary loss of potassium was the primary cause of hypokalemia in these patients [24].

6. Hematologic system and COVID-19 infection

The COVID-19 infection has significant impact on hematopoietic system like other viral infections such as varicella, dengue, MERS-CoV, etc [25–33]. The most common haematological changes observed are lymphopenia, neutrophilia and eosinopenia [25]. It has been found that lymphopenia, thrombocytopenia and leucocytosis have been associated with increased severity and fatality in COVID-19 cases [26]. The ACE2 receptor is expressed on lymphocytes and this virus directly infects lymphocytes causing cell lysis [27]. Also the cytokine storm promotes the lymphocyte apoptosis. It has been recommended that the serial assessment of lymphocyte count must be ensued as an indicator of prognostic outcome [28].

The changes in haemostasis tests like prolonged prothrombin time, activated partial thromboplastin time and elevated D-Dimer levels has been found during the COVID-19 infection [29]. Increasing D-dimer levels and formation of microthrombi in peripheral blood vessels have been associated with severe forms of COVID-19 infection [30]. Also increased ESR, CRP and Serum LDH has been found. Liu et al reported that the severity of COVID-19 infection can be predicted by lymphopenia, neutrophilia and high levels of CRP and Serum LDH [31]. These altered coagulation profiles also suggest that this virus stimulates a low grade DIC state and resulting thrombocytopenia due to consumption [32]. Few researchers also believe that virus infect bone marrow hematopoietic cells directly inducing growth inhibition and apoptosis [33].

7. Cardiovascular involvement

The epicenter of COVID-19 infection is pulmonary complication, however, accompanied cardiovascular complications contributes to mortality [34–45].

Cardiovascular complications commonly found to be associated with COVID-19 are myocardial injury, myocarditis, dysrhythmias, heart failure, acute myocardial infarction (AMI) and venous thromboembolic events (VTE). Myocarditis as the cause of death was reported in 7% of 68 fatal COVID-19 of total 150 cases studied [35]. Another study of 191 patients from Wuhan reported 54 deaths; of which 28 (52%) had heart failure, overall prevalence being 23% (44 of 191) [36].

Various mechanisms are postulated for CVS manifestations like destabilization of vascular plaques due to systemic inflammation, viral infection induced increase in cytokine activity leading to increased cardiac demand and direct damage to the heart by utilizing ACE2 receptors of cardiac tissue by virus [37, 38].

Many patients already may have pre-existing cardiovascular disease like coronary artery disease, hypertension and others which leads to greater severity of COVID-19 infection. A meta-analysis of 1527 patients of COVID-19 infection, showed that the prevalence of hypertension and cardiac disease was 17.1% and16.4% respectively, and all of them were more likely to develop more severe illness requiring ICU care [39]. Previous viral infections, including Middle East respiratory syndrome coronavirus (MERS-CoV), have been linked with myocardial injury and myocarditis with increased troponin concentration [40]. Acute cardiac injury can be recognised by increased troponin levels which were reported to be present in 7 to 17 % patients who are admitted with COVID-19. Cardiovascular complications are life threatening; proper monitoring by following trend of troponin level can be useful. Many such patients may require admission to intensive cardiac care unit [30, 36, 41]. Knowing such complication as part of multi-organ involvement is important for clinicians, as it may improve outcomes [42]. Palpitations may manifest as initial symptom in around 7% of patients with COVID-19 [43]. Patients with COVID-19 are also has increased risk of venous thrombo-embolisms (VTEs) [44, 45].

8. Nervous system involvement and COVID-19 infection

With dreadful presentation of SARS-CoV-2 infection with acute respiratory failure requiring ventilatory support, it also has been implicated in activation of prothrombotic pathways leading to cerebrovascular stroke and Central nervous system (CNS) affection in form of parenchymal and vascular inflammatory responses leading to various neurological manifestations [46–55]. The commonly found (80%) early symptom of anosmia and dysgeusia despite absence of nasal congestion and discharge, suggests the involvement of olfactory bulb and tract [47]. The virus may invade CNS through olfactory epithelium and neuro-mucosal interface [48]. There can be neurological dysfunction due to metabolic derangements due to organ failure and hypoxemia in the form of encephalopathy. In one multicenter study conducted in 69 ICUs across 14 countries, it was found that 55% patients with COVID-19 admitted in ICU had delirium [49]. The authors also found high prevalence of acute brain dysfunction in these patients [49]. Also, encephalopathy can be the primary symptom especially in elderly patients [50].

The direct injury to cerebral blood vessels due to invasion of virus into endothelial cells has also been reported in few autopsy findings, with similar findings in other organs – lungs, kidneys, heart and liver [51]. These findings are evidence suggesting direct invasion of nervous system. Patients with COVID-19 infection are at increased risk of cerebrovascular events. Cerebral venous sinus thrombosis, ischemic stroke, subarachnoid hemorrhage and intraparenchymal hemorrhage have been reported, among them ischemic stroke being the most common [52]. Besides the presence of traditional risk factors for vascular thrombosis, COVID-19infection per se is associated with a hypercoagulable state which is reflected by elevated levels of D-dimer [53].

Isolated cases of meningoencephalitis, acute hemorrhagic necrotizing encephalopathy, acute disseminated encephalomyelitis (ADEM) and GBS have also been reported. In one case report of meningoencephalitis in 24-year-old male who presented with seizures and altered mental status, virus was isolated from CSF [54]. There are increasing number of patients with hemorrhagic encephalomyelitis, with MRI features of hemorrhagic lesions in medial temporal lobes, bilateral thalami and sub insular regions [55].

9. COVID-19 and Pancreas; Diabetes

Diabetes is the most prevalent co-morbidity in COVID-19, second only to obesity. If those with diabetes do contract COVID-19, they are indeed likely to develop more severe form of the disease particularly if the diabetes is uncontrolled [56–68]. Data from Wuhan, China confirms that approximately 20% of severe cases of COVID-19 do show diabetes, as co morbidity [36]. According to reports from India, of the first 125 deaths on COVID-19, 56% had diabetes, 47% had hypertension, and over a third had both diabetes and hypertension [57]. An Indian study of 231 patients of COVID-19 infections, 21.2% had co-morbidities of which diabetes mellitus and hypertension was the most common [58]. In some stable diabetic patients with COVID-19, there was rapid worsening of glycaemic control requiring high insulin dose. Possibility of pancreatic affection due to virus is postulated as high level of ACE2 was found in the pancreatic islet beta cells [59–61].

Wang et al demonstrated that 9 of 52 admitted patients in Wuhan with COVID-19 pneumonia developed pancreatic injury as evidenced by abnormality in serum amylase or lipase levels [62]. After viral entry into the beta cells, there is a downregulation of ACE2 leading to increased angiotensin level, which also impairs insulin secretion [63]. Possible mechanisms on pancreatic injury include (i) direct cytopathic effect of SARS-CoV-2 replication, (ii) systemic response to respiratory failure, and (iii) harmful immune response induced by SARS-CoV-2 infection [62].

An important feature of type 2 diabetes is low grade inflammation. There is long term immune system imbalance, metabolic syndrome, or nutrient excess associated with obesity [64, 65]. Also, in individuals with diabetes, there is an exaggeration of pro-inflammatory responses, especially IL-1, IL-6 and TNF-alpha. This may be further worsened in those with severe COVID-19. Prolonged hyperglycaemia alters the host immune system. Dysfunctions in leukocytes, monocyte and macrophage chemotaxis and phagocytosis, and damaged specific immunity have also been reported in subjects with diabetes [66, 67]. Moreover, diabetes shares common features promoting disease progression with infectious disorders such as pro-inflammatory state and endothelial dysfunction [68].

10. COVID-19 and Gastro-intestinal involvement

Though pulmonary manifestations such as fever and cough are the commonly reported presenting symptoms in patients with severe acute respiratory syndrome coronavirus 2 (SARS-CoV-2), the presenting symptoms in other organs such as the GI tract and hepatobiliary, including nausea/vomiting and diarrhoea, were also reported [69–77]. The entry of SARS-CoV-2 in human cell is through protein ACE-2 which is found on the surface of lung alveolar epithelial cells and also on enterocytes of the small intestine [70]. One of the study of 1099 patients with COVID-19 in retrospective analysis showed that the main presenting symptoms were fever (87.9%) and cough (67.7%), followed by diarrhoea (3.7%) and vomiting (5.0%) [69]. Out of all the GI symptoms, there was higher incidence of diarrhoea and abdominal pain present in severe COVID-19 patients than that in patients with mild COVID-19 [69]. In one of the larger studies, systematic review and meta-analysis of 35 studies on GI manifestations, consisting of 6686 patients of COVID-19infection, the three commonest symptoms include nausea and/or vomiting, diarrhoea and loss of appetite with the pooled prevalence of all GI symptoms was 15% [71].

Currently, loss of appetite was reported, ranging from 1.0% to 79% [71]. It can be explained by taste dysfunction up to some extent, which was found in as high as 88.0% in group of 417 mild-to-moderate COVID-19 patients in Europe. Also taste dysfunction almost go hand in hand with olfactory dysfunction with a high prevalence of 85.6% and may further aggravate loss of appetite as identified in the study [47, 72].

Furthermore, SARS-CoV-2 RNA was first detected in a stool specimen from the first reported COVID-19 case in the United States (US) [73]. In a study of Chinese cohort with 73 COVID-19confirmed hospitalised patients, 53.42% of the patients had detected viral RNA in the stools, after the complete clearance from the respiratory tract with undetectable viral RNA but still it had been identified in the stool specimen [74]. SARS-CoV-2 has also been detected in stool samples of the patients in one of the studies without having GI symptoms [75].

Many a times diagnosis of COVID-19 has been missed as initial presenting symptom may be involving GI tract rather than respiratory tract. Many researchers proposed that patients with GI symptoms might have a bad prognosis than those without digestive symptoms, hence clinician had to give importance to patients presenting with GI symptoms such as diarrhoea for early diagnosis [76, 77]. In the same study, rate of severity of disease was also significantly increased in patients with GI symptoms as compared with those without GI symptoms [76]. Pan and colleagues also showed the same result that as the severity of the disease increased, there is worsening of GI symptoms [77].

11. COVID-19 and Skin involvement

Skin manifestations of COVID-19 include a wide variety of skin disorders which may include specific COVID-19 related dermatoses and a variety of other skin disorders that may be worsened by COVID-19 infection [78–85]. Like other viral infections, skin rash is the most common manifestation, which is described as confluent, erythematous, morbilliform, maculopapular rash. Urticarial rash is found in one fifth of the skin manifested cases. Early lesions can be in form of vesicular eruptions which may appear before symptoms also. Pseudo-chilblain like lesions is described as late manifestation in which acral areas will have red vesicles or pustules. Livedo reticularis/racemose-like pattern can appear with COVID-19 symptoms. Purpuric "vasculitic" pattern is associated with severe COVID-19 infection [78, 79]. Acute urticaria is well known to be triggered by viral infections and COVID-19 is no exception [80]. Urticarial vasculitis has also been well demonstrated in a few patients. Urticarial vasculitis differs from urticaria and in that the lesions tend to persist beyond 24 hours and can be painful instead of pruritic [81]. Confluent maculopapular rash is also a well known manifestation of viral infections. Monomorphic vesicular exanthema is often considered an important clue to COVID-19infection. It differs from chicken pox in the fact that chicken pox rash tends to be polymorphic. Chilblain like acral pattern often manifests with cold sensitivity and purplish discoloration of the extremities. This is believed to be a manifestation of hypercoagulability and prothrombotic consequence of COVID-19. Livedo reticularis is believed to be often of similar aetiology. Purpuric lesions are one of the most common manifestations of COVID-19. Purpuric lesions involving the heel known as "COVID-19 heel" is one the specific markers of COVID-19 infection [82–85].

The mutant strains of COVID-19 are believed to cause more extra pulmonary symptoms and thus skin manifestations of COVID-19 too could become more evident.

12. Lung involvement, ARDS and Multiorgan dysfunction

COVID-19 infection may start with influenza like illness with mild symptoms which can progress to severe acute respiratory distress in around 5.6–13.2% patients; a pooled estimate being around 9.4% [86–92]. A systematic review and meta-analysis reported risks of severity and mortality estimated from 18.0 and 3.2%, respectively. If we extrapolate the data of this meta-analysis, additional around 9% will have risk of severe disease other than ARDS [86]. ABG analysis data of critically ill COVID-19 patients showed mixed ABG picture, suggesting multi-organ involvement [87]. If only lung involvement was the cause of severe disease and/or death, ABG picture should have been of respiratory acidosis or in patients with hyperventilation and CO2 washout of respiratory alkalosis which was not the case in this study [87]. Accompanied metabolic acidosis in a mixed ABG pattern can be because of sepsis, AKI, lactic acidosis ketoacidosis which is reported in COVID-19 patients and in sepsis [87–89].

In lungs, diffuse alveolar damage (DAD), a pathological hallmark of ARDS, has been observed in direct viral invasion of cells and lytic effects [90]. In a systemic review by Bao et al. of 2700 patients of COVID-19, most common abnormalities found on HRCT Chest were ground glass opacifications (83%), ground glass opacification with mixed consolidation (58%) and adjacent pleural thickening (52%) followed by interlobular septal thickening (48%) and air bronchograms (46%) [91]. ARDS can be related to inflammatory markers and also to glycaemic variability, and thus ARDS can be one of the spectrums of MODS and may result in a vicious circle of metabolic derangements [92].

13. Cytokine storm as cause of mods

The cytokine storm caused by COVID-19 has been proposed to be associated with the severity of COVID-19 which is multisystem inflammatory syndrome [30, 93, 94]. The early symptomatic presentation of COVID-19 mainly include fever, cough, myalgia, fatigue, or may have dyspnoea. With the progression of disease in later course, dyspnoea may worsen in susceptible host to acute respiratory distress syndrome (ARDS) or multiple organ failure (MOF) [95]. Severe acute respiratory syndrome (SARS) and Middle East respiratory syndrome (MERS) is known to be associated with a cytokine storm like many other infectious diseases [95, 96].

One of the major reasons for the deaths in this infection is suspected to be due to the "cytokine storm" [also called "cytokine storm syndrome"(CSS)]. Cron and Behrens bring the current knowledge of CSS. They define that "cytokine storm" is an activation cascade of auto-amplifying the production of cytokines due to dysregulated host immune response. The triggering factors for the host immune response may be due to infections, rheumatic disorders, malignancy, etc [97]. It is also thought that cytokine storm is a systemic inflammatory response to infections and drugs and leads to excessive activation of host immunity which further leads to activation of pro-inflammatory cytokines [98].

Cytokine Release Syndrome (CRS) is a similar entity which is mainly due to acute systemic inflammatory syndrome characterized by multiple-organ dysfunction (MOD). It has been said that chimeric antigen receptor (CAR)-T-cell therapy would be helpful to differentiate CRS from a cytokine storm [98]. For patients with COVID-19, C-reactive protein (CRP), and other inflammatory cytokines and chemokines are markedly elevated in the intensive care unit (ICU) patients [99, 100]. Many studies showed link between pro-inflammatory cytokines, especially interleukin 6 (IL-6), with the severity of illness in COVID-19 [30, 101–103]. Increased D-dimer levels are also found in severe disease [104]. The higher concentration of cytokines also has a poor prognosis in COVID-19 [102, 105]. Activation of both innate and adaptive immune responses by SARS-CoV-2 infection can lead to dysregulated inflammatory responses which ultimately results into the cytokine storm [106]. Furthermore, the cytokine storm leads to apoptosis of epithelial cells and endothelial cells, and dysfunction of endothelial cells causing vascular leakage and, finally, result in ARDS, MODS and other severe syndromes, and even death [107].

Many therapies are targeted to reduce the cytokine storm which can results in one of the life-saving measures in severely ill COVID-19 infection. Out of many therapies, Corticosteroids, Hydroxychloroquine (HCQ) and chloroquine (CQ) and Tocilizumab (TCZ) (IL-6 Inhibitor) are widely used in the recent past. Corticosteroids inhibit the host inflammatory response and suppress the immune response and pathogen clearance [108]. In a retrospective study of 401 patients infected with SARS-CoV, the rational use of corticosteroids shortened hospital stays and reduced the mortality of seriously ill patients without complications [109]. In view of their in vitro antiviral effects and anti-inflammatory properties, CQ and its analogue HCQ are most potential therapies against COVID-19. CQ and HCQ can reduce CD154 expression in T cells and suppress the release of IL-6 and TNF53 [110]. TCZ, an IL- 6 receptor (IL-6R) antagonist, can inhibit cytokine storms by blocking the IL-6 signal transduction pathway [111].

14. Sepsis and Multi-Organ Dysfunction Syndrome (MODS) in COVID-19

Patho-physiology of SARS-CoV-2 infection is complex and is known to involve activation of the immune and hematologic systems [112–118]. Endotoxin and tumor necrosis factor-alpha (TNF-alpha) trigger the production of interleukin-6 (IL-6) and IL-8, which is followed by the cytokine storm. Further events lead to activation of the coagulation cascade through endothelial and tissue factor (TF) pathways, as well as systemic inflammatory activation [94, 112]. Moreover, SARS-CoV-2 binds to angiotensin-converting enzyme-2 (ACE-2) receptors, which are widely distributed. not only in lung alveolar epithelial cells and oro-nasopharyngeal mucosa but also in the endothelium as well as vascular smooth muscle cells, in the brain, in the gut and in peripheral organs such as liver and kidney [113]. This suggests that the clinical spectrum of COVID-19 is not limited to local pneumonia, but rather represents a multisystem illness with involvement of different organs and potential for systemic complications [113]. It seems that the highly pathogenic SARS-CoV-2 is associated with rapid virus replication and a tendency to infect the lower respiratory tract, resulting in an elevated response of IL-6-induced severe respiratory distress.

Most SARS-CoV-2 infected patients admitted to ICU showed a dysregulated host response characterized by hyperinflammation, alterations in coagulation, and dysregulation in the immune response that further contribute to MODS, like occurs in sepsis [114, 115]. Due to virus infection and to MODS in some cases, many patients with severe COVID-19 meet the Third International Consensus Definitions for Sepsis (SEPSIS-3), which define sepsis as "a life-threatening condition that arises when the body's immune response to infection damages the host's own tissues" [116]. Also, when performing specimen cultures in septic patients from a COVID-19 cohort, about 80% of patients had no bacterial or fungal infection and so viral infection would seem to be the only reason for sepsis which was reported in 50% of their 191 COVID-19 patients. This retrospective study from Wuhan reported Sequential Organ Failure Assessment (SOFA) score of 5·65 on admission [36]. SOFA score may increase on day 3 to 7as reported in one series of 50 patients of bacterial and malarial sepsis [117]. It may be due to release of mediators that there may be upward trend of SOFA score, development MODS and in mortality in sepsis patients who has unfavourable outcome. COVID-19 sepsis which can be called as viral sepsis or secondary sepsis which can be hospital acquired; may worsen the clinical phenotypes of these critically ill COVID-19 patients [118].

15. Co-morbidities, MODS and COVID-19

Co-morbidities like hypertension, diabetes, cardiovascular diseases and respiratory disorders are associated with COVID-19 infection and they serve as additional risk factors for severity and can have deleterious effect [119–122]. Significant difference was noted in COVID-19 outcomes in those who had co-morbidities and those without it [87, 121]. Multi-organ dysfunction could be due to COVID-19 or may be because of resultant deterioration of co-morbidities associated end–organ acute injury [87]. Drugs used for co-morbidities and for COVID-19 can also lead to multi-organ dysfunction [122]. **Table 3** shows list of co-morbidities commonly encountered in COVID-19 patients leading to organ/multi-organ involvement.

	Co-morbidity	Presenting features	Organ involved/ pathological feature	Consequences
1.	Sepsis/Hospital acquired Sepsis	Fever, Shock, Hypotension, decreased output, respiratory failure, Hospital/ventilator acquired pneumonia.	Lungs, Bloodstream infection, Cardiovascular and circulatory collapse, Renal shutdown.	ARDS, Septic shock, AKI, sudden cardiac arrest, and even death.
2.	Diabetes	Unaware of diabetes, Hyperglycemia, Hypoglycemia, Glycemic variability.	Multiorgan, Liver, Diabetic Ketoacidosis, Hospital acquired sepsis	Lactic acidosis, AKI, poor outcome
3	Hypertension	Unaware about hypertensive state, dyspnea, giddiness, headache, vomiting.	Kidneys, cardiovascular system, more chances of severe infection and SARS.	Hypertensive emergency, CVA (hypertensive bleed), AKI, Acute lung injury.
4	Cardiovascular Disease	Fever, palpitations, dyspnea, chest tightness, dry cough, nausea and vomiting.	Multiorgan-Heart, Kidneys, lungs, CNS	Coronary artery disease, Myocardial injury and myocarditis, dysrhythmias, heart failure, venous thromboembolic events (VTE), Cardioembolic stroke, renal infarction.

	Co-morbidity	Presenting features	Organ involved/ pathological feature	Consequences
5	Cerebrovascular disease	Loss of smell (Anosmia) and taste (dysgeusia), headache, dizziness, myalgia, neuralgia, fatigue, delirium, encephalopathy, seizures.	CNS, Spinal cord, Cranial and peripheral nerves.	Cerebral venous sinus thrombosis, ischemic stroke, subarachnoid hemorrhage and intraparenchymal hemorrhage, meningoencephalitis, acute hemorrhagic necrotizing encephalopathy, acute disseminated encephalomyelitis (ADEM) and GBS.
6	COPD/Other respiratory diseases	Fever, cough with expectoration, dyspnea, chest pain, shortness of breath, fatigue.	In lungs, diffuse alveolar damage (DAD), is a pathological hallmark of ARDS.	ARDS, poor prognosis, MODS.
7	Epilepsy	Seizures, fever, altered mental status, status epilepticus.	Hemorrhagic lesions in medial temporal lobes, bilateral thalami and sub insular regions.	Exacerbation of seizures.
8	Chronic Kidney Disease	Hematuria, proteinuria, vomiting.	Kidneys, cardiovascular system.	Metabolic acidosis, hypertension, decreased renal perfusion leading to shock,pulmonary odema,. heart failure.
9	Chronic Liver Disease	Diarrhea, abdominal pain, loss of appetite, vomiting.	In severe infection, liver failure can occur due to hypotension and immune mediated mechanisms which are heightened in COVID-19infection in the form cytokine storm.	Decompensation of hepatitis B infection, alcohol induced hepatitis, primary biliary cholangitis in COVID-19 infection can occur leading to liver failure.

Table 3.
Co-morbidities commonly encountered in COVID-19 patients leading to organ/multi-organ involvement.

16. Drugs used in COVID-19 and cause of MODS

Various drugs are used in COVID-19 which can alter immunity, can cause organ damage like acute liver and kidney injury, may lead to electrophysiological disturbances in heart and can contribute to pre-existing MODS or may become the risk factor [9]. Tocilizumab (TCZ), a monoclonal antibody which inhibits the interleukin-6 receptor may predispose COVID-19 patients to secondary infections [123]. Tocilizumab (TCZ) can cause liver dysfunction, lead to induction and reduction of cytochrome P450 enzyme and can cause allergic reaction apart from secondary infection [124, 125]. Use of HCQ and Azithromycin may be responsible for QT prolongation, which can in turn lead to torsades' de pointes [126]. Use of corticosteroids in COVID-19 patients can also induce secondary bacterial and fungal infections and such patients may need more antibiotic coverage [127]. It is imperative to see the drug contribution in MODS of COVID-19 infections.

17. Fighting the COVID-19 pandemic; key messages

- Human Corona viruses can lead to Severe Acute Respiratory syndrome with other multiple organ involvement.
- Pathogenesis of COVID-19 MODS can be multi-factorial. Virus entry to the cell through human Angiotensin-converting enzyme-2 (ACE 2) receptor plays an important role in lung and in other organ affection. Inflammatory mediators, rouge antibodies, and dysregulated host response also play role in pathogenesis of COVID-19 organ involvement.
- Various organ and systems are involved in COVID-19 infection. Lung can be considered main but Liver, Kidney, Blood, Heart, Brain, Endocrine glands, Gastro-intestinal tract, and Skin are also involved.
- COVID-19 infection may start with influenza like illness, can lead to SARS with or without multiple organ involvement.
- Cytokine storm as cause of MODS which can lead to unfavourable outcome.
- COVID-19 per se is a sepsis syndrome as per recent definition of sepsis as there is dysregulated immune response. Secondary nosocomial sepsis is also not uncommon. Sepsis due to inflammatory mediators can cause MODS.
- Co-morbidities in patient having COVID-19 infection may serve as additional contributor to MODS.
- Drugs used in COVID-19 may be responsible for acute organ injury or predispose to infections which may be responsible for MODS.
- "FIGHTING THE COVID-19 PANDEMIC" is for better tomorrow.

Author details

Jitendra D. Lakhani[1]*, Sajni Kapadia[2], Rohit Choradiya[2], Roop Preet Gill[2] and Som J. Lakhani[3]

1 SBKSMIRC and Dhiraj Hospital, Sumandeep Vidyapeeth University, Pipalia, Gujarat, India

2 Department of General Medicine, SBKSMIRC and Dhiraj Hospital, Sumandeep Vidyapeeth University, Pipalia, Gujarat, India

3 Dermatology, Parul Institute of Medical Sciences and Research, Parul University, Limda, Gujarat, India

*Address all correspondence to: jitendralakhani@doctor.com

References

[1] C.A. Torres, V. Listorti, C. Lupini, G Franzo, M. Drigo, E. Catelli, P.E. Brandão, M. Cecchinato. Gamma and Deltacoronaviruses in quail and pheasants from Northern Italy. Poultry Science. 2017;96(3):717-722.

[2] Wen Wang, Xian-Dan Lin, Wen-Ping Guo, Run-Hong Zhou, Miao-Ruo Wang, Cai-Qiao Wang, Shuang Ge, Sheng-Hua Mei, Ming-Hui Li, Mang Shi, Edward C. Holmes, Yong-Zhen Zhang.Discovery, diversity and evolution of novel coronaviruses sampled from rodents in China. Virology. 2015;474:19-27. DOI: https://doi.org/10.1016/j.virol.2014.10.017.

[3] Drosten,C., GuntherS., PreiserW., vander WerfS., BrodtH.R., BeckerS., RabenauH., PanningM., KolesnikovaL., FouchierR.A., BergerA., BurguiereA.M., CinatlJ., EickmannM., EscriouN., GrywnaK., KrammeS., ManuguerraJ.C., Muller S., RickertsV., SturmerM., ViethS., KlenkH.D., OsterhausA.D., Schmitz H., DoerrH.W. Identification of anovel coronavirusin patients with severeacute respiratory syndrome. N.Engl.J. Med. 2003;348: 1967-1976.

[4] Acute respiratory syndrome. China, Hong Kong Special Administrative Region of China, and Viet Nam. Wkly Epidemiol Rec. 2003 Mar 14;78(11):73-4. English, French. PMID: 12674023.

[5] Bermingham A, Chand MA, Brown CS, Aarons E, Tong C, Langrish C, Hoschler K, Brown K, Galiano M, Myers R, Pebody RG, Green HK, Boddington NL, Gopal R, Price N, Newsholme W, Drosten C, Fouchier RA, Zambon M.Severe respiratory illness caused by a novel coronavirus in a patient transferred to the United Kingdom from the Middle East. Euro Surveill. 2012;17(40):20290. PMID: 23078800.

[6] Egbi OG, Adejumo OA, Akinbodewa AA. Coronavirus infection and kidney disease: a review of current and emerging evidence. Pan Afr Med J. 2020;37:149. DOI:10.11604/pamj.2020.37.149.23655

[7] WHO Report of the WHO-China Joint Mission on Coronavirus Disease 2019 (COVID-19). 2020:16-24. Available from www.who.int.

[8] Mousavizadeh L, Ghasemi S. Genotype and phenotype of COVID-19 : Their roles in pathogenesis. J Microbiol Immunol Infect. 2020;S1684-1182(20):30082-7. Doi:10.1016/j.jmii.2020.03.022

[9] Robba C, Battaglini D, Pelosi P, Rocco PRM. Multiple organ dysfunction in SARS-CoV-2: MODS-CoV-2. Expert Rev Respir Med. 2020;14(9):865-868. DOI:10.1080/17476348.2020.1778470CDC.

[10] CDC: SARS-CoV-2 Variant Classifications and Definitions updated on Apr. 21, 2021; https://www.cdc.gov/coronavirus/2019-ncov/cases-updates/variant-surveillance.html.

[11] Eliezer M, Hautefort C, Hamel AL, Verillaud B, Herman P, Houdart E, Eloit C. Sudden and Complete Olfactory Loss of Function as a Possible Symptom of COVID-19 . JAMA Otolaryngol Head Neck Surg. 2020;146(7):674-675. DOI: 10.1001/jamaoto.2020.0832. PMID: 32267483

[12] Khamsi R. Rogue antibodies could be driving severe COVID-19 . Nature. 2021;590(7844):29-31. DOI: 10.1038/d41586-021-00149-1. PMID: 33469204.

[13] Beyerstedt S., Casaro E.B. & Rangel É.B. COVID-19 : angiotensin-converting enzyme 2 (ACE2) expression and tissue susceptibility to SARS-CoV-2

infection. Eur J Clin Microbiol Infect Dis (2021). https://doi.org/10.1007/s10096-020-04138-6.

[14] Zaim S, Chong JH, Sankaranarayanan V, Harky A. COVID-19 and Multiorgan Response. CurrProblCardiol. 2020;45(8):100618. DOI:10.1016/j.cpcardiol.2020.100618

[15] ACG News Team. American College of Gastroenterology; 2020. Joint GI Society Message on COVID-19 .https://gi.org/2020/03/15/joint-gi-society-message-on-COVID-19 /[Google Scholar]

[16] Wong SH, Lui RN, Sung JJ. COVID-19 and the digestive system. J Gastroenterol Hepatol. 2020;35(5):744-748. DOI: 10.1111/jgh.15047. Epub 2020 Apr 19. PMID: 32215956.

[17] Guo Y.R., Cao Q.D., Hong Z.S., Tan Y.Y., Chen S.D., Jin H.J., Tan K.S., Wang D.Y., Yan Y. The origin, transmission and clinical therapies on coronavirus disease 2019 (COVID-19) outbreak - an update on the status. Mil Med Res. 2020;7(1):11. DOI: 10.1186/s40779-020-00240-0.

[18] Zhang C., Shi L., Wang F.S. Liver injury in COVID-19 : management and challenges. Lancet Gastroenterol Hepatol. 2020;5(5):428-430. DOI: 10.1016/s2468-1253(20)30057-1.

[19] Cheng Y, Luo R, Wang K, Zhang M, Wang Z, Dong L, Li J, Yao Y, Ge S, Xu G. Kidney disease is associated with in-hospital death of patients with COVID-19 . Kidney Int. 2020 May;97(5):829-838. DOI: 10.1016/j.kint.2020.03.005.

[20] Li W., Moore M.J., Vasilieva N. Angiotensin-converting enzyme 2 is a functional receptor for the SARS coronavirus. Nature. 2003;426:450-454.

[21] Pan X.W., Xu D., Zhang H., Zhou W., Wang L.H., Cui X.G. Identification of a potential mechanism of acute kidney injury during the COVID-19 outbreak: a study based on single-cell transcriptome analysis. Intensive Care Med. 2020;46(6): 1114-1116.

[22] Hong X, Chi Z, Liu G, et al. Analysis of early renal injury in COVID-19 and diagnostic value of multi-index combined detection. MedRxiv. 10.1101/2020.03.07.20032599.

[23] De Carvalho H, Richard MC, Chouihed T, Goffinet N, Le Bastard Q, Freund Y, Kratz A, Dubroux M, Masson D, Figueres L, Montassier E. Electrolyte imbalance in COVID-19 patients admitted to the Emergency Department: a case-control study. Intern Emerg Med. 2021 Jan 23:1-6. DOI: 10.1007/s11739-021-02632-z.

[24] Chen D, Li X, Song Q, Hu C, Su F, Dai J, Ye Y, Huang J, Zhang X. Assessment of Hypokalemia and Clinical Characteristics in Patients with Coronavirus Disease 2019 in Wenzhou, China.JAMA Netw Open. 2020 Jun 1; 3(6):e2011122.

[25] Sun S., Cai X., Wang H., He G., Lin Y., Lu B., Chen C., Pan Y., Hu X. Abnormalities of peripheral blood system in patients with COVID-19 in Wenzhou, China. Clin Chim Acta. 2020;507:174-180.

[26] Henry BM, de Oliveira MHS, Benoit S, Plebani M, Lippi G. Hematologic, biochemical and immune biomarker abnormalities associated with severe illness and mortality in coronavirus disease 2019 (COVID-19): a meta-analysis. Clin Chem Lab Med. 2020 Jun 25;58(7):1021-1028. DOI: 10.1515/cclm-2020-0369.

[27] Terpos E, Ntanasis-Stathopoulos I, Elalamy I, Kastritis E, Sergentanis TN, Politou M, Psaltopoulou T, Gerotziafas G, Dimopoulos MA. Hematological findings and

complications of COVID-19 . Am J Hematol. 2020 Jul;95(7):834-847. DOI: 10.1002/ajh.25829.

[28] Tan L., Wang Q., Zhang D., Ding J., Huang Q., Tang Y.Q., Miao H. Lymphopenia predicts disease severity of COVID-19 : a descriptive and predictive study. Signal Transduct Target Ther. 2020;5:33.

[29] Tang N., Li D., Wang X., Sun Z. Abnormal coagulation parameters are associated with poor prognosis in patients with novel coronavirus pneumonia. J ThrombHaemost 2020;18(4):844-847.

[30] Huang C., Wang Y., Li X., Ren L., Zhao J., Hu Y., Zhang L., Fan G., Xu J., Gu X., Cheng Z., Yu T., Xia J., Wei Y., Wu W., Xie X., Yin W., Li H., Liu M., Xiao Y., Gao H., Guo L., Xie J., Wang G., Jiang R., Gao Z., Jin Q., Wang J., Cao B. Clinical features of patients infected with 2019 novel coronavirus in Wuhan, China. Lancet. 2020;395(10223): 497-506.

[31] Liu Y., Yang Y., Zhang C., Huang F., Wang F., Yuan J., Wang Z., Li J., Feng C., Zhang Z., Wang L., Peng L., Chen L., Qin Y., Zhao D., Tan S., Yin L., Xu J., Zhou C., Jiang C., Liu L. Clinical and biochemical indexes from 2019-nCoV infected patients linked to viral loads and lung injury. Sci China Life Sci.2020;63(3):364-374.

[32] Yang M., Ng M.H., Li C.K. Thrombocytopenia in patients with severe acute respiratory syndrome (review) Hematology. 2005;10(2): 101-105.

[33] Yang J., Yang M., Xu F., Li K., Lee S.K., Ng P.C., Tam J.S., Yuen P.M., Fok T.F. Effects of oxygen-induced lung damage on megakaryocytopoiesis and platelet homeostasis in a rat model. Pediatr Res. 2003;54(3):344-352.

[34] Driggin E, Madhavan MV, Bikdeli B, Chuich T, Laracy J, Biondi-Zoccai G, Brown TS, Der Nigoghossian C, Zidar DA, Haythe J, Brodie D, Beckman JA, Kirtane AJ, Stone GW, Krumholz HM, Parikh SA. Cardiovascular Considerations for Patients, Health Care Workers, and Health Systems During the COVID-19 Pandemic. J Am Coll Cardiol. 2020 May 12;75(18):2352-2371. DOI: 10.1016/j.jacc.2020.03.031.

[35] Ruan Q, Yang K, Wang W, Jiang L, Song J. Clinical predictors of mortality due to COVID-19 based on an analysis of data of 150 patients from Wuhan, China. Intensive Care Med. 2020 May;46(5):846-848. DOI: 10.1007/s00134-020-05991-x.

[36] Zhou F, Yu T, Du R, et al. Clinical course and risk factors for mortality of adult inpatients with COVID-19 in Wuhan, China: a retrospective cohort study. Lancet Mar 28 2020;395(10229):1054-62.

[37] Zhang H, Penninger JM, Li Y, Zhong N, Slutsky AS. Angiotensin-converting enzyme 2 (ACE2) as a SARS-CoV-2 receptor: molecular mechanisms and potential therapeutic target. Intensive Care Med Apr 2020;46(4):586-90.

[38] Libby P, Simon DI. Inflammation and thrombosis: the clot thickens. Circulation 2001;103:1718-20.

[39] Li B, Yang J, Zhao F, Zhi L, Wang X, Liu L, Bi Z, Zhao Y. Prevalence and impact of cardiovascular metabolic diseases on COVID-19 in China. Clin Res Cardiol. 2020 May;109(5):531-538. DOI: 10.1007/s00392-020-01626-9.

[40] Alhogbani T. Acute myocarditis associated with novel middle east respiratory syndrome coronavirus. Ann Saudi Med. 2016;36:78-80.

[41] Wang D, Hu B, Hu C, Zhu F, Liu X, Zhang J, Wang B, Xiang H, Cheng Z, Xiong Y, Zhao Y, Li Y, Wang X, Peng Z.

Clinical Characteristics of 138 Hospitalized Patients With 2019 Novel Coronavirus-Infected Pneumonia in Wuhan, China. JAMA. 2020 Mar 17;323(11):1061-1069. DOI: 10.1001/jama.2020.1585.

[42] Mokhtari T, Hassani F, Ghaffari N, Ebrahimi B, Yarahmadi A, Hassanzadeh G. COVID-19 and multiorgan failure: A narrative review on potential mechanisms. J Mol Histol. 2020 Dec;51(6):613-628. doi: 10.1007/s10735-020-09915-3. Epub 2020 Oct 4. PMID: 33011887; PMCID: PMC7533045.

[43] Liu K, Fang YY, Deng Y, Liu W, Wang MF, Ma JP, Xiao W, Wang YN, Zhong MH, Li CH, Li GC, Liu HG. Clinical characteristics of novel coronavirus cases in tertiary hospitals in Hubei Province. Chin Med J (Engl). 2020 May 5;133(9):1025-1031. DOI: 10.1097/CM9.0000000000000744.

[44] Xie Y, Wang X, Yang P, Zhang S. COVID-19 complicated by acute pulmonary embolism. Radiology: Cardiothoracic Imaging 2020;2(2):e200067.

[45] Danzi GB, Loffi M, Galeazzi G, Gherbesi E. Acute pulmonary embolism and COVID-19 pneumonia: a random association. Eur Heart J. 2020 May 14;41(19):1858. DOI: 10.1093/eurheartj/ehaa254.

[46] Helms J, Kremer S, Merdji H, Clere-Jehl R, Schenck M, Kummerlen C, Collange O, Boulay C, Fafi-Kremer S, Ohana M, Anheim M. Neurologic features in severe SARS-CoV-2 infection. New England Journal of Medicine. 2020 Jun 4;382(23):2268-70.

[47] Lechien JR, Chiesa-Estomba CM, De Siati DR, et al. Olfactory and gustatory dysfunctions as a clinical presentation of mild-to-moderate forms of the coronavirus disease (COVID-1919): a multicenter European study. Eur Arch Otorhinolaryngol 277.8 (2020): 2251-2261.

[48] Meinhardt J, Radke J, Dittmayer C, et al. Olfactory transmucosal SARS-CoV-2 invasion as a port of central nervous system entry in individuals with COVID-19 . Nat Neurosci. 2021;24(2):168-175. doi:10.1038/s41593-020-00758-5.

[49] Pun BT, Badenes R, Heras La Calle G, et al. Prevalence and risk factors for delirium in critically ill patients with COVID-19 : a multicentre cohort study [published correction appears in Lancet Respir Med. 2021 Jan 27;:]. Lancet Respir Med. 2021;9(3):239-250. doi:10.1016/S2213-2600(20)30552-X

[50] Kennedy M, Helfand BKI, Gou RY, Gartaganis SL, Webb M, Moccia JM, Bruursema SN, Dokic B, McCulloch B, Ring H, Margolin JD, Zhang E, Anderson R, Babine RL, Hshieh T, Wong AH, Taylor RA, Davenport K, Teresi B, Fong TG, Inouye SK. Delirium in Older Patients With COVID-19 Presenting to the Emergency Department. JAMA Netw Open. 2020 Nov 2;3(11):e2029540. DOI: 10.1001/jamanetworkopen.2020.29540.

[51] Varga Z, Flammer AJ, Steiger P, et al. Endothelial cell infection and endotheliitis in COVID-19 . *Lancet*. 2020;395(10234):1417-1418. DOI:10.1016/S0140-6736(20)30937-5

[52] Perry RJ, Smith CJ, Roffe C, et al. Characteristics and outcomes of COVID-19 associated stroke: a UK multicentre case-control study. J NeurolNeurosurg Psychiatry. 2021;92(3):242-248. DOI:10.1136/jnnp-2020-324927.

[53] Katsanos AH, Palaiodimou L, Zand R, et al. The Impact of SARS-CoV-2 on Stroke Epidemiology and Care: A Meta-Analysis. Ann Neurol.

2021;89(2):380-388. DOI:10.1002/ana.25967.

[54] Moriguchi T, Harii N, Goto J, et al. A first case of meningitis/encephalitis associated with SARS-Coronavirus-2. Int J Infect Dis. 2020;94:55-58. DOI:10.1016/j.ijid.2020.03.062

[55] Poyiadji N, Shahin G, Noujaim D, Stone M, Patel S, Griffith B. COVID-19 -associated Acute Hemorrhagic Necrotizing Encephalopathy: Imaging Features. Radiology. 2020;296(2): E119-E120. doi:10.1148/radiol.2020201187

[56] Chen X, Hu W, Ling J, et al. Hypertension and diabetes delay the viral clearance in COVID-19 patients. Europe PMC. 2020.DOI: 10.1101/2020.03.22.20040774

[57] Infection rate falling in Chennai, 12 Tamil Nadu districts. Times of India. April 19, 2020. Available from https://timesofindia.indiatimes.com/city/chennai/infection-rate-falling-in-chennai-12-tamil nadu-districts/articleshow/75229137.cms. 2020.

[58] Gupta N, Agrawal S, Ish P, Mishra S, Gaind R, Usha G, Singh B, Sen MK, COVID-19 Working Group SH. Clinical and epidemiologic profile of the initial COVID-19 patients at a tertiary care centre in India. Monaldi Arch Chest Dis. 2020 Apr 10;90(1). doi: 10.4081/monaldi.2020.1294. PMID: 32290644

[59] Yang JK, Lin SS, Ji XJ, Guo LM. Binding of SARS coronavirus to its receptor damages islets and causes acute diabetes. Acta Diabetol. 2009;47(3): 193-199.

[60] Bornstein SR, Rubino F, Khunti K, Mingrone G, Hopkins D, Birkenfeld A. Practical recommendations for the management of diabetes in patients with COVID-19 . Lancet Diabetes Endocrinol. 2020;8(6):546-550.

[61] Batlle D, Soler MJ, Ye M. ACE2 and diabetes: ACE2 of ACEs. Diabetes. 2010;59(12):2994-2996.

[62] Wang F, Wang H, Fan J, Zhang Y, Wang H, Zhao Q. Pancreatic injury patterns in patients with COVID-19 pneumonia. Gastroenterology. 2020;159(1):367-37.

[63] Carlsson PO, Berne C, Jansson L. Angiotensin II and the endocrine pancreas: effects on islet blood flow and insulin secretion in rats. Diabetologia. 1998;41(2):127-33.

[64] Guzman-Flores JM, Lopez-Briones S. Cells of innate and adaptive immunity in type-2 diabetes and obesity. Gac Med Mex. 2012;48(4): 381-9.

[65] Shu CJ, Benoist C, Mathis D, et al. The immune system's involvement in obesity-driven type 2 diabetes. Semin Immunol. 2012;24(6):436-42.

[66] Rajagopalan S. Serious infections in elderly patients with diabetes mellitus. Clin Infect Dis. 2005;40(7):990-6.

[67] Dooley KE, Chaisson RE. Tuberculosis and diabetes mellitus: convergence of two epidemics. Lancet Infect Dis. 2009;9(12):737-46.

[68] Badawi A, Ryoo SG. Prevalence of comorbidities in the Middle East respiratory syndrome coronavirus (MERS-CoV): a systemic review and meta-analysis. Int J Infect Dis. 2016;49:129-33.

[69] Guan WJ, Ni ZY, Hu Y, et al. Clinical characteristics of coronavirus disease 2019 in China. N Engl J Med 2020; 382: 1708-1720.

[70] Hamming I, Timens W, Bulthuis ML, Lely AT, Navis G, van Goor H. Tissue distribution of ACE2 protein, the functional receptor for SARS coronavirus. A first step in

understanding SARS pathogenesis. J Pathol Jun 2004;203(2):631-7.

[71] Mao R, Qiu Y, He JS, Tan JY, Li XH, Liang J, Shen J, Zhu LR, Chen Y, Iacucci M, Ng SC, Ghosh S, Chen MH. Manifestations and prognosis of gastrointestinal and liver involvement in patients with COVID-19 : a systematic review and meta-analysis. Lancet Gastroenterol Hepatol. 2020 Jul;5(7):667-678. DOI: 10.1016/S2468-1253(20)30126-6.

[72] Whitcroft KL, Hummel T. Olfactory Dysfunction in COVID-19-19: Diagnosis and Management. *JAMA*. 2020;323(24):2512-2514.

[73] Holshue ML, DeBolt C, Lindquist S, et al. First case of 2019 novel coronavirus in the United States. N Engl J Med 2020; 382: 929-936.

[74] Xiao F, Tang M, Zheng X, et al. Evidence for gastrointestinal infection of SARS-CoV-2. Gastroenterology 2020; 158:1831-1833.e3.

[75] Wang W, Xu Y, Gao R, et al. Detection of SARSCoV-2 in different types of clinical specimens. JAMA 2020; 323: 1843-1844.

[76] Jin X, Lian JS, Hu JH, Gao J, Zheng L, Zhang YM, Hao SR, Jia HY, Cai H, Zhang XL, Yu GD, et al. Epidemiological, clinical and virological characteristics of 74 cases of coronavirus-infected disease 2019 (COVID-19) with gastrointestinal symptoms. Gut. 2020 Jun;69(6):1002-1009. DOI: 10.1136/gutjnl-2020-320926.

[77] Pan L, Mu M, Yang P, Sun Y, Wang R, Yan J, Li P, Hu B, Wang J, Hu C, Jin Y, Niu X, Ping R, Du Y, Li T, Xu G, Hu Q, Tu L. Clinical Characteristics of COVID-19 Patients with Digestive Symptoms in Hubei, China: A Descriptive, Cross-Sectional, Multicenter Study. Am J Gastroenterol. 2020 May;115(5):766-773. DOI: 10.14309/ajg.0000000000000620.

[78] Genovese G, Moltrasio C, Berti E, Marzano AV. Skin Manifestations Associated with COVID-19 : Current Knowledge and Future Perspectives. Dermatology. 2021;237(1):1-12. DOI:10.1159/000512932.

[79] Galván Casas C, Català A, Carretero Hernández G, et al. Classification of the cutaneous manifestations of COVID-19 : a rapid prospective nationwide consensus study in Spain with 375 cases. Br J Dermatol. 2020;183(1):71-77. DOI:10.1111/bjd.19163.

[80] Gunawan C, Angela A, Widysanto A. Urticarial eruption in coronavirus disease 2019 infection: a case report in Tangerang, Indonesia. J Eur Acad Dermatol Venereol. 2020;34(8):e372-e373. DOI:10.1111/jdv.16622

[81] de Perosanz-Lobo D, Fernandez-Nieto D, Burgos-Blasco P, et al. Urticarial vasculitis in COVID-19 infection: a vasculopathy-related symptom?. J Eur Acad Dermatol Venereol. 2020;34(10):e566-e568. doi:10.1111/jdv.16713.

[82] Fernandez-Nieto D, Ortega-Quijano D, Jimenez-Cauhe J, *et al*. Clinical and histological characterization of vesicular COVID-19-19 rashes: a prospective study in a tertiary care hospital. Clin Exp Dermatol 2020; 45: 872– 875. https://doi.org/10.1111/ced.14277.

[83] Mawhirt SL, Frankel D, Diaz AM. Cutaneous Manifestations in Adult Patients with COVID-19 and Dermatologic Conditions Related to the COVID-19 Pandemic in Health Care Workers. Curr Allergy Asthma Rep. 2020 Oct 12;20(12):75. DOI: 10.1007/s11882-020-00974-w.

[84] Marraha, Farah & Faker, Ibtissam&Gallouj, Salim. (2020). A

Review of the Dermatological Manifestations of Coronavirus Disease 2019 (COVID-19). Dermatology Research and Practice. 2020.1-9. 10.1155/2020/9360476.

[85] Gottlieb M and Long B. Dermatologic manifestations and complications of COVID-19 . Am J Emerg Med. 2020;38(9):1715-1721. DOI:10.1016/j.ajem.2020.06.011.

[86] Hu Y, Sun J, Dai Z, et al. Prevalence and severity of corona virus disease 2019 (COVID-19): A systematic review and meta-analysis. J Clin Virol. 2020;127:104371. DOI:10.1016/j.jcv.2020.104371

[87] Lakhani J, Kapadia S, Pandya H, Gill R, Chordiya R, Muley A. Arterial blood gas analysis of critically ill coronavirus disease 2019 patients. AJRID. 2021;6(3):51-63.

[88] Lakhani JD, Chordiya R, Mota T, Trivedi S, Lakhani Sucheta J. Arterial blood gas analysis in patients of sepsis. International Journal of Pharmaceutical Research. 2020;(Supplementary Issue 1):370-378.

[89] Chhetri S, Khamis F, Pandak N, Al Khalili H, Said E, Petersen E. A fatal case of COVID-19 due to metabolic acidosis following dysregulate inflammatory response (cytokine storm). *IDCases.* 2020;21:e00829. DOI:10.1016/j.idcr

[90] Matthay MA, Zemans RL, Zimmerman GA, et al. Acute respiratory distress syndrome. Nat Rev Dis Prim. 2018 DOI: 10.1038/s41572-019-0069-0.

[91] Bao C, Liu X, Zhang H, et al. Coronavirus Disease 2019(COVID-19) CT findings: a systemic review and meta-analysis. J Am Coll Radiol. 2020;17(6):701-709.

[92] Lakhani, J. D., Pandya, H., Jain, A., &Ghadiya, S. (2020). Continuous Blood Glucose Monitoring to Determine the Glycemic Variability in Patients Having SARS CoV-2 Infection with ARDS and Its Bearing on the Severity of the Disease. Journal of Advances in Medicine and Medical Research, 32(16), 51-56. https://doi.org/10.9734/jammr/2020/v32i1630629.

[93] Jiang L, Tang K, Levin M, Irfan O, Morris SK, Wilson K, Klein JD, Bhutta ZA. COVID-19 and multisystem inflammatory syndrome in children and adolescents. Lancet Infect Dis. 2020 Nov;20(11):e276-e288. doi: 10.1016/S1473-3099(20)30651-4. Epub 2020 Aug 17. PMID: 32818434; PMCID: PMC7431129.

[94] Mehta P, McAuley DF, Brown M, et al. COVID-19 : consider cytokine storm syndromes and immunosuppression. Lancet. 2020;395(10229):1033-4.

[95] Huang KJ, Su IJ, Theron M, et al. An interferon-gamma-related cytokine storm in SARS patients. J Med Virol. 2005;75(2):185-94.

[96] Zhou J, Chu H, Li C, et al. Active replication of Middle East respiratory syndrome coronavirus and aberrant induction of inflammatory cytokines and chemokines in human macrophages: implications for pathogenesis. J Infect Dis. 2014;209(9):1331-42.

[97] CronR and BehrensEM. CytokineStormSyndrome.1ed. Cham:SpringerNature Switzerland AG; Springer International Publishing (2019).

[98] Tisoncik JR, Korth MJ, Simmons CP, Farrar J, Martin TR, Katze MG. Into the eye of the cytokine storm. Microbiol Mol Biol Rev. (2012) 76:16-32. DOI: 10.1128/MMBR.05015-11.

[99] Wang D, Hu B, Hu C, Zhu F, Liu X, Zhang J, et al. Clinical characteristics of 138 hospitalized patients with 2019 novel coronavirus-infected pneumonia

in Wuhan, China. JAMA. (2020) 323:1061-9. DOI: 10.1001/jama.2020.1585

[100] Ali N. Elevated level of C-reactive protein may be an early marker to predict risk for severity of COVID-19. J *Med Virol*. 2020;92(11):2409-2411. doi:10.1002/jmv.26097.

[101] Chen G, Wu D, Guo W, Cao Y, Huang D, Wang H, et al. Clinical and immunological features of severe and moderate coronavirus disease 2019. J Clin Invest. (2020) 130:2620-9. DOI: 10.1101/2020.02.16.20023903

[102] Chen L, Liu HG, Liu W, Liu J, Liu K, Shang J, et al. Analysis of clinical features of 29 patients with 2019 novel corona virus pneumonia.ZhonghuaJie He He Hu Xi Za Zhi. (2020) 43:203-8. DOI: 10.3760/cma.j.issn.1001-0939.2020.0005.

[103] Qin C, Zhou L, Hu Z, Zhang S, Yang S, Tao Y, Xie C, Ma K, Shang K, Wang W, Tian DS. Dysregulation of Immune Response in Patients With Coronavirus 2019 (COVID-19) in Wuhan, China. Clin Infect Dis. 2020 Jul 28;71(15):762-768. DOI: 10.1093/cid/ciaa248. Saravanan B, Vasuki S, Pabithadevi BM, Saradha M, Raskin Erusan R, S Alagesan S, Kalyanaraman S. D-dimer: A Marker of Severity in COVID-19 Journal of Clinical and Diagnostic Research. 2020 Nov, Vol-14(11): BC10-BC14

[104] Saravanan B, Vasuki S, Pabithadevi BM, Saradha M, Raskin Erusan R, S Alagesan S, Kalyanaraman S. D-dimer: A Marker of Severity in COVID-19 Journal of Clinical and Diagnostic Research. 2020 Nov, Vol-14(11): BC10-BC14

[105] Zhong-yong C, Wei-bin Y, Qiang W, Guo-lin L. Clinical significance of serum hs-CRP, IL-6, and PCT in diagnosis and prognosis of patients with COVID-19 . Drugs Clin. (2020) 35:417-20. DOI: 10.7501/j.issn.1674-5515.2020.03.005.

[106] Cao X. COVID-19 : immunopathology and its implications for therapy. Nat Rev Immunol. (2020) 269-70. DOI: 10.1038/s41577-020-0308-3.

[107] Channappanavar R, Perlman S. Pathogenic human coronavirus infections: causes and consequences of cytokine storm and immunopathology. Semin Immunopathol. (2017) 39:529-39. DOI: 10.1007/s00281-017-0629-x.

[108] Favalli EG, Ingegnoli F, De Lucia O, et al. COVID-19 infection and rheumatoid arthritis: Faraway, so close! Autoimmun Rev. 2020:102523.

[109] Chen R-C, Tang X-P, Tan S-Y, et al. Treatment of severe acute respiratory syndrome with glucosteroids: the Guangzhou experience. Chest. 2006;129(6):1441-52.

[110] Wu S-F, Chang C-B, Hsu J-M, et al. Hydroxychloroquine inhibits CD154 expression in CD4 T lymphocytes of systemic lupus erythematosus through NFAT, but not STAT5, signaling. Arthritis Res Ther. 2017;19(1):183.

[111] Zhang C, Wu Z, Li JW, Zhao H, Wang GQ. Cytokine release syndrome in severe COVID-19 : interleukin-6 receptor antagonist tocilizumab may be the key to reduce mortality. Int J Antimicrob Agents. 2020 May;55(5):105954. DOI: 10.1016/j.ijantimicag.2020.105954.

[112] Sinha P, Matthay MA, Calfee CS. Is a "Cytokine Storm" Relevant to COVID-19 ? *JAMA Intern Med*. 2020;180(9):1152-1154. doi:10.1001/jamainternmed.2020.3313

[113] Hamming I, Timens W, Bulthius M, et al. Tissue distribution of ACE2 protein, the functional receptor for SARS coronavirus. A first step in

understanding SARS pathogenesis. J Pathol. 2004;203:631-637.

[114] Quah P, Li A, Phua J: Mortality rates of patients with COVID-19 in the intensive care unit: A systemic review of the emerging literature. Crit Care 2020;24:285.

[115] Nedeva C, Menassa J, Puthalakath H: Sepsis: Inflammation is a necessary evil. Front Cell Dev Biol 2019; 7:108.

[116] Singer M, Deutschman CS, Seymour CW, et al: The Third International Consensus Definitions for sepsis and septic shock (sepsis-3). JAMA 2016; 315:801-810.

[117] Desai S, Lakhani JD. Utility of SOFA and APACHE II score in sepsis in rural set up MICU. J Assoc Physicians India. 2013 Sep;61(9):608-11. PMID: 24772695.

[118] Lin GL, McGinley JP, Drysdale SP, et al: Epidemiology and immune pathogenesis of viral sepsis. Front Immunol 2018; 9:2147.

[119] Ejaz H, Alsrhani A, Zafar A, Javed H, Junaid K, Abdalla AE, Abosalif KOA, Ahmed Z, Younas S. COVID-19 and comorbidities: Deleterious impact on infected patients. J Infect Public Health. 2020 Dec;13(12):1833-1839. DOI: 10.1016/j.jiph.2020.07.014.

[120] Yang J, Zheng Y, Gou X, Pu K, Chen Z, Guo Q, Ji R, Wang H, Wang Y, Zhou Y. Prevalence of comorbidities and its effects in patients infected with SARS-CoV-2: a systematic review and meta-analysis. Int J Infect Dis. 2020 May;94:91-95. DOI: 10.1016/j.ijid.2020.03.017.

[121] Guan WJ, Liang WH, Zhao Y, Liang HR, Chen ZS, Li YM, Liu XQ, Chen RC, Tang CL, Wang T, Ou CQ, Li L, Chen PY, Sang L, Wang W, Li JF, Li CC, Ou LM, Cheng B, Xiong S, Ni ZY, Xiang J, Hu Y, Liu L, Shan H, Lei CL, Peng YX, Wei L, Liu Y, Hu YH, Peng P, Wang JM, Liu JY, Chen Z, Li G, Zheng ZJ, Qiu SQ, Luo J, Ye CJ, Zhu SY, Cheng LL, Ye F, Li SY, Zheng JP, Zhang NF, Zhong NS, He JX; China Medical Treatment Expert Group for COVID-19 . Comorbidity and its impact on 1590 patients with COVID-19 in China: a nationwide analysis. Eur Respir J. 2020 May 14;55(5):2000547. DOI: 10.1183/13993003.00547-2020.

[122] Renu K, Prasanna PL, Valsala Gopalakrishnan A. Coronaviruses pathogenesis, comorbidities and multi-organ damage - A review. Life Sci. 2020;255:117839. DOI:10.1016/j.lfs.2020.117839.

[123] Jones G, Ding C. Tocilizumab: a review of its safety and efficacy in rheumatoid arthritis. Clin Med Insights Arthritis MusculoskeletDisord. 2010;3:81-89. Published 2010 Dec 19. DOI:10.4137/CMAMD.S4864.

[124] Chaudhry D, Singh PK. Tocilizumab and COVID-19 . Indian J Crit Care Med 2020;24(9):741-743.

[125] Scott LJ. Tocilizumab: a review in rheumatoid arthritis. Drugs 2017;77(17):1865-1879. DOI: 10.1007/s40265-017-0829-7.

[126] Mercuro NJ, Yen CF, Shim DJ, et al. Risk of QT Interval Prolongation Associated With Use of Hydroxychloroquine With or Without Concomitant Azithromycin Among Hospitalized Patients Testing Positive for Coronavirus Disease 2019 (COVID-19). *JAMA Cardiol.* 2020;5(9):1036-1041. DOI:10.1001/jamacardio.2020.1834

[127] van Paassen, J., Vos, J.S., Hoekstra, E.M. *et al.* Corticosteroid use in COVID-19 patients: a systematic review and meta-analysis on clinical outcomes. Crit Care 24, 696 (2020). https://doi.org/10.1186/s13054-020-03400-9.

Chapter 18

COVID-19 and Catastrophic Antiphospholipid Syndrome

Hisyovi Cardenas Suri, David Jimomila Bening and Benjamín Demah Nuertey

Abstract

One year after the beginning of the epidemic, mortality continues to be high despite several different protocols being tried. Critical patients with Covid 19 in some degree of organ failure and thrombotic events meet the diagnostic criteria of a complete or incomplete catastrophic antiphospholipid syndrome (CAPS) or at least we may need to consider a partial form of it. The findings of autopsies and the involvement of different organs and systems are similar to those of CAPS. Currently the only therapy that has been shown to reduce mortality include steroids, anti-coagulation and an antinuclear antibody. The same therapy has been shown to be effective for CAPS.

Keywords: COVID-19, multiorgan failure, thrombosis, antiphospholipid antibodies, catastrophic antiphospholipid antibodies syndrome

1. Introduction

After the COVID-19 outbreak in December 2019, a clinical picture was identified in most critical patients that was diagnosed as a cytokine storm associated with high mortality. Hypoxemia was also justified in those patients with severe ARDS who did not respond to the usual ventilation maneuvers such as a reflex of pulmonary hypoxic vasoconstriction, which subsequently lost value or there were no more reports in this regard when thrombosis of pulmonary microvasculature was demonstrated.

After more than a year the medical community has been fighting COVID-19 and having published a number of articles perhaps like never before talking about the same subject in such a short time. We continue with almost the same mortality and with many unanswered questions about the fatal presentation with other systemic manifestations of the disease in patients who develop a serious clinical picture [1].

Obesity, hypertension, diabetes mellitus, cancer, and other chronic diseases have been clearly identified as risk factors for developing severe disease with complications. Just as after large studies it has been shown that the use of steroids, anticoagulation and antinuclear antibodies considerably reduce mortality, being the only recommended treatment in critical patients. Antiviral treatment has been shown to help in 'converting' SAR-COV-2 virus positive patient into having a negative PCR result but has not been shown to modify mortality from the disease [2].

Severe and critical cases of COVID-19 generally present with multi-organ failure, evidence of thrombosis, marked elevation of ferritin, cytokine storm, some patients with DIC but this is generally not a frequent event in the final stages of the disease.

Since March 2020, upon seeing this clinical presentation that appeared suddenly with high mortality, we began to raise the possibility initially in The Lancet rheumatologic, later in Expert Review of Respiratory Medicine about the possibility of taking into account the diagnosis of Catastrophic Antiphospholipid Antibody Syndrome (CAPS). However despite several studies having been carried out, especially relating to the presence or absence of antinuclear antibodies in patients with COVID-19, we have not found any that has made this diagnosis even after meeting the criteria, much less has it been treated as such. However, drugs have been used in COVID-19 that have been shown to reduce mortality in that are part of the CAPS therapeutic arsenal, even in children with multisystemic inflammatory syndrome, immunoglobulins have been used with good results [3].

The presence of antiphospholipid antibodies have been reported in patients with COVID-19 with a percentage that ranges from 9–96% depending on severity of condition and the presence of thrombosis. Overall figures are around 54%, however, in few studies its presence is associated with failure of more than three organs, thrombosis, and even elevated ferritin which meets the criteria for making a diagnosis of CAPS [4].

Catastrophic Antiphospholipid Antibody Syndrome or Asherson's syndrome to honor Ronald A. Asherson for his impressive work on this condition was named in 1992 when catastrophic was added to define an accelerated form of the antiphospholipid syndrome (APS). CAPS is a rare phenomenon, according to the CAPS registry, it occurs in around 1% of all antiphospholipid syndromes, however, since it is a little-studied entity and at the same time little known by doctors, we infer that it is underdiagnosed [5].

2. Precipitating factors in CAPS

Infections
Postpartum or recent fetal loss
Minor surgical procedures or surgery
Other: malignancy, medication, anticoagulation withdrawal, and SLE exacerbation.

Although the pathogenesis of CAPS continues to be insufficiently understood, antiphospholipid (aPL) antibodies (Ab) belong to the immunoglobulin (Ig) family and are directed against phospholipid-binding plasma proteins such as Beta2 Glycoprotein1 (B2- GP1), prothrombin, annexin V, PS, PC, etc.

As a consequence of initial damage, anionic phospholipids would be exposed on the cell surface B2-GP1. If there are circulating anti-B2-GP1 Ab, they will bind to this complex, inducing cell activation with the release of tissue factor (TF), adhesion molecules, IL-8, C3b, C5a, among others, such as the activation of leukocytes and platelets. This increases their adhesion to the vascular endothelium, promoting microthrombosis and promoting the release of proteases and free radicals. Multiple vascular occlusion triggers necrosis tissue with excessive release of cytokines. A present marker is ferritin, which is elevated in 71% of CAPS patients and according to a recent study could play a role in the pathogenesis of APS and as a follow-up marker in CAPS [6, 7].

Kitchen postulates that vascular occlusion triggers additional thrombosis ("thrombotic storm"), which leads to increased thrombin and decreased fibrinolysis. As her son proposes the theory of "molecular mimic-cry" (molecular imitation), where on one hand the anti-B2-GP1 Ab when bound to the B2-GP1 of the endothelial cell generate a procoagulant state and on the other hand, certain viruses and bacteria that have an amino acid sequence similar to that of B2-GP1. This therefore favors the synthesis of more Ab. Furthermore, B2-GP1 could activate the immune response through interaction with a membrane receptor TLRs (toll-like) and from this a series of signals are generated, which increase the production of proinflammatory cytokines (TNF, IL-1B, IL-6, IL.8) and FT, PAI-1, PAF, etc. leading to multi-organ failure [8].

3. The criteria for the classification of catastrophic antiphospholipid antibody syndrome

1. Evidence of involvement of three or more organs, systems, or tissues.

2. Development of manifestations simultaneously or in less than a week.

3. Confirmation by histopathology of small-vessel occlusion in at least one organ or tissue.

4. Laboratory confirmation of the presence of antiphospholipid antibodies (lupus anticoagulant or anticardiolipin antibodies) [5].

4. Probable catastrophic antiphospholipid antibody syndrome

1. All four criteria, except only two organs, systems, or tissues are involved

2. All four criteria, except for the absence of laboratory confirmation at least 6 weeks apart because of the early death of a patient never previously tested for aPL before the catastrophic event.

3. Criteria 1, 2, and 4

4. Criteria 1, 3, and 4, and the development of a third event in more than a week, but less than a month, despite anticoagulation.

There are several reports during this pandemic where a high incidence of antiphospholipid antibodies has been demonstrated in patients with COVID-19. In addition, multiorgan failure and the presence of microthrombosis in critical patients have been associated with cytokine storm and the elevated ferritin. From the first reports in Wuhan, elevated ferritin was identified as a marker of severity in critically ill patients with COVID-19. Four well-recognized clinical conditions may be associated with high ferritin levels: the macrophage activation syndrome (MAS), adult-onset Still's disease (AOSD), catastrophic antiphospholipid syndrome (CAPS), and septic shock. The presentation of critical patients with COVID-19 does not meet the criteria to make a diagnosis of any of these diseases, however, they do meet the criteria to make the diagnosis of complete or incomplete CAPS [9, 10].

However a study by the American society of Hematology (ASH) in which they performed an antiphospholipid antibody (aPL) screen in 27 patients with COVID-19. Only four of these patients were positive for lupus anticoagulant. None of these patients were positive for anticardiolipin or anti-β-2 glycoprotein I antibodies. Given the fact that antiphosholipid antibodies may transiently be elevated during acute infections, thrombosis or inflammation, the American Society of Hematology has strongly recommended against routinely testing for these antibodies (aPL) in COVID-19 patients unless clinically indicated by the history.

It is however important to note that most studies that have been published in this regard do not report findings specific for critical patients with COVID-19. Inclusion criteria have been more generalized targeting patients with COVID-19. This could lead to recording lower positivity rate for aPL antibodies. Also, most of these studies have only tested specifically for lupus anticoagulant which is the least sensitive among the different types of antiphospholipid antibodies which could be positive among this group [11].

This recently led Amezcua-Guerra et al. to test a panel of aPL antibodies in blood specimens from 21 patients hospitalized in the intensive care unit due to severe or critical COVID-19. Anticardiolipin, anti-β2 glycoprotein I, antiprothrombin, antiphosphatidylserine, antiphosphatidylinositol and antiannexin V antibodies were measured, each in IgM and IgG isotypes. Subsequently, demographic and clinical data were obtained from electronic medical records. Samples (sera) collected before the SARS-CoV-2 pandemic from 12 healthy individuals, matched for age and sex, were tested as controls. A total of 19 patients (90%) had dyspneoa while on admission, 57% eventually required mechanical ventilation (invasive) during their stay in the hospital. All of these patients had elevated levels of D-dimer, ferritin and C reactive protein at time of presentation.

Out of the 21 patients with COVID-19, 12 of them tested positive for at least one aPL antibody with only 1 of the 12 controls yielding a positive result. Age and number of comorbidities tended to be lower in patients with aPL antibodies. In contrast, levels of D-dimer, ferritin and C reactive protein were higher both on admission and throughout the hospital stay in the patients. Patients who were positive for aPL demonstrated elevated levels of interleukin-6 (>40 pg./mL) [12].

Interestingly, significant levels of circulating anticardiolipin and anti-β-2glycoprotien I antibodies have recently been described in three severely ill COVID-19 patients with multiple cerebral infarctions by Zhang et al. This is suggestive that coagulopathy associated with COVID-19 could be within or close to the spectrum of antiphospholipid syndrome. A higher-than-expected number of thrombotic episodes have been reported involving both veins and arteries (pulmonary thromboembolism, deep venous thromboses, myocardial infarction and stroke even with the use of anticoagulant therapy or prophylaxis [13].

It is now established that vascular changes are well associated with COVID-19. Formation of fibrin thrombi has been observed in some patients. Many patients with severe illness have shown elevated levels of D-Dimers with other clinically relevant findings suggesting thrombotic microangiopathy such as cutaneous changes in the limbs. Autopsy finding of four out of seven patients with COVID-19 showed that thrombi were consistently present in all pulmonary vessels with a diameter of 1 mm- 2 mm. Also, microthrombi were 9 times more likely to be found in the alveolar capillaries of patients with COVID-19 than in patients with influenza [14].

5. Clinical manifestations of CAPS

Renal (70%): usually accompanied by hypertension and acute renal failure.

Pulmonary (65%): severe dyspnea, frank adult respiratory distress syndrome (ARDS), pulmonary emboli, sometimes multiple pulmonary infarction, interstitial infiltrates, and intraalveolar hemorrhage.

Central nervous system (55%): major cerebral infarctions, cerebral sinus thrombosis, encephalopathy and seizures.

Cardiac (50%): typical myocardial infarction, diffuse myocardial involvement with congestive heart failure or valve lesions.

Gastrointestinal (45%): vascular occlusions of mesenteric, portal and inferior vena cava, arterial occlusions accompanied by gangrene of the bowels and splenic infarctions, hepatic involvement and pancreatitis.

Skin (40–45%): livedo reticularis, ulcerations, gangrene, purpura, acrocyanosis or digital ischemia.

Other manifestations: adrenal thrombosis, testicular infarction, necrosis of the prostate gland [7].

The clinical manifestations are described in multiple reports during the coronavirus pandemic including skin involvement, so we believe, according to the evidence, that a high percentage of critically ill patients meet the diagnostic criteria of this entity.

Coagulation disorders were initially thought to be due to diseminated intravascular coagulopathy (DIC), but with the current evidence from all autopsies it has been shown to be due to a procoagulant phenomenon together with a severe inflammatory state. These findings may explain the events of venous thromboembolism observed in some of these patients and support antithrombotic prophylaxis/treatment. The cumulative incidence of thrombotic complications (mostly PE) is high between 25 and 30%.

The incidence of cerebral thrombosis in two weeks is almost 10 times higher in patients with COVID-19 than in the normal population in patients under 50 years of age. In a report of 3 patients with ischemic stroke the association with antiphosphilipid antibodies was 100% [15, 16].

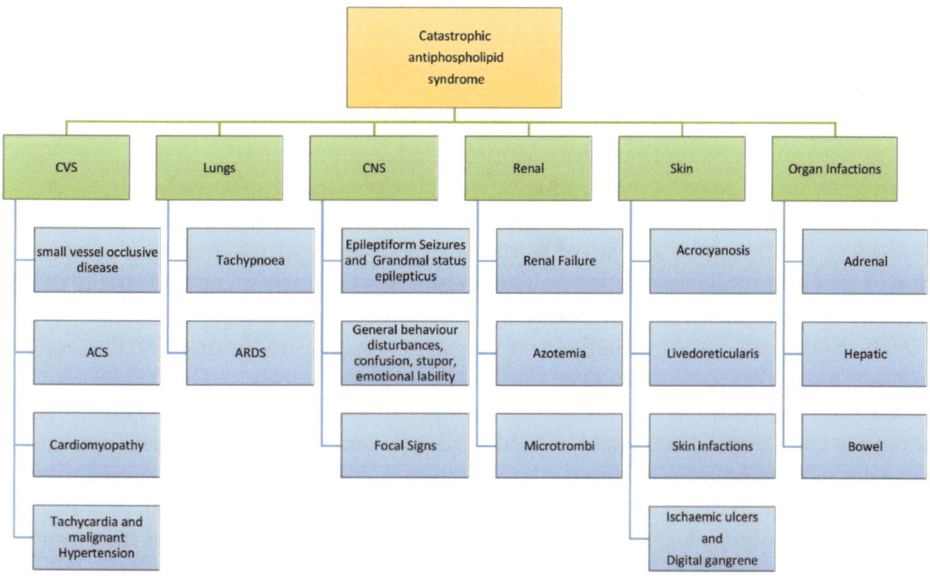

This multisystem inflammatory syndrome is caused by cytokine activation [7]. Cytokines involved include tumor necrosis factor (TNF)-α, interleukin (IL)-1, IL-6, IL-18 and macrophage-migration inhibitory factor. These cytokines are responsible for acute lung inflammation via increasing neutrophil migration and lung vascular permeability, not only for ARDS but also for the cerebral edema, which may be a factor in the initial confusion and deterioration of consciousness in these patients, as well as myocardial dysfunction encountered.

In 6 autopsies performed in a hospital in France it was found that one patient presented a lymphocytic viral pneumonia that could be considered as type L. For five other patients with a phenotype H, the histologic pattern was an acute fibrinous and organizing pneumonia (AFOP), characterized by an extensive intra-alveolar fibrin deposition called fibrin "balls", rather than hyaline membranes. AFOP, a rare form of acute lung injury. This pattern differs from the diffuse alveolar damage (DAD) found in the classic ARDS by the fact that organizing intra alveolar fibrin constitutes the dominant histological finding in AFOP, especially in its subacute presentation by contrast to the fulminant presentation, is a cortico-sensitive pathology.

Kidney histopathology was examined in an autopsy series of 26 patients who died of respiratory failure secondary to COVID-19. All patients had evidence of acute tubular injury (of varying severity); a range of other histopathology findings, such as erythrocyte clusters and pigmented casts, were also present [17].

Myocardial involvement has been described since the first reports adding an increase in the incidence of ACS and arrhythmias in these patients. Reports vary 20–30% of myocardial involvement, even higher percentages of troponin elevation have been found as a marker of myocardial damage [18].

The slightly rarer skin manifestations in this entity, especially when it is secondary to an infectious process, have been reported in two articles, even during the autopsy of these patients with purpuric skin rash. The conclusions of this study were severe COVID-19 may define a type of catastrophic microvascular injury syndrome mediated by activation of complement pathways and an associated procoagulant state.

In the CAPS Registry, CAPS as the initial manifestation of antiphospholipid syndrome occurred in 86.6% of children with infections being the triggering factor in 60.9% of the cases. Cardiac involvement was present in 57.4% of children and included cardiac failure, heart valve lesions, lung 63%, skin 37% and gastrointestinal 17.4% [19, 20].

Infections in children are more frequent than adults, which have been shown to play a role in the theory of "molecular mimic-cry" (molecular imitation) where certain viruses and bacteria that have an amino acid sequence similar to that of B2-GP1 result in an immune response producing antiphospholipid antibodies. B2-GP1 could activate the immune response through interaction with a membrane receptor TLRs (toll-like) and from this a series of signals are generated, which increase the production of proinflammatory cytokines. The medical community recognizes the MIS but most do not agree with the diagnosis of kawassaki disease [16].

Given the data made available from the various studies mentioned earlier, we can say that there is some evidence that critically ill patients with COVID-19 are demonstrating a disease form that meets the criteria for making the diagnosis of complete catastrophic antiphospholipid antibodies syndrome, or at least showing a disease form that is within the spectrum of manifestation of this syndrome. CAPS registry was created in 2000. As of 2012 it had been updated with data from over 400 patients. Not much advancement has been made in the area of this poorly understood syndrome after that. This interesting phenomenon observed during this pandemic which has become the largest public health emergency in recent times calls for more research work in the area of Catastrophic antiphospholipid syndrome. More awareness is required in the medical community in this area [21–23].

Author details

Hisyovi Cardenas Suri[1*], David Jimomila Bening[1] and Benjamín Demah Nuertey[2]

1 ICU Department, Tamale Teaching Hospital, Tamale, Ghana

2 Public Health Department, Tamale Teaching Hospital, Tamale, Ghana

*Address all correspondence to: hisyovics@gmail.com

References

[1] Huang C, Wang Y, Li X, et al. Clinical features of patients infected with 2019 novel coronavirus in Wuhan, China [published correction appears in Lancet. 2020 Jan 30]. Lancet. 2020;395(10223): 497-506. doi:10.1016/S0140-6736(20) 30183-5

[2] Mehta P, McAuley DF, Brown M, et al. COVID-19: consider cytokine storm syndromes and immunosuppression. Lancet. 2020;395(10229):1033-1034. doi:10.1016/S0140-6736(20)30628-0

[3] Zhang Y, Xiao M, Zhang S, et al. Coagulopathy and Antiphospholipid Antibodies in Patients with Covid-19. N Engl J Med. 2020;382(17):e38. doi:10.1056/NEJMc2007575

[4] Helms J, et al. High risk of thrombosis in patients in severe SARS-CoV-2 infection: a multicenter prospective cohort study. Intensive Care Medicine. 2020; DOI: 10.1007/ s00134-020-06062-x

[5] Maria Laura Bertolaccini, OierAteka-Barrutia, and Munther A, Khamashta. Catastrophic Antiphospholipid Syndrome.En: Antiphospholipid Syndrome Handbook. London: Springer; 2010. 47-51.DOI 10.1007/978-1-84628-7

[6] Rossi Andrea. Catastrophic antiphospholipid síndrome. Hematologia. 2014;18 (1): 40-47.

[7] Bowles, L., S. Platton, et al. (2020). "Lupus Anticoagulant and Abnormal Coagulation Tests in Patients with Covid-19." New England Journal of Medicine.

[8] Espinosa G, Cervera R, Asherson RA. Catastrophic antiphospholipid syndrome and sepsis. A common link? J Rheumatol. 2007;34:923-926.

[9] Rosário C, Porat Katz BS et al. Catastrophic antiphospholipid syndrome. HEMATOLOGÍA • Volumen 18 N° 1: 40-47, 2014 2013; 0: 1-9.

[10] Palacios MP y cols. Tormenta trombótica. AnMed (Mex). 2018; 63 (4): 299-305

[11] Panigada M, Bottino N, Tagliabue P, et al. Hypercoagulability of COVID-19 patients in Intensive Care Unit. A Report of Thromboelastography Findings and other Parameters of Hemostasis [published online ahead of print, 2020 Apr 17]. J ThrombHaemost. 2020;10.1111/ jth.14850. doi:10.1111/jth.14850

[12] Castillo-Martínez D, Torres Z, Amezcua-Guerra LM, Pineda C. Are antiphospholipid antibodies just a common epiphenomenon or are they causative of immune-mediated coagulopathy in COVID-19? Clin Rheumatol. 2021 Apr 7:1-5. doi: 10.1007/ s10067-021-05724-5. Epub ahead of print. PMID: 33826045; PMCID: PMC8024929.

[13] Thomas J, et al. Large-Vessel Stroke as a Presenting Feature of Covid-19 in the Young. n engl j med. 2020: e60. DOI: 10.1056/NEJMc2009787

[14] Middeldorp, S.; Coppens, M.; van Haaps, TF; Foppen, M.; Vlaar, AP; Muller, MC; Bouman, CC; Beenen, LF; Kootte, RS; Heijmans, J.; Smits, LP; Bonta, PI; van Es, N. Incidencia de tromboembolismo venoso en pacientes hospitalizados con COVID-19. Preprints 2020, 2020040345 (doi: 10.20944 / preprints202004.0345.v1).

[15] Cervera, R. Update on the Diagnosis, Treatment, and Prognosis of the Catastrophic Antiphospholipid Syndrome. Curr Rheumatol Rep 12, 70-76 (2010). https://doi.org/10.1007/ s11926-009-0073-6

[16] Zhang Y, Xiao M, Zhang S, et al. Coagulopathy and Antiphospholipid

Antibodies in Patients with Covid-19. N Engl J Med. 2020;382(17):e38. doi:10.1056/NEJMc2007575

[17] Copin, M., Parmentier, E., Duburcq, T. et al. Time to consider histologic pattern of lung injury to treat critically ill patients with COVID-19 infection. Intensive Care Med. 2020.https://doi.org/10.1007/s00134-020-06057-8

[18] Hua Su, et al. Renal histopathological analysis of 26 postmortem findings of patients with COVID-19 in China. Kidney Int. 2020. https://doi.org/10.1016/j.kint.2020.04.003

[19] Tao Guo, Yongzhen Fan, Ming Chen, et al. Cardiovascular Implications of Fatal Outcomes of Patients With Coronavirus Disease 2019 (COVID-19). JAMA Cardiol. 2020. doi:10.1001/jamacardio.2020.1017

[20] Magro C, Mulvey JJ, Berlin D, et al. Complement associated microvascular injury and thrombosis in the pathogenesis of severe COVID-19 infection: a report of five cases [published online ahead of print, 2020 Apr 15]. Transl Res. 2020;S1931-5244(20)30070-0. doi:10.1016/j.trsl.2020.04.007.

[21] Betancur, J., Navarro, E., Echeverry, A. et al. Hyperferritinemic syndrome: Still's disease and catastrophic antiphospholipid syndrome triggered by fulminant Chikungunya infection: a case report of two patients. Clin Rheumatol 34, 1989-1992 (2015). https://doi.org/10.1007/s10067-015-3040-9

[22] Ackermann M, Verleden SE, Kuehnel M, Haverich A, Welte T, Laenger F, Vanstapel A, Werlein C, Stark H, Tzankov A, Li WW, Li VW, Mentzer SJ, Jonigk D. Pulmonary Vascular Endothelialitis, Thrombosis, and Angiogenesis in Covid-19. N Engl J Med. 2020 Jul 9;383(2):120-128. doi: 10.1056/NEJMoa2015432. Epub 2020 May 21. PMID: 32437596; PMCID: PMC7412750.

[23] Amezcua-Guerra LM, Rojas-Velasco G, Brianza-Padilla M, Vázquez-Rangel A, Márquez-Velasco R, Baranda-Tovar F, Springall R, Gonzalez-Pacheco H, Juárez-Vicuña Y, Tavera-Alonso C, Sanchez-Muñoz F, Hernández-Salas M. Presence of antiphospholipid antibodies in COVID-19: case series study. Ann Rheum Dis. 2020 Aug 4:annrheumdis-2020-218100. doi: 10.1136/annrheumdis-2020-218100. Epub ahead of print. PMID: 32753426.

Section 3

Diagnosis and Management

Chapter 19

Fighting COVID-19: The Medical Laboratory Involvement

Obeta M. Uchejeso, Jwanse I. Rinpan, Mantu E. Chongs and Maureen O. Ekpere-Ezeugwu

Abstract

The coronavirus disease-19 (COVID-19) virus has infected many people across the globe. The health system particularly medical laboratory has been overwhelmed by the pandemic, and many health professionals including medical laboratory professionals have lost their lives during the fight against the virus. Medical laboratory science is the bedrock of medical practice and the role of medical laboratory science in containing the COVID-19 pandemic cannot be overemphasized as they are also behind the testing of clinical specimens from infected and any recovered patients. As disease detectives, Medical laboratory scientists and other medical laboratory professionals' role in the fight against the COVID-19 pandemic include; diagnosis, monitoring, development of vaccines, testing protocols, testing kits, offering advice to the guide government policy on containment of the virus.: Various methods and techniques such as virological cell culture, genomic sequencing, amplification, polymerase chain reaction (PCR) /gene Xpert systems, immunological testing, biosensors and rapid diagnostic techniques (RDTs) have been employed towards discovery, testing and epidemiology since the onset of COVID-19. The medical laboratory workers and other health workers are so visible at the COVID-19 frontline and are being recognized and applauded for the role played in the recovery of patients affected with the virus. The medical laboratory component is very germane in the COVID-19 vaccine research and vaccination so as to provide pre- and post-vaccination laboratory data.

Keywords: COVID-19, laboratory testing, medical laboratory, involvements, interventions, technologies, medical laboratory scientists

1. Introduction

Medical laboratory is a very important component in public health practice and operation especially in case of COVID-19. Medical Laboratory Science practice involves the analysis of human specimen like body fluids, excretion and various body swabs for the purpose of medical laboratory diagnosis, treatment and research [1] of which coronavirus is the one under study. It is important to note that medical laboratory science can also be called Clinical Laboratory Science or Medical Laboratory Technology depending on the nomenclature in the countries of practice [2].

The historical trend of COVID-19 pandemic [3–6] has adequately placed medical laboratory services in a very critical aspect in containment of the disease across the globe. The medical laboratories play a critical role in the detection, management, disease surveillance and control in provision of accurate health data for national planning and decision making and COVID-19 is not an exception. Timely access and geographical availability of COVID-19 diagnostic testing remains a challenge in the health system and could affect ongoing containment measures [7] for the COVID-19.

The first medical diagnosis made by humans were done by ancient scientists through observation with their physical senses. The ancient Greek attributed all diseases to disorders of bodily fluids called humors, and during late medieval period, then later with the advent of microscope, the microscopy procedure on such specimens have revealed more [8] followed by later technologies, automations, sophistications and molecular testing in the current age.

This chapter shall review the medical laboratory involvement and intervention during COVID-19 era and the ongoing efforts towards supporting laboratory surveillance and response to COVID 19. It will equally show the capacity of medical laboratory perspectives in COVID-19 and provide more information on the medical laboratory testing strategy, towards developing and managing sudden capacities for testing relevant specimens at all levels of health system. Also, the approaches for ensuring laboratory testing sustainability in identifying new and suitable methods consistent with maximizing testing reagents, mobilizing human resources and guide towards implementation of public health measures towards COVID-19 containment, while exploring the recognition and protection policies for medical laboratory professionals during COVID-19 shall be presented.

2. Importance of medical laboratory during pandemic and public health issues

Obeta et al. [1] highlighted some importance of medical laboratory in public health matters to include rapid, accurate and prompt diagnosis for proper treatment and effective monitoring of patients' response to treatment. Medical laboratory provides up to 70% informed decisions regarding patients' hospital admissions and discharge. It guides physicians, nurses and other healthcare workers in choosing the correct laboratory tests and ensure the proper sample collection. Medical laboratory services equally carry out equipment installation, validation and repay in the healthcare laboratories. Medical laboratory component is key in infectious diseases surveillance like Ebola, Tuberculosis, HIV, Malaria and now COVID-19. Quality assurance of a healthcare facility and public health in general is made possible by medical laboratory research towards quality improvement.

Researches [1, 8–10] have shown the main functions of medical laboratory during the COVID-19 pandemic to include the following:

- Establishing appropriate accurate, and sustainable diagnostic testing capacities to respond to COVID-19 needs

- Ensuring surge (sudden) capacity to process a large volume of specimens to cope with COVID-19 epidemiological response needs.

- Conducting virological monitoring of the pandemic at local, state, national, regional and global levels.

- Ensuring timely release of laboratory data and linking data with surveillance data to inform public health decision making and response activities.

- Tracking the genetic evolution of COVID-19 and contributing in research and development of vaccines by characterization of viruses

To achieve adequate COVID-19 monitoring and surveillance, there is need for widespread and continuous testing of not only suspected cases or contacts, but even asymptomatic and apparently healthy population in order to achieve adequate COVID-19 trend monitoring in context of rapid human-to-human spread, and prompt identification of cases.

Undoubtedly, there are many benefits of large-scale population testing for COVID-19 as demonstrated in many high-income countries. For countries that have numerous challenges in their health care delivery system in terms of medical laboratory diagnostics, house-to-house case searching and community contact tracing for infectious diseases surveillance is adequate.

Medical Laboratory plays a crucial role in monitoring co-morbidities, diagnosing complications, assessment of treatment responses and assessing the disease prevalence in the community. Advancement of molecular techniques is mainly relying on understanding the genomic and proteomic composition of COVID-19.

WHO [5, 7] emphasizes "detect, protect and treat" to break the chain of transmission of SARS-COV-2 and COVID-19. Early medical laboratory testing and immediate treatment significantly decrease future COVID-19 cases. Medical laboratory assessment reveals diagnoses, confirms or rules out prognosis based on signs and symptoms, determines severity, monitors treatment responses or complications in COVID-19. The role of medical laboratories is more evident globally today as the battle against COVID-19 rages.

3. Medical laboratory and research towards discovery of COVID-19

On December 31, 2019, China alerted the WHO about the occurrence of several cases of an unusual pneumonia caused by an unknown virus among persons who had either visited or had consumed food from the live animal market in Wuhan city of China, the epicenter of the outbreak. Since then, the infection has spread to other Chinese cities as well as internationally, resulting in the current pandemic. On January 7, 2020, the WHO announced they had identified a new virus. The novel virus was named 2019-COV and was identified as member of the coronaviridae family which also includes SARS and MERS. China announced its first death from the virus on January 23, 2020 as rail and air departure were suspended on January 30, WHO declared the outbreak a global health emergency [4, 5, 7].

The medical laboratory has been duly involved and its involvement ranges from the discovery the pneumonia like virus to the description as SARS and MERS in nature, viral characterization and sequencing and the naming of the viral disease as new coronavirus and COVID-19 [11]. The role of the medical laboratory services from COVID-19 discovery to the management cannot be over emphasized.

4. Challenges and way forward for medical laboratory practice in COVID-19 era

There is no doubt that COVID-19 is new and so are the technologies for testing and research. COVID-19 era is filled with operational differences between the medical laboratory developed protocols and new commercial consumables protocols following the COVID-19 pandemic. However, the implementation of those new protocols is challenging and requires continuous training for the laboratory staff [12]. Another challenge is limited access to COVID -19 reagents. This restricted the number of testing of citizens to those that were having symptoms or at risk as there is fear of exhausting the limited COVID-19 reagents and consumables. In the testing proper, there is delayed

S/N	Challenges	Way forward
1	Misdiagnosis of COVID-19 due to poor training or use of quacks	Adequate training of qualified professionals
2	Poor working environment	Construct modern Medical Laboratory working environment
3	Poor working tools and equipment	Procure modern tools and equipment
4	Unstable power supply	Stabilize power supply and have a standby power supply or an alternative power
5	Poor team work among health professionals	Instill team spirit among practitioners
6	Lack of political will towards medical laboratory practices	Politicians should learn from COVID-19 lockdown to have the will to update medical laboratory facilities as they could be clients in such facilities
7	Corruption	Kill corruption surrounding COVID-19
8	Haphazard quality system	Standardize quality system
9	New technologies and technicalities associated with COVID-19	Imbibe new technologies and technicalities from the producers
10	Paucity of fund in COVID-19 laboratory services	Fund the medical laboratory services to the full with regards to COVID-19 and associated services
11	Unavailability of local testing kits	Give grant and fund research for production of local testing kits
12	Different countries have little no validated rapid kits	Mandate the regulatory bodies to validate more rapid kits to boost testing
13	Poor knowledge and research capacity	Encourage more research in laboratories
14	Non-involvement of medical laboratory component in COVID-19 vaccination	Involve medical laboratory component to give a basal parameter before vaccination and after some days of vaccination to assist in post vaccine research

Table 1.
Challenges and way forward for medical laboratory practice in COVID-19 era.

outbreak detection and reporting of COVID -19 cases maybe due to distance from testing and collection sites and the technicalities involved. Also there is limited access to clinically validated or regulatory approved molecular and serologic tests either through the WHO network, national regulators or through commercial manufacturers [13, 14].

As COVID-19 ravages the world, there are shortages and difficulties in importing large diagnostic kits in the country. There is also poor knowledge and research capacity on COVID-19. Aside from technical difficulties associated with COVID-19 testing, certain seasonal changes might equally affect the number of tests [9]. **Table 1** discusses the challenges and way forward towards offering COVID-19 medical laboratory services.

5. Medical laboratory methods, techniques and technologies applied for COVID-19 testing

The medical laboratory methods and technologies applied in testing COVID-19 includes: neutralization/virological cell culture test, COVID-19 genomic sequencing, nucleic acid testing (NAT) /amplification testing, polymerase chain reaction (PCR), real time PCR (RT- PCR) and Gene Xpert systems, immunological testing, biosensors, rapid diagnostic techniques (RDTs) [15]. These methods are illustrated in **Figure 1**.

Basically, virological cell culture test is the gold standard for virus discovery, pathogenesis research and strategy evaluation but since the emergence of COVID-19, PCR has been adopted as the gold standard and has been in use globally considering the shorter turnaround time. Genomic sequencing uses sophistication to track the

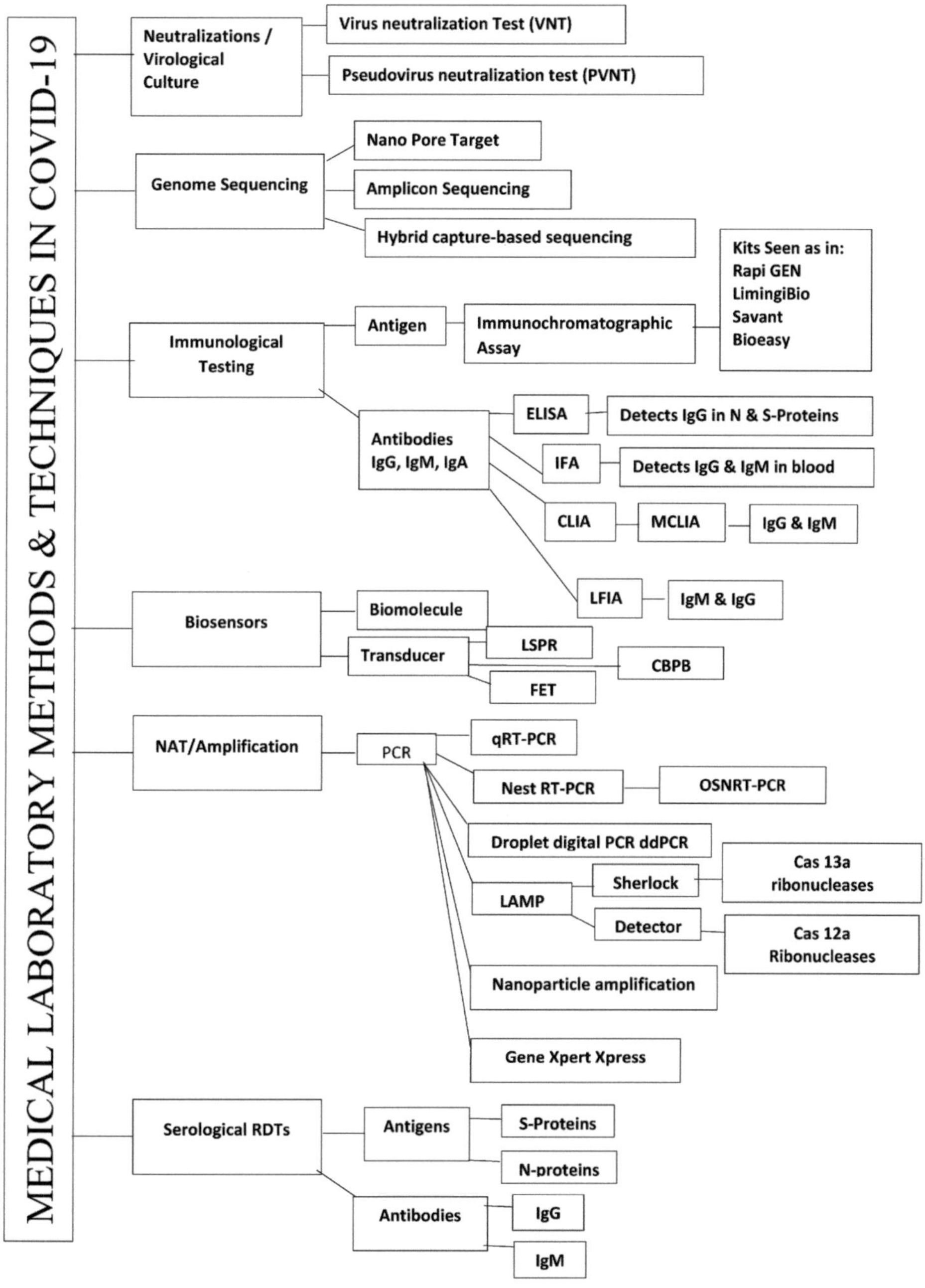

Figure 1.
Diagnostic methods and technologies employed in COVID-19 testing. KEY: CBPB, cell-based potentiometric biose; CLIA, Chemiluminescence immunoassay; ddPCR, droplet digital PCR; E-gene, envelope protein gene; ELISA, enzyme-linked immunosorbent assay; FET, field effect transistor; IFA, Immunoflorescence assay; LAMP, loop mediated isothermal amplification; LFIA, lateral flow immunoassay; LSPR, localized surface plasmon resonance (sensor); MCLIA, magnetic Chemiluminescence enzyme immunoassay; M, membrane protein gene; N-gene, Nucleocapsid protein gene; NAT, nucleic acid testing; PCR, polymerase chain reaction; ORF, open reading frame; OSN-qRT, PCR - one step nested RT-PCR; qRT-PCR, real-time quantification PCR; RDT, rapid diagnostic technique; RdRp, RNA-dependent RNA polymerasegene; S, spike proteins.

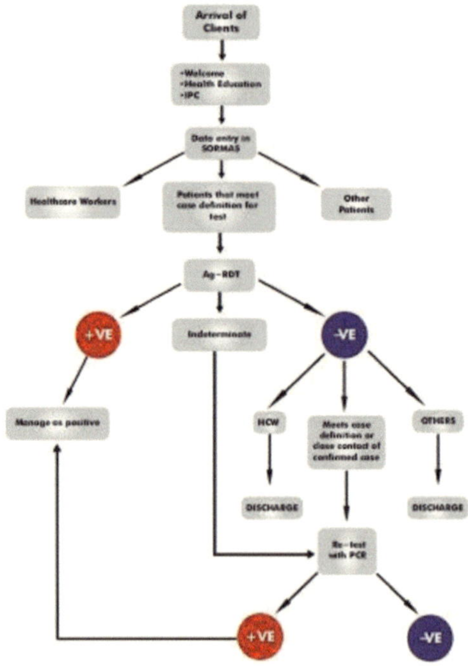

Figure 2.
NCDC medical laboratory testing algorithm in Nigeria while using RDTs.

pandemic and aids vaccine development [16]. Immunological testing is based on the quantification and detection of antigen and antibody interactions. Biosensors use selectivity features of a bimolecular and sensitivity of physiochemical transducers in COVID-19 testing. Rapid Diagnostic Techniques (RDTs) are new technologies which apply some of the above mentioned techniques to achieve shortest turnaround time and accessibility. Although each method has its advantages and disadvantages, it is advisable to employ at least two methods [15, 17–19] for quality medical laboratory testing especially when using RDTs as shown in **Figure 2**.

6. Medical laboratory interventions in COVID-19

As part of the global response to the COVID-19 pandemic, medical laboratory diagnosis has remained the corner stone to this intervention. Molecular assays performed on nasopharyngeal swab or other upper respiratory tract specimen are the most commonly used and reliable test for the diagnosis of COVID-19. A variety of RNA gene targets are used by different molecular assays.

The processes from sample collections, sample transport and actual testing for COVID-19 remains very important including all quality system measures put in place to ensure reliability and sensitivity. The medical laboratory research uses samples from nasopharyngeal swabs, oropharyngeal swabs, throat swabs, saliva, sputum, bronchoalveolar lavage fluid, conjunctival swabs, rectal swabs, whole blood, serum/plasma, stool, and urine [15].

It is evident that medical laboratory parameters have been adequately employed to access diagnosis like increased neutrophil, aspartate aminotransferase, alanine aminotransferase, C-reactive protein, lactate dehydrogenase and urea. There is also decrease in procalcitonin, albumin, and white blood cells like leukocytes, and lymphopenia and eosinopenia have been noted among COVID-19 patients. Also, medical laboratory parameters have been employed in the assessment of the severity of the COVID-19 such as interleukin-6 (IL-6), d-dimer (d-D), glucose, fibrinogen, thrombin time, and C-reactive protein and fibrinogen. Some parameters are predictors during prognosis like IL-6 and D-Dimer, absolute lymphocyte count, lactate dehydrogenase, creatine kinase and absolute monocyte count which can predict whether the patient can be admitted into intensive care unit or not. During treatment, laboratory parameters are used to assess improvement in treatment and complications. For example; reduction in aspartate aminotransferase, alanine aminotransferase, creatine kinase and dehydrogenase shows response to treatment while increased procalcitonin and C-reactive protein indicates liver abnormality, high D-dimer, fibrinogen, prothrombin time predicts thromboembolism and new-onset renal failure [17, 20].

A medical laboratory, irrespective of location, modern, sophisticated or molecular in nature in the aspect of COVID-19 fight, has a huge role to play especially in the local certain where COVID19 testing has not reached. Many in such area may not know their status and no wonder the presence of a knowledgeable Scientist shall corroborate the medical laboratory implications of COVID-19 to be able to approach every client and sample in a safe and professional way.

There is always a manual that help members, states and partners as they set up comprehensive quality assurance measures for COVID-19 testing laboratory network. The guidance emphasizes the use of standardized registration formats as quality tool, Quality control (QC), enrollment of laboratories in external quality assessment (EQA) schemes and issues of external quality assessment performance data for continuous quality improvement of COVID-19 testing laboratories. It is an essential resource for a medical laboratory personnel to be involved in day-to-day testing of COVID-19.

Figures 2 and **3** shows testing Algorithm for Nigeria while using RDTs and approved medical laboratories (75–25 Gene Xpert and 50 PCR Labs) for COVID-19 respectively as released by Nigeria Centre for Disease Control (NCDC).

In medical laboratory testing of COVID-19, each country adopts their protocol based on targeted proteins as it suits them based on available testing techniques and methodology and as well the laboratory set ups and environment. For instance,

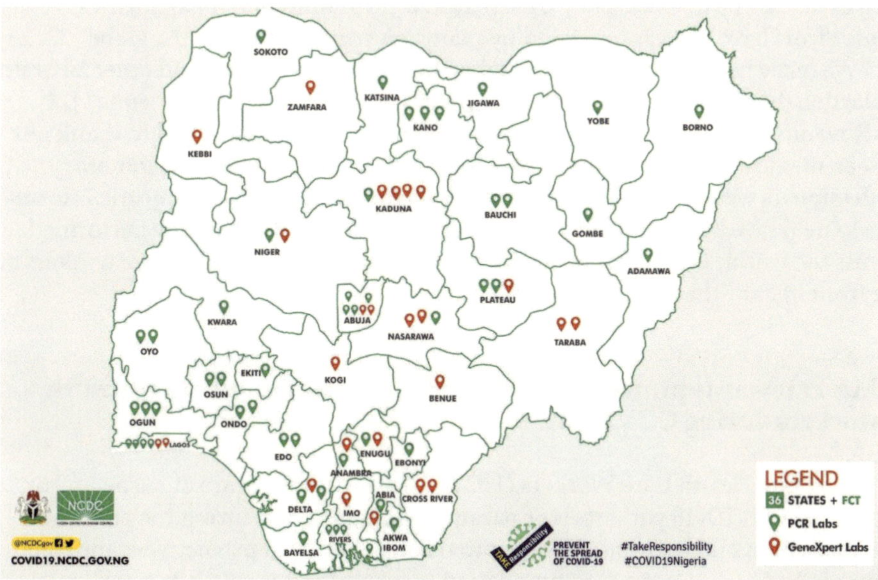

Figure 3.
NCDC approved medical laboratories for COVID-19 as at 23rd February, 2021.

USA protocol for testing targets N (N1, N2, N3) genes and Rp-RNase; China targets ORF 1ab and N-genes, Nigeria targets N-genes and ORF 1ab; Germany RdRp, E and N-genes, Japan and Thailand targets N-genes while Hong Kong targets ORF 1b-nsp-14 and N-genes [15, 17].

7. Recognition of medical laboratory professionals during COVID-19

The world biomedical day of 2020 awareness was solely dedicated to medical laboratory professionals across the globe because of their unique role in COVID-19.

In Nigeria and other countries, the emphasis on Testing is more of the recognition of the medical laboratories and professionals who toil to discover, test, monitor and research further towards COVID-19 elimination. Usually, medical laboratory professionals are not noticed for their great contribution to healthcare. They are rarely seen by people for their heroic contribution to patients' healthcare but cannot be underestimated as they perform series of tests that are crucial to ensuring accurate diagnosis and treatments that can help save patients' lives.

Medical laboratory professionals play a critical role in the diagnostics and testing of COVID-19 which they perform every day. A collaborative committee of 17 medical organizations including American Society for Clinical Laboratory Science (ASCLS), Association of Medical Laboratory Scientists of Nigeria (AMLSN) and American Society of Microbiology (ASM) in the year 2020 helped to coordinate the celebration of annual Biomedical science day in April, 2020 to increase public understanding of and appreciation for clinical laboratory personnel as COVID-19 rages worldwide [21]. Such recognitions usually come from government, organizations or various individuals all over the world.

Laboratory professionals use specialized instruments and techniques to analyze patient samples, such as blood, urine, body fluids, tissues and stool. They may be in a laboratory located in the hospital where the patient may be hundreds of miles away in a reference laboratory, however, no matter their distance to the patient, they produce results that directly affect the patient care. In addition to their day to day activities, laboratory professionals tackle threats to our national security and health such as disease outbreaks. They have played critical roles in fight against COVID-19. These effort have been appreciated by many governments across the globe [22, 23].

"We really need to hail the pathologist, medical technologists, and other laboratory professionals who are becoming unsung heroes of the COVID-19 pandemic" [21].

Now more than ever, is the chance for people all round the world to thank our unseen medical laboratory heroes and heroines. Each year medical laboratory professional's week celebrates the people who provides critical diagnostic information to help save lives and shows appreciation for the vital work they performed. Across the world, everyday people are applauding the brave health care workers on the front lines of the COVID-19 pandemic.

8. Effort towards protection of medical laboratory and other health workers during COVID-19

Protecting Health Care Workers (HCWs) during routine care of suspected or confirmed COVID-19 patients is of paramount importance during the pandemic. The protection ranges from adequate provision of personal protective equipment to provision of temporary accommodation to carter for during testing and treatment of COVID-19 patients outside homes, Life insurance packages, Special Hazard Allowances and other allowances and Commencement of Vaccination among laboratory professionals/healthcare workers. In Nigeria, life insurance to medical laboratory scientists during the COVID-19 was given by the government through the Federal Ministry of Health (FMOH) as seen in **Figure 4** as a clarification that the profession is among the front line healthcare workers targeted in the programme.

Countries may differ in their approach to laboratory and healthcare workers protection and care during the COVID-19 as documented by several authors [24–30] and analyzed in **Table 2**. Such support may involve mental health support provided

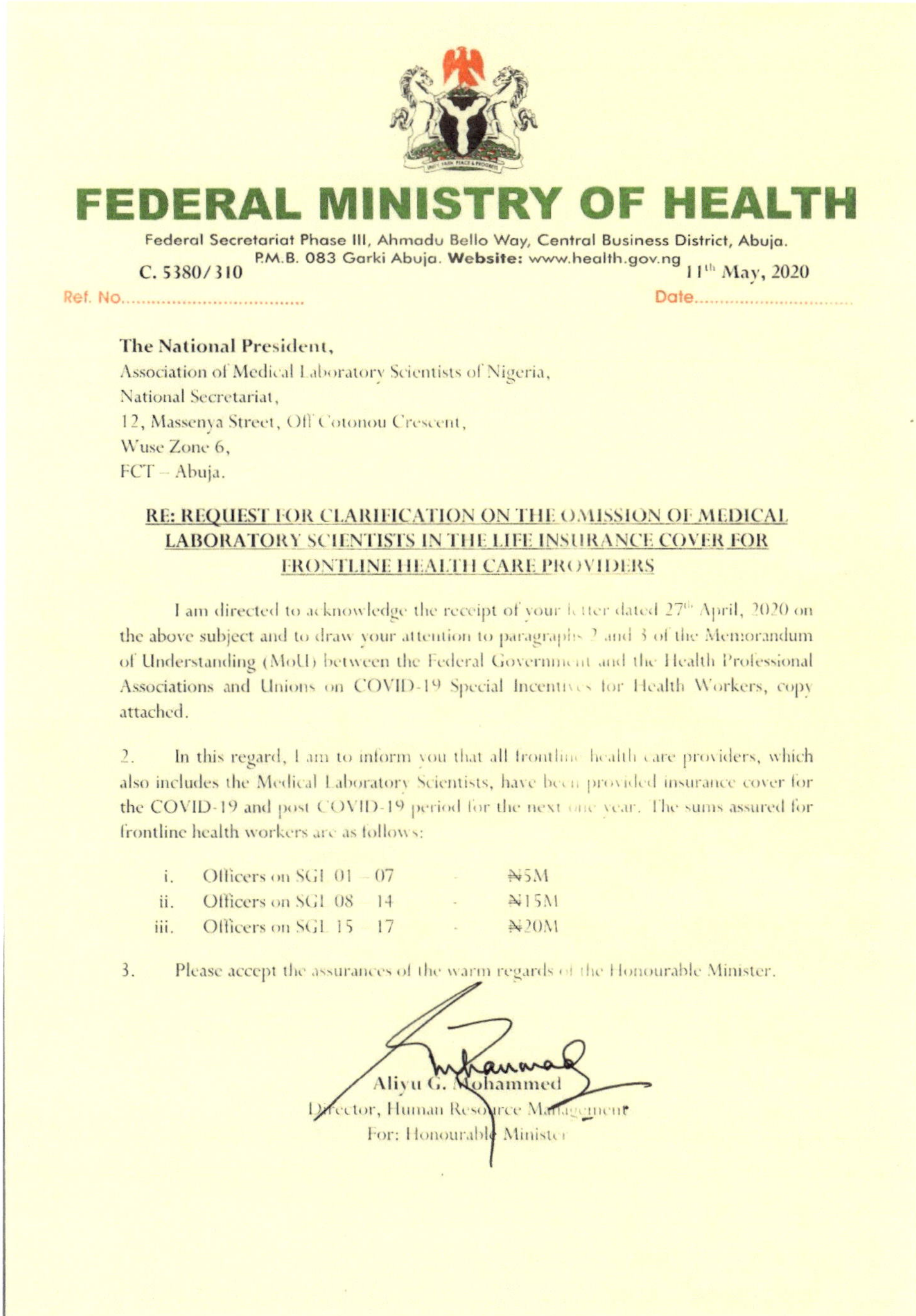

FEDERAL MINISTRY OF HEALTH

Federal Secretariat Phase III, Ahmadu Bello Way, Central Business District, Abuja.
P.M.B. 083 Garki Abuja. Website: www.health.gov.ng

Ref. No. C. 5380/310 — Date 11th May, 2020

The National President,
Association of Medical Laboratory Scientists of Nigeria,
National Secretariat,
12, Massenya Street, Off Cotonou Crescent,
Wuse Zone 6,
FCT – Abuja.

RE: REQUEST FOR CLARIFICATION ON THE OMISSION OF MEDICAL LABORATORY SCIENTISTS IN THE LIFE INSURANCE COVER FOR FRONTLINE HEALTH CARE PROVIDERS

I am directed to acknowledge the receipt of your letter dated 27th April, 2020 on the above subject and to draw your attention to paragraphs 2 and 3 of the Memorandum of Understanding (MoU) between the Federal Government and the Health Professional Associations and Unions on COVID-19 Special Incentives for Health Workers, copy attached.

2. In this regard, I am to inform you that all frontline health care providers, which also includes the Medical Laboratory Scientists, have been provided insurance cover for the COVID-19 and post COVID-19 period for the next one year. The sums assured for frontline health workers are as follows:

i. Officers on SGL 01 – 07 - ₦5M
ii. Officers on SGL 08 – 14 - ₦15M
iii. Officers on SGL 15 – 17 - ₦20M

3. Please accept the assurances of the warm regards of the Honourable Minister.

Aliyu G. Mohammed
Director, Human Resource Management
For: Honourable Minister

Figure 4.
Medical laboratory scientists clarified as frontline health workers covered for life insurance during COVID-19.

S/N	Countries	Government/employee support programme packages												
		Mental health	Salary	Childcare	COVID-19 allowance	Insurance	Food	Transport	Accommodation	CPD Units	Online training	Spiritual/ prayers	Social/ music & dancing	Authors
1	Australia	A	A	A	A	A	A	A	A	NS	A	NS	A	[28]
2	Bulgaria	A	A	NA	A	NS	NS	NS	NA	NS	A	NA	A	[27]
3	Canada	A	A	NA	A	NS	NS	NS	NA	NS	A	NA	A	[24]
4	China	A	A	NS	A	NS	NS	NS	NS	NS	A	NA	A	[30]
5	Denmark	A	A	A	NA	NS	NS	NS	NS	NS	A	NA	A	[27]
6	Finland	A	A	NA	NA	NS	NS	NS	NS	NS	A	NS	A	[27]
7	France	A	A	A	A	NS	NS	NS	NS	NS	A	NS	A	[27]
8	Germany	A	A	A	A	NS	NS	NS	NS	NS	A	NS	A	[27]
9	Ghana	A	A	NS	A	A	NS	NS	A	NS	A	A	A	[29]
10	Israel	A	A	A	NA	NS	NS	A	A	NS	A	A	A	[27]
11	Lithuania	A	A	A	A	A	A	A	A	NS	A	A	A	[27]
12	Malta	A	A	A	A	NS	A	A	A	NS	A	A	A	[27]
13	Nigeria	A	A	NA	A	A	P	NS	A	NA	A	A	A	
14	Romania	A	A	A	A	NS	A	A	A	A	A	A	A	[27]
15	UK	A	A	A	A	NS	A	NS	A	NS	A	NS	A	[27]
16	USA	A	A	A	A	NS	A	NS	A	NS	A	A	A	[24]

KEY: A, Available; NA, Not available; NS, Not sure; P, Partial.

Table 2.
Employee support (assistance) programmes by some countries for COVID-19.

by psychiatrists and psychologists to medical laboratory staff and other healthcare workers working on the frontline which may be in form of counseling or in-house psychologists outreach.

Employee support programme (ESP) or employee assistant programme (EAP) cannot be exhausted and depends on the government, private institutions or the healthcare workers involved. The list may include: mental health, salary, childcare, COVID-19 allowance, insurance, food, transport, accommodation, continuous professional development (CPD) units, online training, spiritual support in form of prayers, social lives using music and dancing and others as may be necessary.

Financial support, payment of salaries and job retention for Medical Scientists and other healthcare workers is a sine qua non, so that healthcare workers who were required to stay at home on preventive quarantine or levels of exposure are protected to receive their basic pay and class/grade allowances. Special allowances for COVID-19 are paid to frontline workers in Nigeria and other countries.

9. Conclusion

No doubt the COVD-19 is now a pandemic and the virus is really testing the resilience of our health delivery system. Medical laboratory science as the bedrock of diagnostic medicine and the role of medical laboratory science in containing any pandemic cannot be relegated to the background, not now or in the future. There is an urgent need to re-strategize in the effort towards fighting COVID-19 especially with regards to medical laboratory diagnosis as well as major component in infectious disease control globally.

All healthcare providers remain in the dark until the release of the medical laboratory test result on any new public health challenge COVID-19 as an example. Quality tools/equipment and conducive working environment provides quality results during public health challenges as noted during this COVID-19 pandemic.

The development of local medical laboratories to international standard are very germane to politicians as COVID-19 discourages medical tourism. Medical laboratories could do better with motivational packages such as recognition, hazard allowances and life insurance policies.

Severe Acute Respiratory Syndrome coronavirus-2 (SARS-COV-2) infection is a global pandemic. Health care workers role in patient management is predisposing and can serve as the means of hospital and community transmission.

Vast majority of health care workers are taking precautionary measures such as avoiding crowded places, washing of hands and the use of personal protective equipment (PPE) against coronavirus infection. This knowledge and attitude of health care workers shows excellent knowledge and possessed a positive attitude and good health practice towards the prevention of COVID-19. It is recommended that health care education of health care workers should continue in order to prevent and control infection.

Medical laboratory testing is very vital in public health emergencies [19] and in COVID-19 in particular thereby encouraging medical laboratory strengthening [31, 32], towards overcoming all laboratory associated challenges in COVID-19 [33–36].

This chapter hereby recommends the following:

a. Healthcare providers should always rely on the medical laboratory testing results in all public health issues and not only on COVID-19

b. There is need to update and quality crosscheck of all COVID-19 testing kits and equipment

c. Adequate construction and update of medical laboratory facilities in use for COVID-19 and other public health issues

d. Institutions involved in COVID-19 should sort for scientific and empirical data for all public health issues and vaccination as guide to public health policies

e. Government should provide and pay good hazard allowances and life insurance to all medical laboratory professionals

f. Train and retrain all medical laboratory professionals to be at the same pace with any upcoming wave of COVID-19

g. Adequate policies should be employed to stem out various challenges affecting optimum performance of various medical laboratories across the globe

h. Knowing fully well that Scientists contributed to the vaccine production research, it should be most appropriate that COVID-19 antibody testing should be carried out on individuals before vaccination to determine status. Not only that, various medical laboratory parameters should be carried out on all that are receiving vaccine before and after vaccine administration to help track changes and monitor health status of individuals who have received the vaccine candidates available currently for COVID-19.

Acknowledgements

The authors wish to acknowledge MLT Ruth Pam Chuwang for initial assistance in the typing of the manuscript.

Conflict of interest

The authors declare no competing interests.

Notes/Thanks/Other declarations

Obeta M. Uchejeso conceptualized the Chapter, All authors contributed equally in the chapter manuscript preparation, editing and approved the final manuscript for submission.

Author details

Obeta M. Uchejeso[1*], Jwanse I. Rinpan[2], Mantu E. Chongs[3] and Maureen O. Ekpere-Ezeugwu[4]

1 Department of Medical Laboratory Management, Federal School of Medical Laboratory Science, Jos, Nigeria

2 Health and Development Support Programme (HANDS), Jos, Nigeria

3 Department of Special Duties, Federal School of Medical Laboratory Science, Jos, Nigeria

4 Department of Pharmaceutical Microbiology and Biotechnology, University of Nigeria, Nsukka, Nigeria

*Address all correspondence to: uchejesoobeta@gmail.com

References

[1] Obeta MU, Maduka KM, Ofor IB, Ofojekwu NM (2019). Improving Quality and Cost Diminution in Modern Healthcare Delivery: The Role of the Medical Laboratory Scientists in Nigeria. International Journal of Business and Management Invention (IJBMI), 08(03) 08-19.

[2] Obeta MU, Maduka MK, Ejinaka OR. (2020). Medical Laboratory Science; the Distortion of Nomenclature across the Globe. New Zealand Journal of Med. Lab. Science. Pg 52

[3] Zhu N, Zhang D, Wang W, et al. (2019). A novel coronavirus from patients with pneumonia in China, 2019. N Engl J Med 2020; 382:727-733.

[4] Etukudoh NS, Ejinaka RO, Olowu FA, Obeta MU, Adebowale OM, Udoudoh M P. (2020). Coronavirus (COVID-19); Review from A Nigerian Perspective. Am J Biomed Sci & Res. - 9(1). DOI: 10.34297/AJBSR.2020.09.001347

[5] WHO (2020). Director-General's opening remarks at the media briefing on COVID-19 – 11March 2020. https://www.who.int/dg/speeches/detail/who-director-general-s-opening-remarks-at-the-media-briefing-oncovid-19---11-march-2020

[6] Nassiri N (2020) Perspective on Wuhan Viral Pneumonia. Adv in Pub. Health, Com and Trop Med: APCTM-106. Kosmos Publishers.

[7] WHO (2020) Laboratory testing for coronvirus disease 2019 (COVID-19) in suspected human cases interim Guidance.

[8] Ozuruoke DFN (2014). History of Medical Laboratory Science: Nigerian Perspective. Pundit Publishers, Lagos

[9] NCDC (2020). Guidance on the Use of Antigen Rapid Diagnostic Kits for Diagnosis of SARS-COV-2 Infection in Nigeria. Accessed on 28th October, 2020 from www.ncdc.gov.ng

[10] Obeta MU, Ejinaka RO, Ofor IB, Ikeagwulonu RC, Agbo E C, Abara US. (2020). "Nigerian COVID-19 (Coronavirus) Patients Update, the Realities with Medical Laboratory Diagnostic Sites." American Journal of Epidemiology and Infectious Disease, vol. 8, no. 1 (2020): 13-15. doi: 10.12691/ajeid-8-1-3.

[11] Sheikhzadeh E, Eissa S, Ismail A, Mohammed Zourob M. (2020). Diagnostic techniques for COVID-19 and new developments. Talanta 220 https://doi.org/10.1016/j.talanta.2020.121392

[12] Bamidele JA and Rana KM (2020) Challenges of healthcare delivery in the context of COVID-19 Pandemic in Sub-Saharan Africa. Iberoamerican Journal of Medicine 02 100-109 http://doi.org/10.5281/zenodo.3755414

[13] MLSCN (2020). Press Release on the pre-market validation of COVID-19 test kits. Accessed on 15th October, 2020 from www.mlscn.gov.ng

[14] WHO (2004). Laboratory biosafety manual, third edition. Geneva: World Health Organization; 2004.

[15] Obeta M. Uchejeso, Nkereuwem S. Etukudoh, Okoli C. Chukwudimma (2021). Nigerian Medical Laboratory Diagnosis of COVID-19; from Grass to Grace as Chapter 5 of Intelligent Computing Applications for COVID-19: Predictions, Diagnosis, and Prevention (Ed.) Saba and Rehman, CRC Press Tailor and Francis Group

[16] Lu R, Zhao X, Li J, Niu P, Yang B, Wu H, Wang W, Song H, Huang B, Zhu N, Bi Y, Ma X, Zhan F, Wang L, Hu T, Zhou H, Hu Z, Zhou W, Zhao L,

Chen J, Meng Y, Wang J, Lin Y, Yuan J, Xie Z, Ma J, Liu WJ, Wang D, Xu W, Holmes EC, Gao GF, Wu G, Chen W, Shi W, Tan W. (2020). Genomic characterization and epidemiology of 2019 novel coronavirus: implications for virus origins and receptor binding, Lancet 395 (10224) 565-574

[17] Tomo S, Karli S, Dharmalingam K, Yadav D, Sharma P. (2020). The clinical laboratory: a key player in diagnosis and management of COVID-19. The Journal of International Federation of Clinical Chemistry and Laboratory Medicine; eJIFCC2020: 31(4) 326-346

[18] Li C, Zhao C, Bao J, Tang B, Wang Y, Gu B. (2020).Laboratory diagnosis of coronavirus disease-2019 (COVID-19). Clinica Chimica Acta 510: 25-46 https://www.who.int/csr/don/05-january-2020-pneumoniaof-unkown-cause-china/en/

[19] Kiros T, Kiros M, Andalem H, Hailemichael W, Damite S, Eyayu T, Getu S, Tiruneh T. (2020). Laboratory Diagnosis of COVID-19: Role of Laboratory Medicine. J Clin Chem Lab Med. 3.142. DOI: 10.35248/clinical-chemistry-laboratory-medicine.20.3.142

[20] Ikeagwolunu RC, Obeta MU, Ugwu IN (2020). Systematic review of laboratory parameters predicting severity and fatality of COVID-19 hospitalised patients New Zealand Journal of Medical Laboratory Science; 74: 165-180

[21] ASM (2020). Celebrating Medical Laboratory Professionals – We Save Lives Every Day. ASM

[22] Darkdaily (2020). Clinical Laboratory Scientist in British Columbia Gets Recognition for Identifying the Province's First Case of COVID-19. https://www.darkdaily.com/clinical-laboratory-scientist-in-british-columbia-gets-recognition-for-identifying-the-provinces-first-case-of-covid-19/

[23] Rohde R. (2020). Beating Pandemics like COVID-19 requires more Medical Laboratory Professionals. https://www.forbes.com/sites/coronavirusfrontlines/2020/04/22/beating-pandemics-like-covid-19-requires-more-medical-laboratory-professionals-this-virologist-explains/amp/

[24] AHA (2020). COVID-19: Caring for Our Health Care Heroes during COVID-19. American Hospital Association

[25] WHO (2020). Health workforce policy and management in the context of the COVID-19 pandemic response; Interim guidance. WHO/2019-nCoV/health_workforce/2020.1

[26] Kirk AK, Brown DF (2003). Employee assistance programs: A review of the management of stress and wellbeing through workplace counselling and consulting. Australian Psychologist 38(2); 138-143 DOI: 10.1080/00050060310001707137

[27] Williams GA, Scarpetti G, Bezzina A, Vincenti K, Grech K, Kowalska-Bobko I, Sowada C, Furman M, Gałązka-Sobotka M, Maier CB. (2020). How are Countries Supporting their Health Workers during COVID-19? Eurohealth; 26(2) 59-64

[28] KPMG (2021). COVID-19 Assistance Programme at a Glance.

[29] AFDB (2020). Ghana COVID-19 RESPONSE SUPPORT PROGRAMME APPRAISAL REPORT RDGW/ECCE/AHHD/ECGF/PGCL DEPARTMENTS accessed on 27th March, 2021 from: https://www.afdb.org/sites/all/libraries/pdf.js/web/viewer.html?file=https%3A%2F%2Fwww.afdb.org%2Fsites%2Fdefault%2Ffiles%2Fdocuments%2Fprojects-and-operations%2Fghana_-_covid-19_response_support_programme_-_project_appraisal_report.pdf#page=1&zoom=auto-13,842

[30] Lu Q, Cai Z, Chen B, Liu T. (2020). Social Policy Responses to the Covid-19 Crisis in China in 2020. International Journal of Environmental Research and Public Health; 17, 5896; doi:10.3390/ijerph17165896

[31] Naidoo D, Ihekweazu C. (2020) Nigeria's efforts to strengthen laboratory diagnostics – Why access to reliable and affordable diagnostics is key to building resilient laboratory systems. Afr J Lab Med. 2020;9(2), a1019 https://doi.org/10.4102/ajlm. v9i2.1019

[32] Bayot ML, & Sanchez RS. (2020). Coronavirus disease (COVID-19) testing using the GeneXpert System: A technical guide on laboratory systems strengthening for COVID-19 pandemic response. 1st Edition. Coach MLB Consulting. Metro Manila, Philippines.

[33] Tang YW, Schmitz JE, Persing DH, Stratton CW. (2020). Laboratory diagnosis of COVID-19: current issues and challenges. J Clin Microbiol 58:e00512-e00520. https://doi.org/10.1128/JCM.00512-20

[34] Abdullahi IN, Emeribe AN, Akande AO, Ghamba PE, Adekola HA, Ibrahim Y, Dangana A. (2020). Challenges of COVID-19 testing services in Africa J Infect Dev Ctries 2020; 14(7):691-695.

[35] Akinyemi KO, Fakorede CO, Anjorin AAA, Abegunrin RO, Adunmo O, Ajoseh SO, Akinkunmi FM. (2020) Intrigues and Challenges Associated with COVID-19 Pandemics in Nigeria. Health, 12, 954-971. https://doi.org/10.4236/health.2020.128072

[36] Enitan SS, Akele RY, Agunsoye CJ, Olawuyi KA, Nwankiti AJ, Oluremi AS, Ofodile CA, Olayanju AO, Alaba OEG, Enitan CB (2020) Molecular Diagnosis of COVID-19 in Nigeria: Current Practices, Challenges and Opportunities. Journal of Infectious Diseases & Case Reports SRC/JIDSCR 116-129. DOI: https://doi.org/10.47363/JIDSCR/2020(1)116.

Chapter 20

Evolution of Diagnostic Methods and Prevalence Detection of COVID-19: A Review

Hemant Bherwani

Abstract

In clinical, research, and public health laboratories, many diagnostic methods are used to detect the coronavirus. Some tests directly detect infection by detecting viral RNA, while others detect the disease indirectly by detecting host antibodies. Several studies on SARS-CoV-2 diagnostic methods have found varying throughput, batching capacity, infrastructure requirements, analytical efficiency, and turnaround times ranging from minutes to hours. Serosurvey studies have been conducted for antibodies to understand, model, and forecast the prevalence of the disease in an area. While on the research and predictive modeling side, sampling and analysis of sewage have been conducted to determine the number of RNA copies and hence the prevalence. Certain studies indicate usefulness of GIS (Geographic Information System) for understanding the pervasiveness of COVID-19 in an area as well. The current chapter deals with the evolution of diagnostic techniques for COVID-19 and discusses use of specific techniques and appropriateness in certain specified conditions. It also focuses on understanding the methods used for assessing the prevalence of COVID-19 in a particular region to extract mitigative strategies from it, either by prediction or management of the affected area.

Keywords: COVID-19, SARS-CoV-2, RT-PCR, GIS, wastewater treatment, biosensors, CRISPR

1. Introduction

Different testing methods are used in clinical, academic, and public health laboratories to diagnose the coronavirus. These methods have different output, batching capacity, analytical result performance, specific requirement of infrastructure setting and worktime. Some tests, such as direct tests, detect viral RNA directly to determine infection, while indirect tests diagnose infection indirectly by measuring host antibodies. The methods that are used for the diagnosis of coronavirus should have enough accuracy and sensitivity to make proper clinical decisions quickly in this pandemic so that the spread of the virus can be controlled [1–3]. A number of experiments were carried out to determine economic loss as well as the urban microclimate [4, 5].

A number of methods that are used for diagnosis have been given an approval from World Health Organization (WHO) and by the US Food and Drug Administration (FDA), while due to the rapid spread of the virus, the Emergency

Use Authorization (EUA) has granted conditional approval to several new methods [1–6]. Several studies on sewage sampling and analysis as well as use of Geographic Information System (GIS) have also been conducted to understand the cause of epidemics, its spread pattern and to predict the occurrence of disease in an area. GIS acts as a useful tool in easing the fight against coronavirus with its advanced features such as mapping, location intelligence and spatial analysis providing a way to the government or public authorities in the determination of active COVID - 19 cases, recoveries, fatalities and even creating containment/hotspots zones [7]. On the other hand the surveillance of wastewater with the help of water based epidemiology [WBE] detects the RNA of the viral genome of SARS-CoV-2 enabling the further mitigation of the virus. The samples of the wastewater are collected and tested from the sewer lines indicating the more accurate location of coronavirus outbreak leading to the reorganization of area of concern [8]. It was also discovered that air plays a significant role in the spread of the SARS-CoV-2 virus, as it is transmitted through air [9].

Apart from the equipment and the method used, the result also depends on collection of sample, use of reagents, and probability of cross-contamination and storage requirements for samples/reagents. While selecting any reliable and fast diagnostic method all these factors should be considered so that a proper decision and immediate action to public health can be made. This chapter focuses on the various types of COVID-19 diagnosis methods presently in use in a comprehensive manner and also the working efficiency of the different methods by checking various parameters such as sensitivity, time of detection, specificity etc. in comparison to other methods. An attempt has been made to discuss the prediction methods used for COVID-19 prevalence detection and analysis. The broad areas focused in the chapter includes diagnosis of COVID-19 and surveillance system for disease prevalence.

2. Diagnosis of COVID-19

Coronavirus is detected by reviewing the affected person's medical history, beginning with the point of contact and progressing through the findings of certain clinical examinations. Various respiratory problems and symptoms like pneumonia also comes under COVID-19 symptoms. Diagnosis methods like reverse transcription – polymerase chain reaction (RT-PCR) are being used now a days. Day by day with passing time many more methods are being developed but are pending for the approval from the regulatory authorities. The diagnostic methods that are studied and discussed in the chapter are shown in **Figure 1** and **Table 1**. These methods have been discussed in detail in the subsequent sections.

2.1 Reverse transcription – polymerase chain reaction (RT-PCR)

RT–PCR is currently the most commonly used laboratory methods for the detection of SARS-CoV-2. This method uses a technique derived from nuclear material to determine the existence of unique genetic material in any pathogen, including viruses. It's also being used to identify other diseases including the Ebola virus and the Zika virus. This method necessitates the collection of samples from body parts where the virus has accumulated, such as the nose or the throat [10]. To extract only the RNA present in the sample, it is treated with different chemicals to remove substances such as proteins and fats. This RNA is a combination of the person's genetic material and, if present, the virus's RNA. The procedure continues with the technique of merging reverse transcription of RNA into complementary

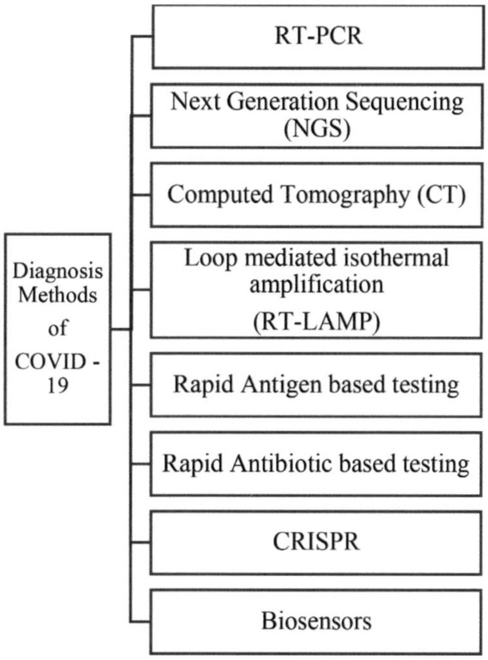

Figure 1.
Diagnosis approaches for COVID-19.

DNA or cDNA, followed by polymerase chain reaction amplification of particular DNA (PCR) [11]. According to various studies, there are several advantages of the real time RT-PCR such as it is very highly sensitive, needs only a small amount of DNA and gives fast results in a duration of three hours as compared to other methods, which usually consumes six to eight hours [12, 13]. It is also the most precise method and gives accurate results after detection. This method, however, does not detect past infection, necessitating the use of other methods to detect, monitor, and study past infections, especially those that may have evolved and spread without causing symptoms. Other disadvantages includes its higher cost due to use of expensive apparatus, which makes it quite uneconomical [14, 15]. The flow process for virus detection using RT-PCR technique is given in **Figure 2**.

2.2 Next generation sequencing (NGS)

The method of determining the nucleic acid sequence – the order of nucleotides in DNA, i.e. the order of the four bases: adenine, guanine, cytosine, and thymine – is known as DNA sequencing [16]. There are several DNA sequencing approaches, one of which is NGS, also known as High-throughput sequencing (HTS). By NGS, in a single experiment it is possible to determine the genomic sequencing of more than 1 million base pairs and hence this method is used for diagnosing inheritable diseases, cancer, and infectious diseases [17, 18]. NGS technology employs array-based sequencing, which utilizes Sanger sequencing techniques to process millions of reactions in parallel, resulting in extremely high speed and throughput at a lower cost [19]. The first step in NGS is library preparation, which involves randomly fragmenting DNA to build libraries, followed by ligation with custom linkers. Amplification is the second step, in which the library is amplified using clonal amplification methods, and PCR Sequencing is the third step, in which DNA is sequenced by using one of the several strategies. This method for diagnosis is specified as it provides all related information and is also highly sensitive. It is helpful in

Method of diagnosis	Working principle	Time required	Cost of treatment per individual	Advantages	Disadvantages	References
RT-PCR	Reverse transcription & amplification	3–4 hrs	Rs 2000 - Rs 2500	Cost effective & rapid small amount of DNA is required	Complex and requires expensive lab apparatus.	[3, 4, 52]
Next Generation Sequencing (NGS)	Capillary electrophoresis	1–2 days	Rs. 25000 – Rs .55000	Highly sensitive, gives quick and accurate results and is more reliable.	Expensive and needs expertise skills	[3, 4]
Computed Tomography (CT)	Chest images by X-Ray technology	1 hr	RS 5700	Rapid identification and higher sensitivity.	Cannot accurately distinguish between COVID -19 & other respiratory diseases	[3, 4, 52]
Loop mediated isothermal amplification (RT-LAMP)	Primer detection and amplification by reverse transcription	30 min	Rs. 200	Very cheap and reliable method, gives quicker analysis.	Requires complex equipment and shows less sensitivity	[3, 4, 53, 54]
Rapid Antigen based testing	Detection of presence of vital proteins (antigens)	15–30 min	Rs.600-Rs.500	Very affordable. High testing speed and sensitivity	May lead to false negatives and hence is not always accurate.	[55]
Rapid Antibiotic based testing	Rapid POC CE-IVD	15–30 min	—	Even a fully recovered person can help other patient free on cost in combating virus and hence supporting humanity.	Depends on the time and speed of the development of antibodies. Positive results of test take 6–7 days.	[36, 37]
CRISPR	Gene Editing technology	10–5 min	Rs.500	Cheap, easily accessible, high speed and aacurate and fast results just within 45 minutes.	Risk of toxicity.	[40, 41]
Biosensors	Mechanism of Receptor and transducer	60–45 min	—	User friendly and detects virus in mass population rapidly	Less accuracy	[43, 44]

Table 1.
Different methods for diagnosis of COVID-19.

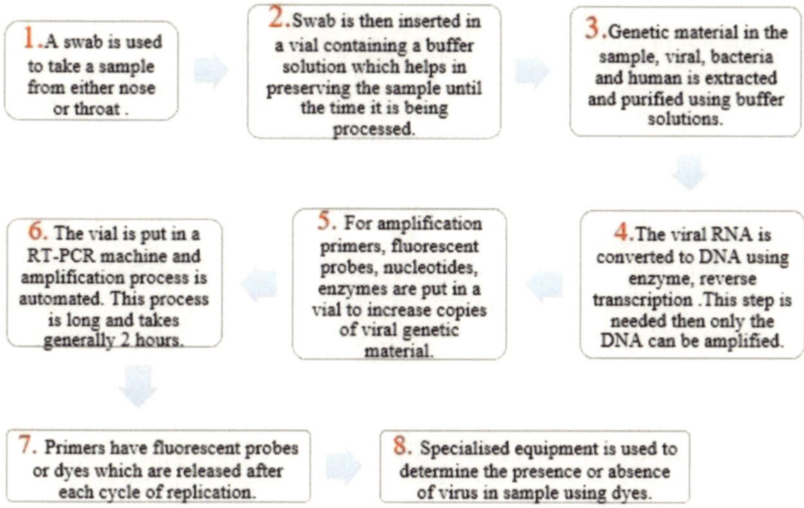

Figure 2.
Working process of RT-PCR method.

identifying secondary infections and has potential tracing. However it is expensive and requires sophisticated laboratory for conducting test.

2.3 Computed tomography (CT)

A computed tomography scan (CT scan) is a medical imaging technique that uses computer-processed combinations of several X-ray measurements taken from various angles to create cross-sectional images of the body, enabling the patient to see inside the body without cutting it open. COVID-19 is a respiratory disease that affects the parenchyma, but several studies claim that extreme cases are linked to a pro-inflammatory cytokine storm that leads to systemic inflammation and sepsis, as well as involvement in other organs such as the cardiovascular system [20]. An integrated Computed Tomography (CT) method may provide useful information on the diagnosis of COVID-19 patients in such circumstances. The expression of acute interstitial lung damage and the subsequent parenchymal changes induced by the cytokine storm triggered by the virus's internalization into the pneumocytes are normal CT findings in patients with COVID-19 [21–23]. During the early stages of the pandemic, CT was commonly used in China to diagnose COVID-19. Although the National Health Commission of China's current recommendations do not include imaging findings in diagnosis of this disease [24]. Furthermore, the American College of Radiology does not consider using a chest CT scan to test for COVID-19 pneumonia as a first-line imaging modality. Patients with symptoms like pulmonary embolism, empyema, or co-infection should get a CT scan, according to the recommendations. Using RT-PCR as a reference standard, several studies have demonstrated the sensitivity of CT. CT scan is being appreciated for its accuracy in results however; extreme precaution must be taken with respect to COVID-19 disease because of a negative CT scan. When compared to RT-PCR, a CT scan of the chest has a sensitivity of 89% and a Likelihood Ratio (LR) of 0.16, according to a study. With an LR+ of 2.81, specificity was moderate (68%) [25].

2.4 Loop mediated isothermal amplification (LAMP)

For the diagnosis of SARS–CoV-2, isothermal polymerase chain reactions methods such as loop-mediated isothermal amplification (LAMP) are supposedly a replacement for the RT-PCR process [26]. As compared to RT - PCR, LAMP is a powerful nucleic acid amplification method that works under isothermal temperature conditions and thus does not involve frequent temperature changes. To allow rapid amplification, this method involves designing assay primers and using a strand-displacing polymerase. LAMP reaction mix includes six primers that target eight different areas of the bacterial or viral genome. Currently RT-LAMP technique is being used for detecting COVID-19. RT- LAMP is a mechanism for auto cycling strand displacement DNA synthesis in which a polymerase uses one pair of inner and one pair of outer primers to carry out a reaction with high strand displacement operation. This method uses six independent sequences at the start and four independent sequences at the end to identify the target sequences. Primer identification of the target genome leads to a strong colorimetric reaction. The nucleic acid sample, 4 (or 6) specially formulated primers, and the best DNA polymerase are all incubated in the same test tube at 60 to 65 degrees Celsius, depending on the optimum LAMP temperature [27]. The ORF1ab gene, S gene, and N gene are among the main areas of coronavirus genomes where the primers are built for this process. ORF1ab is responsible for viral genome replication, while the S gene is required for coronavirus to bind to human ACE2 protein, and the N gene is a nucleocapsid protein found in many coronaviruses [28]. RT- LAMP completes the detection just within 25–30 minutes hence making it more reliable & suitable as compared to the RT-PCR for monitoring. Although it projects lot of gains, it has limitations such as slightly lower sensitivity of RT-LAMP as compared to RT - PCR. Some ongoing research recommended that the addition of guanidine could improve the sensitivity of detection with RT-LAMP [29]. RT-LAMP has a sensitivity of 75% as compared to RT-PCR, but unlike RT-PCR, it does not produce false-positive results, and when the results of RT-PCR and RT-LAMP are combined, diagnostic sensitivity increases to 92–100% [30], proving it to be a good technique.

2.5 Rapid diagnostic test based on detection of antigens

Since antigen tests are simple to perform, they are in high demand for COVID-19 diagnosis. For the evaluation of serious infections in samples, the novel rapid antigen detection test (RADT) is used. This test looks for and detects antigens generated by the SARS-CoV-2 virus in a sample taken from a person's respiratory tract [31, 32]. If adequate concentrations of target antigens are present in the sample, it will merge with particular antibodies fixed on a paper strip attached to a plastic casing within 30 minutes, using either visual or visible. Since the antigens found in the body are only released while the virus is actively replicating, such tests are the best used to detect acute or the early infection. This test depends on factors such as quantity and quality of virus collected from the person's body, duration from onset of one's illness, reagent formulation in a test kit. The test is cost effective, determines results in minutes and reveal an actively infection. They are already being used for influenza, HIV, tuberculosis (TB) and other infectious diseases [33, 34]. Due to the limited data availability for this test currently WHO does not recommend the antigen test keeping in mind the patient's health but encourages more research under this field.

2.6 Rapid diagnostics tests based on detection of antibodies

This is the most common type of test for the diagnosis for COVID-19. The working principle of this test includes the detection antibodies present in blood sample of people infected from COVID-19. It detects two types of antibodies isotopes namely: IgG and IgM [34]. The development of antibodies and their responses varies from person to person accordingly. Some studies show that antibodies response is detected only in 2nd week from the development of COVID-19 symptoms [35] i.e. during the recovery phase. A COVID-19 antibody-based tests can cross-react with other pathogens, including other human coronaviruses [35, 36], resulting in false-positive results. The timing and type of antibody testing determines accuracy. One of the benefits of this testing is that people who have recovered from COVID-19 will donate their plasma, which is then used to cure those who have serious disease and improve their capacity to combat the virus. These tests can be conducted on blood, serum, or plasma samples, with results available in 30 minutes and a positive result after 7–10 days of infection [36, 37].

2.7 CRISPR/Cas

CRISPR (Clustered Regularly Interspaced Short Palindromic Repeats), a rapid approach for diagnosing COVID-19, was recently suggested by scientists and researchers. CRISPR is a family of DNA sequences found in the genomes of prokaryotic organisms including bacteria and archaea that function as an immune system against foreign elements in archaea and bacteria. CRISPR is also used potentially to treat genetic diseases and cancer [38]. This approach employs gene-editing technology, which allows for the detection of the coronavirus in just 5 minutes and the delivery of results in just 45 minutes, attracting a lot of interest. The COVID-19 CRISPR test identifies a 20-base RNA sequence by using a "guide" RNA that is complementary to the target RNA sequence and binds to it in the solution. When guide RNA binds to target RNA, CRISPR tools Cas 13 "Scissors" enzyme activates and cuts apart any nearby single – stranded RNA. Such cuts release a fluorescent particle separately in the test solution. The sample is then hit with a laser light and the released fluorescent particle if lighted up indicating the presence of coronavirus. This method for the diagnosis of coronavirus is currently being used by Sherlock Biosciences, US and in India by Tata group under the brand name 'Feluda'. CRISPR does not require specialized or expensive laboratory apparatus and hence can be perfectly deployed in doctor's office, schools and office buildings. Other advantages of this method include its great programmability and its speed [39]. However, there are certain drawbacks to the CRISPR - Cas9 diagnostic technique, such as off-target effects and unexpected mutations, which are a major worry, particularly when it is used for both therapeutic and diagnostic purposes. Because Cas proteins are obtained from prokaryotic origins, in vivo application of these proteins causes toxic effects in the human cells that contain them, as well as immunological activation and the creation of cas protein specific antibodies, which could obstruct the therapeutic application of CRISPR technology [40, 41].

2.8 Biosensors

Biosensors are new emerging technology for the rapid detection and diagnosis of mass population infected with SARS-CoV-2. Biosensors are made up of chemical or biological receptors that interact with the target analyte directly, as well as a transducer that translates the detection process into a quantitative signal. Biosensors target biological recognition of molecules such as enzymes, nucleic acids or antibodies and contain transducer and a detector detects the interaction with the analyte and generates an output digitally. Biosensors are classified into four types such as electrochemical biosensors, piezoelectric biosensors, thermal biosensors and optical biosensors. In the recent trend of biosensor, RT-LAMP is mediated with Nano particles biosensors (NBS). According to studies, with biosensors, RT-LAMP is less error prone and achieves higher specificity and low false positive result [42].

CRISPR gene editing technology was recently updated as a biological sensor by combining a CRISPR chip with a Field of Effect Transistor (FET) to diagnose COVID-19 in under 40 minutes [40]. Plasmonic Photothermal (PPT) and localized surface plasmon resonance (LSPR), a dual-function plasmonic biosensor, were designed for the ongoing detection of COVID-19 pandemic. For a few covid sequences, the LSPR biosensor has a higher sensitivity, with a detection maximum of up to 0.22 ppm concentration [43]. Biosensors are mostly designed on the basis of surface nucleoproteins. Piezoelectric immune-sensor and thermal biosensor are also being used for detecting the SARS-CoV-2 virus. The electrochemical paper-based biosensor uses the high –ultra charge transfer efficiency AuNPs with magnetic NPs ($Fe_2 0_4$). These biosensors are biodegradable, sensitive, simple and economical [44].

In addition to the methods used to diagnose COVID – 19, some innovative techniques are being used to forecast the source and frequency of the virus's spread so that it can be monitored by implementing some mitigation steps, based on various surveys and studies.

3. Surveillance of COVID-19

3.1 Geographical information system (GIS) based study

GIS is an information system for capturing, gathering, analyzing and managing data into visual form. GIS has brought a new trend of revolution in the field of health and therefore it can be encouraged to be used as a support tool for the tracking of COVID -19 cases during this global pandemic [45]. The world health organization even uses the GIS technology to map and update number of COVID - 19 cases and also lists the deaths occurring all over the world on their dashboard regularly. The spatiotemporal algorithms present in GIS are helpful in identifying the COVID -19 outbreak faster. The algorithms therein are useful in assessing and recording the appropriate number of people infected with the virus. GIS assisted with remote sensing provides the real time aerial and satellite photographs which leads to the evaluation of the disease growth and fluctuations all over the world or in a particular area [46]. The above information captured through GIS is useful in analyzing and locating the area which is worst affected and the areas under risk zone where the virus is likely to spread rapidly in future. Through GIS technique we can became aware of the spread of COVID 19 in advance and hence can take strict decisive actions in areas facing serious COVID circumstances [47]. The ways in which GIS tools can be helpful are summarized in **Figure 3**.

The other ways in which GIS technology can be used for limiting the disease spread includes contact tracing, selection of sites for emergency treatment units and digital mapping that shows location and time-sensitive functions directly related to a spread of virus and hence alert the officials to cancel the particular public event, minimizing the number of persons affected. Web maps are also useful in solving the problem of acute supply of medical appliances signaling the distributors [48]. Researches have used GIS and modeling techniques to understand overlap of environmental parameters such as air pollution, microclimate, and impact on SDGs with COVID-19 prevalence [49]. The parametric and probabilistic modeling along with statistical tools available with GIS have also been used to understand disease prevalence and management in countries [50]. Currently many mobile/android applications are based on GIS technology such as Aarogyasetu (India), COVID-19 symptom trackers, etc. launched by many countries, which are used for contact

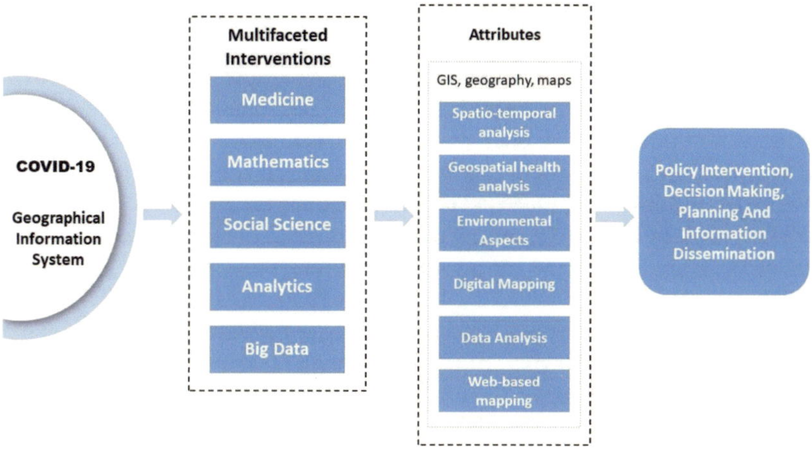

Figure 3.
Role of GIS in disease prevalence mapping, analysis and management.

tracing [51]. These applications are cost efficient, present accurate data and thus are more reliable.

3.2 Wastewater surveillance system

There is growing proof of presence of SARS-CoV-2 in the sewage [51, 52]. Multiple focused researches have been carried out to analyze the presence of virus in wastewater [53]. Many studies have proved wastewater based epidemiology as an eligible and effective tracking tool in detecting SARS-CoV-2 genome at ambient temperature of 45°C giving us a better understanding of the present spreading of the global pandemic. This has led to growing concern in public health authorities for the essential need of the analysis of sewage samples from the sewage treatment plants for computing the presence of viral genome of SARS-CoV-2. While this is a

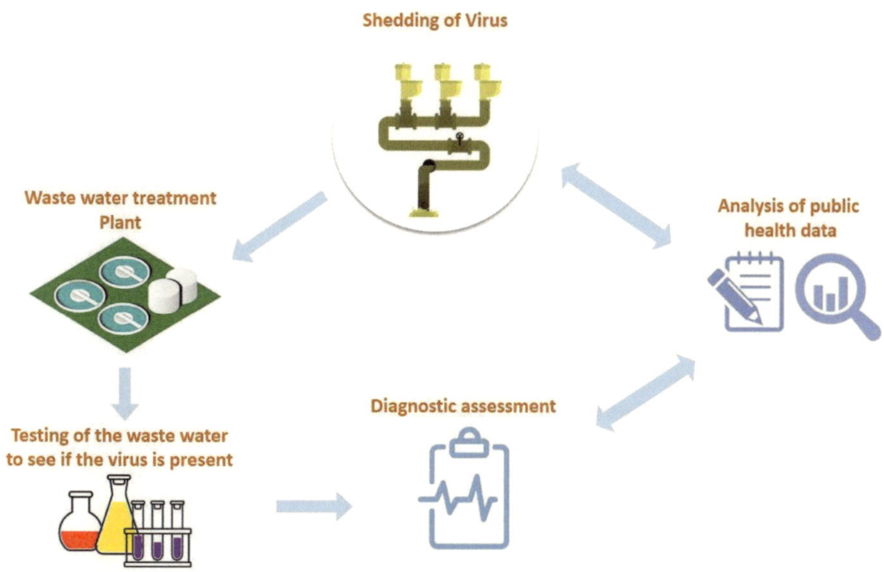

Figure 4.
Analysis of disease prevalence using wastewater samples.

grave concern, it has also presented as an opportunity for the utilization of water-based surveillance system for monitoring and investigating the presence of virus in sewage. The detection of virus in the wastewater samples has created a further possibility that the wastewater containing the virus can also release the same virus into other water bodies such as sea, groundwater, etc. The samples can be collected from drains and sewage treatment plants to understand the load of virus being shed by a particular community [54, 55]. The samples once taken, can be analyzed for load of virus present in it, followed by data analytics to back calculate the disease prevalence in an area. **Figure 4** represent the analysis of wastewater samples for COVID-19 prevalence.

Through wastewater sample analysis, the disease prevalence calculation can serve as an early warning for spreading pandemic in an area. This may give the authorities to act in timely manner for management of proliferation of COVID-19 in the area considered for analysis. Wastewater surveillance comes along with many benefits such as it is an economical method and also acts as a early warning tool signaling the transmission of the disease by neglecting the other epidemiological indicators and gives successful evidences and results [55].

4. Conclusion

Taking into account the present situation of a pandemic it becomes extremely essential to develop a fast, effective, risk-free, and reliable method for diagnosis of COVID-19. There are several diagnostic methods available today for detecting the virus but each method has its pros and cons. Attributes such as accuracy level, complexity of instrumentation, the need for sample preparation & purification, operational and capital cost, time, geo-spatial availability, high technical skills and so on are to be considered before finalizing the best method of testing. The use of RT-PCR diagnosis for the virus is common and widely used everywhere due to its higher accuracy, sensitivity and reliability but due to its expensiveness, it cannot be afforded by lower incomes countries and is also a not suitable method for screening a large population at a time. Many new diagnostic methods such as RT-LAMP and CRISPR based technologies are also emerging which provide rapid, user-friendly, higher specificity & sensitivity, efficient and low-cost diagnosis of SARS-CoV-2 and can be deployed on the airports, office buildings, schools, etc. due to their nature of the simple operation, however, CRISPR has a little risk of contamination associated with it. Rapid serological methods based on antibodies/antigens are proving to be faster tests but not always give faster results and are not recommended because of their limited research. Currently to overcome the COVID-19 pandemic developing rapid, reliable, and novel biosensors for the detection of the virus is of much interest and will prove to be paradigm altering in surveillance, once perfected. The development of new SARS-CoV-2 biosensors is focused on the detection of biomarkers from human hosts, rather than antibodies or immunoglobulins. Developing sensitive, space-friendly, and portable biosensors can prove beneficial for the quick diagnosis of the virus.

With diagnosis, another important aspect is the assessment of disease prevalence in an area. The infection spread of SARS-CoV-2 is rapid and mostly happens through air, hence checking the prevalence of disease only after appearance of symptoms may not help in controlling the spread of virus. For that, advanced tools such as GIS or modeling techniques have to be used which can act as an early warning system. The GIS technology enables the local authorities as well as general public to recognize particular hotspots and take preventive measures in the right time. GIS based platforms and models can help in management of spread of virus through visualization and data analytics. Many tools and techniques use GIS for contact tracing and identification of containment sites. Another way the early warning system can be established is through wastewater sample analysis for analysis of virus. The time lag functions can be developed for various areas through thorough sampling and analysis of wastewater and disease prevalence in the area in order to understand the disease progression and forecast in that area. While this chapter discusses major techniques used for diagnosis and prevalence of COVID-19 among the population, the researchers are continuously working on finding better methods. The chapter comprehensively covers the methods being used currently for targeting and managing the spread of this virus and should helpful in getting an overview related to the tools and techniques being used for the assessment.

Author details

Hemant Bherwani[1,2]

1 CSIR-National Environmental Engineering Research Institute, Nagpur, Maharashtra, India

2 Academy of Scientific and Innovative Research (AcSIR), Ghaziabad, Uttar Pradesh, India

*Address all correspondence to: h.bherwani@neeri.res.in

References

[1] Smith, E. C., & Denison, M. R. (2012), Implications of altered replication fidelity on the Evolution and pathogenesis of coronaviruses, Current opinion in virology, 2(5), 519-524. https://doi.org/10.1016/j.coviro.2012.07.005.

[2] Gupta, A., Bherwani, H., Gautam, S., Anjum, S., Musugu, K., Kumar, N., Kumar, R. (2021). Air pollution aggravating COVID-19 lethality? Exploration in Asian cities using statistical models. Environment, Development and Sustainability, 23(4), 6408-6417.

[3] Cheng MP, Papenburg J, Desjardins M, Kanjilal S, Quach C, Libman M, et al, Diagnostic Testing for severe acute respiratory syndrome–related coronavirus-2: a narrative review, Ann Intern Med. 2020. doi:10.7326/M20-1301.

[4] Bherwani, H., Nair, M., Musugu, K., Gautam, S., Gupta, A., Kapley, A., & Kumar, R. (2020). Valuation of air pollution externalities: comparative assessment of economic damage and emission reduction under COVID-19 lockdown. Air Quality, Atmosphere & Health, 13(6), 683-694.

[5] Bherwani, H., Singh, A., & Kumar, R. (2020). Assessment methods of urban microclimate and its parameters: A critical review to take the research from lab to land. Urban Climate, 34, 100690.

[6] Basant Giri, Shishir Pandey, Retina Shrestha, Krisha Pokharel, Frances S. Ligler, Bhanu B. Neupane (2020), Review of analytical performance of COVID-19 detection methods, Analytical and Bioanalytical Chemistry. .doi:10.1007/s00216-020-02889-x.

[7] Ramesh Kumar, Suman Nagpal, Samander Kaushik, Sanjay Mendiratta, COVID-19 diagnostic approaches: different roads to the samedestination. Virus Dis. 2020; 31(2):97-105. doi:10.1007/s13337-020-00599-7.

[8] Michael-Kordatou, P. Karaolia, D. Fatta-Kassinos, Sewage analysis as a tool for the COVID-19 pandemic response and management: the urgent need for optimised protocols for SARS-CoV-2 detection and quantification, Journal of Environmental Chemical Engineering 8 (2020) 104306, doi:10.1016/j.jece.2020.104306.

[9] Bherwani, H., Gupta, A., Anjum, S., Anshul, A., & Kumar, R. (2020). Exploring dependence of COVID-19 on environmental factors and spread prediction in India. npj Climate and Atmospheric Science, 3(1), 1-13.

[10] Anna See MMed(ORL), Song Tar TohMMed(ORL), FAMS(ORL), 2020, Respiratory sampling for severe acute respiratory syndrome coronavirus 2: an overview, Head and Neck; 42:1652-1656. https://doi.org/10.1002/hed.26232.

[11] Freeman WM, Walker SJ, Vrana KE. 1999. Quantitative RT-PCR: pitfalls and potential. BioTechniques. 26 (1):112-122. doi:10.2144/99261rv01.

[12] Corman VM, Landt O, Kaiser M, Molenkamp R, Meijer A, Chu DK, et al. Detection of 2019 novel coronavirus [2019-NCoV] byreal-time RT-PCR. Eurosurveillance. 2020 25; (3).doi: 10.2807/1560-7917.ES.2020.25.3.2000045.

[13] Vogels CBF, Brito AF, Wyllie AL, et al. Analytical sensitivity andefficiency comparisons of SARS-CoV-2 RT–qPCR primer–probe sets, Nat Microbiology. 2020. doi:10.1038/s41564-020-0761-6.

[14] Cho CH, Lee CK, Nam MH, Yoon SY, Lim CS, Cho Y, Kim YK,

Evaluation of the AdvanSure™ real-time RT-PCR compared with culture and Seeplex RV15 for simultaneous detection of respiratory viruses, Diagnostic Microbiology &Infectectious Disease 2014 May;79(1):14-18. doi: 10.1016/j.diagmicrobio.2014.01.016.

[15] Gaunt E.R., Hardie A, Claas E.C.J., Simmonds P, Templeton K.E., Epidemiology and Clinical presentations of the four human coronaviruses 229E, HKU1, NL63, and OC43 detected over 3 years using a novel multiplex real-time PCR method, Journal of Clinical Microbiology. 2010; 48:2940-2947, doi:10.1128/JCM.00636-10.

[16] Behjati S, Tarpey P.S (December 2013). "What is next generation sequencing?". Archives of Disease in Childhood. Education and Practice Edition. 98 (6): 236-238. doi:10.1136/archdischild-2013-304340.

[17] Harris S.R, Cartwright E.J, Török M.E., et al. Whole-genome sequencing for analysis of an outbreak of methicillin-resistant Staphylococcus aureus: a descriptive study. Lancet Infect Dis. 2013;13:130-136. doi: 10.1016/S1473-3099(12)70268-2.

[18] Brown J.R., Bharucha T. Breuer J., Encephalitis diagnosis using metagenomics: application of next generation sequencing for undiagnosed cases, J Infect. 2018; 76 : 225-240. doi:10.1016/j.jinf.2017.12.014.

[19] Massart S, et al. Virus detection by high-throughput sequencing of small RNAs: large scale performance testing of sequence analysis strategies strategies. Phytopathology 2019;109(3):488-497, doi: 10.1094/PHYTO-02-18-0067-R.

[20] Guzik T.J., Mohiddin S.A., Dimarco A, et.al., 2020, COVID-19 and the cardiovascular system: Implications for risk assessment, diagnosis, and treatment options., Cardiovasc Res; 116(10):1666-1687.doi: 10.1093/cvr/cvaa106.

[21] Felsenstein S., Herbert J.A., McNamara P.S., Hedrich C.M., 2020, COVID-19: Immunology and treatment options. Clin Immunol; 215: 108448. doi: 10.1016/j.clim.2020.108448.

[22] Giamarellos-Bourboulis E.J., Netea M.G., Rovina N. et al. 2020, Complex immune dysregulation in COVID-19 patients with severe Respiratory Failure, Cell Host Microbe; 27(6):992-1000.e3. doi: 10.1016/j.chom.2020.04.009.

[23] Qin C., Zhou L., Hu Z. et al. 2020, Dysregulation of immune response in patients with coronavirus 2019 (COVID-19) in wuhan, China, Clin Infect Dis; 71(15):762-768. doi: 10.1093/cid/ciaa248.

[24] Wu Z., McGoogan J.M. 2020, Characteristics of and important lessons from the coronavirus disease 2019 (COVID-19) outbreak in China: Summary of a report of 72314 cases from the Chinese center for disease control and prevention, JAMA. 323 (13):1239-1242. doi:10.1001/jama.2020.2648.

[25] Hester A. Gietema, Noortje Zelis, Lars J. G. Lambriks, J. Martijn Nobel, Lieke B. van Alphen, Astrid M. L. Oude Lashof, Joachim E. Wildberger, Irene C. Nelissen, Patricia M. Stassen, 2020, CT in relation to RT-PCR in diagnosing COVID-19 in The Netherlands: A prospective study, PLoS One. 15(7): e0235844. doi: 10.1371/journal.pone.0235844.

[26] Hong T.C., Mai Q.L., Cuong D.V., Parida M., Minekawa H., Notomi T., Hasebe F., Morita K. 2004, Development and evaluation of a novel loop-mediated isothermal amplification method for rapid detection of severe acute respiratory syndrome coronavirus, Journal of Clinical Microbiology;

42(5):1956-1961. doi:10.1128/jcm.42.5.1956-1961.2004.

[27] W.E. Huang, B. Lim, C.C. Hsu, D. Xiong, W. Wu, Y. Yu, H. Jia, Y. Wang, Y. Zeng, M. Ji, H. Chang, X. Zhang, H. Wang, Z. Cui, 2020, RT-LAMP for rapid diagnosis of coronavirus SARS-CoV-2. Microb. Biotechnol; 13(4):950-961. doi:10.1111/1751-7915.13586.

[28] Parida, M., Posadas, G., Inoue, S., Hasebe, F., Morita, K., 2004. Real-Time Reverse Transcription Loop-Mediated Isothermal Amplification for Rapid Detection of West Nile Virus, Journal of Clinical Microbiology; 42(1):257-263. doi: 10.1128/jcm.42.1.257-263.2004.

[29] Buck, M. D. et al. (2020). Standard Operating Procedures for SARS-Cov-2 detection by a Clinical Diagnostic RT-LAMP Assay. doi:10.1101/2020.06.29.20142430.

[30] Jürgen Rödel, Renate Egerer, AynurSuleyman, Beatrice Sommer-Schmid, Michael Baier, Andreas Henke, Birgit Edel, Bettina Löffler. 2020, Use of the variplex™ SARS-CoV-2 RT-LAMP as a rapid molecular assay to complement RT-PCR for COVID-19 diagnosis. J Clin Virol; 132: 104616. doi: 10.1016/j.jcv.2020.104616.

[31] Saahir Khan, Rie Nakajima, Aarti Jain, Rafael Ramiro de Assis, Al Jasinskas, Joshua M. Obiero, Oluwasanmi Adenaiye, Sheldon Tai, Filbert Hong, Donald K. Milton, Huw Davies, Philip L. Felgner, 2020, Analysis of serologic cross-reactivity between common human coronaviruses and SARS-CoV-2 using coronavirus antigen micro array. doi: 10.1101/2020.03.24.006544.

[32] Bo Diao, Kun Wen, Jian Chen, Yueping Liu, Zilin Yuan, Chao Han, Jiahui Chen, Yuxian Pan, Li Chen, Yunjie Dan, Jing Wang, Yongwen Chen, Guohong Deng, Hongwei Zhou, Yuzhang Wu, 2020, Diagnosis of acute respiratory syndrome coronavirus 2 infection by detection of nucleocapsid protein. doi: 10.1101/2020.03.07.20032524.

[33] Merckx J, Wali R, Schiller I, Caya C, Gore GC, Chartrand C, Dendukuri N, Papenburg J. 2017, Diagnostic Accuracy of Novel and Traditional Rapid Tests for Influenza Infection Compared With Reverse Transcriptase Polymerase Chain Reaction: A Systematic Review and Meta-analysis. Ann Intern Med. 167(6):394-409. doi: 10.7326/M17-0848.

[34] Venkatesh K, Parija SC, Mahadevan S, Negi VS., 2007, Reverse passive haemagglutination (RPHA) test for detection of mycobacterial antigen in the cerebrospinal fluid for diagnosis of tubercular meningitis. Indian J Tuberc;54:41-48.

[35] Liu Y, Liu Y, Diao B, Ren Feifei, Yue Wang, Jinya Ding, Qianchuan Huang, 2020, Diagnostic indexes of a rapid IgG/IgM Combined Antibody Test for SARS-CoV-2. doi: 10.1101/2020.03.26.20044883.

[36] Zhao J, Yuan Q, Wang H, Liu W, Liao X, Su Y, et al., 2020, Antibody responses to SARS-CoV-2 in patients of novel coronavirus disease 2019.doi: 10.1101/2020.03.02.20030189.

[37] Okba N.M.A, Muller M.A., Li W, Wang C, et al., 2020, Severe Acute Respiratory Syndrome Coronavirus 2–Specific Antibody Responses in Coronavirus Disease Patients, Emerging Infectious Diseases, 26(7), ISSN: 1080-6059, doi: 10.3201/eid2607.200841.

[38] Barrangou R, (2015). The roles of CRISPR-Cas systems in adaptive immunity and beyond. Current Opinion in Immunology. 32:36-41. doi: 10.1016/j.coi.2014.12.008.

[39] Melika Lotfi, Nima Rezaei, 2020, CRISPR/Cas13: A potential therapeutic option of COVID19, Biomedicine &

Pharmacotherapy 113. doi:10.1016/j.biopha.2020.110738.

[40] Broughton J. P., Deng X, Yu G, Fasching CL, Servellita V, Singh J., et al. 2020, CRISPR–Cas12-based detection of SARS-CoV-2, Nature Biotechnology 38, 870-874. doi:10.1038/s41587-020-0513-4.

[41] Hou T, Zeng W, Yang M, Chen W, Ren L, Ai J, et al., 2020, Development and Evaluation of a CRISPR-based Diagnostic for 2019-novel coronavirus. doi: 10.1101/2020.02.22.20025460.

[42] Zhu X, Wang X, Han L, et al., 2020, Multiplex reverse transcription loop-mediated isothermal amplification combined with nanoparticle-based lateral flow biosensor for the diagnosis of COVID-19, Biosensors and Bioelectronics 166, 15, 112437. doi:10.1016/j.bios.2020.112437.

[43] Qiu G, Gai Z, Tao Y, et al. 2020, Dual-functional plasmonicphotothermal biosensors for highly accurate severe acute respiratory syndrome coronavirus 2 detection, : ACS Nano 14, 5268–5277. doi:10.1021/acsnano.0c02439.

[44] Singhal C, Dubey A, Mathur A, et al., 2018, Paper based DNA biosensor for detection of chikungunya virus using gold shells coated magnetic nanocubes. Process Biochemistry 74, Nov, 35-42. doi:10.1016/j.procbio.2018.08.020.

[45] Ivan Franch-Pardo, Brian M. Napoletano, Fernando Rosete-Verges, Lawal Billa, Spatial analysis and GIS in the study of COVID -19. A review, Science of the Total Environment 2020. DOI:10.1016/j.scitotenv.2020.140033.

[46] Sameer Saran, Priyanka Singh, Vishal Kumar, Prakash Chauhan, Review of Geospatial Technology for Infectious Disease Surveillance: Use Case on COVID-19, Journal of the Indian Society of Remote Sensing (2020) 48(8):1121-1138, doi:10.1007/s12524-020-01140-5.

[47] Suleman Sarwar ,Rida Waheed, Sahar Sarwar, Aisha Khan, COVID-19 challenges to Pakistan: Is GIS analysis useful to draw solutions?, Science of the Total Environment 730 (2020) 139089. doi:10.1016/j.scitotenv.2020.139089.

[48] Bherwani, H., Gautam, S., and Gupta, A. (2021). Qualitative and quantitative analyses of impact of COVID-19 on sustainable development goals (SDGs) in Indian subcontinent with a focus on air quality. International Journal of Environmental Science and Technology, 18(4), 1019-1028.

[49] Bherwani, H., Anjum, S., Kumar, S., Gautam, S., Gupta, A., Kumbhare, H. and Kumar, R. (2021). Understanding COVID-19 transmission through Bayesian probabilistic modeling and GIS-based Voronoi approach: a policy perspective. Environment, Development and Sustainability, 23(4), 5846-5864.

[50] Maged N. Kamel Boulos, Estella M. Geraghty, Geographical tracking and mapping of coronavirus disease COVID-19/severe acute respiratory syndrome coronavirus 2 (SARS-CoV-2) epidemic and associated events around the world: how 21st century GIS technologies are supporting the global fight against outbreaks and epidemics, Int J Health Geogr (2020) 19:8. doi:10.1186/s12942-020-00202-8.

[51] Gertjan Medema, Leo Heijnen, Goffe Elsinga, Ronald Italiaander, Anke Brouwer, Presence of SARS-Coronavirus-2 RNA in sewage and correlation with reported COVID-19 prevalence in the early stage of the epidemic in the Netherlands, Environ. Sci. Technol. Lett., 2020, DOI: 10.1021/acs.estlett.0c00357.

[52] Wathore, R., Gupta, A., Bherwani, H., & Labhasetwar, N. (2020).

Understanding air and water borne transmission and survival of coronavirus: Insights and way forward for SARS-CoV-2. Science of the total environment, 749, 141486.

[53] Walter Randazzo, Pilar Truchado, Enric Cuevas-Ferrando, Pedro Simon, Ana Allende, Gloria Sanchez, SARS-CoV-2 RNA in wastewater anticipated COVID-19 occurrence in a low prevalence area, Water Research 181 (2020) 115942, doi:10.1016/j.watres.2020.115942.

[54] Manish Kumar, Arbind Kumar Patel, Anil V. Shah, Janvi Raval, Neha Rajpara, Madhvi Joshi, Chaitanya G. Josh, First proof of the capability of wastewater surveillance for COVID-19 in India through detection of genetic material of SARS-CoV-2, Science of the Total Environment 746 (2020) 141326. doi:10.1016/j.scitotenv.2020.141326.

[55] Jordan Peccia, Alessandro Zulli, Doug E. Brackney, Nathan D. Grubaugh, Edward H. Kaplan, Arnau Casanovas-Massana, Albert I. Ko, Amyn A. Malik, Dennis Wang, Mike Wang, Joshua L. Warren, Daniel M. Weinberger, Wyatt Arnold, Saad B. Omer, Measurement of SARS-CoV-2 RNA in wastewater tracks community infection dynamics, Nature Biotechnology 38, pages 1164-1167(2020), doi: 10.1038/s41587-020-0684-z.

Chapter 21

Usefulness of the Hemogram in COVID-19

Sara Jimeno, Alejandro Peixoto, Sara Velázquez, Paula Sol Ventura, Salvador I. García Adasme and Alejandro López-Escobar

Abstract

SARS-CoV2 infection has devastating consequences on healthcare systems and has caused 3 million deaths by April 2021. Identifying patients at risk of death is a priority. Moderate–severe COVID-19 cases seem to associate a cytokine release that follows endothelial injury, triggering a hyperinflammatory and procoagulant state in which leukocytes and platelets are protagonists. Our group has published some reports about the usefulness of the hemogram in COVID-19. Hemogram-derived ratios, mainly the neutrophil-to-lymphocyte ratio (NLR) and the novelty neutrophil-to-platelet ratio (NPR), obtained on admission and their rate of change during hospitalization, can easily detect patients with high risk of mortality. Hemogram is a tool available to all hospitals and analyzing the hemogram-derived ratios would provide much more information than could be extracted by evaluating the counts in isolation. We now know that in COVID-19 it is essential to start early anti-inflammatory treatment when patient deteriorates and the hemogram could be a good indicator of this situation. More comprehensive studies are needed to determine how useful these hemogram-derived ratios and prognostic scores are. In the next chapter we will present information related to this aspect as well as our group's research on the usefulness of the hemogram in COVID-19.

Keywords: COVID-19, neutrophil-to-platelet ratio, NPR, neutrophil-to-lymphocyte ratio, NLR, hemogram-derived ratios

1. Introduction

COVID-19 is a systemic disease, in which all organs can be affected. Several studies have emphasized an anomalous immune response as the starting point for hypercoagulability phenomena, endothelial damage and macro- and microthrombosis, which would trigger life-threatening consequences in patients. White blood cell populations (monocytes, lymphocytes and neutrophils) play a crucial role in the systemic inflammatory response and platelets have a direct function in the thrombotic response.

Differential blood cell counts can be measured simply, are cost-effective and reliable, and therefore can be used as markers of severity of the immune and inflammatory, and even the procoagulant response. In this context, white blood cells and platelets as circulating biomarkers involved in inflammatory and thrombotic responses could potentially predict clinical outcomes of patients with COVID-19.

Various hemogram parameters, including hemogram-derived ratios, have been used to try to identify patients with worse prognosis for COVID-19. In the following chapter the reader will find information related to this aspect as well as our group's research on the usefulness of the hemogram in COVID-19.

2. Pathophysiological basis for the potential usefulness of the blood count in COVID-19

The clinical presentation of COVID-19, ranges from a mild, self-limited form of the disease to multiple organ failure [1–4]. In the most severe cases, the disease can lead to severe viral pneumonia with dyspnea and hypoxemia that can evolve into severe respiratory distress syndrome, heart failure, obstructive thromboinflammatory syndrome, septic shock and multi-organ failure. This rapidly progressive deterioration causes the disease even fatal in some patients [5–11].

Several studies have emphasized an anomalous immune response as the starting point of an obstructive thrombo-inflammatory syndrome in which all organs can be affected, especially vital organs such as the kidney or the heart, with the incidence of pulmonary embolisms being very high in COVID-19 patients [12–14]. The most severe middle-aged patients suffered more localized lung damage and coagulopathy [14].

Some of the variables that have shown significant correlation with poor outcomes in COVID-19 include male sex, older age, smoking status, and the coexistence of comorbidities such as obesity, hypertension, diabetes, cardiovascular disease, cerebrovascular disease, chronic kidney disease, chronic obstructive pulmonary disease, hepatitis B infections and malignancy [1, 11].

Analytical parameters have also been widely used in early evaluation and monitoring of COVID-19 patients. Many of these parameters, specifically derived from white blood cell or platelet count values, provide information on both immunological status and hemostasis in response to SARS-CoV-2 infection.

In fact, the host's inflammatory response to SARS-CoV-2 infection appears critical in clinical evolution of COVID-19, and blood cell interactions are essential in the pathophysiology of inflammation, immune responses and hemostasis in this setting.

These interactions are complex, and it is often difficult to discriminate the specific roles of each cell type in the different phases of the same disease. Platelets are the main mediators of hemostasis while leukocytes are responsible for the immune responses.

White blood cell populations (monocytes, lymphocytes and neutrophils) are the main protagonists in the systemic inflammatory response to severe infection, injury, trauma and shock and therefore can be used as markers of this response [15]. Neutrophils are the most abundant white blood cells in circulation and represent the first line of innate immune defense, playing a fundamental role [7]. Furthermore, when this cell type is active, it has migratory capacity from the venous system to the affected organ or systems [11].

Accumulating evidence suggests that a portion of patients presenting with severe COVID-19 may have an underlying hyperinflammatory response that drives a cytokine release storm resulting in multiorgan failure and death [16]. A novel form of microvascular obstructive thromboinflammatory syndrome has been proposed as the pathophysiology underlying this hyperinflammatory response. Following SARS-CoV-2 infection, CD4+ T lymphocytes are rapidly activated to become pathogenic T helper 1, cells that produce cytokines that stimulate inflammatory CD14 + CD16+ monocytes generating IL-6 expression and accelerating the inflammatory process [17]. The inflammatory response may stimulate neutrophil production and even accelerate lymphocyte apoptosis.

Autopsies of patients affected by COVID-19 revealed a significant infiltration of neutrophils in the pulmonary capillaries with extravasation towards the alveolar lumen. This existence of acute capillaritis together with the presence of tracheal neutrophilic mucositis demonstrates the existence of a general inflammation of the airways [7].

Neutrophils can release large amounts of oxygen free radicals, which induce cell damage and release of viral particles from cells. Antibody-dependent cells can directly destroy the virus by exposing the viral antigen and thus activating cell-specific and humoral immunity. Neutrophils are also capable of producing large amounts of cytokines and signaling molecules such as endothelial growth factors (VEGF). Two of these factors, VEGF-A and VEGF-C, present significantly higher values in COVID-19 patients [11]. The accumulation of neutrophils associated with endothelial cell infection in COVID-19 disease induces endothelitis in different organs, thus contributing to systemic damage due to hypoxic microcirculation failure [7]. Increased neutrophils is an important risk factor and is closely related to increased patient severity, the development of acute respiratory syndrome (ARDS), and death in COVID-19 patients [18].

Infected pulmonary macrophages produce TNF-α and interleukins that cause T-cell apoptosis and lymphocyte recirculation, with massive recruitment into inflamed tissues [19, 20]. In addition, it is known that SARS-CoV-2 can directly infect lymphocytes, which have the angiotensin-converting enzyme 2 (ACE 2) receptor, so the virus can cause a decrease in their count, especially TCD8 + and TCD4 + lymphocytes [21, 22]. This triggers global lymphopenia, common in patients with severe COVID-19. It has been shown that the lower the lymphocyte count and the longer the duration of lymphopenia, the more severe the condition of infected patients and the worse the prognosis [19, 20].

Dysregulated immune cell responses are thought to play a notable role in the severity of disease [23]. Severe inflammatory responses result in a weak adaptive immune response, which translates into an imbalance of the immune response.

Several studies have shown that patients with COVID-19 who have higher levels of inflammatory cytokines and chemokines have greater disease severity, suggesting the involvement of cytokine storm in severe forms of the disease [1, 24]. This uncontrolled cytokine production, which increases as the infection worsens, provides the setting for SARS-CoV-2 pathogenesis leading to viral sepsis, tissue damage, disseminated intravascular coagulation, shock and even multi-organ failure. Proinflammatory cytokines induce apoptosis in lung epithelial cells, dendritic cells and macrophages, which impairs the pulmonary microvascular barrier and alveolar gas exchange. They increase vascular permeability, as well as the amount of fluid and inflammatory cells in the alveoli, causing dyspnea and respiratory failure [24, 25].

It has been hypothesized that an endothelial thromboinflammatory syndrome is triggered after alveolar viral damage [26]. SARS-CoV-2 uses the cell surface ACE 2 receptor to enter the interior of cells. ACE 2 is expressed in several organs, including endothelial cells [21, 22]. It has been reported that SARS-CoV-2 can infect genetically modified human blood vessel organoids in vitro, and the involvement of endothelial cells in the vascular beds of different organs has also been demonstrated in necropsies performed on deceased COVID-19 patients [27, 28].

Endothelial cell damage may be an important trigger of cytokine discharge, and moderate and severe COVID-19 cases appear to be associated with a large release of cytokines, leading to a hyperinflammatory and procoagulant state. Such inflammation, associated with the disproportionate cytokine storm, spreads widely through the systemic circulation, affecting different organs with high mortality [29].

This procoagulant state is associated with thromboembolic phenomena, such as deep vein thrombosis and pulmonary thromboembolism, which carry a worse prognosis. Anatomopathological studies of the lungs of patients with COVID-19 have shown frequent and systematic findings of thrombotic microangiopathy and hemorrhage [30, 31].

This new form of microvascular obstructive thromboinflammatory syndrome has been proposed as the pathophysiological basis underlying this hyperinflammatory response. This endothelial thromboinflammatory syndrome can progressively involve the microvascular bed of several vital organs, leading to multiple organ failure and death [26].

In addition, individuals with pre-existing endothelial dysfunction and therefore with a more active base inflammatory state, could lead to worse evolution in COVID-19. It has been observed that those patients affected by COVID-19 and with cardiovascular diseases had a greater probability of suffering myocardial injuries than those who did not present this type of previous injuries. Furthermore, those patients with chronic obstructive pulmonary disease (COPD) had a greater probability of suffering pulmonary coinfections and septic shock. Moreover, patients with previous kidney disease are also susceptible to developing COVID-19-induced worsening of kidney disease. The presence of these comorbidities may have increased mortality independently of COVID-19 infection as a result of the worsening of comorbidities induced by the viral infection rather than by the direct damage produced by SARS-CoV-2 [14].

In this context, white blood cells and platelets would have a direct role in this inflammation and in the thrombotic response; therefore, circulating biomarkers representing inflammation and immune status could potentially predict clinical outcomes of COVID-19 patients [11, 32].

Following these findings, routine blood tests and differential white blood cell counts are easy to obtain at most healthcare centers and are affordable and cheap markers for predicting a worse prognosis in COVID-19.

Several studies have reported the results of blood tests in patients with COVID-19, and most severe cases present low lymphocytes counts, higher leukocytes counts and hemogram-derived ratios, as well as lower percentages of monocytes, eosinophils and basophils [24]. Some of these inflammatory markers have been evaluated and found to correlate with worse prognosis, including peripheral white blood cell count and hemogram-derived ratios.

3. Hemogram-derived ratios in COVID-19

The hemogram-derived ratios are parameters which amplify the value of neutrophils, platelets and lymphocytes and could be useful to predict prognosis and severity of the disease. Several hemogram-derived ratios as neutrophil-to-lymphocyte ratio (NLR), derived NLR ratio (dNLR) (neutrophil count/leukocyte count−neutrophil count), platelet-to-lymphocyte ratio (PLR) and lymphocyte-to-monocyte ratio have been used as inflammatory markers of COVID-19 [11, 32–34].

3.1 Neutrophil-to-lymphocyte ratio (NLR)

An available marker of great value for measuring the inflammatory status of an individual is the NLR, an easily measurable parameter that is obtained from a routine blood test. It is the ratio of the absolute neutrophil count to the absolute lymphocyte count of a routine blood count [33, 35, 36].

It has been proposed as a prognostic marker of severity in many pathologies such as oncological processes, septic shock, infectious diseases, intracranial hemorrhage and cardiovascular disease among others [35, 36].

Moreover, NLR appears to be an indicator of endothelial dysfunction and an important predictor of cardiovascular mortality [23, 24].

The endothelial dysfunction could be one of the aggravating factors of SARS-CoV-2 disease and would explain the evolution of the disease towards multiple organ failure [37–40]. Several studies have been published, incorporating NLR as a marker of poor prognosis in patients with COVID-19 [8, 11, 33, 41, 42].

The normal values of this quotient in an adult population, excluding the geriatric population, are around 0.78 and 3.5. When the NLR result exceeds the normal maximum value, the probability of the disease going from a mild–moderate to a severe state dramatically increases.

A higher NLR value at admission is related to mortality in COVID-19, since high values have been observed at the beginning of admission in patients who did not survive [37]. This is because in more severe patients, the inflammatory response stimulates neutrophil production and therefore the neutrophil count is higher, while this response accelerates lymphocyte apoptosis and the lymphocyte count is low, and therefore the NLR value increases.

Our group has investigated the usefulness of this ratio being one of the first groups to publish on the implications of this ratio and its relationship with worse prognosis in COVID-19. In a small cohort of patients, we demonstrated how the evolution of NLR in terms of rate of increase and Peak NLR was associated with worse outcomes in COVID-19 with higher risk of ICU admission or death [38].

Subsequently, in a cohort of more than 2000 patients, we demonstrated that NLR is associated with in-hospital mortality as it is higher at baseline hospital admission and maintains significance after multivariable adjustment [43].

Moreover, patients requiring ICU admission had significantly higher NLR values at the time of hospital admission [44].

3.2 Platelet-to-lymphocyte ratio (PLR)

Some studies demonstrate the ratio of platelet count to lymphocyte count, called PLR, as a reliable marker of immune-mediated, metabolic, prothrombotic and neoplastic diseases.

Its use in combination with other complementary hematological ratios, in particular NLR, provides additional information on the degree of disease activity and helps to monitor the response to anti-inflammatory treatments. It could even help in the early detection of comorbidities that develop in the course of disease treatment [45–47].

PLR primarily reflects the level of systemic inflammation that translates megakaryocyte activity in the hematopoietic tissue of the bone marrow, an important component in thrombosis. It also plays a very important role in the inflammatory response by promoting the recruitment of neutrophils and other inflammatory cells to the site of injury.

This ratio reflects both aggregation and inflammatory pathways and is therefore considered by some authors to be more valid for predicting inflammatory pathology than platelet or lymphocyte counts alone [11]. However, relationship between PLR and mortality has been less explored.

It has been postulated that PLR may reflect the degree of cytokine release, which could be a useful indicator of the clinical course of COVID-19 patients [48]. SARS-CoV-2 infection causes a cytokine storm in body fluids, aggravating the patient's inflammatory response and stimulating platelet release. Some authors consider that platelet number and its dynamic changes during the course of COVID-19 and treatment may correlate with cytokine storm, and consequently, with disease severity and prognosis [48].

Our group has also investigated the usefulness of this ratio in COVID-19 and we observed that patients who died presented significantly higher PLR compared with patients who survived at admission [43], like patients requiring ICU admission [44], but they did not maintain significance after more complex model of multivariable adjustment.

3.3 Systemic immune-inflammation index (SII)

The systemic immune-inflammation index (SII) is a hemogram-derived ratio defined as the count of neutrophils multiplied by the count of platelets and divided by the count of lymphocytes.

SII has recently been proposed as a prognostic indicator in the follow-up of patients with sepsis [49] and cancer patients [50, 51] as an index defining the instability in the inflammatory response.

This quotient derived from the hemogram has also been studied by our group in patients affected by COVID-19 and, like PLR, SII on admission is significantly higher in COVID-19 patients who died and required admission to the ICU, but it did not maintain statistical significance after multivariate adjustment [43, 44].

3.4 Neutrophil-to-platelet ratio (NPR)

The modulatory interaction between neutrophils and platelets has previously been described [52] and based on the biological plausibility of higher total neutrophils count and lower total platelets count observed among the most severe COVID-19 cases compared to more mild ones, we have investigated the utility of a novel parameter, the neutrophil–platelet ratio (NPR).

NPR is the ratio between the count of neutrophils (x 10^9 cells/L) and the count of platelets (x 10^{11}cells/L), and may be useful in signaling a combination of hyperinflammatory response and microvascular occlusion that has been identified in moderate to severe COVID-19 cases [26, 53].

We hypothesize that a damaged and activated endothelium may increase the permeability and release of cytokines that would initiate chemotaxis of inflammatory cells and also recruit other blood cells.

In this context, activated platelets and neutrophils play a determining role in microvascular occlusion during the thromboinflammatory phase of the disease [54]. These findings were observed in the most severe COVID-19 cases who died, especially higher neutrophil and lower platelet counts.

Our results have shown that NPR levels were significantly associated with in-hospital mortality due to COVID-19 and their association remained significant even after multivariable adjustment.

Also, higher levels of NPR at admission are related to higher risk of ICU admission in COVID-19 patients [43, 44].

We are the first group in the world reporting the usefulness of this hemogram-derived ratio in a disease and we believe that this novel finding merits further investigation.

3.5 Incorporation of rates of change of hemogram-derived ratios

Our group has also studied the rate of change in the ratios derived from the blood count during the first days of hospitalization in patients affected by COVID-19.

The rate of increase has been shown to be a useful marker of severity and is associated with mortality.

Undoubtedly, these rates of change could be affected by the course of COVID-19 and the treatments applied, but we hypothesized that some of these rates could be a valuable parameter in the control of patients without additional risk factors to assess modifying the treatment [38, 43, 44].

3.6 Incorporation of hemogram-derived ratios into clinical judgment nomograms

In most cases, the first assessment for a COVID-19 case takes place in the emergency department, where it is routine clinical practice to carry out a full blood panel.

Based on the usefulness of the hemogram-derived ratio, we have developed the Risk Score for Predicting In-Hospital Mortality in COVID-19 (RIM Score COVID) [53].

We have developed four models: two with NLR, the ratio more widely reported, and two with NPR, the novel hemogram-derived-ratio proposed by our group. No significant differences were found between NLR and NPR models; however, models using the NPR ratio showed more robustness in more complex multivariate analyses.

The RIM Score COVID includes following variables at hospital admission: age, sex, oxygen saturation, level of C-reactive-protein, NPR and NLR.

The AUC of models including NLR and NPR were evaluated for predicting in-hospital mortality by COVID-19 and both performed similarly in the validation cohorts: NLR 0.856 (95% CI: 0.818–0.895), NPR 0.863 (95% CI: 0.826–0.901).

Moreover, we have developed two models incorporating the rate of changes of both hemogram-derived ratios during the first week after admission, called Velocity of NLR (VNLR) and Velocity of NPR (VNPR).

The accuracy of the models were also evaluated for predicting in-hospital mortality by COVID-19 and the predictive ability of in-hospital mortality in both models improved slightly in the validation cohorts with respect to the values obtained at admission: VNLR 0.885 (95% CI: 0.885–0.919), VNPR 0.891 (95% CI: 0.861–0.922).

According to our results, the RIM Score COVID models are useful for predicting the risk of in-hospital mortality from COVID-19.

The proposed RIM Score is a simple and widely available tool that can help identify patients at risk of fatal outcomes.

The parameters used in the nomogram are objective, easy to obtain and reproducible in most healthcare facilities without additional cost or need for additional laboratory equipment.

These assessments provide a highly accurate predictive value of in-hospital mortality risk from COVID-19 [53].

4. Conclusions

The hemogram is an easily measurable, readily available, cost-effective and reliable test that could be very useful in establishing the risk of in-hospital mortality on hospital admission and in guiding therapeutic decisions in patients with COVID-19.

In this sense, the hemogram is a tool available to all healthcare centers that do not have the technical and material means to perform complex immunological studies, which usually involve late results.

The combination of hemogram parameters and blood cell count ratios in COVID-19 patients could be a useful combined indicator of host immune and inflammatory status.

The ratios derived from the hemogram at the time of hospital admission and its increasing trend during the first days of hospitalization have shown their value in identifying patients with COVID-19 who have a worse evolution and could be useful as prognostic markers of the disease.

The NLR and the novelty NPR have been shown to be independent markers of mortality and worse prognosis in patients with COVID-19. These ratios should be included in future prospective studies and it would be advisable to start using them by physicians in the first evaluation of patients with COVID-19 in the emergency department to demonstrate their clinical utility.

Acknowledgements

We would like to thank all the authors who have participated in previous publications of our group:

Dr. Marina Bucar, Dr. José M. Castellano, Dr. Mario Miranda, Dr. Isabel Llana, Prof. Rodrigo Madurga, Dr. Justo Menéndez, Santiago Ruiz de Aguiar, Dr. Rafael Suárez del Villar, Dr. Paula Touza.

Conflict of interest

Salvador I. Garcia-Adasme has received private founds by HM Hospitales to course his doctoral studies in CEU International Doctoral School – CEINDO, CEU-San Pablo University.

The remaining authors declare no conflicts of interest.

Author details

Sara Jimeno[1,2,3], Alejandro Peixoto[3], Sara Velázquez[2,4,5], Paula Sol Ventura[2,6,7], Salvador I. García Adasme[8] and Alejandro López-Escobar[2,9,10]*

1 Pediatrics Department, HM Hospitales, Madrid, Spain

2 Fundación de Investigación HM Hospitales, Madrid, Spain

3 Facultad de Medicina, Universidad CEU San Pablo, Madrid, Spain

4 Anaesthesiology Department, Hospital Universitario HM Sanchinarro, Madrid, Spain

5 Anaesthesiology Department, Hospital Universitario Santa Cristina, Madrid, Spain

6 Pediatrics Department, Hospital Universitario HM Nens, Barcelona, Spain

7 Fundació Institut d'Investigació en Ciències de la Salut Germans Trias i Pujol (IGTP), Barcelona, Spain

8 Nurse School, Universidad CEU San Pablo, Madrid, Spain

9 Pediatrics Department, Hospital Vithas Madrid La Milagrosa, Madrid, Spain

10 Clinical Research Unit. Fundación Vithas. Grupo Vithas, Madrid, Spain

*Address all correspondence to: lopezea@vithas.es

References

[1] Huang C, Wang Y, Li X, Ren L, Zhao J, Hu Y, et al. Clinical features of patients infected with 2019 novel coronavirus in Wuhan, China. The Lancet 2020;395(10223):497-506.

[2] Chen N, Zhou M, Dong X, Qu J, Gong F, Han Y, et al. Epidemiological and clinical characteristics of 99 cases of 2019 novel coronavirus pneumonia in Wuhan, China: a descriptive study. The Lancet 2020;395(10223):507-513.

[3] Wang D, Hu B, Hu C, Zhu F, Liu X, Zhang J, et al. Clinical characteristics of 138 hospitalized patients with 2019 novel coronavirus–infected pneumonia in Wuhan, China. JAMA 2020;323(11):1061-1069.

[4] Guan WJ, Liang WH, Zhao Y, Liang HR, Chen ZS, Li YM, et al. Comorbidity and its impact on 1590 patients with COVID-19 in China: a nationwide analysis. Eur Respir J 2020;55(5):10.1183/13993003.00547-2020.

[5] Covino M, Sandroni C, Santoro M, Sabia L, Simeoni B, Bocci MG, et al. Predicting intensive care unit admission and death for COVID-19 patients in the emergency department using early warning scores. Resuscitation 2020;156:84-91.

[6] Zhou F, Yu T, Du R, Fan G, Liu Y, Liu Z, et al. Clinical course and risk factors for mortality of adult inpatients with COVID-19 in Wuhan, China: a retrospective cohort study. The lancet 2020;395(10229):1054-1062.

[7] Fois AG, Paliogiannis P, Scano V, Cau S, Babudieri S, Perra R, et al. The systemic inflammation index on admission predicts in-hospital mortality in COVID-19 patients. Molecules 2020;25(23):5725.

[8] Liang W, Liang H, Ou L, Chen B, Chen A, Li C, et al. Development and validation of a clinical risk score to predict the occurrence of critical illness in hospitalized patients with COVID-19. JAMA Internal Medicine 2020;180(8):1081-1089.

[9] Shang Y, Liu T, Wei Y, Li J, Shao L, Liu M, et al. Scoring systems for predicting mortality for severe patients with COVID-19. EClinicalMedicine 2020;24:100426.

[10] Yamada T, Wakabayashi M, Yamaji T, Chopra N, Mikami T, Miyashita H, et al. Value of leukocytosis and elevated C-reactive protein in predicting severe coronavirus 2019 (COVID-19): a systematic review and meta-analysis. Clinica Chimica Acta 2020;509:235-243.

[11] Yang A, Liu J, Tao W, Li H. The diagnostic and predictive role of NLR, d-NLR and PLR in COVID-19 patients. Int Immunopharmacol 2020;84:106504.

[12] Cespedes MdS, Souza, José Carlos Rosa Pires de. Coronavirus: a clinical update of Covid-19. Revista da Associação Médica Brasileira 2020;66(2):116-123.

[13] Galloway JB, Norton S, Barker RD, Brookes A, Carey I, Clarke BD, et al. A clinical risk score to identify patients with COVID-19 at high risk of critical care admission or death: an observational cohort study. J Infect 2020;81(2):282-288.

[14] Wang P, Sha J, Meng M, Wang C, Yao Q, Zhang Z, et al. Risk factors for severe COVID-19 in middle-aged patients without comorbidities: a multicentre retrospective study. Journal of translational medicine 2020;18(1):1-12.

[15] Zahorec R. Ratio of neutrophil to lymphocyte counts-rapid and simple parameter of systemic inflammation and stress in critically ill. Bratisl Lek Listy 2001;102(1):5-14.

[16] Mehta P, McAuley DF, Brown M, Sanchez E, Tattersall RS, Manson JJ. COVID-19: consider cytokine storm syndromes and immunosuppression. The Lancet 2020;395(10229):1033-1034.

[17] Zhou Y, Fu B, Zheng X, Wang D, Zhao C. Pathogenic T cells and inflammatory monocytes incite inflammatory storm in severe COVID-19 patients. National Science Review 2020;7(6):998-1002.

[18] Hu H, Du H, Li J, Wang Y, Wu X, Wang C, et al. Early prediction and identification for severe patients during the pandemic of COVID-19: A severe COVID-19 risk model constructed by multivariate logistic regression analysis. Journal of Global Health 2020;10(2).

[19] Merad M, Martin JC. Pathological inflammation in patients with COVID-19: a key role for monocytes and macrophages. Nature Reviews Immunology 2020;20(6):355-362.

[20] Mehta AK, Gracias DT, Croft M. TNF activity and T cells. Cytokine 2018;101:14-18.

[21] Maggi E, Canonica GW, Moretta L. COVID-19: unanswered questions on immune response and pathogenesis. J Allergy Clin Immunol 2020;146(1):18-22.

[22] Mehra MR, Desai SS, Kuy S, Henry TD, Patel AN. Cardiovascular disease, drug therapy, and mortality in Covid-19. N Engl J Med 2020;382(25):e102.

[23] Joly BS, Siguret V, Veyradier A. Understanding pathophysiology of hemostasis disorders in critically ill patients with COVID-19. Intensive Care Med 2020;46(8):1603-1606.

[24] Qin C, Zhou L, Hu Z, Zhang S, Yang S, Tao Y, et al. Dysregulation of immune response in patients with COVID-19 in Wuhan, China. Clinical Infectious Diseases 2020; 71(15):762-768.

[25] Gubernatorova E, Gorshkova E, Polinova A, Drutskaya M. IL-6: relevance for immunopathology of SARS-CoV-2. Cytokine Growth Factor Rev 2020;53:13-24.

[26] Ciceri F, Beretta L, Scandroglio AM, Colombo S, Landoni G, Ruggeri A, et al. Microvascular COVID-19 lung vessels obstructive thromboinflammatory syndrome (MicroCLOTS): an atypical acute respiratory distress syndrome working hypothesis. Crit Care Resusc 2020;22(2):95.

[27] Monteil V, Kwon H, Prado P, Hagelkrüys A, Wimmer RA, Stahl M, et al. Inhibition of SARS-CoV-2 infections in engineered human tissues using clinical-grade soluble human ACE2. Cell 2020;181(4):905-913.

[28] Varga Z, FlamAJ, Steiger P, Haberecker M, Andermatt R, Zinkernagel AS, et al. Endothelial cell infection and endotheliitis in COVID-19. Lancet 2020 May 2;395(10234):1417-1418.

[29] Channappanavar R, Perlman S. Pathogenic human coronavirus infections: causes and consequences of cytokine storm and immunopathology. Seminars in immunopathology 2017;39(5):529-539.

[30] Carsana L, Sonzogni A, Nasr A, Rossi RS, Pellegrinelli A, Zerbi P, et al. Pulmonary post-mortem findings in a series of COVID-19 cases from northern Italy: a two-centre descriptive study. The Lancet infectious diseases 2020;20(10):1135-1140.

[31] Fox SE, Akmatbekov A, Harbert JL, Li G, Brown JQ, Vander Heide RS. Pulmonary and cardiac pathology in African American patients with COVID-19: an autopsy series from New Orleans. The Lancet Respiratory Medicine 2020;8(7):681-686.

[32] Teuwen L, Geldhof V, Pasut A, Carmeliet P. COVID-19: the vasculature unleashed. Nature Reviews Immunology 2020;20(7):389-391.

[33] Liu Y, Du X, Chen J, Jin Y, Peng L, Wang HH, et al. Neutrophil-to-lymphocyte ratio as an independent risk factor for mortality in hospitalized patients with COVID-19. J Infect 2020;81(1):e6-e12.

[34] Liu J, Liu Y, Xiang P, Pu L, Xiong H, Li C, et al. Neutrophil-to-lymphocyte ratio predicts critical illness patients with 2019 coronavirus disease in the early stage. Journal of Translational Medicine 2020;18:1-12.

[35] Guthrie GJ, Charles KA, Roxburgh CS, Horgan PG, McMillan DC, Clarke SJ. The systemic inflammation-based neutrophil–lymphocyte ratio: experience in patients with cancer. Crit Rev Oncol 2013;88(1):218-230.

[36] Forget P, Khalifa C, Defour J, Latinne D, Van Pel M, De Kock M. What is the normal value of the neutrophil-to-lymphocyte ratio? BMC research notes 2017;10(1):12.

[37] Mousavi SA, Rad S, Rostami T, Rostami M, Mousavi SA, Mirhoseini SA, et al. Hematologic predictors of mortality in hospitalized patients with COVID-19: a comparative study. Hematology 2020;25(1):383-388.

[38] Jimeno S, Ventura PS, Castellano JM, García-Adasme SI, Miranda M, Touza P, et al. Prognostic implications of neutrophil-lymphocyte ratio in COVID-19. Eur J Clin Invest 2021:e13404.

[39] Lv Z, Wang W, Qiao B, Cui X, Feng Y, Chen L, et al. The prognostic value of general laboratory testing in patients with COVID-19. J Clin Lab Anal 2020:e23668.

[40] Moradi EV, Teimouri A, Rezaee R, Morovatdar N, Foroughian M, Layegh P, et al. Increased age, neutrophil-to-lymphocyte ratio (NLR) and white blood cells count are associated with higher COVID-19 mortality. Am J Emerg Med 2021;40:11-14.

[41] Zeng F, Li L, Zeng J, Deng Y, Huang H, Chen B, et al. Can we predict the severity of coronavirus disease 2019 with a routine blood test? Polish archives of internal medicine 2020;130(5).

[42] Mo P, Xing Y, Xiao Y, Deng L, Zhao Q, Wang H, et al. Clinical characteristics of refractory COVID-19 pneumonia in Wuhan, China. Clinical Infectious Diseases 2020.

[43] López-Escobar A, Madurga R, Castellano JM, de Aguiar SR, Velázquez S, Bucar M, et al. Hemogram as marker of in-hospital mortality in COVID-19. J Invest Med 2021.

[44] Velázquez S, Madurga R, Castellano Vázquez JM, et al. Hemogram rate as prognostic markers of Care Unit Admission in COVID-19. MC Emergency Medicine. 2021. DOI: 10.21203/rs.3.rs-403472/v1.

[45] Abdel Galil SM, Edrees AM, Ajeeb AK, Aldoobi GS, El-Boshy M, Hussain W. Prognostic significance of platelet count in SLE patients. Platelets 2017;28(2):203-207.

[46] Lood C, Tydén H, Gullstrand B, Nielsen CT, Heegaard NH, Linge P, et al. Decreased platelet size is associated with platelet activation and anti-phospholipid syndrome in systemic lupus erythematosus. Rheumatology 2017;56(3):408-416.

[47] Gasparyan AY, Ayvazyan L, Mukanova U, Yessirkepov M, Kitas GD. The platelet-to-lymphocyte ratio as an inflammatory marker in rheumatic

diseases. Annals of laboratory medicine 2019;39(4):345-357.

[48] Qu R, Ling Y, Zhang Y, Wei L, Chen X, Li X, et al. Platelet-to-lymphocyte ratio is associated with prognosis in patients with coronavirus disease-19. J Med Virol 2020;92(9):1533-1541.

[49] Pedersen S, Ho Y. SARS-CoV-2: A storm is raging. J Clin Invest 2020;130(5).

[50] Hu B, Yang XR, Xu Y, Sun YF, Sun C, Guo W, et al. Systemic immune-inflammation index predicts prognosis of patients after curative resection for hepatocellular carcinoma. Clin Cancer Res 2014 Dec 1;20(23):6212-6222.

[51] Zhang Y, Sun Y, Zhang Q. Prognostic value of the systemic immune-inflammation index in patients with breast cancer: a meta-analysis. Cancer Cell International 2020;20(1):1-12.

[52] Lisman T. Platelet–neutrophil interactions as drivers of inflammatory and thrombotic disease. Cell Tissue Res 2018;371(3):567-576.

[53] López-Escobar A, Madurga R, Castellano JM, Velázquez S, Suárez del Villar R, Menéndez J, et al. Risk score for predicting in-hospital mortality in COVID-19 (rim score). Diagnostics 2021;11(4):596.

[54] Li J, Kim K, Barazia A, Tseng A, Cho J. Platelet–neutrophil interactions under thromboinflammatory conditions. Cellular and molecular life sciences 2015;72(14):2627-2643.

Chapter 22

COVID-19 Vaccine: A Way Out of Crisis

Aman Sachdeva and Arup Saha

Abstract

COVID-19 pandemic has taken toll on the entire globe at physical, emotional and administrative level; straining each and every aspect to its fullest. As on April 19/2021, COVID-19 has infected more than 140 million people around world with around 3 million deaths worldwide. Covid-19 vaccine has emerged as an important direction to walk the world out of this crisis. This chapter covers the basic aspects and principles of vaccination and Immunology and its application in COVID-19 pandemic. This chapter further covers the different type of vaccines being developed, their dosage schedule and route of administration, common adverse events and myths related to them.

Keywords: COVID-19, Pandemic, vaccine

1. Introduction

Immunization is a global health and development success story, saving millions of lives every year. Vaccines reduce risks of getting a disease by working with your body's natural defenses to build protection. When you get a vaccine, your immune system responds. Immunization is a key component of primary health care and an indisputable human right. It's also one of the best health investments money can buy. Vaccines are also critical to the prevention and control of infectious-disease outbreaks. They underpin global health security and will be a vital tool in the battle against antimicrobial resistance. The two terms vaccination and immunization has been used synonymously over the time but the two terms differ in their meaning [1].

"Vaccination" as per definition is defined as the process of administering the biochemical product referred to as vaccine in the human body whereas "Immunization" is defined as the process by which body develops immunity against the disease [2].

Vaccines train the immune system to develop antibodies and protect against the disease. As per World Health Organization (WHO) there are number of vaccines which had been developed against number of diseases namely Diphtheria, hepatitis B, measles, mumps, pertussis, polio and many more. On similar grounds, to tackle the menace of COVID-19, various vaccines have been developed [3].

2. Types of vaccines

Vaccines are of different types depending on the property of the pathogen/agent used in vaccine [4, 5].

a. **On basis whether agent is live or killed.**

i. Live attenuated vaccine.

ii. Inactivated vaccine.

b. **On Basis whether part/entire agent used**

i. Whole cell vaccine.

ii. Subunit vaccine.

c. **On basis of Component of agent used.**

i. Nucleic acid based vaccines.

ii. Protein based vaccines.

iii. Polysaccharide vaccines.

iv. Toxoid vaccines.

v. Conjugate vaccines.

d. **Newer type of vaccines**

i. Viral vector based vaccine.

ii. Recombinant vaccines.

1. **Live attenuated vaccine:** These are the type of vaccines which contain weakened form of the pathogen. Immunogenicity of the pathogen is maintained while lowering the virulence and thus the disease-causing potential.

2. **Inactivated vaccine:** This type of vaccine contain pathogen in killed form. The pathogen is inactivated chemically or by other means thus removing the disease-causing potential of the vaccine. These vaccines are safer as compared to live attenuated vaccines as per the disease-causing potential of the vaccine.

3. **Whole cell vaccine:** In this type of vaccine agent is used in its complete form either live attenuated or killed.

4. **Subunit vaccine:** This type of vaccine uses a part of the agent rather than using the whole agent. This type of vaccine induces high and specific immune response as compared to other type of vaccines.

5. **Nucleic acid-based vaccine:** These vaccines employ the genetic material as the active component of the vaccine. Based on the genetic material used, these can be either DNA based vaccine or RNA based vaccines. Further on the type of RNA used vaccines can be further divided into mRNA based and others. Most of the nucleic acid-based vaccines are of mRNA type.

6. **Protein and polysaccharide-based vaccine:** These vaccines use the protein part and polysaccharide portion of the agent as active component respectively.

7. **Toxoid vaccine:** Toxoid vaccines are special type of subunit vaccines in which the toxins produced by the disease-causing agent is chemically inactivated and the resulting toxoid is then used as active component of the vaccines. These

Sr.No.	Characteristics	Primary Immune Response	Secondary Immune Response
1	Definition	Primary Immune Response is the reaction of the immune system when it contacts an antigen for the first time.	Secondary Immune Response is the reaction of the immune system when it contacts an antigen for the second and subsequent times.
2	Appearance	Appears mainly in the lymph nodes and spleen.	Appears mainly in the bone marrow and then, in the spleen and lymph nodes.
3	Occurrence	This occurs in response to the primary contact of the antigen.	This occurs in response to the second and subsequent exposure to the same antigen.
4	Antibody Peak	The antibody level reaches its peak in 7–10 days.	The antibody level reaches its peak in 3–5 days.
5	Affinity of Antibody	Low affinity to their antigens.	High affinity to their antigens.
6	Responding Cells	Naive B cells and T cells	Memory B cells
7	Antibodies	Both thymus-dependent and thymus-independent antibodies are involved in the primary immune response.	Only thymus-dependent antibodies are involved in the secondary immune response.
8	Lag Phase	Long (4–7 days)	Short (1–4 days)
9	Types of Antibodies	A large amount of IgM and a small amount of IgG are produced during the primary immune response.	A large amount of IgG, a small amount of IgM are produced during the secondary immune response.
10	Amount of Antibody	Few antibodies are produced in the primary immune response.	100–1000 times more antibodies are produced in the secondary immune response.
11	Strength of the Response	The primary immune response is usually weaker than secondary immune response.	The secondary immune response is stronger.
12	Antibody level	Antibody level declines to the point where it may be undetectable.	The antibody level tends to remain high for longer time.

Table 1.
Differences between primary and secondary immune responses.

types of vaccines usually require booster doses after some interval to boost up the immune response.

8. **Conjugate vaccine:** This type of vaccines is subgroup under subunit vaccine. In these types of vaccines, a weaker antigen is combined with a stronger antigen in order to boost immune response for weaker antigen.

9. **Viral vector vaccine:** These vaccines use the modified version of different viruses as vector. Several different types of viruses have been used as vectors; adenoviruses being most commonly used [4].

3. Immunological response to vaccine

Immune response is divided into two types:

1. Primary immune response.

2. Secondary immune response.

The differences between these two have been described in **Table 1** [6].

4. Immunological responses to different type of COVID-19 vaccines

Inactivated vaccine: the genetic material is inactivated or destroyed in inactivated vaccine which after ingested by antigen presenting cell stimulate the helper T cells which in order stimulate B-cell to produce antibodies as described in **Figure 1** [7].

Example: COVAXIN (Bharat Biotech).

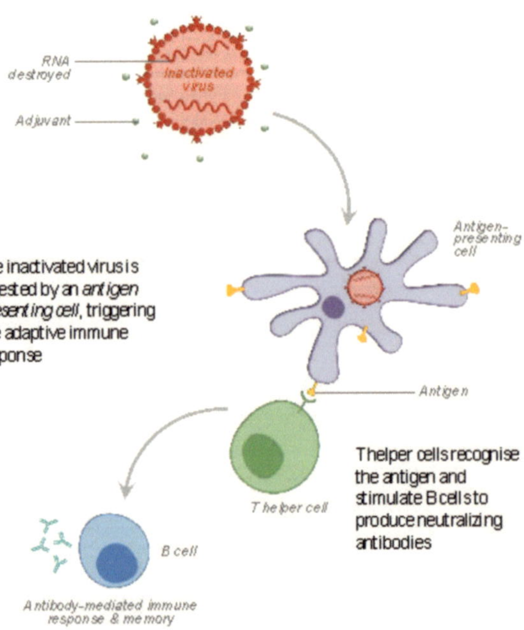

Figure 1.
Inactivated vaccine.

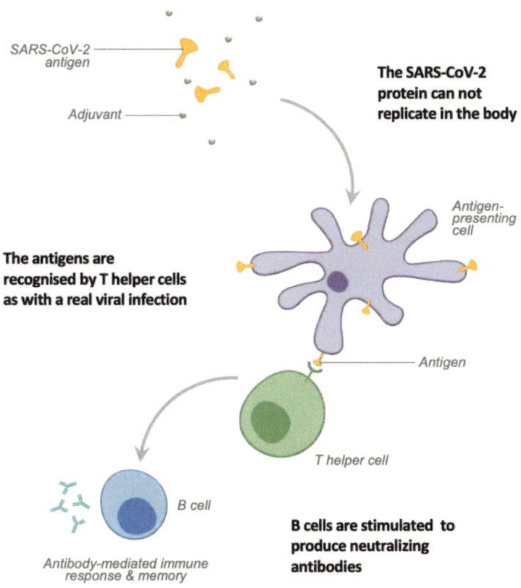

Figure 2.
Subunit vaccine.

Subunit Vaccine: In this vaccine only a part of the agent imitates like real infection and stimulate helper T cells which in turn stimulates B cells to produce antibodies as described in **Figure 2**.

Example: Novavax (protein subunit).

Viral vector Vaccine: these vaccines use non-coronavirus vector modified to carry gene coding for the SARS-COV-2 antigen. This antigen gets expressed on the cells infected gets ingested by antigen presenting cell which then project the complex to helper T cells which then activates both the B-Cells and Cytotoxic T cell as described in **Figure 3**.

Example: AstraZeneca-oxford vaccine and Sputnik-V (Gamaleya Research Institute).

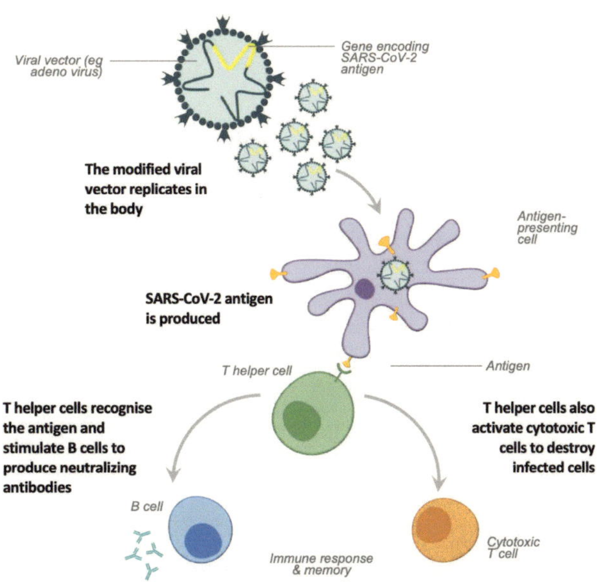

Figure 3.
Viral vector vaccine.

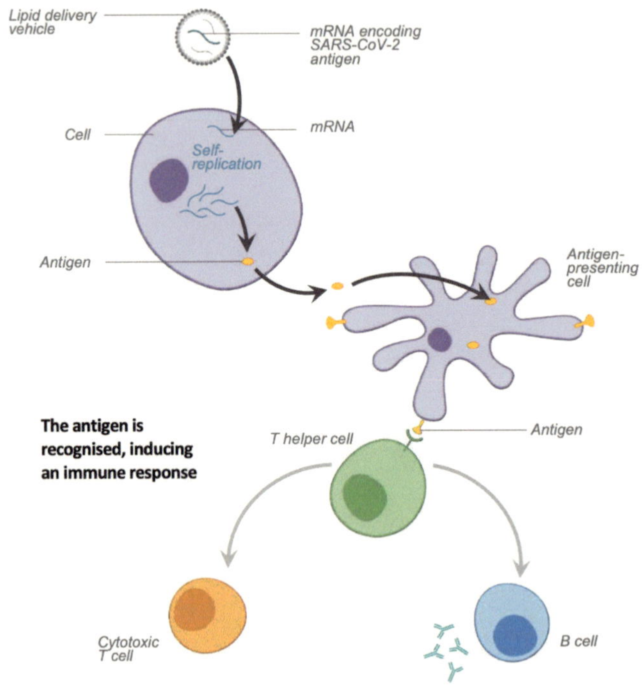

Figure 4.
RNA Vaccine

RNA Vaccine: RNA vaccines are antigen-coding strands of messenger RNA (mRNA) delivered inside a lipid coat. Once inside cells, the mRNA is translated into the protein antigen, which is secreted. The antigen is recognized, inducing an immune reaction. It induces T-helper and cytotoxic T-cells, and antibodies. mRNA also recognized by cells as 'pathogen' stimulating strong immune response as described in **Figure 4**.

Example: Pfizer/BioNTech and Moderna vaccine.

5. COVID-19 vaccines at glance

From February to June 2021, at least seven different vaccines across three platforms have been rolled out in countries [8–10]. Vulnerable populations in all countries are the highest priority for vaccination. At the same time, more than 200 additional vaccine candidates are in development, of which more than 60

Sr. No.	Name of vaccine/manufacturer	Type of vaccine	Age group	Efficacy
1.	Pfizer BioNTech	mRNA	Above 16 years	95.3%
2.	AstraZeneca	Viral vector	Above 18 years	63.09%
3.	Sputnik-V	Viral vector	Above 18 years	91.6%
4.	Moderna	mRNA	Above 18 years	94.1%
5.	Janssen/Johnson & Johnson	Viral vector	Above 18 years	66.3%
6.	Covaxin	Inactivated	Above 18 years	78%

Table 2.
Covid-19 vaccines rolled out in different countries for vaccination.

are in clinical development. COVAX is part of the ACT Accelerator, which WHO launched with partners in 2020. Some of the vaccines which have been rolled out are described in **Table 2**.

6. Dosage and schedule for vaccination

Most COVID-19 vaccines are designed for a two-dose schedule. Two dose vaccination works by mimicking natural immunity. After a first vaccine dose, the immune system needs time to generate a response and to create memory cells that will recognize the pathogen if it is encountered again. The person is considered immune from COVID-19 disease 14 days after the second dose of vaccine in two dose vaccine schedule. All these vaccines are administered Intramuscularly in the deltoid muscle as described in **Table 3**.

7. Vaccine storage and cold chain maintenance

Delivering vaccines to all corners of the world is a complex undertaking. It takes a chain of precisely coordinated events in temperature-controlled environments to store, manage and transport these life-saving products. This is called a cold chain. Vaccines must be continuously stored in a limited temperature range – from the time they are manufactured until the moment of vaccination. This is because temperatures that are too high or too low can cause the vaccine to lose its potency

Sr. No.	Name of vaccine	Dose	Dosage schedule	Route
1	Pfizer BioNTech	0.3 ml	0 + 21 days	Intra-muscular
2	AstraZeneca	0.5 ml	0 + 28 days (second dose can be taken as late as 8–12 weeks)	Intra-muscular
3	Sputnik-V	0.5 ml	0 + 21 days	Intra-muscular
4	Moderna	0.5 ml	0 + 28 days	Intra-muscular
5	Covaxin	0.5 ml	0 + 28 days	Intra-muscular
6	Janssen/Johnson & Johnson	0.5 ml	Single dose	Intra-muscular

Table 3.
Dosage schedule of COVID-19 vaccines.

COVID-19 vaccine	Storage temperature requirement
Pfizer BioNTech	-80°c to -60°c
AstraZeneca	$+2^{o}$c to $+8^{o}$c
Janssen/Johnson & Johnson	$+2^{o}$c to $+8^{o}$c
Sputnik-V	$+2^{o}$c to $+8^{o}$c (Dry form) -18.5^{o}c (Liquid form)
Moderna	$+2^{o}$c to $+8^{o}$c (for 30 days) -50°c to -15°c
Covaxin	$+2^{o}$c to $+8^{o}$c

Table 4.
Cold chain temperature requirements for COVID-19 vaccine.

(its ability to protect against disease). Once a vaccine loses its potency, it cannot be regained or restored. This cold chain temperature differs for different vaccines. Any fault in the cold chain maintenance could lead to wastage of vaccine. Storage condition requirements for various type of vaccines are described in **Table 4**.

8. Adverse effects and contraindications of COVID-19 vaccine

Vaccination is the process of administering foreign agent in the body which is usually associated with various adverse effects which are mostly of mild intensity but may cause severe adverse events in some [11].

Some of the known adverse events following immunizations are fever, pain and swelling at injection site, fatigue, chills, and headache. Some of the vaccine recipients may experience some severe adverse events like Anaphylactic reaction but the incidence of this is rare.

Contraindication to COVID-19 vaccine include severe allergic/anaphylactic reaction to any ingredient of the vaccine or to the first dose of vaccine. COVID-19 vaccine is also contraindicated in pregnant women or those suspected to be pregnant due to paucity of data in this group.

9. Myths related to COVID-19 vaccine

Myths preventing people from taking the vaccine are many and will be mentioned in another chapter, however one of these is:

COVID-19 vaccine was thought to cause infertility in women due to the resemblance of spike protein to the protein syncytin secreted by placenta. This was proved to be myth as the two protein have large difference in amino acid sequences hence ruling out the concern of infertility.

Author details

Aman Sachdeva* and Arup Saha
Pt. B.D. Sharma PGIMS, Rohtak, Haryana, India

*Address all correspondence to: amnsch96@gmail.com

References

[1] World Health Organisation. Vaccines and Immunization. Available from: https://www.who.int/health-topics/vaccines-and-immunization#tab=tab_1 [last accessed on April 27,2021].

[2] Centers for disease control and prevention. Vaccines and immunizations. Available from: https://www.cdc.gov/vaccines/vac-gen/imz-basics.htm [last accessed on April 27 2021].

[3] World Health Organization. Vaccine preventable diseases. Available from: https://www.who.int/southeastasia/our-work/vaccine-preventable-disease [last accessed on April 27 2021].

[4] U.S. Department of Health and Human services. Vaccine types. Available from: https://www.vaccines.gov/basics/types [last accessed on April 27, 2021].

[5] World Health Organization.Types of vaccine. Available from: https://vaccine-safety-training.org/types-of-vaccine-overview.html [last accessed on April 27,2021].

[6] Parija S.Textbook of Microbiology and Immunology. 3rd ed. Elsevier;2016.

[7] World Health Organization. Update on COVID-19 vaccines and immune responses. Available from: https://www.who.int/docs/default-source/coronaviruse/risk-comms-updates/update52_vaccines.pdf?sfvrsn=b11be994_4 [last accessed on April 27,2021].

[8] Centers for disease control and prevention. Different COVID-19 vaccines. Available from: https://www.cdc.gov/coronavirus/2019-ncov/vaccines/different-vaccines.html [last accessed on April 27, 2021].

[9] Logunov DY, Dolzhikova IV, Zubkova OV, et al. Safety and immunogenicity of an rAd26 and rAd5 vector-based heterologous prime-boost COVID-19 vaccine in two formulations: Two open, non-randomised phase 1/2 studies from Russia. Lancet 2020; **396:** 887-897.

[10] Food and Drug Administration. Pfizer-BioNTech COVID-19 Vaccine. Available from: https://www.fda.gov/emergency-preparedness-and-response/coronavirus-disease-2019-covid-19/pfizer-biontech-covid-19-vaccine [last accessed on April 27,2021].

[11] World Health Organization. Coronavirus disease (COVID-19): Vaccine safety. Available from: https://www.who.int/news-room/q-a-detail/coronavirus-disease-(covid-19)-vaccines-safety [last accessed on April 27,2021].

Chapter 23

Myths: Barriers to Fighting the COVID-19 Pandemic

Olabode Omotoso, Teibo John and Gbenga Ojo

Abstract

Myths are widely dispersed but false ideologies or misconceptions. With the thousands of deaths recorded daily and the negative toll of the novel coronavirus disease (COVID-19) on public health, national economy, and human interaction, it remains surprising how people are still being swayed by conspiracy theories. Due to the novelty of the disease, the quest for an answer, what works, and what does not work gave room for the propagation of misinformation, especially on social media. Identifying and debunking myths is very important in managing disease outbreak, since myths can negatively influence the response of people to preventive and containment strategies. Major proponents of COVID-19 myths have promoted their falsehood on the guise that it is a biological weapon engineered to control the world population. Others have also falsely claimed the use of antibiotics or other antiviral drugs in the treatment of COVID-19 and that COVID-19 is no worse than the common flu or it is just the disease of the elderly. This has promoted refusal to take up the COVID-19 vaccine and increased non-adherence to the preventive guidelines. Myths have been a major stumbling block to curtailing the menace of COVID-19. All hands must be on deck to fight this.

Keywords: Myths, COVID-19, preventive, debunk, curtail, media

1. Introduction

Myths are widely proposed false ideas or misconceptions. Since the start of the novel coronavirus disease (COVID-19), several misconceptions have arisen. Belief in the misconceptions could debar certain individuals from adhering to the preventive guidelines leading to the rapid spread of the disease, low vaccine uptake and ultimately, unnecessary deaths. A myth is a story that was told in an ancient culture to explain a practice, belief, or natural occurrence. It is a story that is believed by many people but is not true. Myth is currently commonplace even among the populace, it is confusing and detrimental to the immense efforts put towards fighting the ravaging pandemic [1]. To say that certain stories are in circulation from ancient cultural beliefs from some 'god' or deity imposed/inflicted punishment is contrasting to the facts and reality of the COVID-19 [2].

Ab initio of the COVID-19, which is gradually becoming an endemic, so many myths about the unprecedented outbreak have risen, though untrue, it has facilitated the spread of the virus to about 219 countries, continents, territories and communities with varying belief systems, ways of life and communal practice. However, as unrealistic as this is, it is widely believed by many. Unverified facts which have turned into truth for many have become insurmountable barriers

IntechOpen

against the fight raised against COVID-19. Several myths ranging from the cause of the disease to those susceptible to it, to the assumed cure and even overrated known means of management exist in the premise of the COVID-19. These myths have blurred the line between management and cure, facilitated the rapid spread and even claimed the lives of many with millions of deaths recorded daily on a global scale. The pandemic has a negative toll on public health, national economy, and human interaction, it remains surprising how people are still being swayed by myths and conspiracy theories.

Knowing some of these myths would reveal the ignorance of many and shed more light on the real path to combating the disease [2]. First, if we agree that myths are propagated and perpetuated by ignorance, we must seek knowledge to terminate them, which is where the role of professionals is key in this fight. What we have known since the upsurge of the disease will help rather than what is assumed. Those known facts will then point out false stories or beliefs that must be eradicated.

Because it is safer to move from known to unknown in solving a problem, and there have been stories with unverified sources which are unknown, it is better to consider those facts that have been verified by professionals over the past few months to distinguish between mere myths and facts. In this chapter, we would highlight several myths that have been propagated around it stating how those myths have been a barrier in the fight against the pandemic and what are the reasons or factors responsible for the propagation of these myths, the aftermath and implication of the COVID-19 myths, how to curtail and debunk the myths with evidence or facts and general recommendations and conclusions.

2. Common myths about COVID-19

Myths and misinformation are non-validated concepts or ideologies that are believed by a group of people. Identifying and debunking myths is very important in managing a disease outbreak since myths can negatively influence the response of people to preventive and containment strategies [3]. Within few months of the viral outbreak, it has spread across all continents and has claimed millions of lives. As of June 02, 2021, 22:35 GMT, the death toll due to COVID-19 has reached 3,683,305 deaths from 171,331,780 confirmed cases in 219 countries across the globe [4]. This has brought untold hardship, pressure, and pain to countless individuals across the globe.

The COVID-19 is a novel disease that caught everyone unawares. Due to the novelty of the virus, everyone was looking for an answer as to the origin of the virus, how it spreads, preventive mechanisms, and its mechanism of action, treatment or management of infection and symptoms and how best to curtail its menace. The quest for an answer, what works, and what does not work gave room for the propagation of information and misinformation about the pandemic, most especially on the social media space. Several efforts have been put in place by public health experts, researchers, governments, social response workers, and virtually everyone to understand and curtail the menace of the COVID-19 pandemic. The development, approval and administration of COVID-19 vaccines have brought a sort of relief and hope for almost everyone. Despite this, there are still thousands of confirmed cases and reported deaths on daily basis. Due to the high human-human transmission rate of the virus, the WHO instituted guidelines to help curtail the spread of the virus such as the washing of hands with soap frequently, the use of alcohol-based hand rubs and many more (**Figure 1**).

Since the outset of the pandemic, myths and misinformation about the pandemic have served as a stumbling block or hindrance to the populace acceptance of

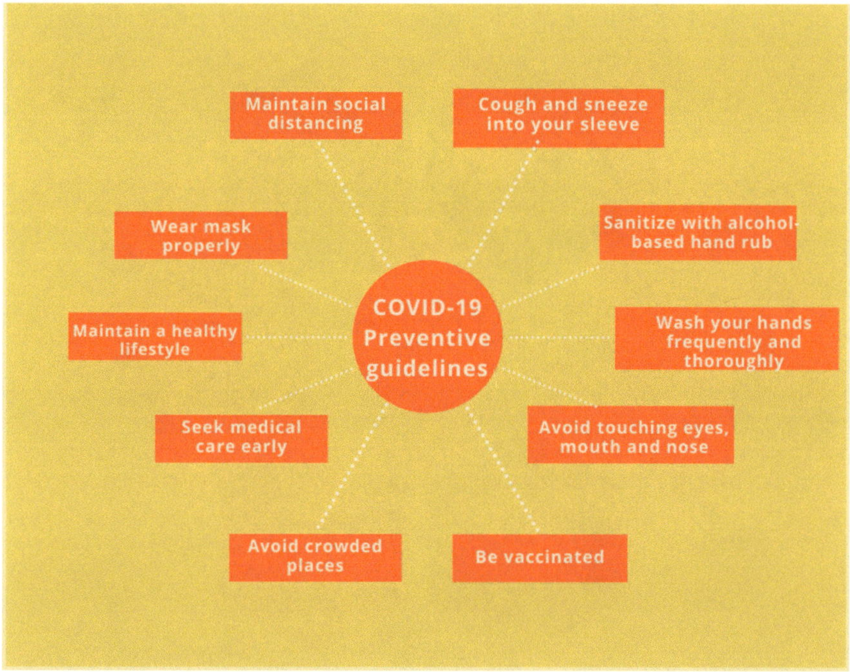

Figure 1.
Instituted preventive guidelines against COVID-19.

instituted guidelines that can reduce the risk of infection. A study [3] on healthcare workers in South Africa identified that myths and misinformation influenced the public's response negatively to the COVID-19 screening campaign. It is quite worrisome that despite the safety rate and promising action of the COVID-19 vaccines, many individuals have decided neither to adhere to the preventive guidelines nor to accept the vaccines. Such individuals do not only put themselves at risk but other thousands of innocent people in their community. Here we highlight common myths and misinformation about the pandemic and their implication in the fight against the pandemic (**Figure 2**).

2.1 COVID-19 is a hoax

Conspiracy theorists, religious fanatics, pseudoscience and science denialists have always been present in the online space looking for means to peddle their belief to unsuspecting individuals [5]. Policies like travel restrictions and total lockdown gave room for much reliance on social media and the internet for information, especially about COVID-19. The novelty of the pandemic and the quest for information has given them a ground to catch many individuals unawares and get them to believe their claim. This has posed a major challenge to the fight against COVID-19 by its generation of fake cure claims, dismissal of public health expert's advice, stigmatization and spread of fear among many others [3, 6]. This is further aggravated when this misinformation is propagated by celebrities and influential people [3]. Major proponents of this claim have promoted their falsehood on the guise that COVID-19 is a biological weapon that was intentionally engineered in a laboratory to control the world population or a means for government and/or public-private enterprise for selfish gains. This is a major stumbling block to curtailing the menace of COVID-19. This has promoted refusal to uptake the COVID-19 vaccines and non-adherence to the preventive guidelines [6].

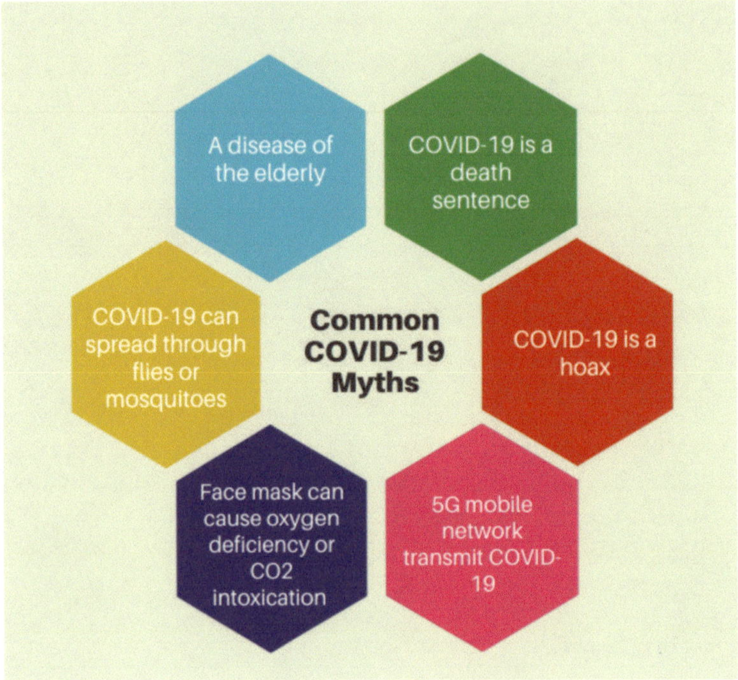

Figure 2.
Common myths about the COVID-19.

2.2 COVID-19 is a death sentence

Although there is a high transmission rate of the virus, it is good to note that the death rate due to COVID-19 is very low compared to other infections due to coronaviruses (MERS in 2012 and SARS in 2002) and other diseases like HIV/AIDS, cancer, and neurodegenerative diseases. Most COVID-19 infected patients will have no or mild symptoms and recover without any professional medical assistance or care. With appropriate care, most infected patients would recover. Most COVID-19 related deaths have been reported in infected patients who are elderly or those who have a weak immune system due to co-morbid health condition like cardiovascular disease, diabetes, chronic respiratory disease, hypertension, HIV/AIDS, cancer etc. As shown in **Table 1**, the death rate increases across all age group among infected patients with underlying health conditions compared to those without co-morbidities.

Age	Number of deaths	Share of deaths	With underlying condition	Without underlying condition
0–17 years	3	0.04%	3	0
18–44 years	309	4.5%	244	25
45–64 years	1581	23.1%	1343	59
65–74 years	1683	24.6%	1272	26
≥ 75 years	3263	47.7%	2289	27
Total	6839	100%	5151	137

Table 1.
Comparison of COVID-19 death rate across age group.

2.3 COVID-19: a disease of the elderly

There have been several reports of young people who get infected and even die due to COVID-19. As earlier mentioned, COVID-19 seems to be more lethal in older people. However, anyone can get infected and develop severe symptoms including young people. The risk for severe symptom from COVID-19 increases with age, those with immune-compromising conditions and a weak immune system, which are more peculiar to older people. Severe illness implies the infected patient will require hospitalization, a ventilator, and professional medical care. Data from **Table 1** provided by New York City Health [7] as of April 14, 2020, shows the disparity in the death rate among the different age group.

As shown in **Table 1**, anyone can be infected with COVID-19 and not only elderly people, although the mortality rate increases with increasing age.

2.4 Shielded by extreme weather conditions

There have been several proponents that the virus cannot survive in a very hot or cold region [8]. Regardless of the temperature or weather condition in the environment, the normal body temperature ranges from 36.5–37°C. More so, there has been a report of COVID-19 infection across all continents (even in countries with hot or cold weather condition).

2.5 Chloroquine, dexamethasone, vitamins and minerals for treating COVID-19

At present, there is no proven cure for COVID-19 [5] rather several vaccines have been developed with promising effectiveness. The best intervention, for now, is vaccination with any of the available approved COVID-19 vaccines. The use of micronutrients (Zinc, vitamins C and D) is well advised to improve the immune system and in promoting overall health. However, there is no evidence of their effectiveness as a treatment option against COVID-19. Dexamethasone, a corticosteroid, at a daily 6 mg dose has been shown to improve the health of some COVID-19 patients on ventilators. However, it showed no improvement for infected patients who had mild symptoms. Chloroquine is a potent antimalarial and rheumatoid arthritis drug, clinical trials have shown no impact in it preventing COVID-19 infection or death [9]. Hence, caution should be taken against stockpiling and self-medication, especially without professional oversight. Garlic and turmeric contain phytochemicals that have antimicrobial properties with promising health benefits. However, there is no supporting evidence of its ability to prevent COVID-19 [8, 10].

2.6 Drinking very cold or hot drinks can prevent infection

Most infected patients will recover with little or no medical care. Taking lots of liquids with essential nutrient composition can help stay well hydrated, improve the immune system, and ensuring a balanced diet. However, there is no approved or proven drink (whether hot or cold) to protect against or cure COVID-19 infection [8, 10].

2.7 Strong disinfectant can protect against infection

Drinking hand sanitizers, ethanol, methanol, or strong disinfectants in a bid to protect against COVID-19 infection can result in very serious health complication [5, 8]. Frequent handwashing with soap and water under running water or rubbing with an alcohol-based hand rub has been recommended as important preventive guidelines. These are meant to be used on the hand and not to be drunk or bathed with as they can result in eye irritation and skin damage. Rinsing the nose with saline has not also shown to offer protection against COVID-19.

2.8 COVID-19 can spread through flies or mosquito bite

COVID-19 is primarily transmitted through exposure to droplets from an infected person or touching a contaminated surface area. Proper handwashing after touching a contaminated surface can offer protection. It is likewise important to avoid touching body parts (eyes, nose and mouth) with unwashed hands and to frequently disinfect surface areas that are often touched or handled. Mosquitoes are vectors for fever. No evidence has linked COVID-19 transmission to either house flies or mosquitoes [5].

2.9 The use of antibiotics

Antibiotics are a potent treatment option for bacterial infection. COVID-19 is caused by a virus, not bacteria. Antibiotics are only recommended for some COVID-19 patients that develop a bacterial infection.

2.10 Face mask can cause oxygen deficiency or carbon dioxide intoxication

Many proponents of this misinformation have held on to this to dissuade people from adhering to the use of face mask. The use of a face mask can be discomforting. When properly worn, a face mask does not result in either oxygen deficiency or CO_2 intoxication. It is advised that face mask be properly worn, not to be worn during exercise activities or when swimming and disposable masks should not be reused.

2.11 Use of thermal scanners and hand dryers

High fever is one of the common symptoms of COVID-19. Thermal scanners can detect people who have high body temperature or fever but not COVID-19 [10]. It takes about 1–14 days for the virus to incubate and to show observable symptoms, hence, thermal scanners may not detect high fever in asymptomatic patients. There are diverse types and causes of fever. It is important to seek proper medical care or go for testing when a very high fever is observed. Hand dryers cannot kill COVID-19 but are only recommended for use to dry hands after thorough and frequent hand washing.

2.12 5G Mobile network transmitted COVID-19

5G mobile network is an advancement in information technology. Viruses like SARS-CoV-2 cannot be transmitted via mobile networks, wireless internet or radio waves as being propagated [5]. Interestingly, COVID-19 transmission has been reported in many countries with no 5G mobile network.

2.13 Pneumonia vaccines offer protection

Pneumonia vaccines (Haemophilus influenza type B vaccine and pneumococcal vaccine) do not offer immunity or protection against COVID-19 [10]. Despite the novelty of the virus, researchers and public health experts have been able to design vaccines that have passed clinical trials and approved for use against the COVID-19.

Though there has been cause for alarm over the new emerging variants of the SARS-CoV-2, existing studies show the effectiveness of these vaccines to a great extent.

3. Factors responsible for myth propagation

3.1 Ignorant belief and assumption

It is appalling that being the 21st century as it is, traditional archaic beliefs are still held in high esteem in certain parts of the world and these beliefs are spread quickly across the globe. Most of these ignorant beliefs are generated from underdeveloped sources, and because most people who reside in these settlements have poor or low technological advancement, and they turn a deaf ear to latest information about the pandemic and are unwilling to adapt to change.

3.2 Fake news or false information peddled via the media

Since the outbreak of the pandemic, there has been the circulation of several untrue information about it reaching people from trusted platforms. Many believed the information and tried to work with it, they then discovered it was false, consequently, there has been a guard against subsequent information targeted at fighting the pandemic. This has limited what can be done to alleviate the situation, the news then proceeds to become myths [6].

3.3 Socioeconomic vulnerability

This is another barrier to the fight that generates myths. The belief that the disease only affects the rich, especially those who are rich enough to travel via air route, is a factor that leads to myths. Most of the population in underdeveloped and developing countries are so poor that they prioritize their struggle to get food and basic means of livelihood to being sick or even death.

Most of these impoverished populaces believe that food comes first, then health, therefore the disease keeps moving as they move about seeking the basic means of livelihood they cannot afford and do not have access readily to face masks, sanitizers and soap for disinfection, with this condition, the myth is sustained. An earlier study [11] reveals two main categories of perceived facilitators of COVID-19 spread in Ethiopia, they are behavioral non-adherence (55.9%) and lack of enablers (86.5%). Behavioral non-adherence was illustrated by fear of stigma (62.9%), not seeking care (59.3%), and hugging and shaking (44.8%). Perceived lack of enablers of precautionary measures includes staying home impossible due to economic challenges (92.4%), overcrowding (87.6%), inaccessible face masks (81.6%) and hand sanitizers (79.1%). Perceived inhibitors were categorized into three factors: two misperceived, myths (31.6%) and false assurances (32.9%) and one correctly identified; engagement in standard precautions (17.1%).

3.4 Poor housing facility/overcrowding

The popular belief that coronavirus does not survive in hot places is backed up by this condition. Probably due to financial constraint or outright ignorance of its dire consequences in the future, many housing facilities like slums used in underdeveloped and developing countries are promoting factors for the spread of COVID-19. These houses encourage neighbor-hood spread rapidly standing in the way of the fight against COVID-19. As people stay on in such an environment, the propagation of the myth is sustained.

3.5 Disobedience/unhealthy curiosity

Some people are just simply disobedient to authority while others are curious to know what would happen if they do not keep the precautions. Because of this, the startup stories that suit them just buttress their act of disobedience. Either of these is unhealthy or are strong barriers to putting a stop to the spread of the disease.

3.6 Illiteracy or low level of education

Some people find it difficult to interpret information received and to comply with safety precautions because of low levels of education. They go about with untrue stories that contradict what is proven. Education breaks the barrier of ignorance, interprets possible consequences to the mind and facilitates easy adherence to precautions, the reverse is the case with a low educated person, thereby posing a barrier to fighting the pandemic.

Studies have shown that those with low levels of education have often misunderstood or taken with levity the public health guidelines which have prompted the spread of the virus. An earlier report [12] showed that men; black persons; those with lower health literacy, co-morbidities; those living below the poverty level; and persons who were unmarried, unemployed, or retired were less likely to make changes because of the coronavirus.

3.7 Government or leadership failure

Due to the previous failure on the part of the leaders, several myths have been generated to counteract the efforts being put into the fight against COVID-19, some just as a way of rebellion or some created as a belief of punishment for those leaders who are infected. These have caused many of the populace not to focus on their health but instead be on the lookout for the victim among the government officials that would be reported to have the virus or being dead because of the virus.

3.8 Belief in history repeating itself

As a result of the Spanish flu of 1918 which is a major pandemic that happened 102 years ago, many historian manic believed history was simply repeating itself and there is no major effort that prevents the escalating potential of the pandemic with the slogan "whatever would be would be". This hampers the initial effort that needed to be put in place in curtailing the spread and sensitization of the populace early enough.

4. Perspective and conclusion

From the hitherto discussed, one fact has been established. That the emergence of myths poses a great danger to the prevention and the halting of further spread of the COVID-19. Whether orchestrated by the different factors we have highlighted or because of other truisms our purview did not cover, fake news, a mythical approach to the novel virus is and has been detrimental to efforts to curtail it both nationally and globally. Combating the menace of misinformation must be a course of action any worthy academics must take seriously. That is what we have done here.

However, from another point of view, some may argue that how can we say for certain that what we generally refer to as unfounded myths about the coronavirus are unfounded? What exactly convinced us of their falsity? Is it because these other views regarded as myths are unpopular or because we have some facts indicating their falsity? Is it not possible that the majority can be wrong? These are questions with far-reaching implications. The history of science is replete with examples whereby the whole scientific community was wrong, and the so-called lonely voices of dissidents were right. In some moments of history, only conspirators were promoting heliocentricity, the real science of the time was touted as geocentricity. It is dissenting voices of the likes of Galileo, Copernicus, Newton, Einstein etc. that has sometimes proven what we have previously known to be false as true. Some may argue then that, it is possible that what seems to be legends of superstitious origin today may come to be flawless truth when further evidence appears. As the American writer Richard Rorty noted, declaring a viewpoint as true or false, one myth and another fact, are ways we condemn or praise views that we like or disagree with not that one is true or false [13]. Going by this, it can be argued then that since we do not have enough knowledge about the coronavirus, it will be too early to classify some views as fake, true, false or myths.

Nonetheless, we must correct any position or postulation presented in the fashion previously stated for two reasons. First, comparing scientific disagreement exemplified in the likes of Galileo, Newton or Einstein can and must not be likened to COVID-19 myths. The reason is conspirators and fake news peddlers have not given any evidence for their theories. They start and end with them postulating it. In the case of scientific dissidents like Galileo, evidence was presented, and, in the end, the truth prevailed. In the case of COVID-19 conspirators, it is not the case that evidence is not enough they are non-existent. Hence, they do not belong to the same category as the moment in which scientific postulation disagrees with known facts.

Secondly, although we do not possess enough knowledge on the COVID-19, it remains a fact that we know a lot already and based on what we currently know, conspirators can be declared false and mythical engagement as cheer falsity. We do not need to know everything about everything to distinguish between what is true or false. One does not need to be in New York to state that it is true that it is in the United States of America and that it is the most populated State therein. In like fashion, scientific knowledge is always open-ended. The reason, a future scientist will retest and re-examine the findings of their predecessors. So, any view that states we cannot distinguish between what is true or false because we do not know all there is to know about COVID-19 is unfounded, illogical, and naïve. We can never know everything about something. Future evidence will either validate or invalidate our present knowledge but based on the authority of our present knowledge, we can always make an informed decision about what is true or false. Given what is presently available, therefore, some views as we have earlier highlighted cannot be vindicated of their mythical nature.

Conclusively, the emergence of fake news and misinformation about the novel coronavirus places a very stringent task on our shoulders. It is the task of always soliciting the truth. Just as the influx of true findings on the virus is enormous, the continuous appearance of convincing conspiracies has crossed a barrier of obscurity into a limbo zone of our postmodern kitsch. Notwithstanding, the question we must always ask when faced with any postulation, comments, theory, or information on COVID-19 is "where are the evidence?" Swallowing any theory either politically motivated or culturally and religiously infused is detrimental not only to individual survival but also to the overall interest of our ailing world. Myth, to be candid, is an amorphous concept rejecting classification either of truth or falsity, but when evidence is lacking or are incoherent, we can assertively declare not just that they are false but more so that they are dangerous and must be tenaciously fought into oblivion.

Conflict of interest

The authors declare no conflict of interest.

Author details

Olabode Omotoso[1]*, Teibo John[2] and Gbenga Ojo[1]

1 University of Ibadan, Ibadan, Nigeria

2 University of Sao-Paulo, Ribeirao Preto, SP, Brazil

*Address all correspondence to: olabodeomotoso@gmail.com

References

[1] Sola Morales S. Myth and the Construction of Meaning in Mediated Culture. Kome. 2013;1(2).

[2] Sahoo S, Padhy S, Ipsita J, Mehra A, Grover S. Demystifying the myths about COVID-19 infection and its societal importance. Asian J Psychiatr. 2020;54.

[3] Schmidt T, Cloete A, Davids A, Makola L, Zondi N, Jantjies M. Myths, misconceptions, othering and stigmatizing responses to Covid-19 in South Africa: A rapid qualitative assessment. PLoS One [Internet]. 2021;15(12 December):1-20. Available from: http://dx.doi.org/10.1371/journal.pone.0244420

[4] Coronavirus Death Toll and Trends - Worldometer [Internet]. [cited 2021 Jun 2]. Available from: https://www.worldometers.info/coronavirus/coronavirus-death-toll/

[5] 9Myths and Misconceptions About COVID-19 [Internet]. Nationwide Children's Hospital. 2020 [cited 2021 Mar 20]. Available from: https://www.nationwidechildrens.org/family-resources-education/700childrens/2020/05/9-myths-and-misconceptions-about-covid-19

[6] Aiyewumi O, Okeke MI. The Myth That Nigerians Are Immune To Sars-Cov-2 And That Covid-19 Is A Hoax Are Putting Lives At Risk. J Glob Health. 2020;10(2):1-4.

[7] Coronavirus Disease 2019 (COVID-19) - NYC Health [Internet]. [cited 2021 Apr 27]. Available from: https://www1.nyc.gov/site/doh/covid/covid-19-main.page

[8] Myths Demystified Coronavirus [Internet]. Babylon. 2020 [cited 2021 Apr 5]. p. 1-12. Available from: https://www.babylonhealth.com/coronavirus/myths

[9] Coronavirus disease (COVID-19) [Internet]. [cited 2021 Apr 27]. Available from: https://www.who.int/emergencies/diseases/novel-coronavirus-2019

[10] 12Myths about COVID-19 [Internet]. WHO. 2020 [cited 2021 Apr 3]. Available from: https://www.who.int/docs/default-source/searo/thailand/12myths-final099bfbf976c54d5fa3407a65b6d9fa9d.pdf

[11] Kebede Y, Birhanu Z, Fufa D, Yitayih Y, Abafita J, Belay A, et al. Myths, beliefs, and perceptions about COVID-19 in Ethiopia: A need to address information gaps and enable combating efforts. PLoS One [Internet]. 2020;15(11 November):1-18. Available from: http://dx.doi.org/10.1371/journal.pone.0243024

[12] Wolf MS, Serper M, Opsasnick L, O'Conor RM, Curtis L, Benavente JY, et al. Awareness, Attitudes, and Actions Related to COVID-19 Among Adults With Chronic Conditions at the Onset of the U.S. Outbreak: A Cross-sectional Survey. Ann Intern Med. 2020;173(2): 100-109.

[13] Rorty R. Contingency, Irony and Solidarity. In Cambridge University Press; 1989.

Chapter 24

Myths Surrounding Covid-19 Vaccine Candidates: A Guide to Fight Back

John Zizzo

Abstract

The Covid-19 pandemic has propelled public health officials into the socio-political sphere due to the need for constantly updated information on behalf of the public. However, many individuals choose to acquire health information/guidance from indirect sources, including social media, news organizations, and general word of mouth. As a result, myths and false narratives about various essential health topics, including vaccine characteristics and protective measures, can circulate un-verified between millions of individuals with little recourse. These can further widen the "gap" between public knowledge and current research, resulting in lower vaccine uptake (vaccine hesitancy) and protective measure adherence. Such actions have profound implications as nations attempt to achieve herd immunity and end the pandemic once and for all. Thus, it is vital that public health officials, health providers, researchers, and the general public be able to differentiate common Covid-19 myths from facts and be prepared to approach such interactions via sound reasoning and research-based evidence. This chapter will serve as a guide to accomplish just that.

Keywords: Covid-19 vaccine, vaccine hesitancy, herd immunity, myths, mRNA technology, clinical trial

1. Introduction

Before the Covid-19 pandemic, vaccine hesitancy was a term reserved for individuals, primarily in developed countries, in which there is a significant refusal or delay in uptake despite vaccine availability/access. In this instance, the term minute might be misleading since vaccine hesitancy is in no way a monolith. Indeed, vaccine hesitancy can take many forms and stems from multiple etiologies. However, never in the past decade had individuals' choices and personal convictions regarding a vaccine had such a profound effect on the perceived ability of entire nations to effectively control a pandemic at large [1].

This "rise to fame" and increased recognition in the public health community was borne out of the realization that multiple vaccine candidates were nearing the later stages of clinical trials in the fall of 2020. After nearly nine months of social protective measures and economic turmoil, a clear disparity had been recognized between the rapid vaccine production process and public knowledge/acceptance toward eventual vaccine uptake. For instance, the first vaccine (Pfizer) against

Covid-19 was given emergency use authorization on December 11, 2020, in the U.S. A week later, a second vaccine (by Moderna) was also approved. However, unlike traditional vaccine rollouts, the U.S. government had pre-purchased hundreds of millions of doses from multiple manufacturers via Operation Warp Speed, hoping to speed up the initial delivery to essential frontline workers and high-risk individuals [2]. The program was considered an overnight success as over 6 million doses of each vaccine was shipped within a week of authorization, enough to vaccinate the entire U.S. healthcare worker population. Within a few weeks, reports began emerging that only 68% of healthcare workers, the supposed most informed subset of the population, had chosen to receive the vaccine when offered to them [3]. To put this in perspective, annual influenza vaccine uptake in the U.S. stands at around 81% [4]. One might ask, what separates the two numbers? The answer is, of course, much deeper than surface level; however, one question has been proposed and proven highly appropriate in post-roll out public opinion polling: where was the vaccine marketing campaign? After all, the U.S. spent over $12 billion on vaccine candidates undergoing clinical trials before a single jab was given [2]. The first official Covid-19 vaccination information campaign was not announced until January

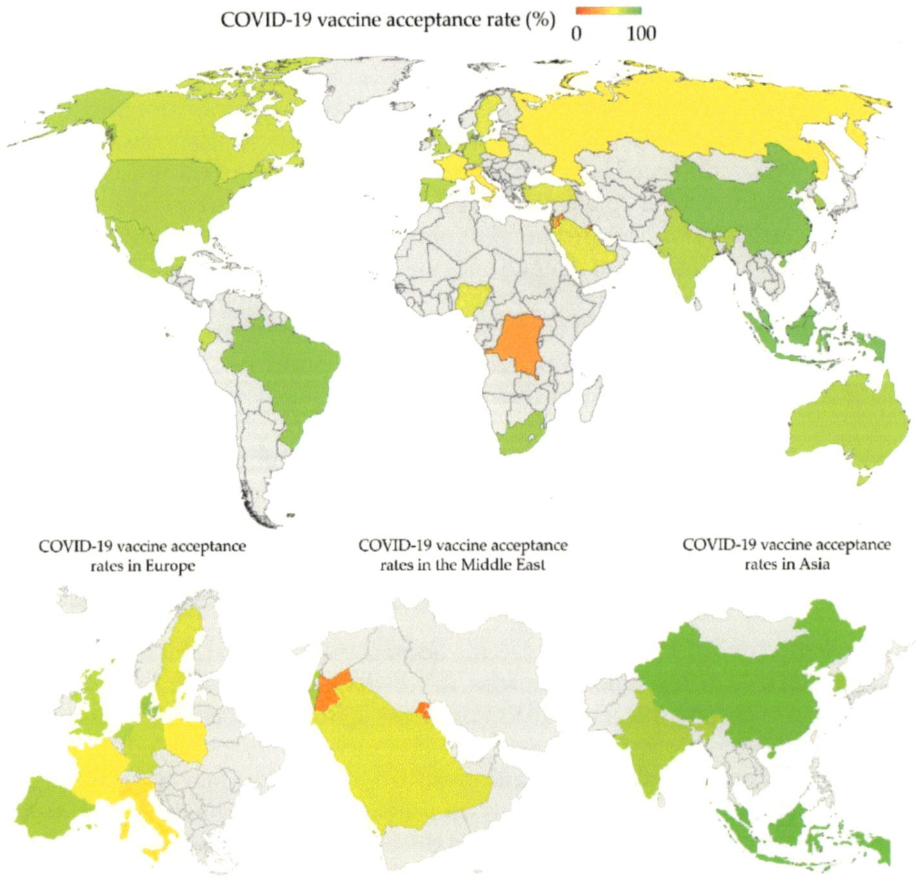

Figure 1.
*"COVID-19 vaccine acceptance rates worldwide. For countries with more than one survey study, the vaccine acceptance rate of the latest survey was used in this graph. The estimates were also based on studies from the general population, except in the following cases where no studies from the general public were found (Australia: parents/guardians; DRC: healthcare workers; Hong Kong: healthcare workers; Malta: healthcare workers)." Source: Reproduced from "**Figure 2:** COVID-19 vaccine hesitancy worldwide: A concise systematic review of vaccine acceptance rates" by Malik Sallam. Licensee MDPI, Basel, Switzerland. Made available under the CC by 4.0 license.*

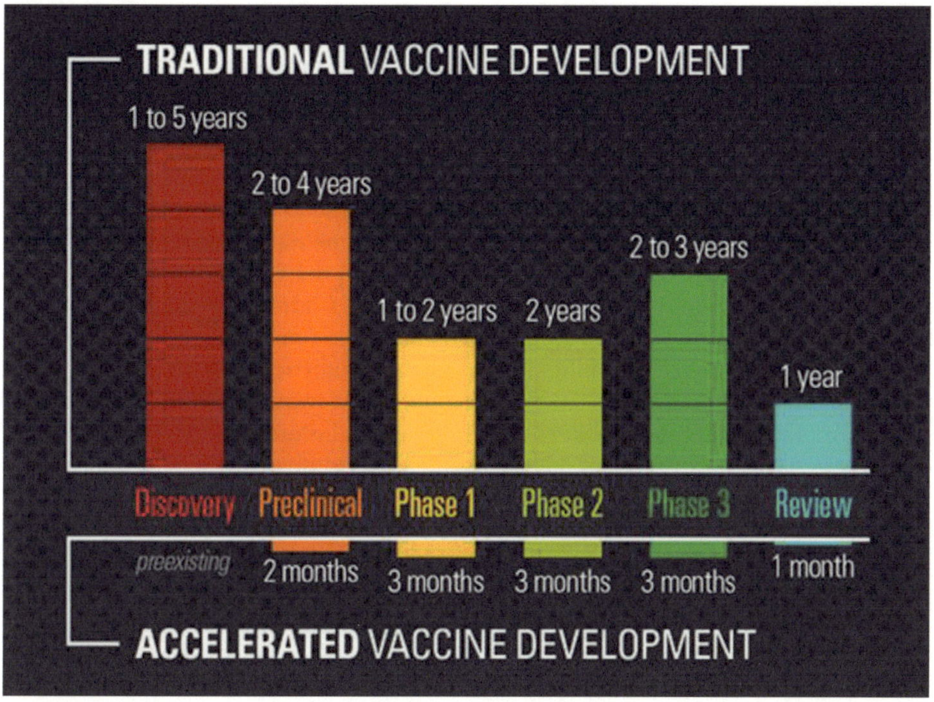

Figure 2.
Traditional vs. (accelerated) Covid-19 vaccine development timeline. Source: GAO analysis of Food and Drug Administration (FDA), pharmaceutical research and manufacturers of America, and Operation Warp speed information. / GAO-21-319.

27, 2021, over a month after the first vaccine approval. Multiple analyses of the U.S. vaccine timeline have dubbed this period, between the late summer of 2020 and early spring of 2021, the "lost time" in the fight against the Covid-19 pandemic [5].

Thus, a question emerges. What could have been done to quell the impending rise of vaccine-hesitant individuals (**Figure 1**)? Here we find a great model in annual influenza immunization campaigns. The initiatives are backed by decades of research showing that a multi-disciplinary collaboration consisting of providers, public agencies, and private sector companies is needed to adequately address questions and instill confidence in individuals regarding upcoming vaccines. The word upcoming is critical in this context, as the marketing campaign is kicked off months BEFORE the first jab is expected to be given. Consequently, a logical time to begin educating individuals on the developing Covid-19 vaccines likely would have been months before the first approval. Unfortunately, the movement did not catch enough support, and we may never know the difference this may have made on vaccine hesitancy levels during the rollout.

During this "lost time," as mentioned, very little data exists surrounding vaccine hesitancy levels via traditional cross-sectional studies/surveys. Most statistics cited are taken from public opinion polling, which asked individuals their opinion on various aspects of the pandemic and, specifically, whether they intended to receive a Covid-19 vaccine if and when it is approved. To continue with the U.S. example, a poll taken in July 2020 showed that only 42% of Americans were considering getting vaccinated, with lower rates among minority groups, who are disproportionately affected by Covid-19 in both hospitalization and mortality rates [6]. Fast forward to November, and that number had not changed. However, the percentage of anticipated uptake among Black Americans had gone down [7]. Hence, we have our disparity: billions of dollars and public resources were given to vaccine development, while virtually no attention was given to promoting the vaccine among its intended populations.

But what could have caused this? How did millions of individuals in one of the most developed nations in the world with access to social media, news outlets, and governmental information not warm to the greatest vaccine development feat in modern history? Well, aside from the missing vaccine marketing campaign, other factors must have been at play to erode public confidence and stall optimism in the wake of the surging pandemic. Of these factors, one was very preventable and remains a global barrier to vaccine administration: myths. That is, myths surrounding virtually every aspect of vaccine production, trials, administration, and long-lasting effects. Such myths, circulated at large with the rise of unverified outlets (e.g., social media), have the ability to reach a mass audience with little recourse. A potent example lies in the fact that one false statement from a well-known celebrity can potentially reach hundreds of millions of viewers before any official rebuttal or correction is offered. Therein lies the challenge in combatting myths, reliant on the public's level of trust in public health officials compared to those spouting such research-lacking claims [8]. To accomplish this on an individual level, like all delicate encounters, requires both first-hand knowledge and effective communication techniques. While the latter two are character traits that may or may not be improved (see Section 2), the first is an area that deserves a review.

2. Addressing vaccine myths

Before diving in, it is worth reiterating that countering vaccine hesitancy, similar to the definition itself, is not a one-size-fits-all approach. The knowledge laid out below will provide a foundation for providers and the general public alike to interact with and have fruitful conversations regarding common misconceptions. However, there are extraneous principles that are important and necessary to follow to maximize such opportunities. A 2018 study out of the Thomas J. Long School of Pharmacy and Health Sciences identified several successful strategies that can be used to improve confidence and decrease hesitancy levels in recipients. Even more impressive is that the study involved pharmacy students rather than licensed medical providers, decreasing the likely power differential and knowledge gap seen in clinical practice [9].

The first viable strategy found was that of rapport. For example, a commonplace argument for vaccine aversion is that "vaccine side effects are worse than the disease itself." Instead of trying to ramble off a dozen facts and figures, a better solution was found in asking patients to boil the fear down to a specific side effect (e.g., headaches, diarrhea, etc.). Once this was done, the student could dig even deeper to determine if the patient had personally suffered or had a family history of suffering from such symptoms. From here, rapport could be established, and a risk–benefit analysis consisting of actual data would be much more appropriate than trying to combat the entire notion that vaccines should be "side-effect free." Now, this may seem like a "no brainer." However, one may not know as much as they think about their friend's/family member's health if they only interact once a year. Thus, it may be wise to take a deeper dive, regardless of relationship, before countering their pre-existing vaccine perceptions.

Once rapport has been established, a winning strategy is to start with the positives rather than harping on rare side effects and complications. A popular starting point would be explaining vaccine-driven herd immunity and how community protection is the basis for eradication/control of nearly all major outbreaks. Next, a solid turning point would be to suggest that they resist looking to unqualified personnel (on social media, television, etc.) and talk to an actual expert on the topic, such as their physician or pharmacist. Another important goal is to evaluate an individual's level of knowledge about the vaccine. Studies have shown that greater education simply about the vaccine itself and how it works can lower levels of hesitancy [10]. Thus, they do not need to walk away agreeing with you; simply informing them about how the vaccine works (mRNA technology, viral vector, etc.) is a step forward in our book. Then, it is important to assess their current risk–benefit stage. Two popular dimensions used are an individuals' perceived likelihood of harm and perceived consequence severity if that harm were to occur [11]. Narrowing this down, similar to establishing rapport, is key to addressing underlying fears/aversions. Consequently, it is also important to establish their "best-case scenario." They likely want the same endpoint for society (eradication/negligible transmission). Using this as common ground and talking about realistic paths toward getting there is an excellent segway into discussing current research projections.

Two factors that cannot be ignored are that of socio-cultural pressure and religious convictions. Unfortunately, these are very hard to change in the long-term, much less in the course of a single conversation. Leveraging the idea of social responsibility, where an individual has a sort of role to play in achieving herd immunity for the betterment of those around them, has proven effective. However, a fine line should not be crossed so as to force down a specific belief on individual behavior [12].

These research-driven strategies may or may not be enough to build your communication arsenal the next time a patient, friend, or loved one mentions hesitancy toward vaccination. However, striving for rapport, providing judgment-free educational information, and being knowledgeable about all components of vaccine development and administration is a recipe for success in this fight toward ending the Covid-19 pandemic and future pandemics to follow. Speaking of knowledge, perhaps you are wondering what myths exactly are circulating about Covid-19 vaccines. If so, let us address your eagerness (not hesitancy).

3. High-yield vaccine myths to know

Recent studies have identified five common myths surrounding Covid-19 vaccines [13, 14]. Let us break them down one by one, separating fact from fiction.

3.1 Myth #1: getting the Covid-19 vaccine will give you Covid-19

To date, no vaccine authorized or in development in the U.S. contains the live SARS-CoV-2 virus. Thus, receiving a Covid-19 vaccine cannot and will not cause Covid-19 infection. However, symptoms seen in common viral infections can arise due to the body's immune response to the vaccine's mechanism of action. Symptom presentation and timelines can vary among different vaccine types and recipient demographics. Generally, the most common symptoms seen in Covid-19 vaccinated individuals are injection site pain, fever, muscle pain, fatigue, and/or headaches. These are a completely normal and benign response as the immune system detects the vaccine components and begins adapting to fight off an actual Covid-19 infection, should that individual get exposed. These side effects typically occur within 24–48 hours post-vaccination. Experts often refer to this as a "good sign" that your immune system is building a response to battle future infections. While this period generally contains a mild presentation, there are steps you can take to alleviate side effects that arise. The first is to use an ice pack or damp cloth to reduce injection site pain/soreness. Next is to take an over the counter (OTC) pain reliever such as acetaminophen. Finally, finding ways to de-stress (e.g., taking off of work, self-care routine) is always a good idea to strengthen your immune system [15].

3.2 Myth #2: vaccine development was rushed and unreliable

In this instance, it is helpful to begin by confirming one of the assumptions of this myth: that the Covid-19 vaccine was developed in record time [16]. Yes, there is some merit to this assumption. However, the other two assumptions are where this myth fails to hold water: that corners were cut, and safety was inherently not ensured as in traditional vaccine development/supervision. There are two possibilities in this discussion that are important to recognize before diving in: (1) the individual holds this distrust regarding all vaccines (or at least the idea is not confined to the Covid-19 vaccine development) or (2) the individual solely holds this belief surrounding Covid-19 vaccine production. If the former, then the individual needs to be counseled about basic vaccine development facts as a whole. If the second is the case, then the argument becomes much more straightforward: how did/does Covid-19 vaccine development compare to previous vaccines? For this, we can look to historical data and the "usual" timeline, step by step (**Figure 2**). So how exactly are vaccines made?

3.2.1 Discovery (1-5 years)

The discovery phase generally consists of learning all aspects of the microbe we are trying to combat (e.g., structure, mechanism of action, etc.) Once SARS-CoV-2 was identified as a type of coronavirus, researchers were able to sequence its genome. From here, the spike protein was selected as a unique target based on its function allowing the virus to penetrate host cells and cause infection. Additionally, the spike protein had been targeted before against the Middle East respiratory syndrome (MERS) coronavirus. This precedent allowed the discovery phase to be accelerated to weeks or months rather than years.

3.2.2 Preclinical (2-4 years)

The preclinical stage generally consists of sifting through potential antigens (such as the spike protein) and deciding which will produce the best immune response and long-lasting protection. This is determined by assessing the safety of candidates for each antigen in cell and tissue cultures as well as in live animal testing. Traditionally, studies are performed on rats and mice; however, the rise of transgenic "humanized" mice, genetically modified with human genetic components, has aided in generalization toward human bodily responses. Researchers must also determine appropriate dosing and delivery form (e.g., injection, pill, etc.). Once this has been completed, the candidate vaccine moves on to the clinical stages. And how did this notoriously tedious process happen so quickly in the case of Covid-19? One example was found in March 2020, when Janssen reported that their novel technology platform, used in its Ebola and novel RSV and HIV viral vector vaccines, was effective against Covid-19. Thus, decades of research on the platform's delivery mechanism, ideal thresholds, and animal study proof-of-concept were utilized to jumpstart the development timeline.

3.2.3 Phase I clinical trial (1-2 years)

The main goal of a Phase I trial is to show that the vaccine is safe in humans and how the body receives it. A small group of volunteers is enrolled. Careful attention is given to signs of adverse events, such as toxicity, organ damage, and death. After the trial is completed, data is analyzed and submitted to the FDA for approval to begin Phase II trials. The FDA has the ability at any point to intervene if one or more serious adverse events are found. If a treatment has already been shown to work for a different condition, the Phase I trial can be shortened or accelerated to Phase II since the vaccine has proven safe in human patients. As was the case with Covid-19, multiple manufacturers were able to combine Phase I and Phase II trials since the steps can be done in parallel without compromising oversight. The experience with the delivery system used for Ebola in Janssen's case is a key example.

3.2.4 Phase II clinical trial (2 years)

Phase II trials primarily focus on narrowing down the ideal dosage to maximize effectiveness and limit side effects. A larger patient population is used. Patients are assigned to multiple groups with varying doses, delivery methods, or controls to compare outcomes. All treatments given have been previously tested (including placebo or current vaccine standard), and this step is meant to pick a "best" scenario. When the trial concludes, the results of each group are compared to determine if the vaccine is better than current treatment/vaccine resources and, if so, ideal dosing/delivery. This is a major checkpoint whereby the FDA can either discontinue the study due to adverse events/ineffectiveness or push it through to Phase III trials.

3.2.5 Phase III clinical trial (2-3 years)

The main hallmark of a Phase III trial is its size, typically around 3,000 participants. Enrolling this many patients with a disease can be a drawn-out process depending on disease prevalence and geographical distribution, often lasting several years. Perhaps the most remarkable feat of the Covid-19 clinical trial race was the ability of vaccine studies to enroll record numbers of patients in record time. Take, for instance, the Pfizer Phase III trial, which recruited over 43,000 participants in just four months. This magnificent accomplishment was able to both shave off precious time and instill greater confidence in the public and scientific community due to the sheer sample size. After all, the number of participants was over ten times greater than that of a typical vaccine candidate. One might argue that this was an invaluable marketing strategy given the shortened development timeline. While this is likely true, it is important to realize that corners were not cut in enrolling patients either. On the contrary, pharmaceutical manufacturers worked with epidemiologists to ensure that the patient population recruited for the studies was representative of the target population for vaccine administration. In layman's terms, groups that are typically hard to reach in general studies (e.g., underserved groups, those at highest risk of transmission) were given priority in enrollment efforts. Once all trial data is compiled, a New Drug Application (NDA) is filed with the FDA, asking for consideration to bring the vaccine to market.

3.2.6 FDA approval/review (1 year)

One cannot understate the amount of administrative burden and patience that goes into reaching this point, much less achieving FDA authorization. A common question asked by patients after witnessing the Covid-19 spectacle is, "Why can't we approve everything this fast?" An excellent question, indeed, given the abundance of vaccines needed for incurable diseases. To answer this, let us talk about what goes into the FDA's decision once an NDA hits its desk. The first component a manufacturer must prove is that the vaccine is safe and effective throughout all clinical trial data. From here, the decision moves toward logistics. Is there a manufacturing process in place? Can this process consistently meet the needs of the general public? Are the batches equivalent to clinical trial data in terms of effectiveness and safety? If all of these boxes are checked, then approval is a possibility. Several panels meet to consider the vaccine data submitted for approval and licensure/regulation grants. The reason for the year timeline is based on a variety of factors. First, a large percentage of applications are incomplete, with required studies missing. Next, a candidate is put on a priority ranking list in which drugs are reviewed based on global need. Then, the FDA must meet with sponsors to ensure no corners were cut and that transparency was insured. Finally, an in-depth manufacturing analysis must be conducted to ensure that the vaccine distribution can meet the global needs of world populations (especially underserved and at-risk groups).

As another wonder of Covid-19 vaccine development, two decisions were made that cut the necessary FDA review period down to less than three weeks: parallel review and anticipatory manufacturing. Since the Covid-19 pandemic was logically considered priority #1, all possible resources were given to evaluate and approve/reject clinical trial data upon submission. Additionally, trial transparency and adverse reaction monitoring was performed concurrently to ensure proper oversight. These cut the typical six-month to one-year delay off of the majority of pre-NDA phases. Anticipatory manufacturing, the production of unapproved vaccines in anticipation of approval, was a previously unproven idea that investing in potential candidates would be cost-effective in the long run and shave previous months or even years off the vaccine distribution timeline. Consequentially, this could save millions of lives by slowing the pandemic morbidity and mortality. This gamble has proven largely successful in the early months of vaccine rollout, and specific examples can be found under the "Introduction."

3.2.7 Manufacturing (6 months-3 years)

As mentioned, anticipatory manufacturing was the key to jumpstarting the vaccine production timeline. Currently, AstraZeneca/Oxford is producing an astounding 200 million doses of their Covid-19 vaccine per month. To give perspective, during the H1N1 outbreak, AstraZeneca was able to produce only 17 million doses of their H1N1 vaccine. That represents a roughly twelve-time increase in production compared to the previous pandemic [17]. While this is not a perfect comparison given differing circumstances, it is both probable and likely that the jumpstart in production and massive funding overhauls contributed to maximizing vaccine production.

3.2.8 Phase IV clinical trial (optional)

Phase IV trials are studies of adverse serious events and safety hazards that arise once a vaccine is approved and made available on the market. The FDA carefully monitors such instances through MedWatch, a service allowing providers, patients, and the trial sponsor to report a suspicious event. At any point, additional Phase IV trials may be commissioned by the FDA or sponsor to examine vaccine effects for varying benefits, risks, and patient populations [18].

3.3 Myth #3: the only way to reach herd immunity and end the pandemic is by letting the virus spread

Herd immunity has risen to prominence in both the scientific community and the general public due to its unique role in infectious disease outbreaks. To set the record straight, herd immunity is the only proven method of definitively preventing the spread of infectious diseases to the point of being statistically irrelevant. This is achieved by a large percentage of the population, called the herd immunity threshold, being protected from infection (**Figure 3**). Consequently, the unprotected (e.g., uninfected individuals, individuals who cannot or choose not to get vaccinated) also become protected due to the interrupted transmission chain. This part, in most cases, is largely understood. Where the record gets bent is in HOW herd immunity is reached. It is important to understand that there are two routes by which herd immunity can be achieved: natural infection and vaccines [19].

3.3.1 Natural infection

When enough individuals in the population have recovered from a specific disease and developed lasting antibodies against future infection, herd immunity can theoretically be reached. However, the issue with this myth's underlying assumption is that relying on natural infection alone ignores two common deviants: reinfection and health toll.

While admittedly, the evidence for reinfection risk is limited given the novel nature of the pandemic, there have been clear instances of Covid-19 reinfection in the community. This phenomenon is dependent on an individual's antibody levels and appears to heighten in risk between six months to a year. Significant reinfection incidence can substantially harp a community's progression toward herd immunity due to waning antibody responses.

While a community could theoretically remove all protective measures and allow the disease to run rampant until herd immunity is achieved, this would allow the full brunt of the disease to affect the community. In layman's terms, this means that millions of individuals could suffer and potentially die unnecessarily. In July 2020, experts predicted that approximately 70% of the U.S. population would need to recover from Covid-19 infection to slow disease spread. Underlying this number was the reality that more than five million individuals could perish before this feat was achieved. As you can probably guess, such a situation is unacceptable, and hence social protective measures were mandated/strongly encouraged until vaccines could fill their role in ending the pandemic [20].

3.3.2 Vaccines

As mentioned, a strong antibody response against the target disease is key to achieving herd immunity. Vaccines remain the quickest and most efficient way of promoting antibody responses on a mass scale. Unlike natural infection, vaccine-driven immunity does not require illness to achieve protection. Herd immunity has been successfully reached against contagious diseases, including rubella, polio, smallpox, diphtheria, and many more. In the long run, vaccines offer a great way to protect newborns and immunocompromised individuals from disease without suffering from the disease itself. While vaccine-driven immunity is the gold standard in fighting back against pandemics such as the Covid-19 pandemic, it is not without faults. Several barriers remain in the fight against Covid-19 that need to be solved before the world can declare victory. First, vaccine hesitancy, as we hashed out in detail before, is a predominant risk to vaccine uptake. If individuals choose not to get vaccinated, herd immunity becomes much harder to reach. Please see "Introduction" for more details. Next is the issue of protection duration. While preliminary studies have shown adequate antibody levels for at least six months post-infection, the exact antibody level drop-off timeline is unknown. Thus, protection from vaccination may be insufficient and require a "booster" dose down

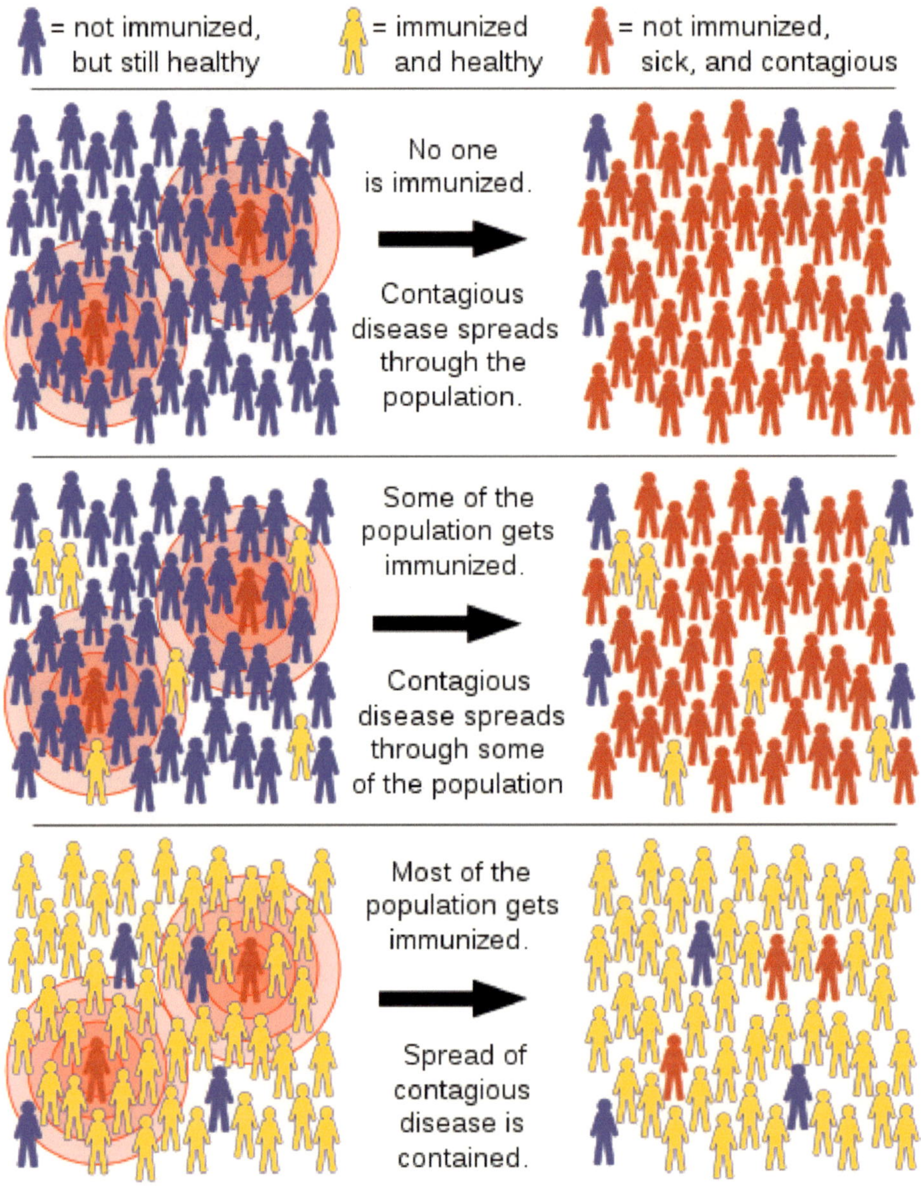

Figure 3.
"The top box shows an outbreak in a community in which a few people are infected (shown in red) and the rest are healthy but unimmunized (shown in blue); the illness spreads freely through the population. The middle box shows a population where a small number have been immunized (shown in yellow); those not immunized become infected while those immunized do not. In the bottom box, a large proportion of the population have been immunized; this prevents the illness from spreading significantly, including to unimmunized people. In the first two examples, most healthy unimmunized people become infected, whereas in the bottom example only one fourth of the healthy unimmunized people become infected." Source: Reproduced from Tkarcher under the creative commons attribution-share alike 4.0 international license.

the road. Additionally, new variants of the Covid-19 virus may be less efficiently targeted by the existing vaccines and require uptake of new vaccines specially made to counter such variants. Finally, outbreak control, while traditionally thought of on a community level, relies on limited transmission in surrounding regions as well. Thus, uneven vaccine distribution and resulting low transmission rates around an area can impact the ability of that area to contain the virus assuming individuals travel to and from [21].

3.4 Myth #4: mRNA technology is brand new

Perhaps the easiest myth to explain, let us state the historical fact: mRNA technology is not new, much less to fighting a pandemic. In fact, mRNA technology was pursued in vaccine research for quick response to a novel pathogen, such as Covid-19. The first studies using mRNA technology were in the 1990s. At the time, experts widely recognized that conventional vaccine types (e.g., live attenuated, subunit, etc.) were not always sufficient to combat pathogens capable of evading the adaptive immune response. Additionally, development and large-scale deployment were obstacles in the face of pandemic-speed response. Early reports showed that the introduction of mRNA could stimulate protein production and therefore antibody production via a disease-specific immune response. While early trials did hit roadblocks due to toxicity and delivery failures, recent advances such as RNA carriers and synthetic delivery have made mRNA engineering much more efficient. Before the Covid-19 pandemic, mRNA technology had been used in vaccine trials for cancer and other diseases for over a decade. However, the Covid-19 vaccines by Moderna and Pfizer/BioNTech are the first mRNA vaccines to receive FDA emergency use authorization. The crucial point here is that the technology is not experimental, has been excruciatingly vetted (see Myth #2), and will likely be a mainstay in vaccine development for future pandemics [22].

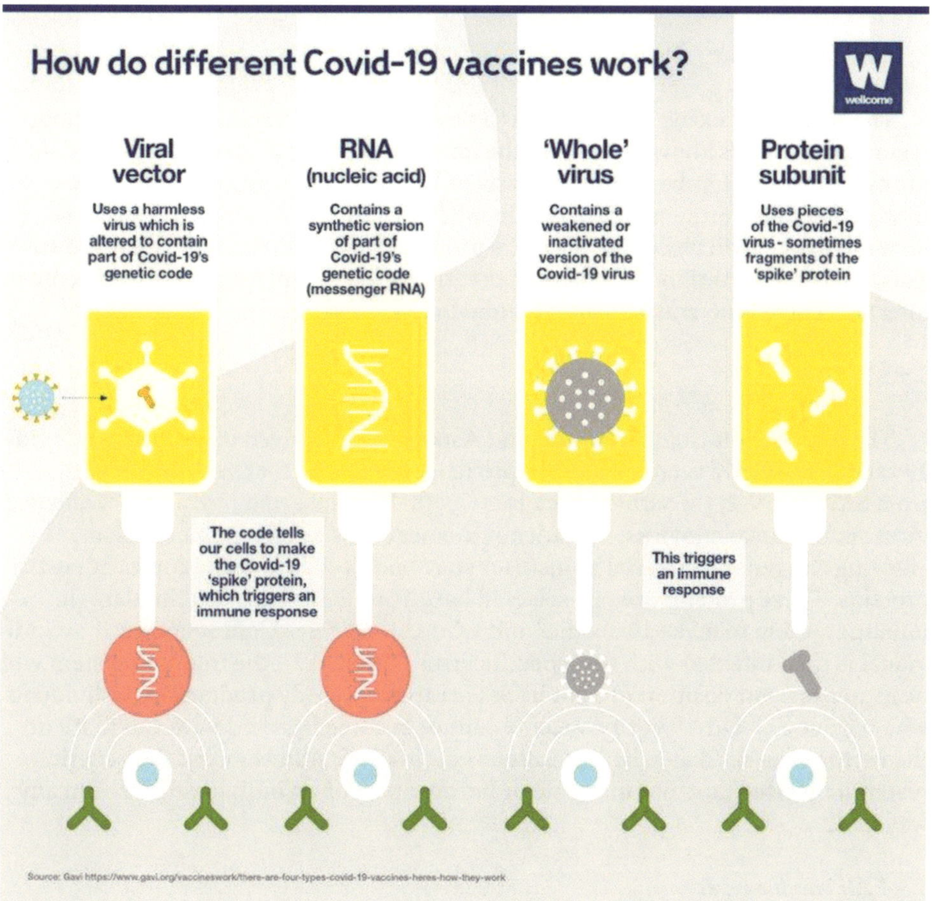

Figure 4.
A diagram showing the mechanism by which various Covid-19 vaccines/vaccine candidates induce an immune response. Source: Reproduced from Gavi https://www.gavi.org/vaccineswork/there-are-four-types-covid-19-vaccines-heres-how-they-work under creative commons attribution 2.0. Licensee the Wellcome Trust: https://wellcome.org/.

3.5 Myth #5: Covid-19 vaccines can alter your DNA

This is a common misconception, likely stemming from the fact that certain vaccines utilize parts of viruses/bacterium as a vector or stimulus to jumpstart the immune system [23]. To give context, we first need to explain the different types of vaccines in use/development against Covid-19 (**Figure 4**).

3.5.1 mRNA

The Pfizer/BioNTech and Moderna Covid-19 vaccines utilize mRNA technology. mRNA is a messenger bridge between DNA and protein synthesis. This process is of high relevance since Covid-19 virus surface proteins, particularly the spike protein, were identified early on. Thus, genetically engineered mRNA can be produced capable of instructing one's cells to make a partial piece of the spike protein that is completely harmless. By introducing raised levels of the spike protein fragments, the immune system will respond by making antibodies to the foreign particles. Upon infection with Covid-19, the body will have a large supply of antibodies ready to crush the virus. While the mRNA does influence body cells to produce protein fragments, it is rapidly degraded and does not enter the cells or influence DNA components [22].

3.5.2 Protein subunit

The Novavax vaccine is classified as a protein subunit vaccine. In this method, segments of a virus known to trigger the immune system are carefully selected. In the case of Covid-19, the vaccine consists of harmless spike proteins (cf. mRNA to stimulate spike protein production in mRNA vaccines). Once introduced, the immune system will recognize the spike proteins and mount an immune response. This will result in antibody formation, creating a reserve if that individual becomes infected. There is no effect on an individual's DNA [24].

3.5.3 Vector

The Janssen/Johnson & Johnson and AstraZeneca/University of Oxford Covid-19 vaccines utilize a vector-driven approach. This means that genetic material from SARS-CoV-2, the virus that causes Covid-19, is inserted into a live, weakened virus such as an adenovirus. The adenovirus serves as a delivery mechanism, allowing the genetic material to instruct your body's cells to make copies of certain proteins. These proteins are pre-selected based on their ability to stimulate the immune system to make antibodies and white blood cells. Consequently, if an individual is then infected with that specific virus (Covid-19), the immune system will be in an excellent position to fight back via rapid antibody production. Individuals who receive a Covid-19 vector vaccine cannot become infected with Covid-19 or the vector virus used as a direct result of vaccination. Additionally, the genetic material inserted does not integrate or become part of an individual's DNA in any way [25].

3.5.4 All vaccine types

In summary, none of the vaccines currently used against Covid-19 have the ability to alter an individual's DNA. Therefore, any such claim is a gross misrepresentation of both molecular processes and modern vaccine technology.

4. Conclusion

The Covid-19 pandemic has brought vaccine hesitancy to the forefront of both public conversation and health marketing research. While global vaccine development succeeded in launching several candidates against Covid-19, the missing link in such race was arguably a collaborative, targeted immunization campaign to inform and raise optimism toward the coming vaccines [2]. As a result, precious months were lost during a pandemic in which over three million lives have been lost [26]. Now, a few months after the initial vaccine rollout, nations are facing a declining yet formidable cohort of individuals who remain skeptical and/or averse to vaccine uptake due to a variety of factors [7]. This poses a serious challenge to communities attempting to reach herd immunity and crush the pandemic once and for all. Healthcare providers enjoy a unique position in society, capable of swaying public opinion through both direct and indirect interactions. Additionally, businesses, religious organizations, and loved ones represent promising avenues of outreach that should be empowered to combat vaccine hesitancy in their respective spheres [2]. While communication setting, skills, and personal relationship all play a role in one's ability to "fight back" against hesitancy, knowledge has a direct correlation with success in this endeavor. Thus, recognizing common myths surrounding Covid-19 vaccine candidate development, production, and administration is key to having fruitful discussions capable of persuading individuals to reconsider vaccination [9]. Herd immunity is closer than ever; it is up to us to band together and defeat misconceptions with research-backed knowledge, humility, and understanding. Together, we can and will crush the Covid-19 pandemic and any that dare to follow.

Acknowledgements

The author thanks Ms. Kathryn Wells for invaluable feedback regarding earlier drafts of this manuscript. The author is also grateful to the original authors of the various figures reproduced under their respective licenses.

Conflict of interest

The author declares no conflict of interest.

Notes/Thanks/Other declarations

Research surrounding the Covid-19 vaccine candidates, vaccine hesitancy response, and public optimism is fast-changing. All data used and studies cited were current at the time of this writing. For up-to-date information, please visit the World Health Organization and/or Centers for Disease Control and Prevention.

Author details

John Zizzo
University of Miami Miller School of Medicine, Miami, FL, USA

*Address all correspondence to: jjz41@med.miami.edu

References

[1] MacDonald NE, Hesitancy SWGoV. Vaccine hesitancy: Definition, scope and determinants. Vaccine. 2015;33(34):4161-4164. doi: 10.1016/j.vaccine.2015.04.036.

[2] Zizzo J. The Missing Link in the Covid-19 Vaccine Race. Hum Vaccin Immunother. 2021;17(5):1326-1328. doi: 10.1080/21645515.2020.1831859.

[3] Prevention CfDCa. About COVID-19 Vaccine Delivered and Administration Data. In: Diseases DoV, editor. cdc.gov: U.S. Department of Health & Human Services; 2021.

[4] Kelly DA, Macey DJ, Mak DB. Annual influenza vaccination. Hum Vaccin Immunother. 2014;10(7):1930-1934. doi: 10.4161/hv.29071.

[5] Dror AA, Eisenbach N, Taiber S, Morozov NG, Mizrachi M, Zigron A, et al. Vaccine hesitancy: the next challenge in the fight against COVID-19. Eur J Epidemiol. 2020;35(8):775-779. doi: 10.1007/s10654-020-00671-y.

[6] YouGov. Yahoo! News Coronavirus - July 30. 2020.

[7] YouGov. Yahoo! News Presidential Election - October 26. 2020.

[8] De Vito EL. [Eight persistent COVID-19 myths and why some people still believe them]. Medicina (B Aires). 2020;80 Suppl 6:112-6.

[9] Vyas D, Galal SM, Rogan EL, Boyce EG. Training Students to Address Vaccine Hesitancy and/or Refusal. Am J Pharm Educ. 2018;82(8):6338. doi: 10.5688/ajpe6338.

[10] Jarrett C, Wilson R, O'Leary M, Eckersberger E, Larson HJ, Hesitancy SWGoV. Strategies for addressing vaccine hesitancy - A systematic review. Vaccine. 2015;33(34):4180-4190. doi: 10.1016/j.vaccine.2015.04.040.

[11] Dubé E, Laberge C, Guay M, Bramadat P, Roy R, Bettinger J. Vaccine hesitancy: an overview. Hum Vaccin Immunother. 2013;9(8):1763-1773. doi: 10.4161/hv.24657.

[12] Koslap-Petraco M. Vaccine hesitancy: Not a new phenomenon, but a new threat. J Am Assoc Nurse Pract. 2019;31(11):624-626. doi: 10.1097/JXX.0000000000000342.

[13] Organization WH. Coronavirus disease (COVID-19) advice for the public. Mythbusters2021.

[14] Prevention CfDCa. Myths and Facts about COVID-19 Vaccines. In: Diseases DoV, editor.: U.S. Department of Health & Human Services; 2021.

[15] Izda V, Jeffries MA, Sawalha AH. COVID-19: A review of therapeutic strategies and vaccine candidates. Clin Immunol. 2021;222:108634. doi: 10.1016/j.clim.2020.108634.

[16] Office USGA. OPERATION WARP SPEED. 2021.

[17] Sparrow E, Wood JG, Chadwick C, Newall AT, Torvaldsen S, Moen A, et al. Global production capacity of seasonal and pandemic influenza vaccines in 2019. Vaccine. 2021;39(3):512-520. doi: 10.1016/j.vaccine.2020.12.018.

[18] Hoft DF, Brusic V, Sakala IG. Optimizing vaccine development. Cell Microbiol. 2011;13(7):934-942. doi: 10.1111/j.1462-5822.2011.01609.x.

[19] Randolph HE, Barreiro LB. Herd Immunity: Understanding COVID-19. Immunity. 2020;52(5):737-741. doi: 10.1016/j.immuni.2020.04.012.

[20] Fontanet A, Cauchemez S. COVID-19 herd immunity: where are we? Nat Rev Immunol. 2020;20(10):583-584. doi: 10.1038/s41577-020-00451-5.

[21] Metcalf CJE, Ferrari M, Graham AL, Grenfell BT. Understanding Herd Immunity. Trends Immunol. 2015;36(12):753-755. doi: 10.1016/j.it.2015.10.004.

[22] Pardi N, Hogan MJ, Porter FW, Weissman D. mRNA vaccines - a new era in vaccinology. Nat Rev Drug Discov. 2018;17(4):261-279. doi: 10.1038/nrd.2017.243.

[23] Chen WH, Strych U, Hotez PJ, Bottazzi ME. The SARS-CoV-2 Vaccine Pipeline: an Overview. Curr Trop Med Rep. 2020:1-4. doi: 10.1007/s40475-020-00201-6.

[24] Al-Kassmy J, Pedersen J, Kobinger G. Vaccine Candidates against Coronavirus Infections. Where Does COVID-19 Stand? Viruses. 2020;12(8). doi: 10.3390/v12080861.

[25] Amanat F, Krammer F. SARS-CoV-2 Vaccines: Status Report. Immunity. 2020;52(4):583-589. doi: 10.1016/j.immuni.2020.03.007.

[26] (CSSE) CfSSaE. Covid-19 Dashboard. April 25 ed: Johns Hopkins University & Medicine; 2021.

Chapter 25

Covid-19 Vaccines and Institutional Trust

Fermín Jesús González-Melado and María Luisa Di Pietro

Abstract

Major public and private laboratories entered into a race to find an effective Covid-19 vaccine. With the arrival of the vaccines, governments have to implement vaccination programs to achieve the necessary immunization levels to prevent further transmission of the disease. In this context, the ethical dilemma of compulsory vaccination *vs*. voluntary vaccination has been raised. Underlying this dilemma lies the problem of the ethical models on which the political decisions of governments in health matters based. The chapter proposes and argues the need to base health policy decisions on an ethical "first person" model, based on personal responsibility, that allows us to move from a normative ethic to an ethic of responsible behavior. This change in the ethical model, together with certain proposals for political action, will help us to restore institutional trust, so that the necessary levels of collective immunity against Covid-19 can be achieved through the voluntary vaccination of the citizens.

Keywords: Covid-19, vaccination, ethics of responsibility, prevention, institutional trust

1. Introduction

While we are still suffering the effects of the Covid-19 pandemic, the major public and private laboratories have entered into a race to find an effective vaccine against Covid-19. A vaccine capable of generating immunity is the only tool that can stop the spread of the virus. As of April 20, 2021, 13 vaccines have been approved and used, and there other 60 vaccine development projects worldwide [1]. The development of these vaccines has posed some serious ethical problems. Some groups were carrying out safety and efficacy tests on animals and humans in parallel, when the normal procedure would be to carry out the tests in animals and, once safety and efficacy have been proven, to carry them out in humans [2, 3]. Other groups had planned to inject the virus directly into healthy volunteers to test the efficacy of the vaccines [4]. In April 2020, the best forecasts spoke of a vaccine by the end of the year, and others by mid-2021 [5]. As we have already said, by mid-April 2021, we have 13 vaccines that are being applied all over the world. The truth is that each country, when the vaccines arrive, will face two successive scenarios: at first, two or three vaccines will arrive which have passed the safety and efficacy clinical trials, but with a limited production that will not allow the vaccination of the entire population; later, when the safety and efficacy of the first vaccines have been verified in the vaccinated population, the production of the most effective and safe vaccines will be increased, and the mass vaccination of the population can be considered [6].

In the first moment, when there is a shortage of available vaccine units, the ethical dilemma that arises is: whom to vaccinate? When there is a shortage of health resources, decisions must be made according to the principle of distributive justice, and the criteria for inclusion (prioritization) of the groups of users who can access vaccination will have to be determined.

In the second stage, when vaccine production has increased, mass vaccination of the population will be considered. In regard to the implementation of mass vaccination, two basic ethical dilemmas arise: the first is that of "free vaccination" *vs.* "paid vaccination"; the second is that of "non-compulsory vaccination" *vs.* "compulsory vaccination". In the case of vaccination against Covid-19, it is clear that the concern will focus on mass immunization, and as a rule, governments will carry out vaccination at no direct cost to citizens, thus eliminating the first dilemma. In this context, the only ethical dilemma that will arise will be compulsory *vs*. non-compulsory vaccination.

In this chapter, we aim to demonstrate that underlying these dilemmas are a series of ethical models on which the political decisions of governments about health matters are based. From there, we propose and argue the need for a "first-person" ethical model, based on responsibility, which allows us to move from a normative ethics to an ethics of responsible moral behavior, and which, together with certain proposals for political action, will succeed in recovering institutional confidence so that the necessary levels of collective immunity against Covid-19 can be achieved through the mass and voluntary vaccination of citizens.

2. Whom to vaccinate?

In the midst of a veritable forest of vaccine research projects, three are leading the way [7]. Therefore, a first scenario is presented with three or four approved vaccines with relative safety and efficacy, enough to reduce mortality, infections and the need for hospitalization. Thereafter, it will be necessary to initiate worldwide production of them in unprecedented quantities. Some centers expect to produce 100 million vaccines per year, while the alliance between various international organizations is talking about achieving 2 billion doses per year. Despite all these efforts to expand production, it is certain that, initially, there will not be enough vaccine for everyone, and governments will have to decide whom to vaccinate as a priority.

Given the lack of availability of health resources, in this case vaccines, *the principle of equal access* to them cannot be applied. The *principle of equity* then appears. Equity is *distributive justice* understood not as the equal distribution of resources, but as justice in relation to needs, especially in the distribution of risks and benefits in society. Following this principle, at least two groups appear in the risk/benefit ratio, and should be the target of the first group of available vaccines: health professionals and users of the health system over 70 years of age.

During the first wave of the Covid-19 pandemic, we have seen in different countries that a large number of health workers has been infected. The infection of such workers has had important consequences for the management of hospitals and the care of patients [8]. Those over 70 years of age have the highest mortality rate from Covid-19 [9]. During the first wave, in some European countries, 66% of deaths officially attributed to COVID were in this population group. The specific case of nursing homes [10] was particularly dramatic, as stated by the WHO [11]. In this sense, the elderly over 70 years of age and those living in nursing homes, as well as their caregivers, should be included in the priority group from the first moment of vaccination.

3. Compulsory vaccination?

Both in the first stage, of priority vaccination of risk groups, and in the second stage, that of mass vaccination once the production problems have been overcome, the possibility of compulsory vs. voluntary vaccination will be raised. Compulsory vaccination is an ethically controversial decision because it affects individual rights, including the individual's right to self-determination about health matters. Consider the case of a healthcare professional who refuses to be vaccinated when the government wants to force all healthcare workers to be vaccinated. Would a government be obliged to assume the responsibility for possible side effects caused by such mandatory vaccination? It is clear that if, for example, a government forces health professionals to be vaccinated, the legal responsibility would be that of the government, which would be obliged to pay the corresponding indemnities in the event that these vaccinations produce serious side effects for the health of those vaccinated. On the other hand, it has been shown that, even in situations of serious infections, merely recommending a vaccine, instead of making it mandatory, has not produced good immunization results [12]. In the event that there are people who refuse to be vaccinated against Covid-19, can a government force them to be vaccinated? [13].

3.1 Ethical models in national health systems

Behind the question of whether or not vaccination should be obligatory lies a much broader debate, one that refers to the ethical model of reference when making political decisions about public and community health issues. The first model is that of a normative ethics (a third-person ethics) that defends the legal obligatory nature of vaccination. The second model is that of virtue ethics (a first-person ethics), which defends the individual protagonist in making decisions about his or her health, taking into consideration the realization of the common good of society through the realization of the personal good. We propose that when making public health policy decisions in regard to Covid-19, it is possible to move from a normative ethics to a virtue ethics, through an ethics of personal responsibility [14].

The objective of a normative ethics, or a third-person ethics, is the search for and establishment of a series of rules or moral norms to be observed when carrying out certain individual actions. Human action is thus governed by norms that disregard the subject who acts and express his own existence. The object of investigation of this ethics is neither how one "should" live nor what would be the desirable lifestyle, but only whether a certain action is licit or illicit from the observation of an external judge: the "third person".

However, any conscious choice on the part of the individual, such as whether or not to be vaccinated against Covid-19, must be based on so-called " the first-person ethics", i.e., the search for the good of human life in its globality and complexity. Ethics would thus come to be configured as a kind of "discussion" on different lifestyles and different ways of living, and only secondarily on individual actions, with the aim of establishing what is the best life to lead and to desire.

3.2 "Responsibility" as an alternative

An appropriate way to move from a third-person ethics to a first-person ethics is a new reading of Hans Jonas' "ethics of responsibility" [15]. Jonas presents the personal responsibility and duty towards the children we have begotten, and who would perish without the care they need, as the clearest example we find in everyday morality of a non-reciprocal elementary responsibility and duty, which are spontaneously recognized and practiced. Jonas locates the origin of the idea of responsibility not in the relationship between autonomous adults, but in this relationship with offspring in need of protection. For Jonas, parental care for children is the archetype of responsible action. This archetype does not need to be deduced from principles, but is implanted in all of us by nature.

Along with parental responsibility, Jonas posits politics as another fundamental form of responsibility. Political responsibility and parental responsibility, although different, have the most in common. Jonas posits five elements in which these responsibilities coincide: *totality, object, sentiment, continuity*, and *future*. This last common element, the future, shows that in both parental and political responsibility, tomorrow is included in today's concerns. In the context of total responsibility, every individual act that is concerned with the immediate also includes, as its object, the future existence of that child or that community. In this sense, personal responsibility cannot be determining but *enabling*; it must prepare the ground for the future and keep the greatest number of options open. It is a matter of keeping open the future of the subject for whom one is responsible, be it the future of the child, or of the individual who is part of the social community.

4. The concept of prevention

For this to be possible, governments and health authorities must change the concept of prevention that they normally use. In regulatory ethics, which would support, for example, mandatory vaccination against Covid-19, the concept of prevention is identified with *risk reduction*. In this sense, a health system will achieve better prevention when the risk of contracting the disease is lower. In the case of vaccination against Covid-19, this will occur when the greatest possible number of individuals is vaccinated. This is an argument that, from a normative ethical point of view, would justify vaccinating as many people as possible against Covid-19 on a compulsory basis.

However, from the point of view of a normative ethics, all preventive medicinal measures, including vaccination against Covid-19, run the risk of becoming a set of *obligations* and *prohibitions* for citizens. These obligations and prohibitions can increase frictions between political decisions and the individual autonomy, and can increase personal frustrations, because these preventive measures are perceived only as an instrument for the good of society. Even worse, they can also potentially lead to a lack of motivation in regard to everything else related to one's own health.

We propose a different concept of preventive medicine. For us, prevention consists in *the acquisition by the individual of ethical behaviors* - this is the novelty with respect to the thought of Hans Jonas - that allow the development of the person towards a "first-person ethics" in the attainment, in general, of his or her own good, and in the particular case, of that which, as Descartes had already observed, is the "greatest" of one's goods: health.

If citizens move from this perspective of personal responsibility in the pursuit of the collective health, compulsory vaccination against Covid-19 would be unnecessary: if the efficacy and the medical and social value of the new Covid-19 vaccines are guaranteed, and citizens are properly informed, vaccination would be, so to speak, a "moral responsibility," a moral duty [16], and vaccination would be one more among the actions that direct the individual towards the achievement of both individual and community health. We believe that, through a first-person ethics, it is possible to create an alternative based on personal responsibility, one that, together with a series of legal actions of a political nature that we will enunciate below, allows effective protection of the entire community and, at the same time, guarantees the expression of personal autonomy. For example, in order to institute confinement, a regime of sanctions was established by the government (normative ethics), but what has allowed confinement to have a high success rate has been the concept of prevention based on personal responsibility, exercised by the citizens according their own determination to cooperate, in a responsible manner, with the prevention measures (first-person ethics).

5. Is there a right to not be vaccinated?

The principle of respect for the autonomy of the individual, enshrined in the Spanish Patient Autonomy Law [17], allows the individual to refuse a treatment and, therefore, also to refuse vaccination [18]. It is clear, therefore, that an individual has the right to choose not to be vaccinated. It is also true that some legislation in democratic countries contemplates the possibility of compulsory vaccination in exceptional circumstances. For example, in Spain, Organic Law 3/1986, of April 14, 1986, on *Special Public Health Measures*, allows the approval of exceptional measures, such as compulsory vaccination, when there is a specific risk to the health of the population, such as an epidemic outbreak [19]. Knowing all this, we cannot forget that vaccination is a treatment applied to healthy people who are not suffering from a disease. Moreover, in the case of Covid-19, a large part of the population, those under 20 years of age and without previous health complications, has a very low percentage of serious complications. Therefore, the medical justification for vaccination, in many cases, would not be based so much on the protection of the individual as on the protection of the community (herd immunity) [20].

Before promoting compulsory vaccination protocols against Covid-19, the question which should be asked is: why is the percentage of individuals vaccinated voluntarily so low even in pandemic situations, as demonstrated with the H1N1 virus? Or, in other words, why does a person refuse a vaccine that could save his or her life?

In August 2017, France's health minister reported a decision to mandate vaccination against 11 diseases for minors starting in 2018. This measure was taken due to alarming data on low vaccination rates for diseases such as measles among the population of France [21]. In Spain, where vaccination is not compulsory, vaccination rates are among the best in Europe in the child population (between 95 and 98% for childhood vaccines), dropping slightly with those administered during adolescence (especially in booster doses). The lowest data belong to seasonal influenza vaccination (54% in 2018).

The French case is not unique in Europe. Other European countries are seeing their vaccination rates decrease year after year [22]. Several factors have led to a change in the perception that part of the population has about vaccines [23]: a feeling that the economic and business motives of large pharmaceutical companies which put pressure on public institutions and governments are more important than healthcare [24]; the belief that user deaths are directly related to vaccines rather than mere coincidences [25]; the sometimes alarmist communication of risks and side effects in the media [26]; healthy individuals are, in general, more fearful of the risk caused by vaccines than of the use of the drugs that treat that disease, because the decline in the number of diseases against which vaccines are given has distorted the perception - through ignorance - of the seriousness of many of them (this was seen during the measles outbreak in European countries two years ago) [27]; there is a certain distrust in scientific knowledge, which seem to change and be surpassed with each new discovery [28].

In the specific case of Covid-19, the two scenarios given above will give us different situations in regard to public trust. On the one hand, the first vaccines to be put into circulation will not necessarily be the most effective or the safest. This may lead some people to doubt whether or not to administer the vaccine. On the other hand, at the second stage, that of mass vaccination, the efficacy data of previous vaccines will be available, and the vaccine with the best safety and efficacy data can be administered, thus increasing the population's trust in the vaccines. In the scenarios described above, we may find different vaccines in different countries or even in different regions within the same country. In addition, trust in vaccines will depend on the evolution of the *fake news* that promote conspiracy theories about Covid-19 and vaccines against the virus. All these factors will affect the levels of trust/distrust of the population towards institutions and towards vaccines against Covid-19.

6. The problem of institutional trust

Public trust in public health systems is critical, and affects the development and maintenance of individual, community and societal health and well-being. This is why health professionals, and especially politicians, need to take the concept of "institutional trust" seriously [29] if they want to improve both the commitment to health among the general population and their public health systems.

Both theoretical and empirical literature show that contemporary societies are built on very low levels of trust [30, 31]. In our societies, there are two types of trust: interpersonal and institutional. Interpersonal trust appears as the result of past interactions by which people learn to make decisions about future interactions; i.e., the individual, from his past experiences, learns whether or not to trust someone else in the future. "Institutional trust" refers to the trust placed by individuals in a system or institution such as a government, a political party, a non-governmental organization, or a particular public or private organization. Institutional trust is based on personal experiences, especially negative ones, that the person has had throughout his or her life, not so much with the institution, but with the people who represent the institution [32]. Research shows that in crisis situations, interpersonal trust tends to increase and institutional trust decreases [33].

Institutional trust is one of the most important concerns when carrying out mass vaccination campaigns [34], not so much because users distrust the public health system, but because they distrust government recommendations [35]. Maintaining institutional trust is critical for mass immunization programs against Covid-19. A clear example of this problem is the low levels of vaccination during the H1N1 pandemic; the lack of trust in the institutions involved in vaccination during the H1N1 pandemic led to an increase in vaccination skepticism. This, together with conspiracy theories, and speculation that the response to the pandemic by governments had been influenced by the commercial interests of big pharma, led to a disastrous failure in immunization levels in most countries [24]. It is clear that in the current period, both interpersonal and institutional trust have undergone changes. Studies point to an increase in interpersonal trust and a decrease in institutional trust during the Covid-19 pandemic [36]. It is necessary to increase the levels of institutional trust when vaccination processes are initiated, both at the first moment, when vaccination is restricted to risk groups, and at the second moment, when vaccines are available for the rest of the population. The recovery of institutional trust will be a key element in achieving vaccination levels that allow herd immunity.

7. Proposals for political action

From a first-person ethics based on personal responsibility, at least two changes are needed before the relevant governments will consider mandatory mass vaccination programs against Covid-19.

The first change is to *rediscover the leading role of each citizen in prevention policies, and more specifically in health decisions*. It is not up to the government to decide for the individual; it is up to the individual himself to evaluate whether, when he makes the decision not to vaccinate himself, he does so with the aim of preserving his health and the health of the community. From this point of view, from an ethics of the first person, the subject will understand that it is his moral responsibility to be vaccinated against Covid-19, because vaccination is a valid instrument in the objective of achieving the good of "health" at both the individual and community level.

The second change focuses on the role of governments. It is *the responsibility of governments to promote prevention policies based on the ethics of individual responsibility* in order to increase institutional trust and, therefore, a reduction in the possible distrust towards vaccination against Covid-19. It is clear that when a person decides not to be vaccinated, it is not with the intention of transmitting the disease, but out of fear and mistrust that the vaccine will be useful for his or her health. For this reason, responsible governments must implement a series of initiatives aimed at reinforcing institutional trust:

- ensure a policy of correct scientific information on the efficacy and safety of vaccines against Covid-19. John M. Barry wrote: "In the next influenza pandemic ... the single most important weapon against the disease will be a vaccine. The second most important will be communication" [37];

- provide for the preparation of well-trained health professionals to offer vaccination to users of health systems, especially family physicians and pediatricians;

- eliminate socioeconomic barriers to allow access to the Covid-19 vaccination program for the entire population;

- prepare an adequate disease control system, both at regional and national level, and;

- provide for a responsible agency, at the political and scientific level, for the introduction, distribution and follow-up in the public health system of the new Covid-19 vaccine(s), both at the first moment of vaccination, of populations at risk and at the second moment, when the vaccine becomes available to the rest of the population.

These are all concrete actions that we propose to increase the population's institutional trust when vaccine(s) against Covid-19 are presented. These measures will help each individual to assume his or her personal responsibility both in the first scenario, of priority vaccination (health professionals + risk groups), and in the second moment, in the mass vaccination campaign. These measures will make it possible to guarantee the necessary immunization levels against Covid-19 with voluntary vaccination.

8. Conclusions

Before the responsible governments, both at the national and regional levels, promote vaccination campaigns against Covid-19, in the different scenarios that are foreseen in the future, it will be necessary to increase the levels of institutional confidence in the population, in order to guarantee the success of vaccination program(s). Only in this way will it be possible to achieve the desired levels of immunization in the population during this pandemic situation. This will only be possible if, together with the concrete measures that we have proposed to be implemented by the different governments, a concept of prevention is promoted which encourages individual ethical behavior aimed at achieving the good of health for both the individual and for his or her community. This concept of prevention, based on individual responsibility, must include all preventive measures in the spread of Covid-19, including vaccination measures. The success of future vaccination programs against Covid-19 will depend on the assumption of this ethic of responsibility, not only by individuals, but also by the various governments involved.

Acknowledgements

We thank Dr. José Manuel Moreno Villares for his review of the final version of the manuscript and his suggestions for the final draft of the text.

Conflict of interest

The authors declare no conflict of interest.

Author details

Fermín Jesús González-Melado[1]* and María Luisa Di Pietro[2]

1 Department of Moral Theology and Bioethics, High Center for Theological Studies (Badajoz), Pontifical University of Salamanca, Salamanca, Spain

2 Hygiene Section, University Department for Life's Sciences and Public Health, Università Cattolica del Sacro Cuore, Rome, Italy

*Address all correspondence to: fjgonzalezme@upsa.es

References

[1] Craven J, Covid-19 vaccine tracker. Regulatory Affairs Professionals Society (RASP) Published online on April 15, 2020: https://www.raps.org/news-and-articles/news-articles/2020/3/covid-19-vaccine-tracker [Accessed 20/4/2021].

[2] Boodman E. Researchers rush to test coronavirus vaccine in people without knowing how well it works in animals. Published online https://www.statnews.com/2020/03/11/researchers-rush-to-start-moderna-coronavirus-vaccine-trial-without-usual-animal-testing/ [Accessed 20/4/2021].

[3] Plotkin SA, Caplan A. Extraordinary diseases require extraordinary solutions. Vaccine. 2020; 38:3987-3988. DOI:10.1016/j.vaccine.2020.04.039.

[4] Eyal N, Lipsitch M, Smith PG. Human challenge studies to accelerate coronavirus vaccine licensure. J Infect Dis. 2020;221:1752-1756. DOI: 10.1093/infdis/jjaa152.

[5] Kelly-Linden, J. University of Oxford Covid-19 vaccine. The Daily Telegraph. Published online on April 29, 2020: https://www.telegraph.co.uk/global-health/science-and-disease/oxford-vaccine-trial-coronavirus/ [Accessed 20/4/2021].

[6] Shumeni, L. COVID-19 vaccine development lab, production department completed in Wuhan. Goblal Times. Published online on July 2, 2020: https://www.globaltimes.cn/content/1193263.shtml [Accessed 20/4/2021].

[7] World Health Organization. Draft landscape of COVID-19 candidate vaccines. Published online on July 2, 2020: [https://www.who.int/publications/m/item/draft-landscape-of-covid-19-candidate-vaccines] [Accessed 20/4/2021].

[8] O. Guell, "España es el país con más contagios entre el personal sanitario", *El País*. Published online on April 25, 2020: [https://elpais.com/sociedad/2020-04-24/espana-es-el-pais-con-mas-contagios-entre-el-personal-sanitario.html [Accessed 20/4/2021].

[9] Coronavirus: case fatality rate by age. Published online https://ourworldindata.org/mortality-risk-covid [Accessed 20/4/2021].

[10] RTVE noticias. "Radiografía del coronavirus en residencias de ancianos: más de 19.000 muertos con Covid-19 o síntomas compatibles". Published online on May 22, 2020: [https://www.rtve.es/noticias/20200528/radiografia-del-coronavirus-residencias-ancianos-espana/2011609.shtml [Accessed 20/4/2021].

[11] Europa Press. La OMS calcula que 55.000 ancianos han muerto con covid-19 en geriátricos de Europa. elPeridodico. Published online April 23, 2020: https://www.elperiodico.com/es/sociedad/20200423/oms-calcula-55000-ancianos-muerto-covid-19-geriatricos-europa-7938134] [Accessed 20/4/2020].

[12] Doganis D, Tsolia M, Dana H, et al. Compliance with immunization against H1N1 influenza virus among children with cancer. Pediatr Hemat Oncol. 2020;30;149-153. DOI: 10.3109/08880018.2012.753961.

[13] Wiwanitkit S, Wiwanitkit V. Compulsory vaccination: a topic to be discussed. Cuad Bioet 2013; 80: 127.

[14] Di Pietro ML, Refolo P, González-Melado FJ. Sobre la 'responsabilidad' de la vacunación. Cuad Bioet. 2012;78:323-336.

[15] Jonas H, Das Prinzip Verantwortung. Versus einer Ethik für die technologische Zivilisation,

Shurkamp, Frankfurt am Main 1979. English translation: The imperative of Responsibility. In Search for an Ethics for the Technological Age. The University of Chicago Press. Chicago, 1984.

[16] Refolo P, González-Melado FJ, Di Pietro ML. Sulla 'doverosità morale' dell'uso di vaccini. Clin. Ter. 2015:162;38-42.

[17] Ley 41/2002, de 14 de noviembre, básica reguladora de la autonomía del paciente y de derechos y obligaciones en materia de información y documentación clínica. BOE núm. 274, de 15/11/2002. Reference BOE-A-2002-22188. Published online: https://www.boe.es/buscar/act.php?id=BOE-A-2002-22188.

[18] Miller BL, Autonomy, in Post SG (ed.), Encyclopedia of Bioethics, Thomson, New York 2003, 246-251, p. 247.

[19] Ley Orgánica 3/1986, de 14 de abril, de Medidas especiales en materia de salud pública. BOE núm. 02, de 29/04/1986. Reference BOE-A-1986-10498. Published online: https://www.boe.es/buscar/act.php?id=BOE-A-1986-10498.

[20] Ludvigsson JF. Systematic review of COVID-19 in children shows milder cases and a better prognosis than adults. Acta Paediatr. 2020;109:1080-1095. DOI: 10.1111/apa.15270.

[21] Perez Avila, M. La caída en las tasas de vacunación provoca un fuerte brote de sarampión en Europa. El Mundo. Published online on August 5, 2017: https://www.elmundo.es/ciencia-y-salud/salud/2017/08/05/596e4743468aebb30b8b46a9.html [Accessed 20/4/2021].

[22] Dawson, A. Herd protection as a public good: vaccination ad our obligation to others, in Dawson A, Werweij M. Ethics prevention and public health, Clarendon Press, Oxford, 2007, p.160-178.

[23] Larson HJ, Cooper LZ, Eskola J, et al. Addressing the vaccine confidence gap. Lancet. 2011;378:526-535. DOI: 10.1016/S0140-6736(11)60678-8.

[24] Yaqub O, Castle-Clarke S, Sevdalis N, Chataway J. Attitudes to vaccination: a critical review. Soc Sci Med. 2014;112:1-11. DOI: 10.1016/j.socscimed.2014.04.018.

[25] Lon Z, Puliyel JM. Introducing prevalent vaccine in the EPI in India: a counsel for caution. Indian J Med Res. 2010; 132:1-3.

[26] Campbell P. Understanding the receivers and the reception of science's uncertain messages. Philos Trans A Math Phys Eng Sci. 2011;369:489-4912. DOI: 10.1098/rsta.2011.0068.

[27] Doteval L. The return of measles to Europe highlights the need to regain confidence immunization. Acta Paediatr. 2019;108: 8-9. DOI: 10/1111/apa.14621.

[28] Clements CJ, Ratzan S. Misled and confused? Telling the public about MMR vaccine safety. J Med Ethics. 2003;29:22-26.

[29] Ward PR. Improving Access to, use of, and outcomes from public health programs: the importance of building and maintaining trust with patients/clients. Front Public Health 2017;5:22. DOI: 10.3389/fpubh.2017.00022.

[30] Row R, Calnan M. Trust relations in health care – the new agenda. Eur J Public Health. 2006;16:4-6. DOI: 10.1093/eurpub/ckl004.

[31] Gilson T. Trust and the development of health care as a social institution. Soc Sci Med. 2003;56:1453-1468. DOI: 10.1016/S0277-9536(02)00142-9.

[32] Giddens A. The consequences of modernity. Polity Press, Cambridge, 1990.

[33] Evaristi H., Kouvo Antti, Venetoklis T. Social and institutional trust in times of crisis: Greece 2002 – 2011. Social Indicators Research. 2019;141: 1207-1123. DOI: 10.1007/s11205-018-1862-y.

[34] Browlie J, Howson A. "Leaps of faith" and MMR: an empirical study of trust. Sociology. 2005;39: 221-239. DOI: 10.1177/0038038505050536.

[35] American Academy of Arts and Science. *Public trust in vaccines: defining a research agenda.* Cambridge (MA). American Academy of Arts and Sciences, 2014. Published online : https://www.amacad.org/publication/public-trust-vaccines-defining-research-agenda [Accessed 20/4/2021].

[36] Lee J, Sniderman B, Marquad B, et al. Embedding trust into Covid-19 recovery. Four dimensions of stakeholder trust. Deloitte insights. Published online April 23, 2020: https://www2.deloitte.com/uk/en/insights/economy/covid-19/building-trust-during-covid-19-recovery.html [Accessed 20/4/2021].

[37] Barry JM. Pandemics: Avoiding the mistakes of 1918. Nature. 2009;459: 324-325. DOI: 10.1038/459324a.

Chapter 26

Pharmacotherapy for COVID-19: A Ray of Hope

Mayank Kapoor, Prasan Kumar Panda and Vivek Mohanty

Abstract

Most viral infections have limited treatment options available and the same holds for COVID-19, its causative agent being the SARS-CoV-2 virus. Drugs used in the past against Severe Acute Respiratory Syndrome (SARS) or Middle East Respiratory Syndrome (MERS) viruses, which belong to the same family of viruses as the novel Coronavirus included ribavirin, interferon (alfa and beta), lopinavir-ritonavir combination, and corticosteroids. There remains controversy regarding their efficacy to date, except for the last one. Hence, large-scale multicentric trials are being conducted involving multiple drugs. Chloroquine and hydroxy-chloroquine were initially taking the race ahead but have now been rejected. Remdesivir was a promising candidate, for which the FDA had issued an emergency use authorization, but now is not recommended by the WHO. Convalescent plasma therapy had promising results in the early severe viremia phase, but the PLACID trial made an obscure end. Only corticosteroids have shown demonstrable benefits in improving mortality rates among severe COVID-19 cases. Many new modalities like monoclonal antibodies and tyrosine kinase inhibitors are discussed. In this chapter, we review the therapeutic drugs under investigation for the COVID-19 treatment, their mode of action, degree of effectiveness, and recommendations by different centers regarding their use in current settings.

Keywords: antiviral, monoclonal antibody, coronavirus disease 2019, dexamethasone, immunomodulator, ivermectin, remdesivir

1. Introduction

Because of the high rate of infectivity of the COVID-19 virus, the global burden associated with the disease, and its impact on the economies of different countries, efforts are being made to find a possible cure for the disease as soon as possible [1]. As with most viral infections, limited options are available for the treatment of COVID-19. Since there is no efficient therapy available for the same, given the public emergency, efforts are ongoing to find drugs helpful in COVID-19 infection. Drugs used in the past against Severe Acute Respiratory Syndrome (SARS) or Middle East Respiratory Syndrome (MERS), which also belong to the group of Beta coronaviruses, included ribavirin, interferon, lopinavir-ritonavir, and corticosteroids [2]. Most randomized controlled trials (RCTs) performed to test the effectiveness of these drugs have not shown any satisfying results, apart from corticosteroids. Many RCTs are still undergoing, the results of which are awaited. Studies about the virus-induced host immune response and viral processing within target cells have led to several potential therapeutic targets.

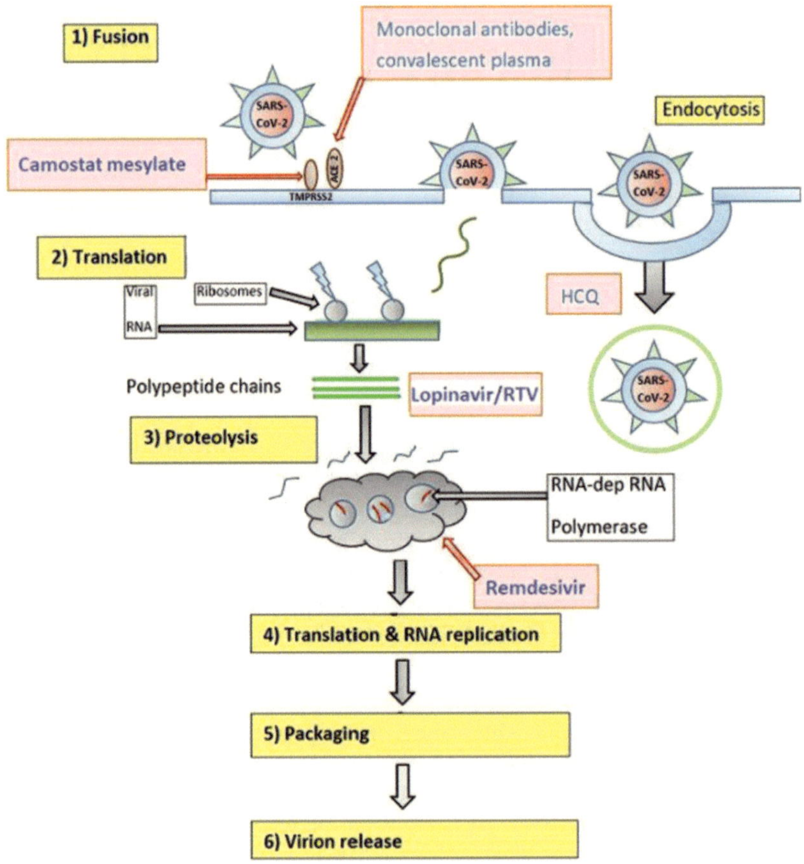

Figure 1.
Site of action of different possible pharmacotherapeutics used in COVID-19 treatment.

Drug	Mode of action	Effectiveness	Recommendation
Corticosteroids	Immunosuppressant	Decreased death rate in ARDS, no effect in non-ARDS	WHO, CDC, and IDSA recommendations
Remdesivir	RdRp inhibitor	Decreases recovery time	FDA approval in October, WHO issued a conditional recommendation against use in November, IDSA suggests the use
Convalescent plasma	Anti-COVID 19 antibodies	No benefit	FDA EUA issued
Monoclonal antibodies	Directed against COVID spike proteins	Benefit in Mild cases, no benefit in hospitalized cases	FDA EUA issued for OPD patients
Azithromycin	Immunomodulation	No benefit	No recommendation, but widely used
Ivermectin	Viral IMPα/β1(Importin) mediated nuclear import inhibition	Benefit in prophylaxis	NIH: Insufficient data for or against the use
Melatonin	Pineal gland hormone, anti-inflammatory	Benefit in critical patients	No recommendation

Drug	Mode of action	Effectiveness	Recommendation
Tocilizumab	IL-6 R inhibitor	Reduces inflammatory markers	Single-dose in addition to dexamethasone in critical patients with rapid progression of respiratory failure may be given: NIH
Favipiravir	Inhibits RNA polymerase	Faster viral clearance, improved imaging findings	No recommendation yet
Ribavirin	Inhibits RNA polymerase	No concrete evidence	No recommendations yet
Chloroquine/ Hydroxy-chloroquine	Increases endosomal pH, interfere with glycosylation of receptor, immunomodulator	Benefit in clinical parameter & virological clearance	Removed from Solidarity trial, no other recommendation
Lopinavir/ Ritonavir	Protease inhibitor: SARS-Cov-2 3CL pro	Not significant	Removed from Solidarity trial, no other recommendation
Interferon	Immunomodulation	No concrete evidence	Removed from Solidarity trial, no other recommendation
Tyrosine Kinase inhibitors	Inhibit STAT phosphorylation, decrease hyperimmune state	No concrete evidence	Use with remdesivir if corticosteroids are contraindicated: NIH/IDSA

RdRp: RNA dependent RNA polymerase; ARDS: Acute respiratory distress syndrome; WHO: World Health Organization; CDC: Centers for Disease Control and Prevention; FDA: Food and Drug Administration; IDSA: Infectious Disease Society of America; EUA: Emergency Use Authorization; NIH: National Institute of Health; Il-6 R: Interleukin-6 receptor; STAT: Signal transducer and activator of transcription.

Table 1.
Summary of various pharmacotherapeutics being considered for COVID-19 treatment.

We hereby discuss the potential therapeutic drugs under investigation for the COVID-19 treatment, their modes of action (**Figure 1**), degree of effectiveness, and recommendations (**Table 1**) by different centers regarding their usage in the current settings.

2. Review of pharmacotherapy

2.1 Chloroquine/hydroxychloroquine

The first studied drugs for COVID-19 were chloroquine and hydroxychloroquine (HCQ). Chloroquine was found to be effective against Avian influenza A H5N1 virus in animal models [3, 4] and also had demonstrable activity resulting in in-vitro inhibition of SARS-CoV [5]. COVID-19 infection showed high pandemicity in countries where malaria is the least prevalent and least pandemicity where malaria is highly prevalent. This observation led to the concept that chloroquine may be beneficial in COVID-19 since it is used as an anti-malarial. The mechanism of chloroquine action depends on the pathogen involved. Chloroquine increases the endosomal pH and interferes with the glycosylation of cellular receptor [Angiotensin Converting Enzyme (ACE) II] of SARS-CoV [6]. It also inhibits quinone reductase-2, which is involved in sialic acid biosynthesis. There is inhibition of MAO-kinase, virion assembly, and processing of M protein [7]. Besides its antiviral activity, it also has immunomodulatory effects that may be synergistic. HCQ was found to be equally effective as chloroquine, although a study concluded that HCQ was more effective and less toxic than chloroquine [8]. Chloroquine inhibitory actions against SARS-CoV were equal whether the primate cells were treated before or after exposure. This suggested that chloroquine could have both prophylactic and therapeutic applications [9]. One of the first studies performed to study the effect of chloroquine was done in the Chinese population. In this trial, patients in the study group who received chloroquine had reduced symptom duration, radiological improvement, and earlier seroconversion to the virus-negative state compared to controls [10]. Following this study, the National Health Commission of the People's Republic of China included chloroquine in its guideline for the management of pneumonia due to Covid-19. In a study conducted by Gautret et al. in France, chloroquine treatment group had significant clearing of the nasopharyngeal swab viral load compared to the control [11]. The virological clearance day-6 post inclusion (primary outcome) with HCQ vs. controls was 70% vs. 12.5% ($p < 0.001$). The virological clearance at day 6 in HCQ plus azithromycin, HCQ and control arms were 100%, 57.1%, and 12.5% respectively ($p = 0.001$) thus suggesting synergistic action of azithromycin to HCQ. Gradually the side effect profile of HCQ, that is QTc prolongation with concomitant use of Azithromycin, lead the American Heart Association (AHA) to recommend withdrawal/withholding these drugs in patients with QTc ≥ 500 millisecond (either baseline or developing during treatment). On 28 March 2020, Food and Drug Administration (FDA) had issued Emergency Use Authorization (EUA) for Chloroquine/HCQ. However, the Centers for Disease Control and Prevention (CDC) on April 7 issued a statement stating no drugs or other therapeutic measures were approved by the US FDA to prevent or treat COVID-19. In April, the FDA issued a Drug Safety Communication cautioning against the use of HCQ or chloroquine for COVID-19 outside the hospital setting or a clinical trial due to the risk of heart rhythm problems. In June 2020, it was announced by World Health Organization (WHO) that the HCQ arm of the Solidarity Trial (Multi-national trial including remdesivir, HCQ, lopinavir/ritonavir, and lopinavir/ritonavir with interferon beta-1a) would be stopped [12]. This was keeping in view the lack of any mortality benefit of HCQ. Hence in June itself, FDA revoked the EUA of HCQ and chloroquine [13]. The pre-exposure prophylaxis benefit of HCQ needs further research.

2.2 Lopinavir/ritonavir

The combination of lopinavir/ritonavir was considered as an option for the treatment of Covid-19 during initial pandemic days. Lopinavir is an HIV-1 protease inhibitor, which is combined with ritonavir to increase its half-life through cytochrome p-450 inhibition. Both anti-HIV drugs interact with residues at the active site of SARS-CoV 3C-like protease, suggesting the mechanism of action in COVID-19 [14]. Its role was first evaluated in the treatment of SARS where patients treated with lopinavir/ritonavir for 14 days combined with ribavirin for 21 days. They had a milder disease in form of less diarrhea, fever, lymphadenopathy, the incidence of nosocomial infections, viral loads, demonstration of virus in the fecal sample by reverse transcription-polymerase chain reaction (RT-PCR), and 21 days adverse outcomes [15]. The combination was tested for MERS-CoV. It was postulated that the lopinavir/ritonavir combination may inhibit the 3C-like protease of MERS-CoV and may affect apoptosis in human cells. Results revealed that treatment with lopinavir/ritonavir led to clinical, radiological, and pathological improvement. Those animals treated with this combination had the lowest mean viral load detected by RT-PCR in lung and other extrapulmonary tissue [16]. There was only a single case report of a man being treated and recovered with a combination of lopinavir/ritonavir, ribavirin, and interferon-α for the MERS [17]. Based on this data, an urgent RCT was done to study the efficacy of lopinavir/ritonavir in the Wuhan province of China [18]. The analysis revealed no significant difference in terms of time for clinical improvement and mortality at 28 days. The median time for clinical improvement was just one day shorter in the lopinavir-ritonavir group compared to the standard care group. In July 2020, WHO discontinued the lopinavir/ritonavir arm of the solidarity trial due to a lack of any mortality benefit [19]. It causes QTc prolongation, just like HCQ [20].

2.3 Azithromycin

Azithromycin is a broad-spectrum antibiotic belonging to the macrolide group, having anti-inflammatory properties also. It is commonly used for treating atypical respiratory pathogens. Azithromycin's anti-viral efficacy against some RNA viruses has also been described. Its efficacy has been demonstrated in-vitro against Zika virus and rhinovirus, as well as SARS-CoV-2 [21, 22]. As described, azithromycin also has immunomodulatory effects and can decrease acute exacerbations of chronic airway disease. Owing to its wide availability, excellent safety profile, and easy availability, azithromycin is one of the commonest drugs being used in the COVID-19 pandemic also. The Lancet reported the result of the COALITION II trial, [23] which was an open-label randomized trial evaluating azithromycin in addition to the standard of care (including HCQ), against the standard of care alone in severe COVID-19 patients. Azithromycin demonstrated no benefit in clinical outcome including clinical status or mortality, as compared to the standard of care alone (OR 1·36 [95% CI 0·94–1·97], p = 0·11). There was no increase in adverse events with azithromycin. In a study published in NEJM, HCQ alone or in combination with azithromycin had no demonstrable improvement in clinical status at 15 days compared with standard care in mild to moderate COVID-19 admissions [24].

2.4 Ivermectin

Ivermectin is a commonly used drug for various parasitic infestations including head lice, scabies, strongyloidiasis, ascariasis, and lymphatic filariasis. It is a macrocyclic lactone, which is derived from streptomyces avermitilis [25]. Its mechanism of activity against SARS-CoV-2 is believed to be via viral IMPα/β1 (Importin) mediated nuclear import inhibition. This leads to a decrease in the multiplication of the virus and hence the viral load [26, 27]. Ivermectin and doxycycline combination also inhibit viral entry and increases viral load clearance by the targeting of multiple viral proteins [28]. A recent study from India demonstrated that 2-dose ivermectin prophylaxis (300 micrograms/kg) within a gap of 3 days led to a 73% reduction in the number of COVID-19 infections among healthcare workers [29]. In studies conducted in Bangladesh also, the ivermectin-doxycycline combination was demonstrated to be highly effective in virological clearance in mild to moderate COVID-19 patients [30, 31]. National Institute of Health (NIH) stated in January 2021 that there was insufficient data to recommend either for or against the use of ivermectin for the treatment of COVID-19 [32].

2.5 Melatonin

Melatonin is a hormone, which is synthesized from tryptophan in the pineal gland of the body and also by mostly all the organs of the body, as its production is associated with mitochondria. Higher levels of melatonin have positive roles in health and aging. Melatonin promises to be a great adjunctive drug for viral infections owing to its anti-inflammatory, anti-apoptotic, immunomodulatory, and antioxidant activities [33]. Sirtuin-1 (SIRT1) is the proposed mediator of melatonin's anti-inflammatory action. This is via inhibition of high mobility group box-echromosomal protein-1 (HMGB-1), leading to down-regulation of the polarization of macrophages towards pro-inflammatory type [34]. It inhibits the over-activity of the innate immune system. Hence, theoretically, the cytokine storm induced by COVID-19 can be suppressed by melatonin. But the use of melatonin in COVID-19 is still very sparse, with only a few studies evaluating the same, hence further research is warranted [35]. Owing to melatonin's anti-inflammatory, anti-oxidant, and anti-viral actions, its role in critical illness caused due to COVID has been studied. Melatonin has easy availability, is not expensive, and has an excellent safety profile [36]. A trial (EudraCT: 2020–001808-42) is ongoing for the identification of the doses of melatonin that may prove effective in this disease. It is a phase II, single-center, double-blind, RCT to address the efficacy and safety of intravenous melatonin in COVID-19 ICU patients [37].

2.6 Remdesivir

Remdesivir is a 1′-cyano-substituted adenosine nucleotide analog prodrug, which was found to be effective against several RNA viruses. It was initially developed in 2017 by Gilead science for the treatment of the Ebola virus [38]. It has demonstrated extensive antiviral activity & effective treatment of lethal Ebola and Nipah virus infections in nonhuman primates [39]. Subsequently, it was investigated for SARS-CoV and MERS-CoV. Studies have shown that Remdesivir inhibits viral replication in human airway epithelial cell culture by affecting the early stages of viral replication through viral RNA synthesis inhibition, as an RNA-dependent RNA polymerase (RdRp) inhibitor [39]. This may be due to the absence of Exon-mediated proofreading in viruses sensitive to Remdesivir [40]. One of the first trials of Remdesivir was performed by the Gilead sciences center in hospitalized patients with confirmed SARS-CoV-2 having oxygen saturation < 94% or a need for oxygen support. Till 28 days of follow-up, the cumulative incidence of clinical improvement was 84% (95% CI 70–99) by Kaplan–Meier analysis and it was less among patients receiving invasive ventilation compared to non-invasive ventilation [41]. In another randomized, double-blind, placebo-controlled, multicentre trial at 10 hospitals in Hubei, China, Remdesivir use was not associated with any difference in time to clinical improvement [42]. In February 2020, WHO cast a vote of confidence for remdesivir, indicating that it has great potential. In April 2020, the US National Institute of Allergy and Infectious Diseases (NIAID), announced that a clinical trial in >1,000 people showed that those taking remdesivir recovered in 11 days on average, compared with 15 days for those on a placebo, even adding that remdesivir may become a standard for COVID treatment [43]. US FDA had issued a EUA for remdesivir for severe COVID-19 disease. On 22nd October 2020, the FDA approved remdesivir for use in adult and pediatric patients (≥12 years, ≥40 kg) requiring hospitalization [44]. In October 2020 itself, an interim analysis of the WHO-led, open-label, randomized SOLIDARITY trial demonstrated that 301 (11·0%) of 2743 patients who received remdesivir and 303 (11·2%) of 2708 patients who received standard care died by day 28 (Kaplan–Meier rate ratio 0·95, 95% CI 0·81–1·11; p = 0·50) [45]. The ACTT-1 study had also reported a 29-day mortality of 11·4% in patients receiving remdesivir as compared to 15·2% in placebo (hazard ratio 0·73, 95% CI 0·52–1·03) [43]. Hence in November 2020, WHO issued a conditional recommendation against remdesivir utilization in hospitalized patients, regardless of their disease severity. This was because they could not find evidence of remdesivir improving survival and other outcomes in the patients [46]. Infectious Disease Society of America (IDSA) still suggests the use of remdesivir in severe and critical patients, as does NIH [47, 48].

2.7 Tocilizumab

Tocilizumab is an Interleukin-6 (IL-6) Receptor inhibiting monoclonal antibody. Studies have shown that infection with the SARS virus leads to a cytokine storm with the release of inflammatory cytokines like IL-6, Tumor Necrosis Factor- α (TNF $-\alpha$), and IL-12 [49]. Further research done on MERS-CoV showed IL-6, IL-1β, and IL-8 were elevated in these patients. In patients with confirmed COVID-19 infection who were admitted to ICU, levels of IL-2, IL-6, IL-7, IL-10, granulocyte-colony stimulating factor (G-CSF), interferon-γ-inducible protein (IP10), monocyte chemoattractant protein (MCP1), macrophage inflammatory protein 1 alpha (MIP1A), and TNF-α levels were found to be high, suggesting possible cytokine storm [50]. The first trial involving tocilizumab was performed in China in February 2020. The National Institute for Infectious disease had recommended tocilizumab in moderate to severe infections and IL-6 levels >40 pg/mL (or D-dimer levels >1000 ng/mL). However, it is not recommended by the CDC. In an RCT published in JAMA, in moderate-to-severe pneumonia, tocilizumab did not reduce the WHO Clinical Progression Scale scores. The proportion of patients with non-invasive or invasive ventilation or death at day 14 was 36% with usual care and 24% with tocilizumab. There were no differences in 28 days mortality. This meant tocilizumab could decrease the requirement for mechanical and non-invasive ventilation or death by day 14 but not mortality by day 28 [51, 52]. An RCT published by NEJM in October 2020, which included patients fulfilling at least two of the following: fever, pulmonary infiltrates, or the need for oxygen therapy to maintain oxygen saturation more than 92%, concluded that tocilizumab was not effective in preventing intubation or death in moderately ill hospitalized patients with Covid-19 [53]. Sarilumab, another IL-6 receptor antagonist was being tested in a multicentre trial for hospitalized patients with severe COVID-19 [54]. It was concluded that at 28 days, clinical improvement and mortality in severe COVID-19 were not significantly different between sarilumab and standard of care [55]. Preliminary results from the Randomized, Embedded, Multifactorial Adaptive Platform Trial for Community-Acquired Pneumonia (REMAP-CAP) were released in a non-peer-reviewed report. REMAP-CAP is the largest trial to date investigating the use of IL-6 inhibitors in COVID-19. In February 2021, after reviewing the evidence from REMAP-CAP and other trials, the NIH Panel revised the recommendations on the use of tocilizumab and sarilumab, stating there was insufficient data to recommend either for or against the use of these drugs. But given the REMAP-CAP trial, some members suggested administering a single dose of tocilizumab (8 mg/kg of actual body weight, max 800 mg) in addition to dexamethasone in the ICU patients having high oxygen requirements/invasive and non-invasive mechanical ventilation and exhibiting rapid progression of respiratory failure [56]. The number of patients receiving sarilumab in the REMAP-CAP trial was too low to assess the efficacy.

2.8 Convalescent plasma

There was a hypothesis that plasma collected from the persons who have recovered from Covid-19 may contain antibodies against SARS-CoV-2, which may be used as a treatment tool. A case series was done in China where 5 critically ill patients with confirmed Covid-19 and Acute respiratory distress syndrome (ARDS) were selected [57]. They received two consecutive transfusions of 200 mL to 250 mL of convalescent plasma (total dose: 400 mL) with a SARS-CoV-2-specific antibody (IgG) titer more than 1:1,000. After receiving the plasma, the SOFA score of the patients decreased and ventilator parameters of the patients (pO2/FiO2 ratio) of the patient improved, and viral load decreased by day 12. ARDS resolved in four patients by Day 12 and 3 were weaned off the ventilators by 2 weeks. Further trials are needed the study the effectiveness of convalescent plasma. FDA is encouraging people who have fully recovered from COVID-19 for at least two weeks to donate plasma. FDA had issued guidance providing recommendations to health care providers & investigators on administration and study of COVID-19 convalescent plasma during the public health emergency. FDA issued a EUA for convalescent plasma on August 23, 2020, although convalescent plasma did not show any stoppage of progression to severe COVID-19 or all-cause mortality in the PLACID trial [58, 59]. In a trial published in NEJM in November 2020, in 228 patients receiving convalescent plasma and 105 receiving placebo at 30 days, there was not any significant difference among the clinical outcome distribution (odds ratio [OR], 0.83 (95% CI, 0.52–1.35; P = 0.46). Mortality in the plasma group was 10.96% as compared to 11.43% in the placebo group [risk difference 0.46% points (95% CI, −7.8 to 6.8) [60].

2.9 Favipiravir

Favipiravir (FPV) is a purine nucleotide that inhibits viral RNA polymerase. It was initially used against Ebola but later found to have in-vitro activity against other RNA viruses. The EC50 (concentration of a drug that gives half-maximal response) of FPV against SARS-CoV-2 in vitro in Vero E6 cells was found to be 61.88 μM/L [6, 61]. A study investigated the effect of FPV vs. lopinavir/ritonavir on the treatment of COVID-19. FPV was independently associated with faster viral clearance and a higher improvement rate in chest imaging. These findings suggest that FPV has significantly better treatment effects on COVID-19 in terms of disease progression and viral clearance as compared with lopinavir/ritonavir [62]. In an RCT on moderate to severe COVID patients, FPV was compared with umifenovir (Arbidol) by measuring the clinical recovery at 7 days [63]. Results showed no significant differences between the 2 groups. At present, there are no recommendations for the use of FPV in Covid-19 patients. Just like HCQ & lopinavir/ritonavir combination, it also causes QT prolongation [20].

2.10 Ribavirin

Ribavirin, a guanine analog, inhibits viral RNA dependent RNA polymerase (RdRp). It has demonstrable activity against many coronaviruses, but when used against SARS-CoV it was found to have less effectiveness in vitro requiring higher doses with combination therapy. When used with interferon in the treatment of MERS-CoV, no benefits were observed in terms of clinical outcomes or the rate of virus clearance [64]. Ribavirin also causes dose-dependent hematological toxicity & transaminase elevation when used in SARS patients and being a teratogen, is contraindicated in pregnancy [65, 66]. A recent trial showed ribavirin not being associated with better negative conversion times for the SARS-CoV-2 test and not being associated with improved mortality rates [67]. Due to its lack of demonstrable efficacy against other coronaviruses and high toxicity profile, it has got a limited role in the treatment of Covid-19. However, its combination with other antivirals is being tried in the SEV trial, the result of which is yet to be published [68].

2.11 Interferons

Studies with interferon-β had shown its activity against MERS. Most studies involved combination therapy with lopinavir/ritonavir or ribavirin. However, there was no concrete evidence showing its effect on SARS- CoV-2 in-vitro and the lack of clinical trials precluded the justification for its use in Covid-19 patients and hence there are no recommendations regarding its use [69]. In a study, it was shown that early triple antiviral therapy with lopinavir/ritonavir, ribavirin, and interferon beta-1b was safe and superior to lopinavir-ritonavir combinations alone in alleviating symptoms and shortening the duration of viral shedding and hospital stay in patients with mild to moderate COVID-19 [70]. In a trial utilizing interferon β-1a, clinical response time was not significantly different between interferon and the control groups (9.7 ± 5.8 versus 8.3 ± 4.9 days, respectively, P = 0.95). On day 14, 66.7% versus 43.6% of patients in the interferon group and the control group respectively was discharged (OR, 2.5; 95% CI, 1.05–6.37). The 28-day overall mortality was significantly less in the interferon than the control group (19% versus 43.6%, respectively, P = 0.015). Early administration significantly decreased mortality (OR, 13.5; 95% CI, 1.5–1.18) [71]. Another trial testing interferon β-1b showed its effectiveness in reducing the clinical improvement time without any serious adverse events in severe COVID-19 patients. ICU admission and invasive ventilation need also decreased following administration of interferon β-1b [72]. The Lancet Respiratory Medicine showed the results of an RCT of nebulized interferon beta-1a in 101 adults admitted to the hospital with COVID-19. It demonstrated better odds of clinical improvement than placebo (OR 2·32 [95% CI 1·07–5·04]; p = 0·03). No significant difference was there in the hospital discharge odds by day 28 [73]. Recently, the SOLIDARITY trial also showed no benefit of interferon therapy [74].

2.12 Corticosteroids

ARDS is a leading cause of mortality in Covid-19 pneumonia. Cytokine storm plays a key role in the pathogenesis of ARDS in Covid-19 patients and thus immunosuppression may have a role in the treatment of such patients [75]. Glucocorticoids modify the inflammation-mediated lung injury and hence can alter progression to respiratory failure and death. Studies on SARS and MERS showed that corticosteroids did not show any improvement in overall survival but showed delayed viral clearance from the respiratory tract and other steroid-related complications like Hyperglycaemia & Psychosis [76]. A retrospective study was carried out in Covid-19 patients in China who had developed ARDS. Those who received steroids had decreased death rates compared to those who did not [77]. In another study in non-ARDS patients, corticosteroid treatment did not influence virus clearance time, hospital length of stay, or duration of symptoms in mild COVID-19. Another study reported that early application of low-dose corticosteroid improves the treatment effect, presenting as improvement of hypoxia and fever, shortening disease course, and accelerating focus absorption [78]. Steroids are now the only therapy showing mortality benefit in COVID-19 severe disease. RECOVERY trial has concluded that dexamethasone 6 mg given once daily for up to 10 days decreased 28-day mortality in patients with COVID-19 on respiratory support. But a careful decision has to be made regarding severity as patients not requiring oxygen showed no benefit but had a possibility of harm with corticosteroid therapy. In the dexamethasone group, the incidence of death was less than the usual care group among patients receiving invasive mechanical ventilation (29.3% vs. 41.4%; rate ratio, 0.64; 95% CI, 0.51–0.81) and those receiving oxygen without invasive mechanical ventilation (23.3% vs. 26.2%; rate ratio, 0.82; 95% CI, 0.72–0.94). No benefit was demonstrated among those who were receiving no respiratory support at randomization (17.8% vs. 14.0%, rate ratio, 1.19; 95% CI, 0.91–1.55) [79]. Subsequent RCTs also confirmed the same. Hence, all guidelines advocated steroids as first-line therapy in severe COVID-19. In due course, specific dose, route, and duration of therapy will be answered.

2.13 Monoclonal antibodies

Various novel monoclonal antibodies are under investigation for COVID-19. In a study published in NEJM, it has been described that LY-CoV555 (bamlanivimab) (also known as LY3819253), is a potent anti-spike neutralizing monoclonal antibody [80]. It binds to the receptor-binding domain of SARS-CoV-2. It was extracted from the convalescent plasma obtained from a COVID-19 patient. The protection of bamlanivimab against SARS-CoV-2 in primates has been reported [81]. In the interim analysis of data, patients receiving LY-CoV555 reported fewer hospitalizations and a lesser symptom burden than placebo receivers. In November 2020, it got the FDA EUA [82]. According to FDA, bamlanivimab reduced COVID-19 related hospital admissions in patients who are at high risk for disease progression [83]. This authorization came even after the company making the drug, Lilly, had announced in October 2020 that it was holding the trial in the hospital admitted patients as it not showing any benefits in them (ACTIV-3 trial). Remaining studies of bamlanivimab remain ongoing, including ACTIV-2 trial which includes the newly diagnosed mild to moderate COVID-19 patients; BLAZE-1, including recently diagnosed COVID-19 patients in the ambulatory (non-hospitalized) setting, studying bamlanivimab as monotherapy and in combination with etesevimab; and BLAZE-2, a phase 3 study for COVID-19 prophylaxis. Based on BLAZE-1 data, Lilly had submitted a request for EUA for bamlanivimab for the treatment of recently diagnosed mild to moderate COVID-19 patients to the FDA [84]. FDA reported 3% hospitalizations and emergency room visits in bamlanivimab treated patients compared to 10% in placebo. The FDA has approved bamlanivimab for patients age ≥ 12, and at high risk for progressing to severe covid-19 or hospital admission. However, it is emphasized that bamlanivimab should not be given to in-hospital COVID-19 patients or those requiring oxygen therapy; as such monoclonal antibodies may worsen outcomes in these patients. Another potential antibody treatment for COVID-19, REGN-COV2, a combination of two monoclonal antibodies casirivimab and imdevimab (REGN10933 and REGN10987), also faced some issues among inpatients with high oxygen requirements. In November 2020, the FDA issued EUA to monoclonal antibodies casirivimab and imdevimab (REGN10933 and REGN10987- against spike proteins of SARS-CoV-2) to be administered together for the treatment of mild to moderate COVID-19 in adults and pediatric patients (≥12 years of age) [85]. Although, in this case also, Regeneron Pharma had to halt its antibody cocktail trial in the admitted patients due to safety concerns, hence it was approved for non-admitted patients only [86]. Interestingly, US President Donald Trump had also received this regime when he tested positive for COVID-19 [87]. Astra Zeneca's COVID-19 Long-Acting AntiBody (LAAB) combination AZD7442 trial has also advanced into Phase III [88]. On February 9, 2021, the FDA has issued a EUA for bamlanivimab plus etesevimab for the management of mild to moderate COVID-19 in outpatients at high risk for disease progression. The data come from a randomized, double-blind, placebo-controlled clinical trial in 1,035 non-hospitalized adults with mild to moderate COVID-19, at high risk for progression to severe disease. Hospitalization or death occurred in 36 (7%) of placebo recipients compared to 11 (2%) patients treated with bamlanivimab 2,800 milligrams and etesevimab 2,800 milligrams administered together, demonstrating a 70% reduction [89].

2.14 Janus kinase (JAK) inhibitors

The kinase inhibitors are being proposed as a novel modality of COVID-19 treatment. The rationale behind this being the prevention of phosphorylation of key proteins that are involved in the signal transduction that in turn leads to immunological activation and inflammation. This includes the cellular responses to the pro-inflammatory cytokines like IL-6 [90]. JAK inhibitors interfere with the phosphorylation of signal transducer and activator of transcription (STAT) proteins [91, 92]. These proteins are in turn involved in cell signaling, growth, and survival. The immunosuppression may reduce the hyperactive immune state induced by COVID-19. Moreover, JAK inhibitors like baricitinib have a theoretical direct antiviral activity via interference with viral endocytosis. This can prevent viral entry in the cells [93]. NIH has recommended that in the rare circumstances where corticosteroids cannot be used, baricitinib in combination with remdesivir may be used for the treatment of hospitalized, non-intubated patients requiring oxygen supplementation. IDSA guidelines also suggest the use of this combination in hospitalized severe COVID-19 patients [47]. Use of baricitinib without remdesivir is not recommended, except in a clinical trial [94]. As for the use of baricitinib in combination with corticosteroids, there is still insufficient data. Both baricitinib and corticosteroids cause immuno-suppression; hence, there is an additive risk of infection.

2.15 Other miscellaneous drugs with a possible therapeutic effect

In the pathogenesis of Covid-19, ACE 2 receptors play an important role by facilitating the entry of the virus into the cell [1, 95]. Thus it could be a possible therapeutic target with the use of ACE-inhibitors and ARB [1, 96]. However, there is a concern that the use of these drugs to stop virus replication may increase the expression of ACE-2 receptors and paradoxically worsen the infection. However, no in-vitro studies are available which show either definite detrimental or protective effect of these agents. As a result, the current guidelines state to continue these drugs in patients who are already taking them [97].

Umifenovir (also known as Arbidol) is an antiviral agent with a unique mechanism of action targeting the S protein/ACE2 interaction and inhibiting membrane fusion of the viral envelope [98]. It is approved in Russia for prophylaxis and treatment of influenza. Of particular interest is its demonstrable in-vitro activity against Covid-19 [99]. In an observational study in China, patients treated with umifenovir for a median duration of 9 days had a higher discharge rate and lesser mortality [100]. But as with other agents, the lack of RCT limits the justification for its use in Covid-19. However, ACE targeting therapy is a promising one [1].

Camostat mesylate is an agent used in the treatment of pancreatitis. It inhibits host serine protease, TMPRSS2.3, and has been shown to prevent viral cell entry in-vitro and thus could be a target for future studies [101].

Nitazoxanide, an anti-helminthic with a relatively favorable safety profile has shown in-vitro activity against SARS-CoV and MERS [102]. Besides it also has additional immunomodulatory action & thus can be used in trials in Covid-19 patients as a therapeutic option.

Many non-allopathic pharmaceuticals are also in pipeline as promising COVID-19 therapy. In June 2020, yoga guru Baba Ramdev announced that his company Patanjali Ayurved had launched a drug called 'Coronil' that could cure COVID-19 [103]. However, no scientific basis for this claim is produced until now.

3. Conclusion

The Global pandemic with COVID-19 is on. Drug therapy holds the key to the treatment and containment of the disease. Hence, large-scale multicentric trials are ongoing involving multiple drugs. Until now, no therapy is absolutely effective in the treatment of the patient as infection and death rates continue to mount all over the world. Corticosteroids have shown a significant effect on reducing the mortality in severe COVID-19 patients. It is hoped that the results of the ongoing trials will open further opportunities towards understanding the disease process and designing safe and effective treatments.

Conflict of interest

The authors declare no conflict of interest.

Author details

Mayank Kapoor, Prasan Kumar Panda* and Vivek Mohanty
Department of Internal Medicine, All India Institute of Medical Sciences (AIIMS), Rishikesh, India

*Address all correspondence to: motherprasanna@rediffmail.com

References

[1] Kapoor M, Dhar M. A look into Possible New Treatment Modality for COVID-19: ACE 2 [Internet]. 2020. Available from: https://www.omicsonline.org/open-access/a-look-into-possible-new-treatment-modality-for-covid-19-ace-2.pdf

[2] Zumla A, Chan JFW, Azhar EI, Hui DSC, Yuen KY. Coronaviruses-drug discovery and therapeutic options. Nat Rev Drug Discov. 2016;15(5):327-47.

[3] Yan Y, Zou Z, Sun Y, Li X, Xu KF, Wei Y, et al. Anti-malaria drug chloroquine is highly effective in treating avian influenza A H5N1 virus infection in an animal model. Cell Res. 2013;23(2):300-2.

[4] Vincent MJ, Bergeron E, Benjannet S, Erickson BR, Rollin PE, Ksiazek TG, et al. Chloroquine is a potent inhibitor of SARS coronavirus infection and spread. Virol J. 2005;2:1-10.

[5] Keyaerts E, Vijgen L, Maes P, Neyts J, Ranst M Van. In vitro inhibition of severe acute respiratory syndrome coronavirus by chloroquine. Biochem Biophys Res Commun. 2004 Oct 8;323(1):264-8.

[6] Wang M, Cao R, Zhang L, Yang X, Liu J, Xu M, et al. Remdesivir and chloroquine effectively inhibit the recently emerged novel coronavirus (2019-nCoV) in vitro. Cell Res. 2020;30(3):269-71.

[7] Colson P, Rolain JM, Raoult D. Chloroquine for the 2019 novel coronavirus SARS-CoV-2 [Internet]. Vol. 55, International Journal of Antimicrobial Agents. Elsevier B.V.; 2020 [cited 2020 Nov 20]. p. 105923. Available from: https://www.ncbi.nlm.nih.gov/pmc/articles/PMC7134866/

[8] Liu J, Cao R, Xu M, Wang X, Zhang H, Hu H, et al. Hydroxychloroquine, a less toxic derivative of chloroquine, is effective in inhibiting SARS-CoV-2 infection in vitro. Cell Discov [Internet]. 2020;6(1):6-9. Available from: http://dx.doi.org/10.1038/s41421-020-0156-0

[9] Shukla AM, Archibald LK, Shukla AW, Mehta HJ, Cherabuddi K. Chloroquine and hydroxychloroquine in the context of COVID-19 [Internet]. Vol. 9, Drugs in Context. Bioexcel Publishing LTD; 2020 [cited 2020 Nov 20]. Available from: /pmc/articles/PMC7192209/?report=abstract

[10] Gao J, Tian Z, Yang X. Breakthrough: Chloroquine phosphate has shown apparent efficacy in treatment of COVID-19 associated pneumonia in clinical studies [Internet]. Vol. 14, BioScience Trends. International Advancement Center for Medicine and Health Research Co., Ltd.; 2020 [cited 2020 Nov 20]. p. 72-3. Available from: www.biosciencetrends.com

[11] Gautret P, Lagier JC, Parola P, Hoang VT, Meddeb L, Mailhe M, et al. Hydroxychloroquine and azithromycin as a treatment of COVID-19: results of an open-label non-randomized clinical trial. Int J Antimicrob Agents [Internet]. 2020 Jul 1 [cited 2021 Mar 4];56(1). Available from: https://pubmed.ncbi.nlm.nih.gov/32205204/

[12] Coronavirus disease (COVID-19): Hydroxychloroquine [Internet]. [cited 2020 Nov 26]. Available from: https://www.who.int/news-room/q-a-detail/coronavirus-disease-covid-19-hydroxychloroquine#

[13] FDA cautions against use of hydroxychloroquine or chloroquine for COVID-19 outside of the hospital setting or a clinical trial due to risk of heart rhythm problems | FDA [Internet]. [cited 2020 Nov 26]. Available from: https://www.

fda.gov/drugs/drug-safety-and-availability/fda-cautions-against-use-hydroxychloroquine-or-chloroquine-covid-19-outside-hospital-setting-or

[14] Nutho B, Mahalapbutr P, Hengphasatporn K, Pattaranggoon NC, Simanon N, Shigeta Y, et al. Why are lopinavir and ritonavir effective against the newly emerged coronavirus 2019? Atomistic insights into the inhibitory mechanisms. Biochemistry [Internet]. 2020 [cited 2020 Nov 20];59(18):1769-79. Available from: https://dx.doi.org/10.1021/acs.biochem.0c00160

[15] Chu CM, Cheng VCC, Hung IFN, Wong MML, Chan KH, Chan KS, et al. Role of lopinavir/ritonavir in the treatment of SARS: Initial virological and clinical findings. Thorax [Internet]. 2004 Mar 1 [cited 2020 Nov 20];59(3):252-6. Available from: www.thoraxjnl.com

[16] De Wilde AH, Jochmans D, Posthuma CC, Zevenhoven-Dobbe JC, Van Nieuwkoop S, Bestebroer TM, et al. Screening of an FDA-approved compound library identifies four small-molecule inhibitors of Middle East respiratory syndrome coronavirus replication in cell culture. Antimicrob Agents Chemother [Internet]. 2014 Aug 1 [cited 2020 Nov 20];58(8):4875-84. Available from: http://dx.doi.org/10.1128

[17] Kim UJ, Won EJ, Kee SJ, Jung SI, Jang HC. Combination therapy with lopinavir/ritonavir, ribavirin and interferon-a for Middle East respiratory syndrome. Antivir Ther. 2016;21(5):455-9.

[18] Cao B, Wang Y, Wen D, Liu W, Wang J, Fan G, et al. A Trial of Lopinavir–Ritonavir in Adults Hospitalized with Severe Covid-19. N Engl J Med [Internet]. 2020 May 7 [cited 2020 Nov 20];382(19):1787-99. Available from: https://www.nejm.org/doi/full/10.1056/NEJMoa2001282

[19] WHO discontinues hydroxychloroquine and lopinavir/ritonavir treatment arms for COVID-19 [Internet]. [cited 2020 Nov 26]. Available from: https://www.who.int/news/item/04-07-2020-who-discontinues-hydroxychloroquine-and-lopinavir-ritonavir-treatment-arms-for-covid-19

[20] Naksuk N, Lazar S, Peeraphatdit TB. Cardiac safety of off-label COVID-19 drug therapy: a review and proposed monitoring protocol. Eur Hear journal Acute Cardiovasc care [Internet]. 2020 May 6 [cited 2020 Nov 20];9(3):215-21. Available from: http://journals.sagepub.com/doi/10.1177/2048872620922784

[21] Retallack H, Di Lullo E, Arias C, Knopp KA, Laurie MT, Sandoval-Espinosa C, et al. Zika virus cell tropism in the developing human brain and inhibition by azithromycin. Proc Natl Acad Sci U S A [Internet]. 2016 Dec 13 [cited 2020 Nov 26];113(50):14408-13. Available from: www.pnas.org/cgi/doi/10.1073/pnas.1618029113

[22] Schögler A, Kopf BS, Edwards MR, Johnston SL, Casaulta C, Kieninger E, et al. Novel antiviral properties of azithromycin in cystic fibrosis airway epithelial cells. Eur Respir J [Internet]. 2015 Feb 1 [cited 2020 Nov 26];45(2):428-39. Available from: http://ow.ly/BVw2U

[23] Oldenburg CE, Doan T. Azithromycin for severe COVID-19 [Internet]. Vol. 396, The Lancet. Lancet Publishing Group; 2020 [cited 2020 Nov 26]. p. 936-7. Available from: https://doi.org/10.1056/NEJMoa2019014.

[24] Cavalcanti AB, Zampieri FG, Rosa RG, Azevedo LCP, Veiga VC, Avezum A, et al. Hydroxychloroquine with or without Azithromycin in Mild-to-Moderate Covid-19. N Engl J Med [Internet]. 2020 Jul 23 [cited 2020 Nov

29]; Available from: https://www.nejm.org/doi/full/10.1056/nejmoa2019014

[25] Laing R, Gillan V, Devaney E. Ivermectin - Old Drug, New Tricks?. Trends Parasitol. 2017;33(6):463-472. doi:10.1016/j.pt.2017.02.004

[26] Pandey S, Pathak SK, Pandey A, Salunke AA, Chawla J, Sharma A, et al. Ivermectin in COVID-19: What do we know? [Internet]. Vol. 14, Diabetes and Metabolic Syndrome: Clinical Research and Reviews. Elsevier Ltd; 2020 [cited 2020 Nov 29]. p. 1921-2. Available from: https://www.ncbi.nlm.nih.gov/pmc/articles/PMC7521351/

[27] Caly L, Druce JD, Catton MG, Jans DA, Wagstaff KM. The FDA-approved drug ivermectin inhibits the replication of SARS-CoV-2 in vitro. Antiviral Res [Internet]. 2020 Jun 1 [cited 2020 Nov 29];178:104787. Available from: /pmc/articles/PMC7129059/?report=abstract

[28] Kumar Maurya D. A Combination of Ivermectin and Doxycycline Possibly Blocks the Viral Entry and Modulate the Innate Immune Response in COVID-19 Patients.

[29] Behera P, Kumar Patro B, Kumar Singh A, Kumar RS, Kumar Pradhan S, Kumar Pentapati S, et al. Title: Role of ivermectin in the prevention of COVID-19 infection among healthcare workers in India: A matched case-control study. medRxiv [Internet]. 2020 Nov 3 [cited 2020 Nov 29];2020.10.29.20222661. Available from: https://doi.org/10.1101/2020.10.29.20222661

[30] Alam MT, Murshed R, Bhiuyan E, Saber S, Alam RF, Robin RC. A Case Series of 100 COVID-19 Positive Patients Treated with Combination of Ivermectin and Doxycycline. J Bangladesh Coll Physicians Surg [Internet]. 2020 Jun 12 [cited 2020 Nov 29];10-5. Available from: https://doi.org/10.3329/jbcps.v38i0.47512

[31] Rahman MA, Iqbal SA, Islam MA, Niaz MK, Hussain T, Siddiquee TH. Comparison of Viral Clearance between Ivermectin with Doxycycline and Hydroxychloroquine with Azithromycin in COVID-19 Patients. J Bangladesh Coll Physicians Surg [Internet]. 2020 Jun 12 [cited 2020 Nov 29];5-9. Available from: https://doi.org/10.3329/jbcps.v38i0.

[32] Ivermectin | COVID-19 Treatment Guidelines [Internet]. [cited 2021 Feb 16]. Available from: https://www.covid19treatmentguidelines.nih.gov/antiviral-therapy/ivermectin/

[33] Diao B, Wang C, Tan Y, Chen X, Liu Y, Ning L, et al. Reduction and Functional Exhaustion of T Cells in Patients With Coronavirus Disease 2019 (COVID-19). Front Immunol [Internet]. 2020 May 1 [cited 2020 Nov 29];11:827. Available from: https://www.frontiersin.org/article/10.3389/fimmu.2020.00827/full

[34] Hardeland R. Melatonin and inflammation—Story of a double-edged blade [Internet]. Vol. 65, Journal of Pineal Research. Blackwell Publishing Ltd; 2018 [cited 2020 Nov 29]. Available from: https://onlinelibrary.wiley.com/doi/full/10.1111/jpi.12525

[35] Zhang R, Wang X, Ni L, Di X, Ma B, Niu S, et al. COVID-19: Melatonin as a potential adjuvant treatment. Vol. 250, Life Sciences. Elsevier Inc.; 2020. p. 117583.

[36] Reiter RJ, Abreu-Gonzalez P, Marik PE, Dominguez-Rodriguez A. Therapeutic Algorithm for Use of Melatonin in Patients With COVID-19. Front Med [Internet]. 2020 May 15 [cited 2020 Nov 29];7:226. Available from: https://www.frontiersin.org/article/10.3389/fmed.2020.00226/full

[37] Acuña-Castroviejo D, Escames G, Figueira JC, de la Oliva P, Borobia AM, Acuña-Fernández C. Clinical trial to test the efficacy of melatonin in COVID-19. J Pineal Res. 2020;69(3):2-5.

[38] Tchesnokov E, Feng J, Porter D, Götte M. Mechanism of Inhibition of Ebola Virus RNA-Dependent RNA Polymerase by Remdesivir. Viruses [Internet]. 2019 Apr 4 [cited 2020 Nov 20];11(4):326. Available from: https://www.mdpi.com/1999-4915/11/4/326

[39] Cao Y chen, Deng Q xin, Dai S xue. Remdesivir for severe acute respiratory syndrome coronavirus 2 causing COVID-19: An evaluation of the evidence. Vol. 35, Travel Medicine and Infectious Disease. Elsevier USA; 2020. p. 101647.

[40] Yethindra V. Role of GS-5734 (Remdesivir) in inhibiting SARS-CoV and MERS-CoV: The expected role of GS-5734 (remdesivir) in COVID-19 (2019-nCoV)-VYTR hypothesis. Int J Res Pharm Sci [Internet]. 2020 Mar 6 [cited 2020 Nov 20];11(Special Issue 1):1-6. Available from: https://doi.org/10.26452/ijrps.v11iSPL1.1973

[41] Protocol: Specific Antiviral Therapy in the Clinical Management of Acute Respiratory Infection with SARS-CoV-2 (COVID-19) [Internet]. 2020 [cited 2020 Nov 20]. Available from: https://www.who.int/publications-detail/clinical-management-of-severe-acute-respiratory-

[42] Wang Y, Zhang D, Du G, Du R, Zhao J, Jin Y, et al. Remdesivir in adults with severe COVID-19: a randomised, double-blind, placebo-controlled, multicentre trial. Lancet. 2020 May 16;395(10236):1569-78.

[43] Beigel JH, Tomashek KM, Dodd LE, Mehta AK, Zingman BS, Kalil AC, et al. Remdesivir for the Treatment of Covid-19 — Final Report. N Engl J Med [Internet]. 2020 Nov 5 [cited 2020 Nov 29];383(19):1813-26. Available from: https://www.nejm.org/doi/full/10.1056/NEJMoa2007764

[44] FDA. Available from: https://www.accessdata.fda.gov/drugsatfda_docs/nda/2020/214787Orig1s000Sumr.pdf.

[45] WHO Solidarity Trial Consortium, Pan H, Peto R, Henao-Restrepo A-M, Preziosi M-P, Sathiyamoorthy V, et al. Repurposed Antiviral Drugs for Covid-19 — Interim WHO Solidarity Trial Results. N Engl J Med [Internet]. 2020 Dec 2 [cited 2020 Dec 4];NEJMoa2023184. Available from: http://www.nejm.org/doi/10.1056/NEJMoa2023184

[46] WHO recommends against the use of remdesivir in COVID-19 patients [Internet]. [cited 2020 Nov 29]. Available from: https://www.who.int/news-room/feature-stories/detail/who-recommends-against-the-use-of-remdesivir-in-covid-19-patients

[47] Overview of IDSA COVID-19 Treatment Guidelines [Internet]. [cited 2021 Feb 16]. Available from: https://www.fda.gov/media/143603/download

[48] Therapeutic Management | COVID-19 Treatment Guidelines [Internet]. [cited 2021 Feb 16]. Available from: https://www.covid19treatmentguidelines.nih.gov/therapeutic-management/

[49] Li Y, Chen M, Cao H, Zhu Y, Zheng J, Zhou H. Extraordinary GU-rich single-strand RNA identified from SARS coronavirus contributes an excessive innate immune response. Microbes Infect. 2013 Feb 1;15(2):88-95.

[50] Huang C, Wang Y, Li X, Ren L, Zhao J, Hu Y, et al. Clinical features of patients infected with 2019 novel coronavirus in Wuhan, China. Lancet. 2020 Feb 15;395(10223):497-506.

[51] Hermine O, Mariette X, Tharaux PL, Resche-Rigon M, Porcher R, Ravaud P. Effect of Tocilizumab vs Usual Care in Adults Hospitalized with COVID-19 and Moderate or Severe Pneumonia: A Randomized Clinical Trial. JAMA Intern Med [Internet]. 2020 [cited 2020 Nov 29]; Available from: https:// jamanetwork.com/

[52] Guaraldi G, Meschiari M, Cozzi-Lepri A, Milic J, Tonelli R, Menozzi M, et al. Tocilizumab in patients with severe COVID-19: a retrospective cohort study. Lancet Rheumatol. 2020 Aug 1;2(8):e474-84.

[53] Stone JH, Frigault MJ, Serling-Boyd NJ, Fernandes AD, Harvey L, Foulkes AS, et al. Efficacy of Tocilizumab in Patients Hospitalized with Covid-19. N Engl J Med [Internet]. 2020 Oct 21 [cited 2020 Nov 29]; Available from: https://www.nejm.org/doi/full/10.1056/NEJMoa2028836

[54] Sanofi and Regeneron begin global Kevzara® (sarilumab) clinical trial program in patients with severe COVID-19 - Mar 16, 2020 [Internet]. [cited 2020 Nov 20]. Available from: http://www.news.sanofi.us/2020-03-16-Sanofi-and-Regeneron-begin-global-Kevzara-R-sarilumab-clinical-trial-program-in-patients-with-severe-COVID-19

[55] Della-Torre E, Campochiaro C, Cavalli G, De Luca G, Napolitano A, La Marca S, et al. Interleukin-6 blockade with sarilumab in severe COVID-19 pneumonia with systemic hyperinflammation: an open-label cohort study. Ann Rheum Dis [Internet]. 2020 [cited 2020 Nov 29];79:1277-85. Available from: http://dx.doi.org/10.1136/annrheumdis-2020-218122

[56] Statement on Tocilizumab | COVID-19 Treatment Guidelines [Internet]. [cited 2021 Feb 16]. Available from: https://www.covid19treatmentguidelines.nih.gov/statement-on-tocilizumab/

[57] Shen C, Wang Z, Zhao F, Yang Y, Li J, Yuan J, et al. Treatment of 5 Critically Ill Patients with COVID-19 with Convalescent Plasma. JAMA - J Am Med Assoc [Internet]. 2020 Apr 28 [cited 2020 Nov 20];323(16):1582-9. Available from: https://jamanetwork.com/

[58] Kadlec RP. Convalescent Plasma COVID-19 Letter of Authorization [Internet]. 2020 [cited 2020 Nov 29]. Available from: https://www.govinfo.gov/content/pkg/FR-2020-04-01/pdf/2020-06905.pdf.

[59] Agarwal A, Mukherjee A, Kumar G, Chatterjee P, Bhatnagar T, Malhotra P. Convalescent plasma in the management of moderate covid-19 in adults in India: Open label phase II multicentre randomised controlled trial (PLACID Trial). BMJ [Internet]. 2020 Oct 22 [cited 2020 Nov 29];371. Available from: https://www.bmj.com/content/371/bmj.m3939

[60] Simonovich VA, Burgos Pratx LD, Scibona P, Beruto M V., Vallone MG, Vázquez C, et al. A Randomized Trial of Convalescent Plasma in Covid-19 Severe Pneumonia. N Engl J Med [Internet]. 2020 Nov 24 [cited 2020 Dec 4];NEJMoa2031304. Available from: http://www.nejm.org/doi/10.1056/NEJMoa2031304

[61] Furuta Y, Komeno T, Nakamura T. Favipiravir (T-705), a broad spectrum inhibitor of viral RNA polymerase. Proc Japan Acad Ser B [Internet]. 2017 Aug 2 [cited 2020 Nov 20];93(7):449-63. Available from: https://www.jstage.jst.go.jp/article/pjab/93/7/93_PJA9307B-02/_article

[62] Cai Q, Yang M, Liu D, Chen J, Shu D, Xia J, et al. Experimental Treatment with Favipiravir for COVID-19: An Open-Label Control Study. Engineering. 2020 Mar 18;

[63] Chen C, Zhang Y, Huang J, Yin P, Cheng Z, Wu J, et al. Favipiravir versus Arbidol for COVID-19: A Randomized Clinical Trial. [cited 2020 Nov 20]; Available from: https://doi.org/10.1101/2020.03.17.20037432

[64] Arabi YM, Shalhoub S, Mandourah Y, Al-Hameed F, Al-Omari A, Qasim E Al, et al. Ribavirin and Interferon Therapy for Critically Ill Patients with Middle East Respiratory Syndrome: A Multicenter Observational Study. Clin Infect Dis [Internet]. 2020 May 1 [cited 2020 Nov 20];70(9):1837-44. Available from: https://academic.oup.com/cid/article/70/9/1837/5523209

[65] Stockman LJ, Bellamy R, Garner P. SARS: Systematic Review of Treatment Effects. Low D, editor. PLoS Med [Internet]. 2006 Sep 12 [cited 2020 Nov 20];3(9):e343. Available from: https://dx.plos.org/10.1371/journal.pmed.0030343

[66] Altınbas S, Holmes JA, Altınbas A. Hepatitis C Virus Infection in Pregnancy. Gastroenterol Nurs [Internet]. 2020 Jan 1 [cited 2020 Nov 20];43(1):12-21. Available from: http://journals.lww.com/10.1097/SGA.0000000000000404

[67] Tong S, Su Y, Yu Y, Wu C, Chen J, Wang S, et al. Ribavirin therapy for severe COVID-19: a retrospective cohort study. Int J Antimicrob Agents. 2020 Sep 1;56(3):106114.

[68] Panda PK, Bandyopadhyay A, Singh BC, Moirangthem B, Chikara G, Saha S, et al. Safety and efficacy of antiviral combination therapy in symptomatic patients of Covid-19 infection - a randomised controlled trial (SEV-COVID Trial): A structured summary of a study protocol for a randomized controlled trial [Internet]. Vol. 21, Trials. BioMed Central Ltd; 2020 [cited 2021 Mar 4]. Available from: https://pubmed.ncbi.nlm.nih.gov/33081849/

[69] Totura AL, Bavari S. Broad-spectrum coronavirus antiviral drug discovery. Expert Opin Drug Discov [Internet]. 2019 Apr 3 [cited 2020 Nov 20];14(4):397-412. Available from: https://www.tandfonline.com/doi/full/10.1080/17460441.2019.1581171

[70] Hung IFN, Lung KC, Tso EYK, Liu R, Chung TWH, Chu MY, et al. Triple combination of interferon beta-1b, lopinavir–ritonavir, and ribavirin in the treatment of patients admitted to hospital with COVID-19: an open-label, randomised, phase 2 trial. Lancet. 2020 May 30;395(10238):1695-704.

[71] Davoudi-Monfared E, Rahmani H, Khalili H, Hajiabdolbaghi M, Salehi M, Abbasian L, et al. A randomized clinical trial of the efficacy and safety of interferon β-1a in treatment of severe COVID-19. Antimicrob Agents Chemother [Internet]. 2020 Sep 1 [cited 2020 Nov 29];64(9). Available from: https://doi.org/10.1128/AAC

[72] Rahmani H, Davoudi-Monfared E, Nourian A, Khalili H, Hajizadeh N, Jalalabadi NZ, et al. Interferon β-1b in treatment of severe COVID-19: A randomized clinical trial. Int Immunopharmacol. 2020 Nov 1;88:106903.

[73] Peiffer-Smadja N, Yazdanpanah Y. Nebulised interferon beta-1a for patients with COVID-19. Lancet Respir Med [Internet]. 2020 Nov 12 [cited 2020 Nov 30];0(0). Available from: http://www.ncbi.nlm.nih.gov/pubmed/33189160

[74] Solidarity clinical trial for COVID-19 treatments [Internet]. [cited 2021 Feb 16]. Available from: https://www.who.int/emergencies/diseases/novel-coronavirus-2019/global-research-on-novel-coronavirus-2019-ncov/solidarity-clinical-trial-for-covid-19-treatments

[75] Mehta P, McAuley DF, Brown M, Sanchez E, Tattersall RS, Manson JJ.

COVID-19: consider cytokine storm syndromes and immunosuppression [Internet]. Vol. 395, The Lancet. Lancet Publishing Group; 2020 [cited 2020 Nov 20]. p. 1033-4. Available from: https://www.ncbi.nlm.nih.gov/pmc/articles/PMC7270045/

[76] Arabi YM, Mandourah Y, Al-Hameed F, Sindi AA, Almekhlafi GA, Hussein MA, et al. Corticosteroid therapy for critically ill patients with middle east respiratory syndrome. Am J Respir Crit Care Med [Internet]. 2018 Mar 15 [cited 2020 Nov 20];197(6):757-67. Available from: http://www.atsjournals.org/doi/10.1164/rccm.201706-1172OC

[77] Wu C, Chen X, Cai Y, Xia J, Zhou X, Xu S, et al. Risk Factors Associated With Acute Respiratory Distress Syndrome and Death in Patients With Coronavirus Disease 2019 Pneumonia in Wuhan, China. JAMA Intern Med [Internet]. 2020 Jul 1 [cited 2020 Nov 20];180(7):934. Available from: https://jamanetwork.com/journals/jamainternalmedicine/fullarticle/2763184

[78] Wang Y, Jiang W, He Q, Wang C, Wang B, Zhou P, et al. Early, low-dose and short-term application of corticosteroid treatment in patients with severe COVID-19 pneumonia: single-center experience from Wuhan, China. medRxiv [Internet]. 2020 Mar 12 [cited 2020 Nov 20];2020.03.06.20032342. Available from: https://doi.org/10.1101/2020.03.06.20032342

[79] Dexamethasone in Hospitalized Patients with Covid-19 — Preliminary Report. N Engl J Med [Internet]. 2020 Jul 17 [cited 2020 Nov 30]; Available from: https://www.nejm.org/doi/full/10.1056/NEJMoa2021436

[80] Chen P, Nirula A, Heller B, Gottlieb RL, Boscia J, Morris J, et al. SARS-CoV-2 Neutralizing Antibody LY-CoV555 in Outpatients with Covid-19. N Engl J Med [Internet]. 2020 Oct 28 [cited 2020 Nov 29]; Available from: https://www.nejm.org/doi/full/10.1056/NEJMoa2029849

[81] Jones BE, Brown-Augsburger PL, Corbett KS, Westendorf K, Davies J, Cujec TP, et al. Title: LY-CoV555, a rapidly isolated potent neutralizing antibody, provides protection in a non-human primate model of SARS-CoV-2 infection. bioRxiv [Internet]. 2020 Oct 9 [cited 2020 Nov 29];2020.09.30.318972. Available from: https://doi.org/10.1101/2020.09.30.318972

[82] Coronavirus (COVID-19) Update: FDA Authorizes Monoclonal Antibody for Treatment of COVID-19 | FDA [Internet]. [cited 2020 Nov 29]. Available from: https://www.fda.gov/news-events/press-announcements/coronavirus-covid-19-update-fda-authorizes-monoclonal-antibody-treatment-covid-19

[83] Mahase E. Covid-19: FDA authorises neutralising antibody bamlanivimab for non-admitted patients. BMJ [Internet]. 2020 Nov 11 [cited 2020 Nov 29];371:m4362. Available from: https://www.fda.gov/media/143602/download.

[84] Lilly Statement Regarding NIH's ACTIV-3 Clinical Trial | Eli Lilly and Company [Internet]. [cited 2020 Nov 29]. Available from: https://www.lilly.com/news/stories/statement-activ3-clinical-trial-nih-covid19

[85] Coronavirus (COVID-19) Update: FDA Authorizes Monoclonal Antibodies for Treatment of COVID-19 | FDA [Internet]. [cited 2020 Nov 29]. Available from: https://www.fda.gov/news-events/press-announcements/coronavirus-covid-19-update-fda-authorizes-monoclonal-antibodies-treatment-covid-19

[86] Regeneron halts trial of antibody treatment in seriously ill Covid patients | Financial Times [Internet]. [cited 2020

Nov 29]. Available from: https://www.ft.com/content/42256a8d-0073-4f57-9ac4-d3cc65a8e5c0

[87] President Trump Received Regeneron Experimental Antibody Treatment - The New York Times [Internet]. [cited 2020 Nov 29]. Available from: https://www.nytimes.com/2020/10/02/health/trump-antibody-treatment.html

[88] COVID-19 Long-Acting AntiBody (LAAB) combination AZD7442 rapidly advances into Phase III clinical trials | PharmaShots [Internet]. [cited 2020 Nov 29]. Available from: https://pharmashots.com/press-releases/covid-19-long-acting-antibody-laab-combination-azd7442-rapidly-advances-into-phase-iii-clinical-trials/

[89] Coronavirus (COVID-19) Update: FDA Authorizes Monoclonal Antibodies for Treatment of COVID-19 | FDA [Internet]. [cited 2021 Feb 16]. Available from: https://www.fda.gov/news-events/press-announcements/coronavirus-covid-19-update-fda-authorizes-monoclonal-antibodies-treatment-covid-19-0

[90] Zhang W, Zhao Y, Zhang F, Wang Q, Li T, Liu Z, et al. The use of anti-inflammatory drugs in the treatment of people with severe coronavirus disease 2019 (COVID-19): The experience of clinical immunologists from China [Internet]. Vol. 214, Clinical Immunology. Academic Press Inc.; 2020 [cited 2021 Feb 16]. Available from: https://pubmed.ncbi.nlm.nih.gov/32222466/

[91] Babon JJ, Lucet IS, Murphy JM, Nicola NA, Varghese LN. The molecular regulation of Janus kinase (JAK) activation [Internet]. Vol. 462, Biochemical Journal. Portland Press Ltd; 2014 [cited 2021 Feb 16]. p. 1-13. Available from: https://pubmed.ncbi.nlm.nih.gov/25057888/

[92] Bousoik E, Montazeri Aliabadi H. "Do We Know Jack" About JAK? A Closer Look at JAK/STAT Signaling Pathway [Internet]. Vol. 8, Frontiers in Oncology. Frontiers Media S.A.; 2018 [cited 2021 Feb 16]. Available from: https://pubmed.ncbi.nlm.nih.gov/30109213/

[93] Stebbing J, Phelan A, Griffin I, Tucker C, Oechsle O, Smith D, et al. COVID-19: combining antiviral and anti-inflammatory treatments [Internet]. Vol. 20, The Lancet Infectious Diseases. Lancet Publishing Group; 2020 [cited 2021 Feb 16]. p. 400-2. Available from: https://pubmed.ncbi.nlm.nih.gov/32113509/

[94] Kinase Inhibitors | COVID-19 Treatment Guidelines [Internet]. [cited 2021 Feb 16]. Available from: https://www.covid19treatmentguidelines.nih.gov/immunomodulators/kinase-inhibitors/

[95] Chen Y, Liu Q, Guo D. Emerging coronaviruses: Genome structure, replication, and pathogenesis [Internet]. Vol. 92, Journal of Medical Virology. John Wiley and Sons Inc.; 2020 [cited 2020 Nov 20]. p. 418-23. Available from: https://onlinelibrary.wiley.com/doi/full/10.1002/jmv.25681

[96] Gurwitz D. Angiotensin receptor blockers as tentative SARS-CoV-2 therapeutics [Internet]. Vol. 81, Drug Development Research. Wiley-Liss Inc.; 2020 [cited 2020 Nov 20]. p. 537-40. Available from: https://onlinelibrary.wiley.com/doi/full/10.1002/ddr.21656

[97] Wang W, Zhao X, Wei W. Angiotensin-converting enzyme inhibitors (ACEI) or Angiotensin receptor blockers (ARBs) may be safe for COVID-19 patients. [cited 2020 Nov 20]; Available from: https://doi.org/10.21203/rs.3.rs-51043/v2

[98] Kadam RU, Wilson IA. Structural basis of influenza virus fusion inhibition

by the antiviral drug Arbidol. Proc Natl Acad Sci U S A [Internet]. 2017 Jan 10 [cited 2020 Nov 20];114(2):206-14. Available from: www.pnas.org/cgi/doi/10.1073/pnas.1617020114

[99] Khamitov RA, Loginova SY, Shchukina VN, Borisevich S V., Maksimov VA, Shuster AM. Antiviral activity of arbidol and its derivatives against the pathogen of severe acute respiratory syndrome in the cell cultures. Vopr Virusol [Internet]. 2008 Jul 1 [cited 2020 Nov 20];53(4):9-13. Available from: https://europepmc.org/article/med/18756809

[100] Wang Z, Yang B, Li Q, Wen L, Zhang R. Clinical features of 69 cases with coronavirus disease 2019 in Wuhan, China. Clin Infect Dis [Internet]. 2020 Aug 1 [cited 2020 Nov 20];71(15):769-77. Available from: https://academic.oup.com/cid/article/71/15/769/5807944

[101] Hoffmann M, Kleine-Weber H, Schroeder S, Krüger N, Herrler T, Erichsen S, et al. SARS-CoV-2 Cell Entry Depends on ACE2 and TMPRSS2 and Is Blocked by a Clinically Proven Protease Inhibitor. Cell. 2020 Apr 16;181(2):271-280.e8.

[102] Rossignol JF. Nitazoxanide, a new drug candidate for the treatment of Middle East respiratory syndrome coronavirus. J Infect Public Health. 2016 May 1;9(3):227-30.

[103] Patanjali's Coronil, 1st "proof-based" drug to fight Covid, gets govt nod | Business Standard News [Internet]. [cited 2021 Mar 4]. Available from: https://www.business-standard.com/article/current-affairs/ramdev-releases-paper-on-patanjali-s-1st-proof-based-covid-drug-coronil-coronavirus-treatment-121021900404_1.html

Chapter 27

Home Care as a Safe Alternative during COVID-19 Crisis

Heloisa Amaral Gaspar and Claudio Oliveira Flauzino

Abstract

High mortality rate for the coronavirus disease (COVID-19) has been reported worldwide in nursing home residents, and the global concern about the safety of patients and professionals in these institutions is relevant. A large part of post-acute and chronic patient care in Brazil is performed at home through Home Care (HC) services. The objectives of this chapter are to describe the main measures that can be implemented in patient homes in order to keep professionals, patients, and family members safe and to analyze the safety of choosing the home as the place of care during a pandemic, especially in contrast to the results observed in long-term care facilities. COVID-19 infection data among home care patients, obtained after a year of severe epidemic in Brazil, demonstrate that home care is safe and is associated with a low incidence and low lethality related to the new coronavirus.

Keywords: Home care, safety, pandemic, COVID-19, professional protection equipment

1. Introduction

In Brazil, the first confirmed case of COVID-19 occurred on February 26th. Since then, the number of cases has grown exponentially and, despite recognized underreporting, the country ranked second in the world among countries with the highest number of cases and deaths due to COVID-19 [1, 2].

COVID-19 is a potentially severe acute respiratory infection caused by the novel coronavirus severe acute respiratory syndrome coronavirus 2 (SARS-CoV-2). The clinical presentation is generally that of a respiratory infection with symptom severity ranging from a mild common cold-like illness to a severe viral pneumonia leading to acute respiratory distress syndrome that is potentially fatal. Characteristic symptoms include fever, cough, dyspnea, and loss of taste/smell, although some patients may be asymptomatic. Complications of severe disease include, but are not limited to, multi-organ failure, septic shock, and venous thromboembolism. Symptoms may be persistent and continue for more than 12 weeks in some patients. After the acute phase and especially following hospital discharge patients may present with muscular weakness, oxygen dependency requiring extra-hospital rehabilitation and, still, may need continuous care for complications such as infectious, thrombosis or wounds [3].

1.1 How did the pandemic affect Brazil?

The pandemic struck Brazil in an overwhelming way. The lack of effective preventive measures added up to a poor coordination by the various spheres of

IntechOpen

government, resulting in a favorable environment for viral transmission and the emergence of new variants. The explosion in the number of infections, reaching more than 15 million Brazilians infected, a number that is underestimated due to the low availability of diagnostic tests especially at the beginning of the pandemic, led to the largest health and hospital collapse in the country's history. The ICUs were filled in several states both in the public and private system and patients died while waiting in line for a hospital bed.

In 2021 the country faced, and still faces, a shortage of human resources in hospitals, a shortage of medications, and a severe crisis in the supply of medicinal oxygen.

1.2 How did the pandemic affect patients with comorbidities and those who are more dependent?

Advanced age and the presence of comorbidities are associated with increased mortality due to the new coronavirus. The high prevalence of this combination, associated with physical environments that provide inadequate barriers to infection control, place patients in long-term care facilities at greater risks. Studies show that once the first case in these institutions exists, the possibility to have the infection spread to other patients is quite high [4–6]. There are several reports worldwide about high mortality related to COVID-19 among residents of long-term care institutions (LTCI) with up to 2/3 of patients affected within a period of 3 weeks and mortality reaching levels as high as 72% [7]. Dr. Grabowski's [6] point of view highlights the elevated mortality rates due to COVID-19 among LTCI residents, representing 25% of the deaths from COVID-19 in the US. Percentages are even higher in some US states and European countries such as France and Ireland. The concern with the safety of patients and professionals at these facilities is extremely relevant and compels us to make a deeper reflection.

The HC sector has grown exponentially in the last few decades. Currently it is estimated that approximately one million patients/year from the public and private sectors use HC in Brazil, where much of post-acute care, rehabilitation, and long-term chronic patient care is provided at home. Data from 2019 revealed that the number of patients treated at home was equivalent to 5% of the number of hospital beds in our country [8].

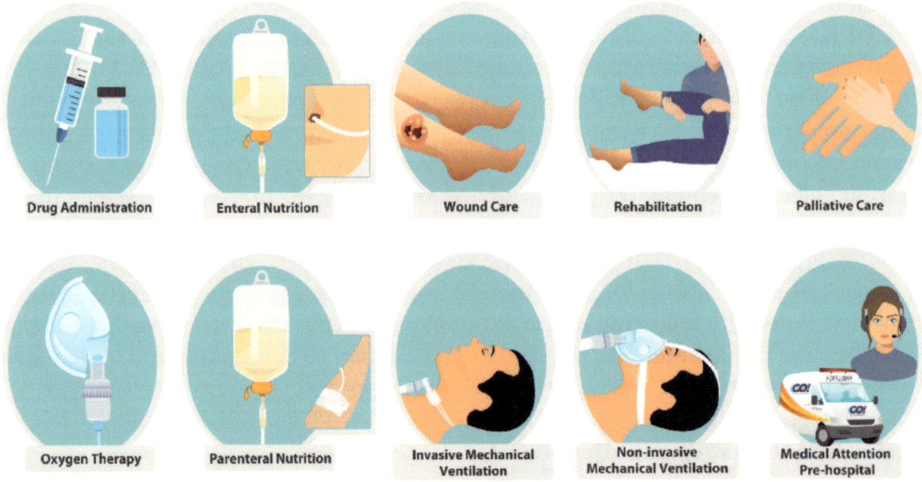

Figure 1.
Most frequent therapies performed by home Care in Brazil.

This modality of treatment includes drug administration, enteral nutrition, wound care, rehabilitation, oxygen therapy, respiratory support, and more complex therapies such as parenteral nutrition and invasive or non-invasive mechanical ventilation (**Figure 1**).

Home care is available in both public and private health sectors and has been distinguished by humanized care, the patient's reintegration into society, and low incidence of infections.

2. What did home care do differently in Brazil?

Home Care providers needed to take additional steps to keep patient care at home and to ensure a safe environment for patients and professionals. Each institution adopted targeted measures and Home Doctor, a private home care company, became a Brazilian reference on this topic. The main measures adopted were as follows:

2.1 Environment measures

With regard to the COVID-19 pandemic, patients in home care have an advantage. As they are naturally in isolation at home, it is possible for them to strictly follow the recommendations of keeping distance from other people, especially those with any suspicious symptoms while staying in a ventilated and clean environment with rigorous hand hygiene and the use of individualized materials (**Figure 2**).

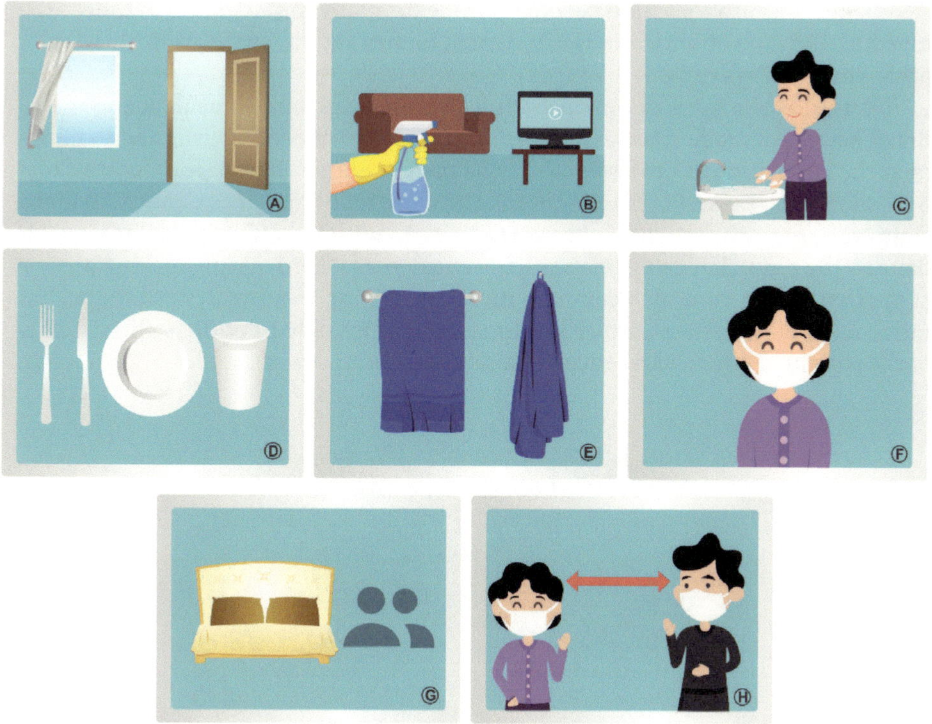

Figure 2.
Main environmental benefits: A - ventilated environment; B - environment cleaned with 70% alcohol; C - strict hand hygiene; D - individualized kitchenware; E - individualized hygiene utensils; F - face mask; G - privative room; and H - social distancing.

Physically, the home environment is the best place to reduce the circulation and spread of the virus and patients in home care take advantage of this evident benefit.

2.2 Professionals and training

Patients under home care are treated by a team of skilled professionals in a directed way in order to receive exactly the assistance needed by a qualified team trained in the use of personal protective equipment (PPE) with rational optimization of the number of home visits depending on the patient's clinical condition.

These professionals receive training on topics related to the pandemic so as to inform professionals regarding the recommended protocols, as well as to provide the emotional and psychological support necessary for caring in this critical scenario (**Figure 3**).

2.3 Personal protective equipment (PPE)

The professionals who work at home care services undergo periodical training about how to use PPE, regarding the criteria of indication, and in the techniques for putting on and taking off the PPE (**Figure 4**).

2.4 Telemedicine

Telemedicine was regulated in Brazil on an emergency basis at the beginning of the pandemic. In this way, home care companies that were not structured for virtual care had to quickly prepare themselves, acquire secure telemedicine platforms, train their employees, guide patients and family members, and implement this resource in practice.

Virtual consultations have become routine for many professionals in order to reduce the flow of professionals in patient homes and the circulation of these professionals (**Figure 5**).

Telemedicine played an important role in home care during the pandemic in Brazil because it made it possible to replace regularly scheduled visits and to minimize the circulation of professionals in the patient homes. It also showed itself to be a valuable resource for more rigorous and close follow-up of patients with more complex clinical conditions and patients infected with COVID-19. The monitoring done by the physician using telemedicine enabled a faster decision-making process at the first sign of clinical decompensation, optimizing treatment, reaching a rational use of scarce ambulance resources, and ultimately providing a better care of the patient at home with reduced levels of hospitalization.

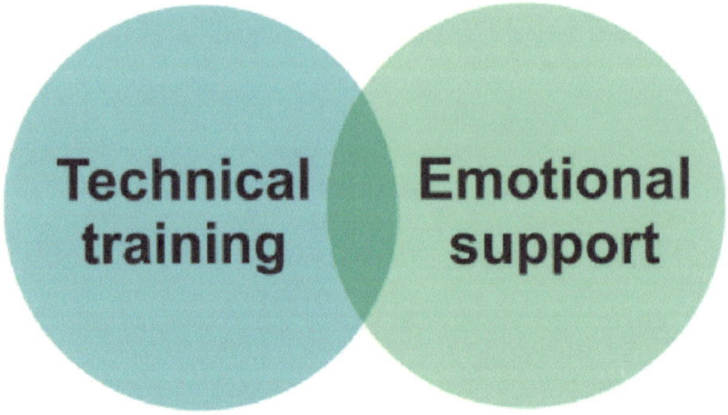

Figure 3.
Two training spheres.

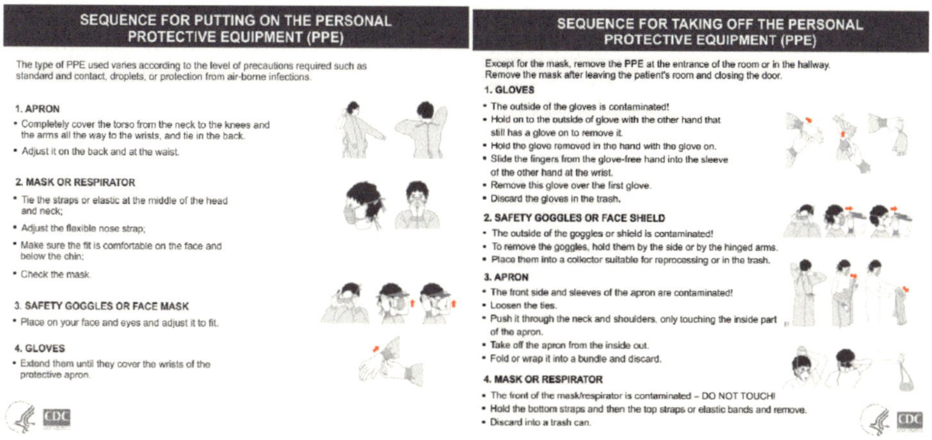

Figure 4.
Definition of PPE use and training protocol regarding putting on and taking off PPE.

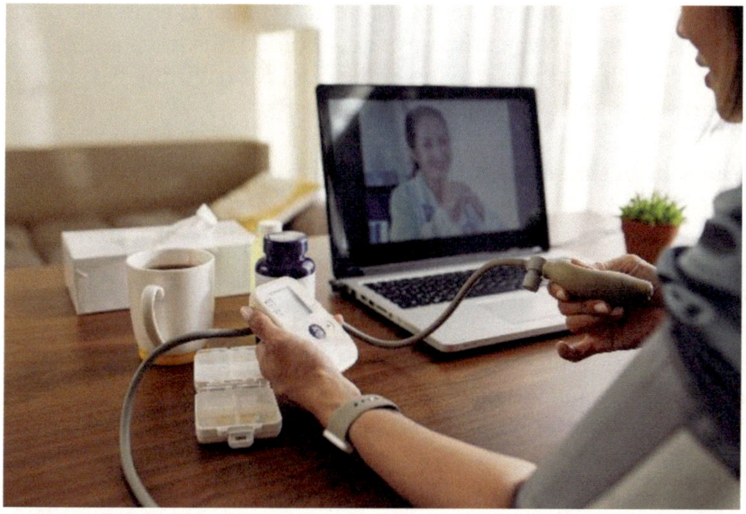

Figure 5.
Teleconsultation.

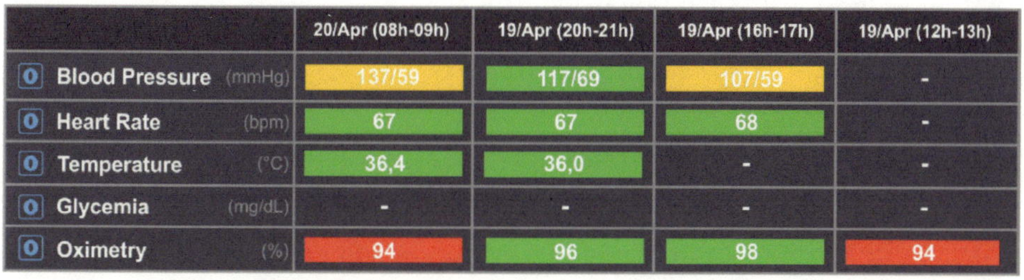

	20/Apr (08h-09h)	19/Apr (20h-21h)	19/Apr (16h-17h)	19/Apr (12h-13h)
Blood Pressure (mmHg)	137/59	117/69	107/59	-
Heart Rate (bpm)	67	67	68	-
Temperature (°C)	36,4	36,0	-	-
Glycemia (mg/dL)	-	-	-	-
Oximetry (%)	94	96	98	94

Figure 6.
A COVID-19 patient remote monitoring (blood pressure, heart rate, temperature, glycemia, oxygen saturation).

2.5 Remote devices for monitoring

Vital signs such as blood pressure, heart rate, temperature, and pulse oximetry can be measured by the patient using Bluetooth wireless devices, which are transmitted in real time to a monitoring center (**Figure 6**).

Additionally, patients using mechanical ventilation may have their ventilation monitored remotely through equipment with this real-time transmission feature. This resource, which had already been utilized on a smaller scale for home care in Brazil, began to be used more widely during the pandemic. It allows real-time visualization of patient ventilation monitoring so that decompensations are quickly identified, allowing adjustments to be made in an agile manner, and consequently improving patient care and optimizing the deployment of resources to the home (**Figure 7**).

2.6 Use of oxygen concentrator

In Home Care, it is classically recommended to use oxygen concentrators instead of oxygen cylinders in order to reduce the risks related to the physical factors of explosion and of shortages due to delayed cylinder substitution. During the pandemic, the scarcity of oxygen and gas cylinders for recharging was intense in Brazil, but Home Care treatment managed to safely keep oxygen therapy in the homes due to having oxygen concentrators in most households. There was no need for hospitalization of patients because of lack of oxygen. All patients were able to be safely maintained under home oxygen therapy and, additionally, more patients under oxygen therapy could be transferred to home care, contributing to the availability of hospital beds for more severe patients (**Figure 8**).

2.7 What have been the results of home care during the COVID-19 pandemic?

During the first year of the pandemic (from March 2020 to March 2021), one of the largest home care providers in Brazil treated a total of 4,500 patients at home and registered only 179 confirmed cases of COVID-19 among patients who were already receiving home care during this period, 91 (50,8%) in women and 88 (49,2%) in men, with a mean age of 61.1 years [9]. COVID-19 had an incidence of 3.9% in the population studied, which is below the Brazilian incidence of 6%. There were 56 (31.2%) hospitalizations with 21 (11.7%) hospital deaths and 4 (2.2%) cases of home death, which represents a lethality of 13.9% (25 total cases of death). The number, clinical outcomes, and geographical distribution of the confirmed COVID-19 cases were reported daily to all healthcare teams through a case panel [10].

Apart from COVID-19, more than 2,500 patients per day were treated at home, which allowed hospital beds to be dedicated to critically COVID-19 patients and contributed to reduce total hospital occupancy.

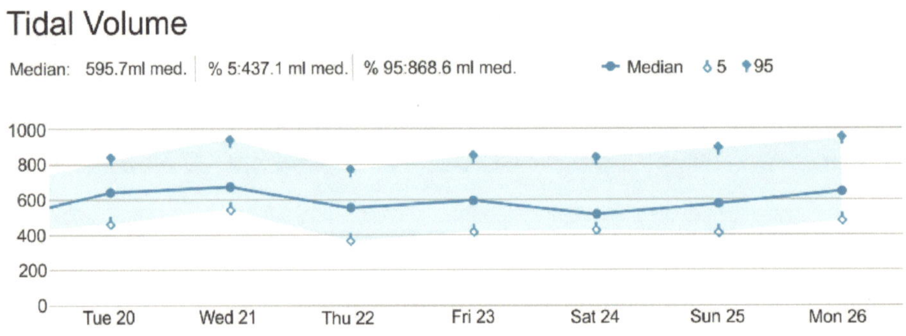

Figure 7.
Image representing remote monitoring of the mechanical ventilation of a patient under home care.

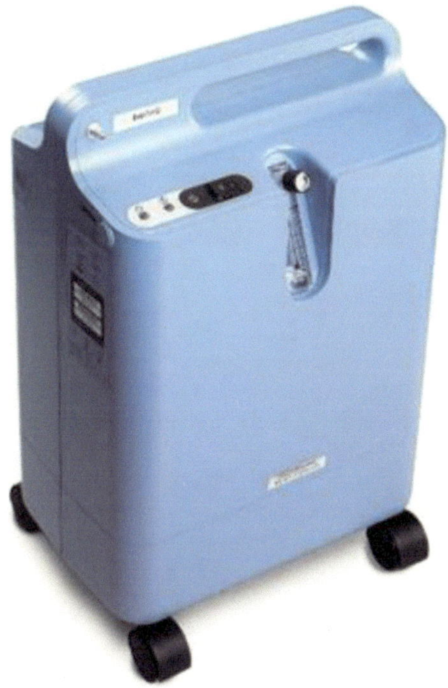

Figure 8.
Oxygen concentrator.

On the other hand, acute COVID-19 patients with mild and moderate symptoms were taken care of at their homes, and also patients in the recovery phase of the disease were admitted for rehabilitation after hospital discharge. During this 1-year period, 64 new patients with a diagnosis of mild or moderate COVID-19 were successfully treated at home and 123 post-COVID patients were admitted to home care after hospital discharge to receive rehabilitation therapy and treatment for complications.

Home care assumed an important role in avoiding hospitalization of non-critical, suspected, or confirmed cases of COVID-19 and in providing care to patients through home monitoring of oximetry, oxygen supplementation, home medical support, daily medical telephone monitoring, and the provision of a medical emergency center available daily round-the-clock.

3. Conclusion

Home care in Brazil has undergone a profound transformation as a result of the pandemic. Significant and rapid technological advances were needed and training of the team became crucial. This, associated with the physical benefits of distancing by staying at home, boosted home care, which played a key role in treating COVID-19 and non-Covid-19 patients during the pandemic, resulting in liberating hospital beds and contributing to the sustainability of the Brazilian Health System in this catastrophic health crisis.

COVID-19 infection data in home care patients obtained after a year of severe epidemic in Brazil demonstrate that home care is safe environment for patients and professionals with low incidence and lethality related to SARS-CoV-2.

Author details

Heloisa Amaral Gaspar[1*] and Claudio Oliveira Flauzino[2]

1 Home Doctor, Medical Manager, São Paulo, Brazil

2 Home Doctor, CEO, São Paulo, Brazil

*Address all correspondence to: heloisa.gaspar@homedoctor.com.br

References

[1] World Health Organization. Infection prevention and control during health care when COVID-19 is suspected [Internet]. 2020. Available from: https://www.who.int/publications-detail/infection-prevention-and-control-during-health-care-when-novel-coronavirus-(ncov)-infection-is-suspected-20200125 [Accessed: 2021 04 20].

[2] Ministry of health. Brazil confirms first case of coronavirus. [Internet]. 2021. Avaible from: https://agenciabrasil.ebc.com.br/en/saude/noticia/2020-02/brazil-confirms-first-case-coronavirus [Accessed: 2021 Apr 20].

[3] BMJ Best Practice: Coronavírus disease 2019 (COVID-19). [Internet]. 2021. p. 3-266. Available from: https://bestpractice.bmj.com/info/ [Accessed: 2020 03 19]

[4] Kemenesi G, Kornya L, Tóth G, Kurucz K, Zeghbib S, Somogyi B, Zöldi V, Urban P, Herezeg R, Jakab F. Nursing homes and the elderly regarding the COVID-19 pandemic: situation report from Hungary. GeroScience [Internet]. 2020. p. 1093-1099. Available from: https://doi.org/10.1007/s11357-020-00195-z [Accessed: 2021 04 30]

[5] Comas-Herrera A, Zalakaín J, Litwin C, Hsu AT, Lemmon E, Henderson D, et al. Mortality associated with COVID-19 outbreaks in care homes: early international evidence. Available from: https://ltccovid.org/2020/04/12/mortality-associated-with-covid-19-outbreaks-in-care-homes-early-international-evidence/ [Accessed: 2021 04 30]

[6] Grabowski DC, Mor V. Nursing home care in crisis in the wake of COVID-19. JAMA. 2020. DOI: 10.1001/jama.2020.8524.

[7] McMichael TM, Currie DW, Clark S, Pogosjans S, Kay M, Schwartz NG, et al; Public Health–Seattle and King County, EvergreenHealth, and CDC COVID-19 Investigation Team. Epidemiology of Covid-19 in a long-term care facility in King Country, Washington. N Engl J Med. 2020. DOI: 10.1056/nejmoa2005412

[8] Censo NEAD 2019/2020: Censo NEAD FIPE de Atenção Domiciliar. [Internet]. 2020. 4-59. Available from: https://www.neadsaude.org.br/wp-content/themes/nead/nead-digital/Censo-NEAD-FIPE-2019-2020/index.html [Accessed: 2021 04 30]

[9] Gaspar HA, Oliveira CF, Jacober FC. Home care as a safe alternative in post-acute and long-term care during covid-19 crisis. Oral apresentation at World Hospital at Home Congress 2021. Available from https://virtualmeeting.kenes.com/VirtualMeeting/whahc21/

[10] Gaspar HA, Oliveira CF, Jacober FC, Deus ER, Canuto F. Home Care as a safe alternative during the COVID-19 crisis. Rev Assoc Med Bras (1992). 2020 Nov;66(11):1482-1486. doi: 10.1590/1806-9282.66.11.1482.

Chapter 28

Tackling COVID-19 through the One Health Approach

Ayodele Oluwaseun Ajayi, Olawale Peter Odeleye and Oluwabukola Atinuke Popoola

Abstract

The Covid-19 pandemic is currently ravaging the globe with enormous morbidity and mortality. This pandemic, caused by the SARS-CoV-2 started from China and has spread across the globe. Initial reports indicated that the SARS-CoV-2 initially emerged among animals from where they transfer to humans. Different strategies deployed to curtail the pandemic have yielded little result. Therefore, the One-Health concept may compliment existing strategies. The One Health places emphasis on the between the animal-human-ecosystem interface and how this can be used to tackle public health problems, including the COVID-19 pandemic. One Health Surveillance will involve tracking viral pathogens in animals to access risk of transfer to humans. It will also stimulate targeted approaches for prevention and treatment of viral zoonotic infections. There should be an integrated and interdisciplinary One-Health surveillance that should incorporate veterinary, medical or public health and environmental scientists to synergise surveillance effort to track emergence of infectious diseases in the future.

Keywords: Surveillance, One-Health, COVID-19, SARS-CoV-2

1. Introduction

The One Health is an interdisciplinary concept that encompasses animal health, human health and the ecosystem with huge emphasis on how public health problems can be solved at the interface between these entities [1–3]. The interface between humans, animals and the ecosystem are intricately interconnected to the extent that whatever happens in any of these entities most likely affects others [4]. Therefore, the concept of One Health relies on the understanding that human health, animal health and the environment are intricately linked together and they can be affected simultaneously [5]. Historically, the nature of the intricate interactions between animals, humans and the ecosystem have continued to shape human events and local or global public health [6].

There has been a historical consensus that some factors that affect human health can be traced to animal factors and origins [7]. Humans have coexisted with animals and this has formed the basis for studying the human-animal interface [8, 9]. For example, it has been confirmed that close to 70% of all infectious diseases have zoonotic origins [10–12]. It has also been implied in some scientific contexts that the control of aetiological agents in animals could prove effective in controlling such agents within the human population to improve public health [13, 14].

Another imperative of the One Health is the growing interconnectedness between the ecosystems of humans, animals and the environment, which may include wildlife, urban areas and farming systems [15, 16]. The increasing anthropological activities of humans have diminished the delineation between these ecosystems and have increased the frequency of contact between animals and humans [17]. Humans now stand at increased risk of having contact with animals that have been displaced from their original ecosystems. This has further increased the risks of emerging and re-emerging infectious diseases and their attendant burdens on humans and global economy [18]. Some infectious diseases that were hitherto absent in human populations are now common due to the increased contact of humans with animals [19].

It has also been noted that some environmental factors affect the health of humans and animals [20]. The increasing anthropogenic activities have led to a distortion of the delicate natural environmental balance [21]. Intense industrial activities release greenhouse gases into the environment, leading to climate change and increased risk of respiratory problems among humans and animals. The activities of chemical and pharmaceutical industries have also been linked with the release of chemicals into the environment, particularly soil and water; and they can be absorbed by humans, animal and plants [22]. For instance, some studies have confirmed the residual amounts of antibiotics found in urine of animals are partly due to the release of pharmaceutical wastes into the environment [23]. Several pathogens, particularly viruses and bacteria, have been confirmed to be carried by environmental reservoirs and matrixes from where they can be transmitted to humans and animals to cause diseases [24]. One of the fallouts of globalization is the increased speed and frequency of travels by different channels of transportation, namely air, sea and land. This has facilitated the massive movement of humans and animals across transcontinental boundaries [25]. Unfortunately, humans that carry active infectious diseases serve as reservoir through which infectious pathogens can be transmitted or transferred across international boundaries [26, 27]. In addition, massive demand for protein and animal products increases the number of animals that are transported across international borders with increased risk of transfer of resident zoonotic flora and pathogens across international boundaries [28]. This factor has contributed to the increased interface between animals and humans.

It is within this context that different countries and international organizations, particularly the World Health Organization, (WHO), Organization for Animal Health (OIE) and Food and Agricultural Organization (FAO) agreed on a global consensus that some problems of global importance can be tackled through the One Health approach [29]. It places emphasis on multi-sectoral collaborations and frameworks to solve pertinent global health problems, both nationally and internationally. They also encourage different countries to come up with their One Health policies with a view to enhance the quality of their public health. Many countries across the globe have responded to this challenge and institutionalized One Health into their surveillance systems to improve public health. For instance, the African Center for Disease Control has incorporated the One Health framework into its activities with a view to tackle the periodic problem of emerging infectious diseases within the continent.

2. Brief review of zoonotic viruses and their epidemiology

Zoonotic infections are those infections that originate from animals and are transmitted through the agency of animals or insects to humans [30, 31]. It has since been on record that the vast majority of emerging infectious diseases have zoonotic origins [32, 33]. It has also been established that many viruses have animals as their reservoirs and some even exist as part of the natural flora of the animals. Many animals that have served as proven reservoirs of viruses include bats, dogs, primates, and many other exotic species of animals [34]. It has been recognized that the knowledge of viruses and their natural hosts or ecosystems is important to effectively recognize measures to combat zoonotic infections, including those caused by viruses [35]. Such knowledge will enable scientists determine the possible viral flora of such animals, detect any seasonal changes in the carriage of such viruses that may negatively impact public health and allow medical practitioners, veterinary physicians and epidemiologists to predict possible emergence of viral infections, risks and threats to humans and public health [36–38].

A vast majority of infectious diseases that have significant toll on public health, in terms of mortality and morbidity, have zoonotic origins [39]. Similarly, viral zoonoses contribute a significant proportion of infectious diseases across the globe with significant economic burden running to billions of US dollars annually [37]. Furthermore, Africa and other developing countries appear to have the highest burden of viral zoonotic infections, with significant mortality and morbidity [40, 41]. The diminishing demarcation between the animal wildlife and human ecosystems increases the risk of contact and interaction between humans and animals with consequent increase in the surge of emerging and re-emerging infectious diseases in Africa and across the globe [42]. As stated above, Africa has its fair share of zoonotic viral diseases with well documented mortality and morbidity attributed to them. The following are examples of past or recent wave of zoonotic viral diseases in Africa.

i. **Ebola virus disease:** This is a usually fatal disease caused by the Ebola virus. It has been established that this disease is usually transmitted through contact of apparently healthy individuals with the body fluids of individuals infected with the virus [43, 44]. Earlier and recent reports suggest that the virus was originally found in primates and bats in wildlife from where they were transmitted to humans that came in contact with them [45, 46]. It can also be transmitted from wild animals such as fruit bats and porcupines [47]. The earliest reported case of the diseases was in 1976 in the Democratic republic of Congo [48]. The most pronounced outbreak of this disease was reported in 2014 in Liberia, Sierra Leone and Guinea with combined mortality of approximately 11,000 deaths [49]. The fatal nature and the huge mortality reported in the recent outbreaks draws attention to the zoonotic origin of the disease and how it can be tackled through one health.

ii. **Lassa fever:** This disease is caused by the Lassa fever virus and is endemic mostly in Nigeria and other neighboring countries, including Cote d'Ivoire, Guinea, Central African Republic, Mali, Senegal and Congo [50]. The natural host of the virus is the rodent *Mastomys natalensis,* which is mostly found in tropical environments in West Africa [51]. This rodent is originally resident in the bushes and tropical rainforest but the increasing and massive urbanization in most parts of Nigeria and West Africa dislodge these rodents from their natural habitat, increasing the risk of transmission of this virus to humans [42]. Epidemiologically, the annual incidence of this disease in Africa is estimated at 200,000, with estimated mortality of 500 with 60 million people at risk of contracting the disease [52, 53].

iii. **Rabies**: This disease is caused by the Rabies virus and it is found mostly in Africa and Asia [54]. It is a fatal disease with high mortality in endemic regions where the disease is common. Relative to the high mortality associated with this disease, it is estimated that 99% of close to 59000 deaths caused by this disease are originated from dogs [55]. The virus also circulates in wildlife, especially wild bats and racoons where they can also be transmitted to domestic animals that come in contact with them [55]. The strong knowledge of the transmission link of the virus between dogs and humans led the effective control of the disease through vaccination of dogs and this has proven effective till date [56–58].

iv. **Human Arbovirus infections:** This represents the categories of infections that are caused by mosquitoes and ticks that feed on blood and transmit viruses to susceptible hosts during the process [59]. These Arboviruses still present a huge threat to public health especially in developing countries [60]. The morbidity and mortality associated with diseases caused by arboviruses is significant [61]. However, the increasing rate of urbanization and other related anthropogenic forces increase the chance of transmission of arboviruses to humans [62]. The most prominent arboviral infection among humans is the Dengue fever caused by the Dengue virus which accounts for more than 40.000 deaths per annum [63]. Around 2015, the Zika virus infection caused some morbidities and mortalities in Brazil and neighboring countries and still a threat till date [64].

It has been noted that the zoonotic origins, epidemiological burden and transmission cycles of the viral infections emphasize the need for effective control of zoonotic viral infections through the One Health approach, especially in the paradigm of other measures that have been adopted and have not effectively controlled the diseases.

3. Brief review of the COVID-19 pandemic

A new viral disease emerged in China and has since spread to different parts of the world with more than 145 million people infected and more than 3 million deaths. After extensive molecular studies, the etiology of the virus was identified as SARS-COV-2 with innate ability to spread rapidly among humans [65–68]. Furthermore, new variants of the virus were later identified in different countries with enhanced abilities to spread faster than the previous wild types discovered. This implies that more people will be infected and more may likely die of this disease. These new variants therefore appear to have altered the epidemiology of the disease in some parts of the world [69–72].

Different countries, international and scientific organizations responded swiftly to the spread of the pandemic with an array of measures to limit the spread of the disease across national and international boundaries [73, 74]. Such measures included isolation and quarantine, restriction of international flights, social distancing and personal hygiene, which include hand washing and use of nose masks [74–78]. Following global agreement that vaccines may likely end the pandemic, different companies and research organisations have developed vaccines and the largest and unprecedented vaccination drive have since commenced in different countries and millions more people have been projected to be vaccinated over time [79, 80].

However, the different initiatives intended to control the spread of the disease shortly before the vaccines were discovered appeared to have limited effects in controlling the spread of the disease. For instance, strict hand washing remains a challenge in many poor and developing countries due to lack of adequate water supply [78]. Furthermore, the screening measures at international airports only captures symptomatic carriers while asymptomatic carriers can escape the screening routines [77]. Also, most of these measures appear short term and may not be sustained on these long run [81]. Inadequate logistics for distribution of masks and other sanitary materials limit access by people in remote areas. The limited success achieved in limiting the spread of the disease calls for more deliberate and innovative approaches towards controlling the spread and even eliminating the disease.

4. Zoonotic origin of *COVID-19*

The preliminary investigations in China that followed the onset of the pandemic revealed that bats and exotic animals at a popular market are the initial sources of the organisms [82, 83]. It was also hypothesized that the humans that initially came into contact with the animals may have triggered the pandemic [84]. The coronaviruses are a large family of viruses that has been found to be common among animals and wildlife, including bats [82]. The initial strains of the virus were genomically correlated with that of bats. This implies that the virus may have originated from bats, although the exact transmission to animals remains relatively unknown [84]. The extensive zoonotic origin of these types of viruses heightens the risk of their transfer from the wildlife to the human population [85]. The growing urbanization, anthropogenic pressure and climate change encroaches the original wildlife, resulting in the spillover of the viruses as the animals migrate to areas inhabited by humans [86].

5. The imperative of one health surveillance

The initial transfer pattern of the virus from animals and wild life to the environment and humans confirms that the One Health approach can be applied to tackle the spread of the diseases, in view of the outright failure or limited success achieved with other preliminary methods deployed to control the transmission of the disease [81, 87]. Animals serve as the reservoir of the virus from where they can be shed into the environment. Such animals, usually in wildlife, frequently come into contact with humans and they transmit the virus in the process. Furthermore, humans can serve as conduit to transfer to other humans and this scenario is particularly problematic in the case of the SARS-CoV-2 [88]. In addition, humans can also transmit the virus asymptomatically to other humans and the environment [89]. The virus has been found on surfaces, foods and sewages [90].

There is a strong consensus in the global scientific arena that the One Health concept provides a stronger approach to tackle the spread of infectious diseases including those caused by zoonotic viruses. In response, different international organizations have put up strong statements in support of the One Health approach to tackle the current surge of infectious diseases. They further encourage different countries to prioritize this concept and come up with policies to tackle the spread of infectious diseases, which can be extended to the current COVID-19 pandemic.

In major effort to solidify the One Health footprint on global public health, three major international organizations, namely the World Health Organization (WHO), Food and Agricultural Organization (FAO) and the Organization for Animal Health (OIE) produced a joint and strategic framework aimed at reducing infectious diseases at the animal-humans-ecosystem interface. With strong link of the coronavirus with wild life and the environment, viral diseases of zoonotic origins also fall with the scope of infectious diseases that can be tackled through the One-Health policy [91].

Several countries have since keyed into the strategic initiatives and have recognized it as an important approach to tackle the surge of emerging infectious diseases, including the current COVID-19 pandemic. For instance, the African Center for Disease Control has incorporated it into its public health programmes in the continent [29]. The European Union (EU) have since produced its own One Health action plan to tackle different public health problems most especially antibiotic resistance and zoonoses [92]. Similarly, the Asia continent has the One Health Tripartite frame work the comprises of the Asia region of the WHO, FAO and OIE to give full attention to One Heal issues with a view to tackle public health challenges that most especially antibiotic resistance and zoonoses [93].

However, it appears there is no standard approach for tackling COVID-19 as a means to prevent further spread of the pandemic. This can be viewed from the fact that the pandemic is relatively new and it may take some time to design One health policies that will specifically suit the pandemic. One of the key peculiarities of the current pandemic is the easy spread of the COVID-19, compared with the other public health threats that are currently being addressed by One Health. Also, the massive mortality and morbidity of the current pandemic is another peculiarity for which custom made One Health policies should be designed to tackle the current pandemic. Generally, the One Health approach recognizes that scientific expertise should be drawn from disciplines, most especially, medicine, veterinary science and environmental science in order to public health threats including the current COVID-19.

6. Surveillance for infectious diseases

The surveillance for infectious diseases is a very crucial epidemiological tool that serves different purposes in public health. More specifically, infectious diseases surveillance can be used to determine the current prevalence of infectious diseases at a given time. It also assists in the monitoring of changes in infectious diseases trend over time. It helps to determine or reveal risks of emergence of infectious diseases and how such risks can be mitigated. More importantly, infectious diseases surveillance allows targeted policies for prevention and control of infectious diseases within particular groups within a population [94].

Within the COVID-19 pandemic, the extensive surveillance capacities and protocols developed over the years have assisted in tracking the spread of the pandemic and helped to determine the massive threat it has posed in terms of morbidity and mortality [95, 96]. The massive surveillance efforts put forward, most especially by developed countries and China has enhanced targeted policies to tackle the spread of the disease and treatment. For instance, the United Kingdom recently announced massive vaccinations for the entire country. China was able to track sporadic emergence of the diseases and targeted quarantine followed such efforts. In contrast, African countries seem to have limited capacities for surveillance of infectious diseases and this may partly explain the low prevalence of the diseases in Africa.

7. One health surveillance

The paradigm of surveillance for the COVID-19 pandemic within the one health concept is somewhat different. Due to the interdisciplinary nature of one health, surveillance efforts and policies should be designed to encompass human health or population, animal health and the ecosystem. In fact, this surveillance approach has been recognized as a crucial component of One Health and this integrated approach can be used to track emerging and re-emerging diseases. Surveillance efforts targeted at animals and wild life has revealed that coronaviruses, including the SARS-CoV-2 constitute part of the flora of such animals. Although the immediate animal to human transmission of the SARS-CoV-2 could not be established, direct human to human transmission has been established and this has been attributed to the vast majority of the transmission of the virus. The virus has also been found in solid household waste, sewage and hospital droplets and these carry the risk of transmitting the virus to susceptible individuals [97].

8. Conclusion

The One Health concept is a relatively new approach being promoted as a strategy to tackle some public health problems at the human-animal-ecosystem interface. Consequently, its application is gradually gaining traction and some time is needed to really access its benefits. Currently, there are few evidence of the potential and practical benefits of this approach to tackle public health challenges on the scale of those posed by the COVID-19 pandemic.

That notwithstanding, few instances of the immediate, potential and practical benefit of using the One Health approach have emerged. The United States Agency for International development recently developed a PREDICT One Health surveillance system to track potential emergence of pathogenic viruses and their possible spill-over to the human population. The successful application of this project has led to the improvement of our understanding of evolution of viruses on a global scale [98]. Furthermore, another coordinated One Health simulation study using the Rift Valley virus was used to demonstrate the potential applicability and success of this approach. The study concluded that a multidisciplinary investigation using this approach can yield a higher statistical power and reveal complex relationships between regarding the epidemiology of the virus in animal and environmental settings [99].

It is evident from the foregoing that the One Health surveillance initiative can be applied at the human-animal-ecosystem interface to track any emerging infectious diseases. The incorporation of molecular techniques can be used to establish the clonality between the viral strains among animals, humans and the ecosystem. Due to the massive and devastating nature of the COVID-19 pandemic, the One Health surveillance must be globally envisioned in order to effectively track and control the spread of the disease [100].

Author details

Ayodele Oluwaseun Ajayi[1]*, Olawale Peter Odeleye[1]
and Oluwabukola Atinuke Popoola[2]

1 Department of Microbiology, Federal University Oye Ekiti, Ekiti State, Nigeria

2 Genetics, Genomics and Bioinformatics, National Biotechnology Development Agency, Abuja, Nigeria

*Address all correspondence to: ayodele.ajayi@fuoye.edu.ng

References

[1] Davis MF, Rankin SC, Schurer JM, Cole S, Conti L, Rabinowitz P. Checklist for one health epidemiological reporting of evidence (COHERE). One Health 2017; 4:14-21. doi: 10.1016/j.onehlt.2017.07.001.

[2] Mackenzie JS, Jeggo M. The One Health Approach-Why Is It So Important?. Trop Med Infect Dis. 2019; 4(2):88. doi:10.3390/tropicalmed4020088

[3] Chiesa F, Tomassone L, Savic S. A Survey on One Health Perception and Experiences in Europe and Neighboring Areas. Front Public Health. 2021; 9:609949. doi:10.3389/fpubh.2021.609949.

[4] Rabinowitz P, Conti L. Links among human health, animal health, and ecosystem health. Annu Rev Public Health. 2013;34:189-204. doi: 10.1146/annurev-publhealth-031912-114426. Epub 2013 Jan 16. PMID: 23330700.

[5] Trinh P, Zaneveld JR, Safranek S, Rabinowitz PM. One Health Relationships Between Human, Animal, and Environmental Microbiomes: A Mini-Review. Front Public Health. 2018;6:235. doi:10.3389/fpubh.2018.00235

[6] Evans BR, Leighton FA. A history of One Health. Rev Sci Tech. 2014;33(2):413-20. doi: 10.20506/rst.33.2.2298. PMID: 25707172.

[7] Reperant L.A., Cornaglia G., Osterhaus A.D.M.E. The Importance of Understanding the Human–Animal Interface. In: Mackenzie J., Jeggo M., Daszak P., Richt J. (eds) One Health: The Human-Animal-Environment Interfaces in Emerging Infectious Diseases. Current Topics in Microbiology and Immunology, 2012; 365. Springer, Berlin, Heidelberg. https://doi.org/10.1007/82_2012_269

[8] Carter NH, Shrestha BK, Karki JB, Pradhan NM, Liu J. Coexistence between wildlife and humans at fine spatial scales. Proc Natl Acad Sci U S A. 2012;109(38):15360-15365. doi:10.1073/pnas.1210490109

[9] Mekonen, S. Coexistence between human and wildlife: the nature, causes and mitigations of human wildlife conflict around Bale Mountains National Park, Southeast Ethiopia. BMC Ecol 2020;**20:** 51. https://doi.org/10.1186/s12898-020-00319-1

[10] Kruse H, kirkemo AM, Handeland K. Wildlife as source of zoonotic infections. Emerg Infect Dis. 2004;10(12):2067-2072. doi:10.3201/eid1012.040707

[11] Serge Morand, K. Marie McIntyre, Matthew Baylis, Domesticated animals and human infectious diseases of zoonotic origins: Domestication time matters, Infection, Genetics and Evolution, 2014; 24: 76-81, ISSN 1567-1348, https://doi.org/10.1016/j.meegid.2014.02.013.

[12] Haider N, Rothman-Ostrow P, Osman AY. COVID-19-Zoonosis or Emerging Infectious Disease?. Front Public Health. 2020;8:596944. doi:10.3389/fpubh.2020.596944

[13] Rabinowitz PM, Kock R, Kachani M. Toward proof of concept of a one health approach to disease prediction and control. Emerg Infect Dis. 2013;19(12): e130265. doi:10.3201/eid1912.130265

[14] Degeling, C., Johnson, J., Kerridge, I. Implementing a One Health approach to emerging infectious disease: reflections on the socio-political, ethical and legal dimensions. BMC Public Health . 2015;**15:** 1307. https://doi.org/10.1186/s12889-015-2617-1

[15] Milner-Gulland EJ. Interactions between human behaviour and

ecological systems. Philos Trans R Soc Lond B Biol Sci. 2012;367(1586):270-278. doi:10.1098/rstb.2011.0175

[16] Zulkifli I. Review of human-animal interactions and their impact on animal productivity and welfare. J Anim Sci Biotechnol. 2013;4(1):25. doi:10.1186/2049-1891-4-25

[17] Hendry AP, Gotanda KM, Svensson EI. Human influences on evolution, and the ecological and societal consequences. Philos Trans R Soc Lond B Biol Sci. 2017;372(1712): 20160028. doi:10.1098/rstb.2016.0028

[18] National Research Council (US) Committee on Achieving Sustainable Global Capacity for Surveillance and Response to Emerging Diseases of Zoonotic Origin; Keusch GT, Pappaioanou M, Gonzalez MC. (ed). Sustaining Global Surveillance and Response to Emerging Zoonotic Diseases. Washington (DC): National Academies Press (US); 2009. 3p, Drivers of Zoonotic Diseases. Available from: https://www.ncbi.nlm.nih.gov/books/NBK215318/

[19] Cristiano Salata, Arianna Calistri, Cristina Parolin, Giorgio Palù. Coronaviruses: a paradigm of new emerging zoonotic diseases. *Pathogens and Disease*.2019; 77(9): ftaa006. https://doi.org/10.1093/femspd/ftaa006

[20] Acevedo-Whitehouse K, Duffus AL. Effects of environmental change on wildlife health. Philos Trans R Soc Lond B Biol Sci. 2009;364(1534):3429-3438. doi:10.1098/rstb.2009.0128

[21] Rhind SM. Anthropogenic pollutants: a threat to ecosystem sustainability?. Philos Trans R Soc Lond B Biol Sci. 2009;364(1534):3391-3401. doi:10.1098/rstb.2009.0122

[22] Khatri N, Tyagi S. Influences of natural and anthropogenic factors on surface and groundwater quality in rural and urban areas, Frontiers in Life Science. 2015;8:1, 23-39, DOI: 10.1080/21553769.2014.933716

[23] Polianciuc SI, Gurzău AE, Kiss B, Ştefan MG, Loghin F. Antibiotics in the environment: causes and consequences. Med Pharm Rep. 2020;93(3):231-240. doi:10.15386/mpr-1742

[24] Gerba CP. Environmentally Transmitted Pathogens. Environmental Microbiology. 2015;509-550. doi:10.1016/B978-0-12-394626-3.00022-3

[25] Goetz AR, Graham B. Air transport globalization, liberalization and sustainability: post-2001 policy dynamics in the United States and Europe. J Transp Geogr. 2004;12(4):265-276. doi:10.1016/j.jtrangeo.2004.08.007

[26] Mangili A, Gendreau MA. Transmission of infectious diseases during commercial air travel. Lancet. 2005;365(9463):989-996. doi:10.1016/S0140-6736(05)71089-8

[27] Hertzberg VS, Weiss H, Elon L, Si W, Norris SL; FlyHealthy Research Team. Behaviors, movements, and transmission of droplet-mediated respiratory diseases during transcontinental airline flights. Proc Natl Acad Sci U S A. 2018;115(14):3623-3627. doi:10.1073/pnas.1711611115

[28] Goodwin R, Schley D, Lai KM, Ceddia GM, Barnett J, Cook N. Interdisciplinary approaches to zoonotic disease. Infect Dis Rep. 2012;4(2):e37. doi:10.4081/idr.2012.e37

[29] AfricaCDC. One Health [Internet]. 2021. Available from: https://africacdc.org/programme/surveillance-disease-intelligence/one-health/.

[30] Asante J, Noreddin A, El Zowalaty ME. Systematic Review of Important Bacterial Zoonoses in Africa in the Last Decade in Light of the 'One